MAKING THE IMPOSSIBLE POSSIBLE

YOHEI SASAKAWA

Making the Impossible Possible

*My Work for Leprosy Elimination
and Human Rights*

Translated by
LUCY NORTH

HURST & COMPANY, LONDON

First published in the United Kingdom in 2023 by
C. Hurst & Co. (Publishers) Ltd.,
New Wing, Somerset House, Strand, London, WC2R 1LA
Copyright ©Yohei Sasakawa, 2023
All rights reserved.

Distributed in the United States, Canada and Latin America by
Oxford University Press, 198 Madison Avenue, New York, NY 10016,
United States of America.

A Cataloguing-in-Publication data record for this book
is available from the British Library.

ISBN: 9781787389472

Printed in Great Britain by Bell and Bain Ltd, Glasgow

This book is printed using paper from registered sustainable
and managed sources.

www.hurstpublishers.com

CONTENTS

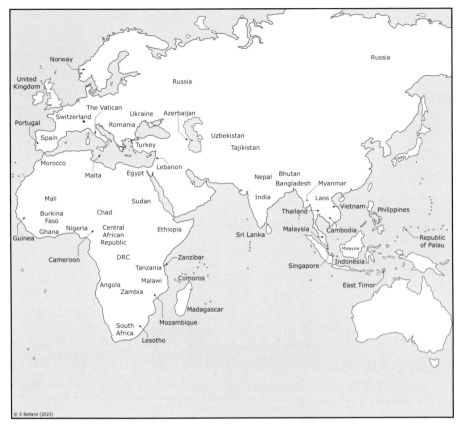

Main countries and regions visited

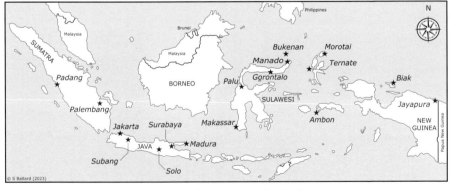

Main states and cities visited in Indonesia

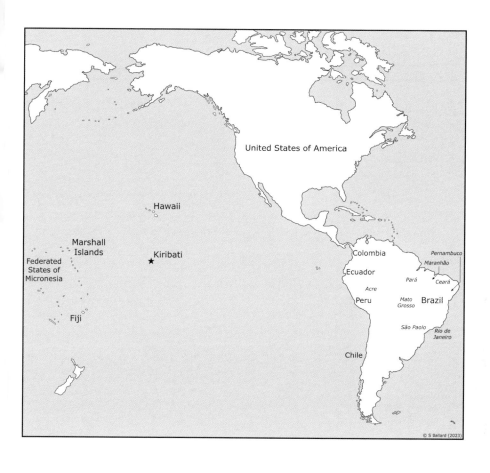

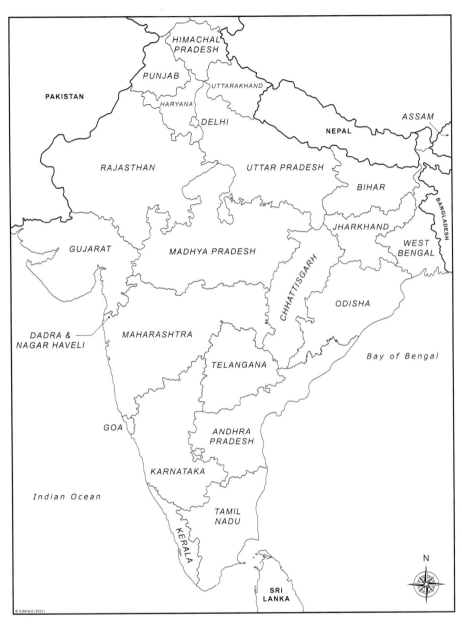

Main states and territories visited in India

FOREWORD

Professor Shigeki Sakamoto
President of the Center for Human Rights Education and Training

A man with a sense of mission—Yohei Sasakawa's struggle against the scourge of leprosy

This book is a record by Mr. Yohei Sasakawa, chairman of the Nippon Foundation and World Health Organization (WHO) Goodwill Ambassador for Leprosy Elimination, of his decades-long fight to eradicate leprosy and stamp out the discrimination attached to the disease. It is a record of the efforts he has undertaken throughout his life to turn his sense of mission into a reality. However, it is not simply a list of his activities and achievements: it is also a store of precious personal recollections that give a vivid picture of the overwhelming passion and commitment to the cause that has taken him traveling all over the globe as he puts his sense of mission into practice. Even now, when he is well into his eighties, an age when one might have expected him to have retired, his energetic endeavors continue unabated.

I had the honor of working closely with Mr. Sasakawa when, in June 2008, the Japanese government introduced a draft resolution to the United Nations Human Rights Council titled "Elimination of Discrimination against Persons Affected by Leprosy and Their Family Members." As a member of the Advisory Committee to the United Nations Human Rights Council, I was in charge of formulating the

Principles and Guidelines that were attached to that draft resolution, which were subsequently adopted.

As he explains in Chapter 1 of this book, Mr. Sasakawa was the first person ever to seek to persuade the United Nations Office of the High Commissioner for Human Rights that the stigma and prejudice incurred by leprosy are an issue of human rights. This he did in July 2003. The issue of leprosy in the context of human rights had never before been raised in the Office of the High Commissioner. Nor had it ever before been discussed by the member nations in the United Nations Commission on Human Rights (later re-organized as the United Nations Human Rights Council).

Mr. Sasakawa has made it his life's work to carry on a project started by his late father Ryoichi Sasakawa, a politician, philanthropist, and one of the pioneers of humanitarian activities in modern Japan, active both before the war and after it, whose dream it was to drive out leprosy from the world and to offer succor to those who suffer under the unwarranted discrimination associated with the condition. As president, and then as chairman of the Nippon Foundation, as WHO Goodwill Ambassador for Leprosy Elimination, and subsequently as Japan's Goodwill Ambassador for the Human Rights of Persons Affected by Leprosy, Yohei Sasakawa has continued to work for this cause with tireless commitment, astonishing ingenuity, and real intelligence.

Reading this book, I am deeply impressed both by the depth of the compassion that Mr. Sasakawa clearly feels for people who are forced to endure great suffering and by the sheer strength of will with which he pushes forward his strategies and tactics for implementation, which are consistently developed on the basis of deep insight into the issues that surround this disease, which for so many centuries has caused such misery to humankind.

As one of Mr. Sasakawa's most outstanding achievements, I must first mention the unprecedented decision he took in 1994 to have the Nippon Foundation provide, for a period of five years starting in 1995, the funding for the provision of free multidrug therapy (MDT) to people affected by leprosy worldwide. This undertaking made possible accelerated efforts against the disease, allowing millions to receive treatment in a timely manner, before the disease had the chance to wreak irreparable damage. It sent out to the world the important message that leprosy could be cured. It was also a salvation to impoverished communities who had previously been unable to afford medication, even if they knew it existed. When the five-year period came to an end, MDT continued to be available at no cost, when the Swiss organization the Novartis Foundation took over its provision.

Another outstanding achievement is the role Mr. Sasakawa took in persuading stakeholders around the world of the importance of the idea of having a benchmark to work toward in the fight against leprosy—the elimination of leprosy as a public health problem, with elimination defined as a disease prevalence rate of less than one case per 10,000 population. Mr. Sasakawa stood at the forefront of this cause, championing it, and built up a huge international network comprising governments, international organizations, healthcare professionals, private foundations, nongovernmental organizations (NGOs), and organizations of persons affected by leprosy, to work toward this common goal. As a result of this collaborative international effort, the number of countries where leprosy is a public health problem, more than 120 in the 1980s, has now, in 2023, decreased to one. Such a positive outcome in the battle of an age-old disease is due in no small part to Mr. Sasakawa's efforts, which often take place behind the scenes.

Mr. Sasakawa has not simply sought to approach the problem of leprosy as a medical issue. He has gone further, and broached leprosy as a social issue as well, pushing for a solution in the international arena to the social discrimination endured by those affected by leprosy and their family members. His first move in this regard was to visit, as a private individual, the United Nations Office of the High Commissioner for Human Rights, in Geneva, where he made a strong case to the Acting High Commissioner for attention to the matter of leprosy-related human rights. The office, moved by Mr. Sasakawa's intervention, offered to help in any way it could, and its advice led to draft proposals and resolutions on leprosy and human rights being put before the United Nations Commission on Human Rights and later before the United Nations Human Rights Council. So began a process that eventually ended in the unanimous adoption in 2010 by the UN

General Assembly of a resolution titled "Elimination of Discrimination of Persons Affected by Leprosy and Their Family Members," accompanied by a set of Principles and Guidelines. The role Mr. Sasakawa played at every step of the way was nothing short of crucial. The final result was testimony to the effectiveness of his tenacity in the face of setbacks, his tactical ingenuity, and his unstinting lobbying activities. After the adoption of the resolution, Mr. Sasakawa then embarked on measures to make sure that governments, international organizations, and private sector organizations in leprosy-endemic countries would put the accompanying Principles and Guidelines into practice, holding symposiums in five regions around the world, and working tirelessly for the appointment of a United Nations Special Rapporteur on the Elimination of Discrimination against Persons Affected by Leprosy and Their Family Members. It was Mr. Sasakawa who came up with the idea for what is now called the "Global Appeal," made every year in January, which gathers endorsements of global leaders, Nobel Peace Prize laureates, and numerous international bodies, with the explicit aim of ending stigma and discrimination against people affected by leprosy—something only he could do because of his vast and impressive network of personal connections. The huge number of interviews and meetings Mr. Sasakawa has had with global leaders and opinion makers listed at the back of this book represents an astonishing network of relationships, an outcome of the passion and commitment with which he has approached eradicating the disease and the discrimination associated with it.

One other area in which Mr. Sasakawa has been uniquely successful is in his efforts to ensure that persons affected by leprosy and their family members—people who previously lived in the shadows, shunned and forgotten—take center stage in the fight against leprosy. As this book will demonstrate, when he goes to leprosy-endemic countries, Mr. Sasakawa makes a point of visiting people affected by leprosy in their communities, joining hands and sharing meals with them, and wherever possible providing support. But he is also concerned to promote their agency and empowerment, and to show them how important it is that they advocate for themselves. As a result, we now see a great many powerful organizations of people affected by leprosy emerging all around the globe. People who were formerly left out of the picture now have the knowhow to take a stand, make their voices heard, and fight to obtain their rights. Only a person with the kind of vision and determination possessed by Mr. Sasakawa could have succeeded so well in ensuring that people affected by leprosy come forward and speak for themselves, so that they can now exert real political influence at the negotiating table.

Mr. Sasakawa's activism and advocacy are not things he undertakes lightly but are carried out consistently on the basis of detailed analysis of trends and developments, and short- and long-term strategies and tactics built on detailed feasibility studies and an accurate understanding of political, economic, and social conditions on the ground. In that sense, this book is also an excellent reference tool for people wishing to tackle other major global issues of our time, with case studies of best practice in identifying and prioritizing issues and of effective implementation. But equally importantly, the book provides an inspiring example, without being in the least sanctimonious, of someone who has lived, and continues to live, a principled and moral life.

What motivates one man to go to such extraordinary lengths on behalf of others? Reading this book, my overriding impression is of a man of compassion and gentleness, someone who has a love and a concern for people who are made to suffer, forgotten and overlooked. This surely developed out of his own painful experiences as a child and adolescent. In the course of these pages, we read how on more than one occasion Mr. Sasakawa was moved to tears on hearing about the often unendurable conditions in which people affected by leprosy have to live their lives, frustrated that he was not able to do more. It is this combination of respect for others and high expectations of himself, as well as his ability to feel other people's pain, that lie at the heart of the activism of this prodigious philanthropist and activist. And driving all of this is without a doubt his own prodigious love for people in general.

Mr. Sasakawa is not a man content to issue commands and pretty speeches from the comfort of an air-conditioned office in a luxurious skyscraper in Tokyo. One of his favorite sayings is: If you want to know the best way to solve a problem, go to where the problem is. Another of his sayings is: Knowledge is inseparable from practice.

Mr. Sasakawa is a man who talks the talk—and walks the walk. In keeping with his favorite sayings, he has been putting his words into practice for over forty years, going to places where leprosy is an issue and getting things done.

I consider it a huge honor to have been able to work by the side of such a man. The experience is something that I will treasure for the rest of my days.

Mr. Sasakawa has now reached the ninety-ninth mile of his 100-mile journey. But as he himself points out, the last mile of a journey is often the longest. It is this last mile that he is walking now. As far as Mr. Sasakawa is concerned, there is still much to be done—this is an ongoing quest.

I have every reason to believe that this book will be enjoyed widely, especially by young people, in whose hands our future lies. For anyone involved in international aid, it will serve as a useful textbook, but for the general reader it will surely be an inspiration that will encourage them to develop compassion for their fellow human beings. One final important message that I hope readers will take away is that with a strong sense of mission it is indeed possible to make a lasting difference in the world.

INTRODUCTION

AN ONGOING QUEST

I was born in 1939, which means that I am now eighty-four years of age. In 2019, I made twenty-seven trips abroad for the purpose of humanitarian activities. Between 1982 (when my secretary of forty-five years Taeko Hoshino started to keep a record) and 2019, I made

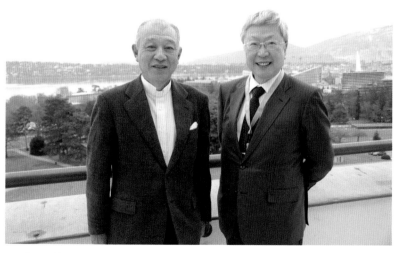

1. The author Yohei Sasakawa (left) with Professor Shigeki Sakamoto (right) at a meeting of the Human Rights Advisory Committee (Geneva, February 2015)

a total of 545 trips, to over 122 destinations. I have now spent 3,354 days traveling, which means that in this thirty-seven-year period I have been abroad for the equivalent of ten years. Of course, some of these trips involved work on other projects in addition to my main one, which is the elimination of leprosy. The focus in this book is on the work I undertook as the World Health Organization (WHO) Goodwill Ambassador for Leprosy Elimination, which started in 2001 and has involved over 200 trips to nearly seventy countries. Nearly all of my destinations have been remote locations where people live in quite desperate conditions. I could just as easily have got things done sitting in an air-conditioned office in Tokyo reading reports drawn up for me by staff on the ground. But it has always been my belief that the place where the problems are happening is also pre-cisely where the solutions will be found. I am also a firm proponent of the Neo-Confucian idea that knowledge is inseparable from prac-tice. I want to be a man of deeds. I became involved in my interna-tional humanitarian work out of a passionate desire to be involved on the front lines until my last breath, and I am the first to admit that my work is done, in that sense, for my own personal satisfaction.

The long history of my battle with the scourge of leprosy can be traced to a story told to me by my father Ryoichi Sasakawa about something he witnessed as a boy that made a deep and lasting impres-sion on him. In his village, there was a lovely young woman, he told me, who the neighborhood suspected had contracted the disease. She was confined to her home and eventually sent away from the village. The feelings he experienced at that time remained with him, and he promised himself that when he grew up he would do everything in his power to drive out leprosy from the world.

In 1962, my father Ryoichi Sasakawa established the organization that became the precursor to today's Nippon Foundation. This was the Japan Shipbuilding Industry Foundation, a public interest incor-porated foundation that engaged primarily in marine- and shipbuild-ing-related activities, and also managed the proceeds (3 percent of the total revenue) made from motorboat racing administered by local municipalities to regenerate sectors that were in need. This was a novel system in Japan at the time, introduced by my father as an early philanthropist—he made no personal profit from this work. The pro-ceeds of boat racing were used in the rebuilding of Japan's shipping and shipbuilding industries, and in the regeneration of facilities to provide social welfare, which had to be totally rebuilt after the war. Once this was achieved, the activities extended to various areas, including health and sanitation, firefighting and natural disaster protection, maritime issues, and eventually to combating starvation and infectious diseases in countries around the globe. It was at this point that my father turned the focus of his activities to alleviating the situation of people affected by leprosy, with the aim of achieving his long-held ambition of eradicating the disease. In 1967, he provided the funding for the construction of a new leprosy center in Agra, India, which marked the start of an effort that continued for the rest of his life. In 1974, my father founded the Sasakawa Memorial Health Foundation (today's Sasakawa Health Foundation), an organization of specialists devoted to tackling leprosy, and thereafter he devoted himself with particular energy and assiduousness to this cause.

In 1974, I accompanied my father on a trip he made to the Republic of Korea to attend the opening ceremony of a leprosy hospital he had funded. I had gone with him on several other trips to hospitals, but this was the first time I had ever set foot inside one. It was there that I had a profoundly moving experience that was to change my life forever. The patients in the wards were still and completely expressionless—they reminded me of wax dolls. A peculiar smell associated with leprosy, the smell of pus, emanated from the wards. I watched as my father touched the hands and faces of the patients, many of whom had open sores, held the patients tightly in his arms, sat with them, and encouraged them to have hope. The patients' faces, however, remained devoid of emotion. All sorts of thoughts poured into my head. These people were living human beings. And thanks to medical treatment, they were going to live. But I had to wonder: What kind of life awaited them? I then turned my thoughts to what made a life truly worth living. It was at this moment that I decided that I should take up humanitarian work and continue what my father had begun.

Leprosy and humankind

Medically speaking, leprosy is an infectious disease that develops from a bacillus called the *Mycobacterium leprae*, which a Norwegian physician named Armauer Hansen (1841–1912) identified in 1873. (Hence its other name, Hansen's disease.) However, as a disease it is only mildly contagious: more than 95 percent of people commonly have a natural immunity to it, and for a person to develop a full-blown case requires certain particular conditions. I myself have hugged thousands upon thousands of people affected by leprosy and touched with my bare hands the sores that are one of the effects of the disease, but never once have I been infected. The first tell-tale signs of the disease are the pale or sometimes reddish lesions, or patches, that appear on the skin. This is accompanied by loss of sensation in the affected areas, so that individuals become unable to feel injuries or burns. If the individuals receive treatment at this stage of the disease, they will recover with no lasting impairment. Left untreated, however, and leprosy will go on to attack the nervous system, which will give rise to injuries, which will then become subject to bacterial infection, giving rise to festering sores. Ultimately this leads to parts of the body becoming disfigured after repeated trauma that is not felt due to sensory loss, resulting in irreversible physical deformity. The resulting physical transformations are what defines leprosy for most of the general population. It is also not uncommon for people affected by leprosy to lose their sight. It is the powerful impression left by these physical deformities that has led to people with leprosy being subject to discrimination since ancient times.

In Japan, the disease was known until relatively recently by the name *rai* or *raibyo*. Both of these names are equivalent to the word "leprosy." The word "leprosy" is still commonly used in English, and it finds its way into medical terminology. One major professional association in the field is named the International Leprosy Association. In Brazil and Japan, however, the term "Hansen's disease" is preferred, and recent years have seen efforts made toward encouraging countries around the world to do the same.

There are references to a disease that seems very like leprosy in the *Sushruta Samhita*, an ancient compendium on diseases and their treatments written in India (probably completed between the third and fourth century) as well as in the *Nihon Shoki*, one of Japan's earliest extant chronicles. At one time, it was thought that leprosy was a disease that originated in Asia. However, recent DNA analysis of the bacillus suggests that leprosy first occurred in Eastern Africa. Nevertheless, it is certainly not a disease only to be found in Asia or Africa. It was once found in nearly every country of the world. In medieval times, leprosy could be found in every land in Europe. In the central regions of Europe, leprosy became a significant problem, but the details of its history thereafter, and how in Western Europe it then changed from being a common disease to a rarer one, remain unclear.

Leprosy was at one time a significant health problem in Japan as well. Data from surveys conducted in the Meiji period (1868–1912) indicate that there were probably nearly 200,000 people with leprosy at the time, which in relation to the population would be equivalent to more than thirty individuals affected by leprosy in every 10,000 persons. Professor Morizo Ishidate (1901–96), the first chairman of the Board of Directors of the Sasakawa Memorial Health Foundation, an emeritus professor of pharmaceutical science at the University of Tokyo, and the first person in Japan to synthesize promin, which is one of the first modern treatments of leprosy, used to recount how as a student in the early 1920s he saw lines of people with leprosy on Ochanomizu Bridge in Kanda, Tokyo, begging. And at the Asakusa Kannon Temple, he reported, the situation was just as dire: lines of people suffering from leprosy, begging, wherever one looked.

In the early twentieth century, no effective cure for leprosy was known, and patients could do little more than wait while the symptoms of the disease got progressively worse. The mistaken notion that the disease was a divine punishment for misdeeds committed in a former life, or that it was hereditary, was entrenched. Among the general population, there was the notion that leprosy was a contagious disease, which led to leprosy patients being forcibly segregated from their communities out of the fear that it would spread to other people. Leprosy patients were often kept hidden from society, which only increased their sorrow and suffering. The deep-rooted belief that leprosy was a hereditary disease meant that family members and even distant relatives of people with leprosy were also made the objects of discrimination and social ostracization. When the Leprosy Prevention Law was passed in Japan in 1931, people with leprosy were mandatorily confined in leprosy settlements, forbidden to have any contact with the outside world; they were also pressured not to have families of their own. Social segregation of people affected by leprosy happened around the globe, endlessly repeated. I remember one Hawaiian woman who was sent to a leprosy settlement on the remote peninsula of Kalaupapa on the Hawaiian island of Molokai giving the following account: "When I was a child, I remember there was a man who was living like a beggar near us. He had leprosy. His family lived in a large, beautiful house nearby, but he was living in a shack. He just sat there, covered in filth, completely still—very rarely emerging. I regret to say, though, that my family was just as indifferent as his. He was eventually detained in hospital, but he was ultimately cured and allowed to go free. It became possible for him to return to his family. But his family didn't want him. 'We don't want you hanging round anywhere near us,' they told him. 'Don't think you can live with us anymore.'"

There must have been countless other tragedies like this one in leprosaria all over the world.

The establishment of a leprosy cure

Until promin was developed for the treatment of leprosy in the United States in 1941, the only therapy for leprosy had been chaulmoogra oil. This was oil extracted from the seeds of a tree in the Achariaceae family, used in traditional medicine in Southeast Asia and India since ancient times. In the nineteenth century, it started being used to treat leprosy in Europe and America, either ingested orally, or applied topically to the skin; in the twentieth century, it was administered intravenously. Nevertheless, the effectiveness of chaulmoogra oil was anything but complete—its effects were ephemeral for the most part, and often there was no alleviation of symptoms at all.

With the introduction of promin, leprosy finally became a fully curable disease. However, it was only possible to administer promin intravenously, and there were significant side effects. Before long, a new drug appeared, the antibiotic dapsone (diaminodiphenyl sulfone or DDS), that could be taken orally. However, the duration of treatment lasted years, making compliance difficult, and when it became clear over time that *Mycobacterium leprae* developed resistance to DDS, an urgent search began for alternative treatment methods. In 1977, it was discovered that when two other antibiotic drugs known to be effective in suppressing leprosy, clofazimine and rifampicin, were used in combination with the drug dapsone, it became possible to suppress the generation of drug-resistant bacteria. This led to the establishment of what has come to be known as multidrug therapy (MDT) as the accepted therapeutic cure to leprosy. It is important to note, however, that each of the drugs comprising MDT have significant adverse effects: in the case of rifampicin, liver and kidney problems, anemia, and attenuation of the effectiveness of concomitantly used drugs; in the case of dapsone, a number of adverse reactions that come under the term dapsone syndrome, as well as headaches, decreased appetite, and liver problems; in the case of clofazimine, bowel blockages, diarrhea, visible skin discoloration, and dry, rough, scaly skin. Further, during treatment of leprosy, and even after the treatment is over, it sometimes happens that the dead leprosy bacilli remaining in the tissues can provoke a reaction in the patient's immune system, resulting in acute inflammatory episodes. These episodes are known as "leprosy reactions," and they involve a variety of presentations including swellings in the skin, pain, and nerve inflammation, as well as the loss of sensation in the hands and feet. A variety of drugs are used to manage leprosy reactions, including corticosteroids, clofazimine, and thalidomide. Here too, early diagnosis and treatment are essential for the prevention of irreversible damage.

Progress in elimination of the disease

The discovery of drugs that could cure leprosy brought about a major advancement in the battle against leprosy, and MDT in particular was a gamechanger. This prompted the WHO to announce in 1991 that it had set a target of the elimination of leprosy as a public health problem globally (applying to countries with populations of over 1 million) by the year 2000, with elimination meaning a disease prevalence rate of less than one case per 10,000 population. But initially, no specific measures were presented for reaching this benchmark. A dearth in funds meant that little if any progress could be made. Further, the reality was that nearly one-third of the world's population had to survive on earnings of less than a dollar a day, which made it impossible for most people affected by leprosy to find a doctor, let alone buy medication.

So it was that I devised a plan to have the Nippon Foundation pay for the drug therapy so that it could be offered at no cost to all those affected by leprosy—globally. At the world's first International Conference on Leprosy Elimination in Hanoi, Vietnam, I announced that the Nippon Foundation would donate $50 million (equivalent to 5 billion yen at the time) to WHO to fund the free distribution of MDT all over the world for five years, starting in 1995. My announcement was initially received with a stunned silence, followed by confused excitement, and then resounding applause. It was at this time that I made a silent promise to myself to devote my life to the battle against leprosy, and to involve myself with the problems and solutions firsthand for the rest of my days.

As a result of this free provision, roughly 5 million patients were estimated to have been cured of leprosy in the period from 1995 to 1999. Sadly, WHO's target of eliminating leprosy as a public health problem worldwide by the turn of the millennium was not ultimately reached; however, there was a widespread reduction in many countries at the national level: in 1995, there were 122 countries where leprosy was a public health problem; in 2000, there were eleven. By 2011, the number had decreased still further, to one country—Brazil. At the turn of the millennium, the Novartis Foundation in Basel, Switzerland, took over the MDT donations. Since the 1980s, we have seen a more than 95 percent reduction in case numbers. According to WHO statistics, the number of newly registered cases in 2018 annually worldwide was just 208,000 persons.

My work as WHO Goodwill Ambassador for Leprosy Elimination and my "Three Key Messages"

In 1999, a number of governments of countries that had yet to achieve the WHO elimination goal, along with WHO and the International Federation of Anti-Leprosy Associations (ILEP), got together and formed an international organization called the Global Alliance for the Elimination of Leprosy (GAEL) in order to better unify their efforts and more effectively continue the fight against leprosy worldwide. In 2001, GAEL held its first meeting in New Delhi, India, but a divergence then emerged in the ideas about policy among some of the stakeholders. The WHO delegate for the region of the Americas and others proposed that to break the deadlock I be appointed GAEL Special Ambassador, and the proposal was ratified. As Ambassador, it was my role to be the public face for the elimination of leprosy on the world stage, to work to strengthen the commitment of political leaders in every country (getting them to make concrete proposals), and to play the part of intermediary between the stakeholders. I was thus required to be both a leader and an intermediary in the anti-leprosy fight. GAEL was dissolved in 2003, but WHO then appointed me as the WHO Goodwill Ambassador for Leprosy Elimination.

When I was entrusted with this role, I considered that I had three main tasks. The first was to meet with world leaders, presidents, prime ministers, and health ministers, so that I could obtain their collaboration in the efforts to fight leprosy. The second was to make use of every kind of media available to me to disseminate accurate knowledge and information about leprosy to as wide an audience as possible. The third was to have as much contact with people at the grass-roots level, to provide as much encouragement as I could to the people working on the front lines, and the people affected by leprosy and their family members, so that I could reflect their voices and views in my dealings with political leaders.

For as long as I can remember, I have made a point of repeating three messages in every meeting, conference, or press conference that I attend. You will come across them any number of times in the chapters that follow. The first message is that leprosy is curable. The second message is that free treatment is available everywhere around the world. And the third message is that discrimination against people affected by leprosy has no place. These messages are very easy to understand. But the third one, the message that discrimination has no place, is extremely difficult to put into practice. The habits of a lifetime and ingrained unconscious attitudes are not easily dispelled. Diseases of a medical nature can be cured with a simple course of medicine, but combating the prejudice and discrimination that exist in wider society requires a Herculean effort.

As one might expect, WHO made the control of leprosy as a public health problem from the medical point of view the core focus of its attention. But I was concerned with the problem of the discrimination and stigma that were connected to leprosy, which I'd become sharply aware of around the turn of the millennium. Until then, I had assumed that when the disease itself disappeared, this would solve the problem of the associated discrimination. However, in fact things are not nearly so simple (I deal with this in Chapter 1). This is what stirred me to start my advocacy efforts with the United Nations Commission on Human Rights (replaced in 2006 by the United Nations Human Rights Council). These efforts involved a great deal of work over a period of several years, but eventually, in September 2010, a resolution on the "Elimination of Discrimination against Persons Affected by Leprosy and Their Family Members" and an accompanying set of Principles and Guidelines for fulfilling the resolution was put before the members of the UN Human Rights Council, where it was passed with unanimous approval. The Japanese government then submitted a motion for the above resolution along with its guidelines to the United Nations General Assembly in December of the same year, and it received unanimous approval from all 193 delegates. This resolution encouraged governments and relevant UN bodies to "give due consideration to the Principles and Guidelines in the formulation and implementation of the [anti-leprosy measures]." A number of people worked closely with me to secure this resolution: Tatsuya Tanami of the Nippon Foundation; Professor Kenzo Kiikuni, one of the founding members in 1974 of the Sasakawa Health Foundation; Chuo University Professor Yozo Yokota; and Professor Shigeki Sakamoto, who at the time was teaching at Kobe University. All of us carried out determined lobbying efforts. The collaborative cooperation and diplomatic efforts of the Permanent Mission of Japan to the International Organizations in Geneva were also absolutely key.

I am always conscious that there is a limit to what I can accomplish as a private individual working on my own, so I make a point of reaching out to opinion leaders and organizations and groups from countries all over the world to help me in my mission to spread the message about the human rights dimension of leprosy. Since 2006, every year we have held an annual campaign to end all leprosy-related stigma and discrimination, which we call the Global Appeal, in which we partner with individuals and organizations in business, politics, and culture to disseminate our message. We launch these Global Appeals on what is now designated World Leprosy Day, on the last Sunday of January.

Incidentally, I was recently very surprised to learn that my three messages, and my motorcycle metaphor too (in which I compare the fight against leprosy to the two wheels of a motorbike—the front wheel symbolizes cure of the disease, the back wheel represents eliminating discrimination; unless both wheels turn together, we will not reach our goal of zero leprosy), and another favorite aphorism, which I originally drew from a classical Chinese source, that the last mile of a 100-mile journey is as arduous as all the others combined, have now become standard turns of phrase among WHO staff and other bodies engaged in the anti-leprosy fight.

Thinking about leprosy makes us think about humanity in all its dimensions

Nowadays in Japan the figures for new cases of leprosy reported annually are low. I imagine that a large portion of people may never even have heard of the disease. But worldwide at least 200,000 new cases are still being reported to WHO annually, and leprosy remains very much a live disease. The count may be higher, with numerous hidden leprosy cases. Certainly, when compared with other major diseases like malaria, AIDS, and tuberculosis, the number of new patients with leprosy may seem small, but in the case of leprosy the extreme prejudice and discrimination means that for patients, diagnosis of the disease means untold emotional pain and suffering. And often people affected by leprosy will remain the object of discrimination and prejudice for the rest of their lives, even after they have been cured. One reason for the prejudice is thought to be the severe physical disfigurements that often occur as the disease progresses (mainly with damage to the limbs, not a direct outcome of leprosy but arising because of damage to the sensory nerves), but another major cause is that religions have often seen leprosy as a disease of impurity and defilement, and a divine punishment for sins. This has exacerbated the prejudice and caused it to become entrenched.

For many decades, before the advent of social media, people with leprosy were often forcibly isolated from their loved ones and placed in facilities on far-off, uninhabited islands, left there with no hope of any communication with the outside world. Such "leprosaria" existed on Robben Island, South Africa, which was where Nelson Mandela spent his imprisonment, Kalaupapa Island in Hawaii, Culion Island in the Philippines, Jerejak Island in Malaysia, Makogai Island in Fiji, a number of islands in the Mediterranean Sea, and other places. They existed in Japan as well: such were the Okinawa Airakuen sanatorium, the Oshima Seishoen sanatorium in Kagawa prefecture, the Oku-Komyoen sanatorium, and the Nagashima Aiseien sanatorium on the island of Nagashima in Setouchi, Okayama prefecture, to name just a few.

Discrimination is alive and well today, and it exists in every nation and region in the world. As long as people hesitate to come forward when they know that they or other members of their family have the disease out of their terror of ostracization and discrimination, this allows their condition to worsen, so that in the end they are left with lasting disabilities; in some cases, the fear engendered by these disabilities results in people being driven out of their communities and shunned by their families. In Nepal, we know of one case where a man developed leprosy and his entire family was forced to move and take up life in a public toilet on the edges of the village. In Indonesia, there was a report in the newspapers of one patient abandoned by his family who was discovered living deep in the mountains, where he had managed to survive by eating snakes and rats. Such tragic stories can be found all over the world. Discrimination becomes a disincentive to getting treatment for the disease, which results in disfigurement, which gives rise to yet more discrimination. It is a horrific vicious circle, and we have to put a stop to it.

I believe that leprosy offers us important lessons for when we think about other kinds of discrimination: the intolerance, for example, that many of us have toward people of different ethnicities and religions. Yet the history of leprosy is not only a negative one of sadness and misery. It can also serve to inspire us, as we learn about the courage and hope with which people have managed to carry on living their lives, persevering in the midst not only of the disease but also the prejudice and discrimination that are connected with it and creating good lives for themselves. That is why I always say that thinking about leprosy means thinking about humanity in all its dimensions.

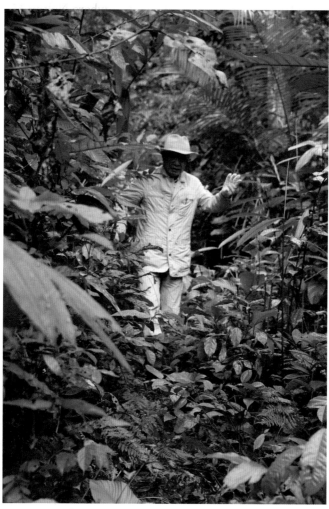

2. The author on a foray in the jungle to meet with persons affected by leprosy in a pygmy village (Cameroon, August 2016)

1

THE OTHER FRONT LINE

THE UN RESOLUTION AND SUBSEQUENT INITIATIVES TO PUSH FOR IMPLEMENTATION

Leprosy and human rights

It is my firmly held belief that if you want to know how to solve a problem, you should go directly to where the problem is—the front line. In my anti-leprosy fight, I have made a point of visiting the front line in every country where leprosy is endemic, and meeting with as many people as possible—men, women, and children, whether currently affected by leprosy or recovered—so that I can hear directly what they have to say and see for myself how they are living their lives.

Around the turn of the millennium, I became sharply conscious that the problem of leprosy is not simply a medical issue but very definitely also a human rights issue—and I developed the view that it was imperative that we get global recognition that the social and economic effects that the disease inflicts on persons affected by leprosy and their family members are a matter of their human rights. In order to obtain this recognition, I decided that it would be effective for me to try to solicit support from the United Nations. Thus it was that the United Nations became one more front line for my anti-leprosy operations.

At time of writing, just over 200,000 new cases of leprosy are still being detected worldwide each year. The figure has remained roughly the same for the last decade. Sixteen million people have now been treated with multidrug therapy (MDT) since 1980. If we include the family members of these individuals, we can be sure that the figure for people who are subjected to unwarranted leprosy-related discrimination must run into several tens of millions. Even when people affected by leprosy have been cured by MDT, they continue to suffer discrimination, encountering barriers to education, marriage, and employment prospects. Moreover, often, this discrimination continues even after their lifetime, and family members encounter similar barriers. I decided it was essential if I wanted to tackle the human rights dimension of leprosy that I use my position as World Health Organization (WHO) Goodwill Ambassador for Leprosy Elimination and formulate a plan of action to take to the United Nations that would lead to the UN requiring governments to take whatever measures were necessary to put an end to this situation. Thus it was that I started my efforts to solicit the support and cooperation of the UN Commission on Human Rights.

At the beginning, however, I had absolutely no idea of the steps that I, a mere private citizen, had to take in order to get the United Nations to deliberate this issue. Everyone around me told me that it would be impossible—easier for the proverbial camel to go through the eye of a needle. But it is an article of faith with me that action is the first step to problem-solving. So I rolled up my sleeves and got down to the task.

The human rights dimension of leprosy: never before addressed by the UN

In July 2003, I paid my first visit to the Office of the UN High Commissioner for Human Rights, in Geneva, Switzerland, to meet with Dr. Bertrand D. Ramcharan, acting High Commissioner at the time (High Commissioner Sérgio Vieira de Mello had just been seconded as the Secretary-General's special representative in Iraq; and in fact was killed by a bomb blast while there), and set out the case for official attention to the human rights dimension of leprosy—

explaining the harrowing circumstances in which people who are affected by leprosy and their families have to live, that such people number in their thousands, and that they are spread throughout the world. Dr. Ramcharan admitted to being astonished at the extent of the problem and acknowledged that the UN had not once given its attention to the issue of the human rights of people affected by leprosy. He agreed that the issue of the discrimination and social stigma that people affected by leprosy have to suffer should indeed be treated as an issue of human rights.

Dr. Ramcharan gave me three pieces of advice at this first meeting. First, he recommended that I put together a "side-event" (an activity organized outside the formal program) at the next session of the UN Sub-Commission on the Promotion and Protection of Human Rights, due to be held one month later, in August, and use this as an opportunity to air the topic to the delegates. Second, he recommended that I meet with Professor Paul Hunt of the University of Essex, England, at that point serving as UN Special Rapporteur on the Right to the Highest Attainable Standard of Health, to ask him for his views. He also recommended that I try to create the opportunity for a meeting to discuss the issues with staff members of the UN High Commissioner's Office.

I immediately got down to putting together, as quickly as I could, a seminar to be hosted by the Nippon Foundation featuring presentations by people affected by leprosy, and other stakeholders, to be held alongside the main program of the fifty-fifth session of the UN Human Rights Sub-Commission in the Palais des Nations in Geneva, in August. Persons affected by leprosy and health specialists from Ethiopia, the United States, and the Philippines took part, the first time they had ever had the opportunity to draw people's attention at the United Nations to the social discrimination endured by persons affected by leprosy and their family members. We were also given permission to hold a panel display in the lobby outside our seminar room of eighteen truly superb photographs taken by Natsuko Tominaga, official photographer to the Nippon Foundation. However, we had great difficulty attracting anybody to come and listen. The delegates all had tight schedules, leaving them little time to attend a seminar like ours given by ordinary citizens who weren't part of any governmental organization. After wracking our brains, we decided to serve food and drinks outside our seminar room, in the hope that we could entice delegates there, and they would listen to our reports while they ate. Two members of our team, Satoshi Sugawara and Natsuko Tominaga, waylaid the delegates as they emerged from the main conference hall for lunch, handed them a seminar pamphlet, and directed them to the table laid with food by our room. We were basically exercising a kind of pushy sales technique. Even so, despite all our endeavors, only about ten or so people—all representatives from NGOs and the media—actually came into the room, which had the capacity for fifty. The delegates to the UN Human Rights Sub-Commission showed no interest whatsoever. Nevertheless, the attendees did pose a few interested questions, and there were reactions of astonishment from people who were learning for the first time the extent of leprosy-related discrimination. At the end of the seminar, I saw several people come up to the speakers, wanting to shake hands with them. All in all, I consider it was a useful opportunity to start attendees thinking seriously about the ways in which people affected by leprosy suffer a violation of their human rights, and to demonstrate that this is a modern-day problem.

I always keep in mind three things whenever I'm engaged in my global activities: to never let my passion slip away; to endure and be patient until the difficulty, no matter how large, is overcome; and to persevere until the desired result is achieved. I decided I wasn't about to let myself be discouraged by a poorly attended seminar. I should think of this as simply the start of a long campaign. In fact, this campaign was to last for the next seven years, during which I continued to hold such seminars alongside annual sessions of human rights bodies at the UN, improving them and making them more effective as I went along.

I then traveled to England, where, following Dr. Ramcharan's advice, I met with Professor Paul Hunt of the Human Rights Centre at the University of Essex to ask for his help. Professor Hunt was serving in the post of UN Special Rapporteur on the Right to the Highest Attainable Standard of Health, with a mandate to study the situation of the right to health around the world. Professor Hunt immediately recognized what I was trying to argue and offered a number of helpful suggestions. First, he recommended that the Nippon Foundation organize a seminar on the discrimination and stigma suffered by people affected by leprosy as a side event at the sixtieth session of the United Nations Human Rights Commission due to take place in March and April the following year, 2004, where we could bring the topic to the attention of the delegates. Professor Hunt suggested that it would be most effective to treat the matter of stigma and discrimination endured by people affected by leprosy in a broader discussion of "health and human rights." If we drew too much attention to leprosy as a discrete issue, he said, there was the risk that this would lead only to the strengthening of the stigma and discrimination associated with the disease. I, however, had misgivings about leprosy-related human rights being treated under the broad category of "the right to health," which would imply that we were simply arguing for better delivery of treatment and medication; it was my contention that leprosy-related human rights ought to be treated as a separate and independent category. This problem—how leprosy should be treated, as a health rights issue, or as a human rights issue—was repeated in many other discussions over the next few years in meetings of the United Nations Human Rights Sub-Commission and other forums.

In March 2004, on the suggestion of Professor Hunt, the Nippon Foundation duly organized a panel discussion titled "Leprosy and Human Rights" as a side event to the sixtieth session of the United Nations Human Rights Commission in the Palais des Nations in Geneva. At this side event, we had direct testimony from representatives of associations of persons affected by leprosy in India, Brazil, and the United States, Professor Paul Hunt, and WHO's health and human rights adviser Helena Nygren-Krug. Again, sadly, very few people attended. Only ten or so seats were filled of the fifty-seat capacity room.

Nevertheless, as a representative of an NGO, I was permitted to give a short (two-minute) speech before the fifty-three delegates of the plenary session of the Human Rights Commission, which I duly did, on "Leprosy and Human Rights." I'm proud to say that this was the first time in history that any oral statement concerning leprosy had ever been made on the floor of the United Nations. Here is the transcript of my speech.

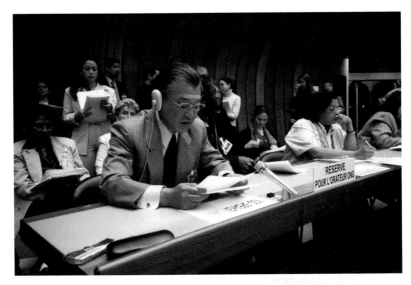

3. A historical first: The author making his oral statement about leprosy to the Human Rights Commission (Geneva, March 2004)

Oral Statement by Yohei Sasakawa
Sixtieth Session of the Human Rights Commission

Mr. Chairperson, I am here to talk to you about leprosy and human rights. If left untreated, leprosy results in serious deformity. Therefore, through the ages, it has triggered fear and loathing. Patients have been isolated. Isolation led to discrimination. Discrimination turned people into pariahs.

Once affected, a person was fated to a lifetime more miserable than death.

Families were terrified of the shame if a member developed leprosy. They kept the leprosy-affected hidden from view. Or they simply abandoned them.

Today, leprosy is treatable. Since the early 1980s, 12 million people have been cured. 116 countries have seen the disease eliminated as a medical issue. Today, there are less than 600,000 known cases.

But, Mr. Chairperson, a problem remains. Discrimination is still rampant. Those cured of leprosy still can't marry. They can't get work. They can't go to school. They are still treated as outcasts. The problem is massive, global in scale.

Many still think leprosy is dangerous or hereditary. Many still see it as a divine punishment. And so millions live in isolation. They have no homes to return to. They are dead to their families.

As WHO Goodwill Ambassador for Leprosy Elimination, I spent 125 days last year traveling to twenty-seven countries. I have seen this damage with my own eyes.

So Mr. Chairperson, why has this never been treated as a human rights issue? This is because these are abandoned people. They have had both their names and their identity stripped away. They cannot cry out for their rights. They are silenced people.

That is why I stand before you today. To draw your attention to these voiceless people.

Mr. Chairperson, leprosy is a human rights issue. I urge the members of this commission to rectify this problem. Develop a resolution. Support worldwide research. And create guidelines that guarantee freedom from discrimination for all affected by leprosy.

Thank you.

Over the next six months (summer 2003–spring 2004), I met a number of times with Professor Yozo Yokota of Chuo University, who was a member of the UN's Sub-Commission on the Promotion and Protection of Human Rights, and discussed matters with him. Professor Yokota was a renowned international authority on human rights and international law who started his career as legal counsel to the World Bank in Washington, DC and had held numerous prestigious posts of high responsibility, including president of the Committee of Experts on the International Labour Organization and president of the Center for Human Rights Education and Training, as well as professorships at the International Christian University (Tokyo), the University of Tokyo, and Chuo Law School, and from 2004 till his untimely death in 2019 he took a keen interest in our efforts to fight for attention to the human rights dimension of leprosy, helping us greatly with our cause.

Professor Yokota suggested that in order to get leprosy taken up as a human rights issue by the UN Human Rights Commission, it would be helpful to create a kind of natural progression: the first step was to get the UN Human Rights Commission delegates to recognize the validity of investigation into the issue of leprosy and to task the

Sub-Commission to conduct research into the matter. The Sub-Commission would then put together a group of health experts and human rights specialists to do this research who would organize a series of workshops in which they would present their findings, which could then be taken with recommendations to the Human Rights Commission, at which point we could then attach principles and guidelines to end stigma and discrimination against persons affected by leprosy and their family members. In order to do this, he told me, I would have to get the support of every nation, and for this it would be essential to seek to convince each and every delegate of the validity of our cause. One way to do this, he suggested, might be to hold luncheons or dinners whenever the Sub-Commission was in session, inviting delegates who might be interested so that we could gather their proposals and ideas. He also advised me to work toward getting officials to appoint a Special Rapporteur, who would ensure that proper research and assessments by the Sub-Commission would be carried out.

2004: The mountain moves

In May 2004, during a visit to Geneva to attend a meeting of the WHO, I was able to put into action the third piece of advice from Dr. Ramcharan and hold a seminar with staff members of the UN Office of the High Commissioner for Human Rights. I prepared a mountain of materials of every kind for my talk. Dr. Ramcharan himself participated in the meeting, but sadly, yet again the event was poorly attended. Our audience consisted of a mere five persons. It seemed to me astonishing that the level of interest was so low— here, of all places, in the Office of the High Commissioner for Human Rights, where one would expect people to care about such things. However, I am not a man to give up. I simply became even more determined.

The following June, on a visit to Brazil to attend a symposium on leprosy control, I went to meet Professor Paulo Sérgio Pinheiro, then affiliated with the University of São Paulo, with whom I had been put in touch by Professor Yokota. Professor Pinheiro was a representative on the UN Sub-Commission for the Promotion and Protection of

Human Rights. I was surprised when he launched into an anecdote relating to the Nippon Foundation. As UN Special Rapporteur on the Situation of Human Rights in Myanmar, he told me, he had once been taken seriously ill far from any city, and the ambulance that had taken him to hospital had the Nippon Foundation's logo on its side. As far as he was concerned, he owed the Nippon Foundation his life. "I should thank you," he told me, looking at me with real appreciation in his eyes. He also mentioned how moving he found the scenes of the medics tending people affected by leprosy in the leprosy settlement in Peru in the biopic about the motorcycle road trip taken by Che Guevara (*Motorcycle Diaries*, showing in Brazil at the time). "It is essential to get a motion passed at the Sub-Commission to look into the human rights dimension of leprosy," he told me. "If that is passed, a member of the Sub-Commission, or one of the Rapporteurs, will be officially tasked with research and assessment. Why not invite members of the Sub-Commission to a working lunch early on in the next session [28 July–15 August]? That would be the best strategy. I will be happy to attend, and I'll mention it to other members. I will get other independent experts on the Sub-Commission, people like Professor Yokota and my friend José Antonio Bengoa Cabello, to join me in tabling the matter to a vote. I will do all I can to support you."

I well remember the joy I felt when I heard him say this. I returned to Japan, reported to Professor Yokota, and initiated arrangements immediately for a working lunch to be held early in the upcoming session.

One month later, on 29 July 2004, the second day of the fifty-sixth session of the UN Sub-Commission for the Promotion and Protection of Human Rights, the Nippon Foundation held a working lunch, which was attended, thanks to the efforts of Professors Pinheiro and Yokota, by twenty-two of the twenty-six delegates on the Human Rights Sub-Commission. At the lunch, Professor Kenzo Kiikuni, chair of the Sasakawa Memorial Health Foundation (the present Sasakawa Health Foundation), and I gave presentations on why leprosy deserved particular attention as a human rights issue and appealed to the Sub-Commission for action. Dr. Ramcharan was also present. I well remember Mr. Soli Jehangir Sorabjee, India's delegate, who was also chairperson of the Sub-Commission, announcing his decision to consider the issue. "Leprosy is an age-old phenomenon that leads to severe human rights violations," he stated. "We will be happy to do something to support your movement." This was followed by expressions of loud agreement from others who were present.

As a consequence of this step, on 9 August 2004, the UN Sub-Commission on the Promotion and Protection of Human Rights unanimously endorsed the resolution to take up the issue of discrimination toward persons affected by leprosy and their family members. Professor Yokota was appointed Special Rapporteur and tasked with leading a fact-finding study on the issue and producing a preliminary working paper that he was required to submit to the fifty-seventh session of the Sub-Commission in the following year. It was still only a preliminary working paper, but at last we were getting traction. The mountain had begun to move.

A world first: statements made by leprosy-affected persons on the floor of the UN

In August 2005, as a response to the findings and recommendations presented by Professor Yokota at the fifty-seventh session of the Sub-Commission on the Promotion and Protection of Human Rights, a further resolution relating to leprosy and human rights was adopted. Professor Yokota had spent the whole of the previous year attending international conferences, workshops, and seminars, in India, Brazil, and Africa, and conducting interviews with people affected by leprosy and their families, as well as doctors, social workers, experts, NGOs, and governmental officials, so that he could produce a detailed report on the discrimination that leprosy patients face on a daily basis and also highlight inadequacies in the legal systems and instances of social stigma. He ended his report with a list of requests for actions to be taken by governments and UN bodies to rectify the situation. Although there were a few on the Sub-Commission who voiced doubts about whether it was fair to single out human rights violations related to leprosy to the exclusion of other diseases, a resolution, dated 11 August 2005, was ultimately passed endorsing the conclusions and recommendations contained in Professor Yokota's report, which included requests for governments to: (1) repeal all existing legislation requiring the forced institutionalization of leprosy patients; (2) provide appropriate relief measures to people affected by leprosy who had previously been forcibly institutionalized in a sanatorium, colony, hospital, or community, and their family members; (3) immediately prohibit discrimination of any type against persons with leprosy and their families; and (4) include education about leprosy in school curricula so as to give correct information about leprosy and people affected by leprosy. Professor Yokota was reappointed in his position of Special Rapporteur. Further, the Sub-Commission recommended that the resolution be adopted by the UN Commission on Human Rights and requested that the UN High Commissioner for Human Rights and the UN Secretary-General provide the Special Rapporteur with all the assistance necessary to enable him to accomplish his task.

The Nippon Foundation had invited quite a few people from countries around the globe to participate in the plenary meeting of the fifty-seventh session of the Sub-Commission on the Promotion and Protection of Human Rights. These included Professor Ujjwal K. Chowdhury, an Indian documentary filmmaker who had made *From Dignity Lost to Dignity Regained*, a film about the struggle for social acceptance and rehabilitation, and the Brazilian filmmaker Andrea Pasquini, who had made a film titled *The Best Years of Our Lives*, featuring heart-rending testimonies from residents of Santo Angelo, one of Brazil's thirty-three leprosy colony hospitals. Also, Dr P. K. Gopal, the president of the International Association for Integration, Dignity and Economic Advancement (IDEA), an association for and of leprosy-affected persons; Nevis Mary, a person formerly affected by leprosy now a clerical worker for the Indian Railways; Kofi Nyarko from Ghana, a board member on IDEA and headmaster of a school for children with special needs; and Amar Timalsina, a board member of The Leprosy Mission, president of IDEA Nepal, and a person formerly affected by leprosy who is now a school principal.

On 5 August 2005, I was given another opportunity to make an oral statement before the members of the UN Sub-Commission on the Promotion and Protection of Human Rights, in the plenary meeting of the fifty-seventh session of the UN Sub-Commission on the

Promotion and Protection of Human Rights, before an audience of representatives, governmental bodies, UN bodies, and NGOs. In the statement, I outlined the prejudice and discrimination faced by people with leprosy and argued for the necessity of taking action to eradicate such inhumane treatment. Here is the text of the speech.

Oral Statement

by

Yohei Sasakawa,

WHO Goodwill Ambassador for Leprosy Elimination;

Chairman, the Nippon Foundation

at

the Fifty-Seventh UN Sub-Commission on the Promotion and Protection of Human Rights

August 2005

Mr. Chairman, last year, this Sub-Commission passed a resolution calling for a report on discrimination against leprosy-affected people. It was the first time in thousands of years that the disease was formally taken up as a human rights issue.

Why did this take so long?

The fact is, people with leprosy have been invisible.

They have had their names and identities taken away from them.

The disease has been their only identity, and they became "leprosy patients," or "lepers."

These people have been made to believe they have no rights.

Just because they have leprosy.

They have been forced into silence.

Because of stigma, because of the myths that have built up, many people are unfamiliar with the facts.

Yes, it is an infectious disease.

Yes, *IF* untreated, it results in deformity.

But the most important fact, Mr. Chairman, is that leprosy is curable.

Nonetheless, this stigma is so strong that even the cured are turned into outcasts.

Even today, they are driven out, forced together, into thousands of isolated leprosy colonies.

This isolation is discrimination's most frightening face.

Unnecessary shame still terrifies the families of those with the disease.

They disowned their loved ones.

But again Mr. Chairman, *today leprosy can be cured*.

Since the early 1980s, I have worked on the front lines of a battle that has cured 14 million people.

This work, my lifework, is more important to me than anything.

But while the discrimination remains, the curing of those 14 million means next to nothing.

Because they have still not regained their stolen lives, their stolen dignity.

Even cured, they are still called "former patients."

Mr. Chairman, why is this?

Do we see this degree of discrimination with tuberculosis? With malaria?

No, Mr. Chairman, we do not.

Only those who have had leprosy continue to be referred to as "former patients."

The problem is massive in scale.

If families are included, nearly 100 million people suffer.

Mr. Chairman, the time to restore their human dignity is long overdue.

Thus, I respectfully end, with a call for an action by this commission that will end all discrimination against those affected by leprosy.

Thank you.

After these brief remarks, I gave the microphone to the four people with lived experience of leprosy from India, Ghana, and Nepal who had accompanied me into the assembly hall, so that they could introduce themselves. I told them that they were the lead actors today—they had thirty seconds each to say something! This was a totally unexpected move, and the atmosphere in the hall changed completely. A stir immediately set in among the delegates, and they all craned their necks to stare at us—some even stood up so that they could get a good look at the speakers' faces. It was actually rather a strange moment.

Despite some nerves, my companions all spoke with great dignity, telling the audience where they were from and the many ways in which they had endured stigma and discrimination even after they were completely cured. All four of them went well over their allotted thirty seconds, but no one told them to hurry and wrap things up. Here were individuals with lived experience of leprosy speaking up for themselves on an international stage. A truly momentous occasion—the first time such a thing had ever happened at the UN. And surely something that would serve as an inspiration to many other people affected by leprosy all over the world.

During the same session, on 4 and 5 August, we held a special presentation on leprosy and human rights featuring the two films on leprosy mentioned earlier, made by Brazilian journalist and filmmaker

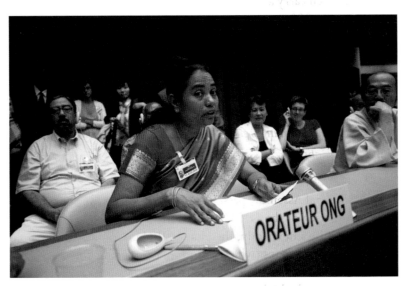

4. Nevis Mary, from India, making her appeal to the plenary session at the author's sudden request (Geneva, August 2005)

Andrea Pasquini and Indian journalist Ujjwal K. Chowdhury, and a panel discussion with the two directors present. The impact of the films, with their vivid, harrowing images, was immediately evident. The witnesses from India, Nepal, and Ghana, and some who had spoken so movingly in the plenary session, again gave presentations, along with members of their families. A lot of what they said seemed to shock people in the audience, many of them experts in the field of human rights and yet clearly learning the facts about leprosy for the first time. For people who weren't able to attend this special presentation with the film directors, we also put on an exhibition of twelve photographs of leprosy patients taken by Nippon Foundation photographer Natsuko Tominaga, along with some text written by people affected by leprosy. This display, which lasted from 2 to 5 August, was held in the lobby space just outside the main conference room of the United Nations building. Security restrictions regarding vehicle access to the Palais des Nations meant that we weren't able to use a van to transport the panels to be used for this display, which we had brought all the way from Japan, inside the grounds. Instead, Satoshi Sugawara and other Nippon Foundation staff had to divide up the panels and each carry a number on their head, covering themselves in sweat, for the 300 meters or so from the Pregny Gate of the Palais des Nations to the conference room. Thanks to their labors, we were able to put on a stunning display, which brought home in vivid detail why it is so important to deal with leprosy from a human rights point of view.

2007: The UN Human Rights Council replaces the UN Commission on Human Rights

In March 2006, we were somewhat taken aback when the United Nations General Assembly passed a resolution calling for the progressive phasing out of the UN Commission on Human Rights and its replacement by a new body, the Human Rights Council, with a total of forty-seven delegates (which would, of course, include Japan). All of the discussions that we had had on the human rights of leprosy-affected persons had taken place at sessions of the Sub-Commission on the Promotion and Protection of Human Rights, the subsidiary body of the Commission, and it had been this Sub-Commission that had tasked Professor Yokota to conduct fact-finding surveys on the discrimination faced by people affected by leprosy and their families. The institutional rearrangements meant that the Sub-Commission was abolished, which left the findings of the surveys undertaken by Professor Yokota at the Sub-Commission's behest essentially hanging. Just when the stage seemed finally set for a resolution on the issue of the human rights of leprosy-affected persons, we were faced with the necessity to return to square one.

So it was that I came to Geneva in September 2007, on a mission to persuade the members of the Human Rights Council, at their sixth session, to allow the issue of leprosy and human rights to be put on the table. I had decided that I would simply have to redouble my efforts.

The UN Human Rights Council was set up in principle as a forum for governmental delegates from nations around the world to meet and discuss matters of concern, but in some discussions and delibera-tions, it was permitted for NGOs who had obtained consultative status to voice their concerns. The Nippon Foundation had obtained such consultative status. I therefore submitted a written request to the Human Rights Council for the issue of leprosy and human rights to be discussed as a formal agenda item and also asked to be allowed to make an oral statement at the plenary session. I asked Dr. P. K. Gopal, president of IDEA India, an organization that works for the rehabilita-tion of people affected by leprosy, to be the person who would make this oral statement. I arranged for a panel exhibition of photographs taken by our photographer Natsuko Tominaga to be held directly opposite the conference room and for leprosy-related leaflets to be distributed. A symposium on leprosy and human rights was also hosted by the Nippon Foundation and the Sasakawa Health Foundation on 25 September. Chaired by Professor Kenzo Kiikuni of the Sasakawa Health Foundation, the symposium had presentations by panelists from three countries. Dr. Arturo C. Cunanan, head of the Culion Leprosy Control and Rehabilitation Program, Culion Sanitarium and General Hospital, the Philippines, provided a struc-tural analysis of discrimination against people affected by leprosy and how it can be eradicated. Dr. P. K. Gopal highlighted the existence of discriminatory legislation in India and cited examples of human rights violations. From Brazil, Artur Custodio, national coordinator of MORHAN (Movement for the Reintegration of Persons Affected by Hansen's Disease), and Dr. Lavinia Schuler-Faccini, a professor at the Federal University of Rio Grande do Sul, described the leprosy situation in Brazil and MORHAN's successes in empowering people affected by the disease. There was also a videotaped message from Professor Yozo Yokota, our former Special Rapporteur, who made a very moving case and appealed to the Human Rights Council to look at the issue of the human rights of people affected by leprosy.

At around this time, the Japanese government, which had become increasingly impressed with the Nippon Foundation's efforts and activities, announced that it would take a stand in the international arena for eradicating leprosy-related discrimination, making it a key plank of its diplomacy. (Shortly before I set off for Geneva, I had indeed been formally appointed the Japanese Government Goodwill Ambassador for the Human Rights of People Affected by Leprosy on 21 September by then Minister for Foreign Affairs Nobutaka Machimura.) One result of this was that Ambassador Ichiro Fujisaki, Japan's permanent representative in Geneva, became committed to taking proactive steps on our behalf. As the Japanese government representative in Geneva and as a member of the Human Rights Council, he told us he would be more than willing to request that the issue of leprosy and human rights be taken up as a formal agenda item in the plenary session.

On the evening of 25 September, we attended a reception hosted by Ambassador Ichiro Fujisaki, as the representative of the Permanent Mission of Japan to the International Organizations in Geneva, and over 140 other guests, which included a number of Human Rights Council members, representatives from WHO, and delegates from NGOs. The UN High Commissioner for Human Rights Louise Arbour gave an opening speech. Many of the people at this reception were human rights experts, and yet the vast majority of them admitted to being entirely unaware of the problem. The general verdict on the short video that we showed on the subject of leprosy and human rights was that it was absolutely eye-opening. Now that they knew what the issues were, they promised they would lend us their support. Realistically, in order to get the Human Rights Council to agree to have the issue discussed as a formal agenda item, much more had to happen: we would have to obtain the assent of nearly all of the member nations. However, this reception was extremely effective in demonstrating to the other nations that we were now operating with the full backing of the Japanese government.

2008: The world's first resolution, unanimously adopted, to end leprosy-based discrimination

Human rights have now become a universally recognized concept. But all too often, finding the right kinds of solutions to human rights issues is no simple matter. Human rights issues are always intertwined with the interests and political positions of the parties concerned. Fortunately, the problem of leprosy transcends matters of politics, ideology, ethnicity, and national borders, and I had high hopes that a good number of nations would support the resolution being put forward by the Japanese government. Nevertheless, I knew that any misreading of politics and political alliances in the Human Rights Council on our part would lead to a failure to get a resolution passed, no matter how valid the contents of our proposal. With this in mind, I decided to call on the diplomatic missions of the twenty-seven principal member nations of the United Nations Human Rights Council to explain the aims of the resolution submitted by the Japanese government and convince them of the need to adopt it.

Two countries especially stand out in my memories of this "pilgrimage of persuasion": Cuba and China. I'd been warned that, for political reasons, both countries would automatically oppose any proposal put forward by the Japanese government. Several people had advised me that it might be a waste of time to approach them, but my thinking is always that the first step to understanding is to have a conversation. I went first to Cuba's mission, where I talked with the ambassador. I opened the conversation with comments about how Mr. Castro's close companion Che Guevara, a physician, had taken a great interest in leprosy; how commendable were the efforts made by Cuba's doctors toward medical care around the world; and how both Fidel Castro and I had been recognized with awards from the WHO in 1998, on the fiftieth anniversary of its establishment. I noticed that tears were welling up in the ambassador's eyes. He extended his hand to me. "As far as this matter that you have brought up is concerned," he told me, "I will take full responsibility for carrying it out. Don't worry about a thing. I assure you."

My next target was China. At the Chinese mission, I recounted how my father Ryoichi Sasakawa had met with Deng Xiaoping and how the two of them had hit it off. I then proceeded to my argument, which was that sickness and disease happen to everyone and afflict all humankind regardless of political persuasion, ideology, or religion. After this preamble, I made my formal request and asked that China give us their support. The Chinese ambassador showed none of the deep emotion expressed by his Cuban counterpart. His response was rather more typically bureaucratic. He said simply that he would relay the message to his country's government.

On 18 June 2008, at the eighth regular session of the United Nations Human Rights Council held at the Palais des Nations, a motion drawn up by the Japanese government was proposed jointly (quite amazingly) by no fewer than fifty-nine member nations of the United Nations calling for the "elimination of discrimination against persons affected by leprosy and their family members." The council chair addressed the participants with a proposal that the motion be adopted by consensus, without voting, and asked if anyone had any objection to the motion. No nation voiced an objection. The motion was thus unanimously approved—and adopted. When the gavel struck, signifying that the motion was going to be put into effect, the sound resonated throughout the hall. This was a huge and historic achievement.

To my astonishment, among the fifty-nine nations that jointly submitted this motion were Cuba and China, two nations that I'd been led to believe, at least at the outset, would automatically oppose any motion put forward by the government of Japan. Both countries had given me indications that they might vote in favor, but in the end they had added their name to the list of countries that submitted the motion itself.

I was told that the passage of this leprosy resolution marked a rare occasion in history when the nations of the world had fully united on an issue to do with human rights—something that, no matter what the specifics might entail, could usually be expected to be greeted by a vote of opposition from somewhere. Even resolutions relating to HIV and AIDS had met with opposition from certain quarters.

The motion passed at the Human Rights Council session also called for the preparation of principles and guidelines for eliminating discrimination against persons affected by leprosy. A request to this effect was sent to the Human Rights Council Advisory Committee, and committee member Shigeki Sakamoto, then professor of international law at Kobe University, was appointed to draw up what came to be formally referred to as the "Principles and Guidelines." Professor Sakamoto, currently at Doshisha University, is an expert in international human rights law and had held a number of distinguished positions, including deputy director of the Japanese Society of International Law, president of the Japanese Association of International Human Rights Law, and president of the Japanese Institute for the Law of the Sea. Following Professor Yokota's death

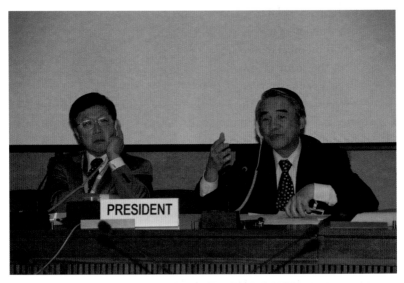

5. Two people who played an essential part in the discussions on leprosy and human rights in the United Nations Human Rights Council: Professor Shigeki Sakamoto (left) and Professor Yozo Yokota (right) (Geneva, January 2009)

in 2019, Professor Sakamoto has also been the president of the Center for Human Rights Education and Training, in Tokyo. The huge contributions made by these two men to my endeavors to take the issue of leprosy discrimination forward have been absolutely key. I am deeply grateful to both of them.

2009: An international meeting on leprosy and human rights, the first to be held at the United Nations

In January 2009, the Office of the United Nations High Commissioner for Human Rights called a meeting, officially termed an "open-ended consultation," to look into the matter of leprosy and human rights, in the Palais des Nations at Geneva.

The consultation was arranged in response to the resolution calling for the elimination of discrimination against people affected by leprosy and their family members that had been passed in June 2008, which had mandated the Office of the High Commissioner for Human Rights to look into what kinds of measures were in place to eliminate leprosy-related discrimination in countries around the world; and convene a meeting to exchange views with stakeholders, agencies, and medical experts. This was nearly five years after I first knocked on the door of the Office of the High Commissioner for Human Rights requesting that the human rights dimension be put on the table for discussion at the UN. Every year since then, I had paid at least one visit to the office to make the same request. Now, finally, it was happening. This was the first time that the UN itself had convened an official meeting on the topic of the human rights of people with leprosy.

More than eighty people took part in this meeting, which brought together representatives of governments, human rights specialists, international bodies, leprosy-related NGOs, people affected by the disease, and experts in other fields, including HIV/AIDS. Mr. Ibrahim Wani, chief of the economic and social issues branch of the Office of the High Commissioner for Human Rights, opened the discussions on the first day with a speech in which he referred to the Universal Declaration of Human Rights. Mr. Wani pointed out that the principle of non-discrimination on the grounds of health was as valid as that on the grounds of race, age, ability, and sex; and also stated that states were obliged to examine both the public and the private sphere in their promotion and protection of human rights. The first session saw presentations from Stefan Trömel of the International Disability Alliance, and Zilda Borges, a leprosy-affected person from Brazil, on aspects of the topic of non-discrimination under international law. In the second session, a number of people, including Denis Daumerie, WHO program officer for neglected tropical diseases, Susan Timberlake of the Joint United Nations Programme on HIV/AIDS, and Professor Yokota, formerly the Special Rapporteur for the now abolished Sub-Commission for the Promotion and Protection of Human Rights, gave presentations on "Leprosy and Human Rights and Health-Related Discrimination." At times, the debate grew very heated indeed. The third session featured Valdenora da Cruz Rodrigues from MORHAN, an NGO for leprosy-affected persons in Brazil; Leulseged Berhane Asres from the Ethiopian National Association of Persons Affected by Leprosy (ENAPAL); Dr. Arturo Cunanan, a doctor at the Culion Sanatorium and General Hospital in

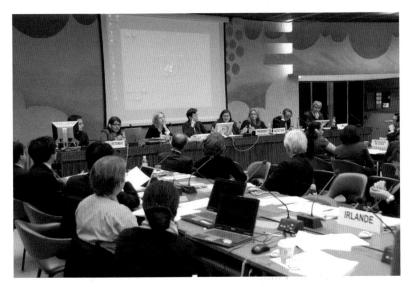

6. The meeting on Leprosy and Human Rights at the Palais des Nations (Geneva, January 2009)

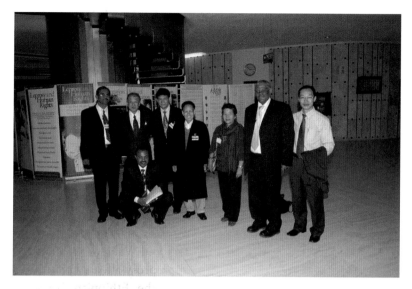

7. With participants at the meeting at the Palais des Nations (Geneva, January 2009)

the Philippines; and Douglas Soutar, general secretary of the International Federation of Anti-Leprosy Associations (ILEP), among others, all of whom made presentations that brought home the depth of discrimination that exists in their countries.

On 16 January, a second day of supplementary discussions took place, hosted by the Nippon Foundation and the Sasakawa Health Foundation, with the idea of looking more closely into the specifics of leprosy-based discrimination and investigating the kinds of issues that might be mentioned in the guidelines. Recent years have seen the growing recognition that people with disabilities should play a central role in deciding how they are supported, and leprosy is no exception. We had set up these discussions with the express purpose of getting UN human rights experts and government representatives to listen to what leprosy-affected persons themselves had to say. Today, they were to be the protagonists. Leprosy-affected individuals from Brazil, Ethiopia, India, the Philippines, China, Ghana, and the Republic of Korea told the audience about their experiences. One or two of them became choked with emotion as they talked, which only brought

37

home more vividly how painfully won their successes were and the depth of discrimination they had been subjected to in their lives.

I was most concerned that the issues of leprosy-related human rights might end up positioned as part of the right for all human beings to have equal access to medical care—in other words, simply as a "right to health." It is of course essential that we work toward a world in which all people in every nation can get access to a doctor and receive appropriate treatment. But to my knowledge, leprosy is the only disease in the world that causes its victims to suffer discrimination even after they have been completely cured. The fact that people get stuck with a label because of an illness that even after they are fully recovered goes on to become an obstacle to opportunity in all other areas of their life—education, employment, marriage—demonstrates that there is a social dimension to the problem that far transcends the parameters of a "right to health"—and has to be seen in terms of a violation of their basic human rights. There is a huge difference implied in the question of whether one sees the issues surrounding leprosy and human rights in terms of a general right to health, or as part of a debate about the violation of an individual's basic human rights. Ultimately, I am glad to say, it was decided that the human rights of people affected by leprosy deserved attention as a discrete issue.

These two days of open-ended consultations and discussions became the basis for the draft of the Principles and Guidelines for the Elimination of Discrimination against Persons Affected by Leprosy and Their Family Members, which had to be drawn up by the Advisory Committee to the Council for Human Rights and submitted to the UN Council for Human Rights for consideration by September that year. The Advisory Committee designated Professor Shigeki Sakamoto, a member of the Advisory Committee, to formulate the draft.

2009–10: Drawing up the Principles and Guidelines, and the United Nations resolution

Later in that same month of January 2009, Professor Sakamoto submitted a "Working Paper on the Elimination of Discrimination against Persons Affected by Leprosy and Their Family Members" to the UN

Advisory Committee to the Human Rights Council at its second session, laying out key objectives together with recommendations for measures for national governments to take in order to achieve the elimination of discrimination to be included in the Principles and Guidelines. The Advisory Committee approved it. Among the key objectives was the suggestion that a paragraph be included that called for an end to the common use of the derisive word "leper" to refer to persons affected by leprosy. At the third session of the UN Advisory Committee to the Human Rights Council in August 2009, Professor Sakamoto had submitted a finalized draft of the Principles and Guidelines for review, and this draft was then approved and submitted to the council for consideration. During that session, several influential members on the Advisory Committee had argued, regarding one clause in the draft of the Principles and Guidelines that recommended the immediate abolition of any law or policy to forcefully hospitalize, segregate, or intern persons affected by leprosy and their family members, that isolation would in some cases be necessary, bearing in mind the communicable nature of the disease. The article was amended during the session acknowledging the possible necessity for isolation. In September 2009, at the twelfth session of the UN Human Rights Council, a resolution was adopted requesting governments, UN specialized agencies, and NGOs to submit their views on the Draft Principles and Guidelines to the Office of the High Commissioner for Human Rights. The Advisory Committee was also requested to take the comments into full consideration in completing the Principles and Guidelines. Comments were submitted from twelve countries (including Japan), WHO, and nine NGOs. Strong opposition to the retention of the clause on isolation was then expressed by the WHO and related NGOs. In view of this opposition, at the fourth session of the Advisory Committee to the Human Rights Council in January 2010, Professor Sakamoto proposed that the clause on "isolation" be deleted, and this was approved. The draft submitted to the Advisory Committee at its fifth session in August 2010 had been further revised to read "isolation either before, during or after treatment should be temporary and should be conducted in the context of public health consideration." This was approved on 5 August 2010. The final Principles and Guidelines were adopted, with some other partial amendments, at the fifteenth regular session of the Human Rights Council in August 2010. It was an extremely complex process, but finally with the tireless efforts of Professor Sakamoto, it did prove possible to get agreement on the content and revised wording.

After this, in November 2010, the Japanese Ministry of Foreign Affairs submitted a draft resolution calling for the Elimination of Discrimination against Persons Affected by Leprosy and Their Family Members, and the adoption of the Principles and Guidelines, with eighty-four co-sponsoring nations, to the Third Committee (Social, Humanitarian & Cultural Issues) of the UN General Assembly, and it was adopted. One month later, on 21 December 2010, this resolution was unanimously adopted at the UN General Assembly in New York. In the resolution was a paragraph urging member states to let their governments know that they should pay due attention to the Principles and Guidelines. According to Professor Sakamoto, the true significance in getting the resolution passed, along with the Principles and Guidelines, lay first in the establishment of standards for the human rights of persons affected by leprosy; and secondly, in that it indicated clearly that the human rights of people affected by leprosy were worthy of protection under international law. This was a truly major advance. It meant that we now had a powerful tool that would help us in our work for the securing of human rights for persons affected by leprosy and for their full reintegration and inclusion into society.

On the actual day that the resolution and the Principles and Guidelines to end stigma and discrimination against people affected by leprosy and their family members was unanimously passed by the 193 nations at the UN General Assembly in New York, I was in Chiang Mai, Thailand. When word came from the Nippon Foundation, I was overcome with emotion. What wonderful news this was—coming at the very end of the year. The memories of all the meetings, the symposiums, the visits, the receptions we had arranged over the past seven years kept running through my mind like the images on a revolving lantern, and for a while all I could do was sit, lost in thought, in my hotel room.

This was an outcome with truly global significance for the fight against leprosy, one that Japan had played a major role in achieving.

I wanted the whole world to know about this epoch-making achievement, a demonstration of what can be done when a private sector organization in Japan, a country that has so often been criticized for following the lead of others in matters of human rights, joins hands with government and works for a common cause.

2011–17: Toward actual implementation of the Principles and Guidelines

The General Assembly's unanimous adoption of the resolution against discrimination of persons affected by leprosy and their family members, along with the Principles and Guidelines, was a momentous event. It had been seven long years since I had made my original appeal to the United Nations High Commissioner for Human Rights in 2003 and realized just how little people were aware of the human rights dimension of leprosy. Every year, I had attended regular sessions of the commission and council, steadily trying to persuade the members in lobbies and side-event rooms. The fact that our seven-year-long efforts had ended in such a spectacular success was due in no small part to the tremendous efforts of the staff at the Nippon Foundation and the Sasakawa Health Foundation. I am well aware of how selflessly and tirelessly they worked, and I will never forget a single moment of our endeavors together.

Even with this achievement, my battle was not at an end. Needless to say, the adoption of resolutions by the UN Human Rights Council and UN General Assembly did not translate into the immediate elimination of the stigma associated with and the discrimination toward persons affected by leprosy and their family members.

To ensure that the resolution we had worked to pass in the United Nations didn't just calcify, or dissipate into mere empty words—in other words, to publicize the resolution and accompanying Principles and Guidelines, and to guide nations in their implementation—I decided to put in place two further initiatives.

The first was a series of international symposiums on leprosy and human rights to be held in the five regions of the world—the Americas, Asia, Africa, the Middle East, and Europe. The second was to form an international working group to look into ways of imple-

41

menting the Principles and Guidelines. I will deal with the symposiums first.

The first international symposium took place in Rio de Janeiro, Brazil, in February 2012. It was preceded a couple of days earlier by the launch of the seventh Global Appeal to end stigma and discrimination against people affected by leprosy (to be dealt with later) in São Paulo, endorsed that year by the World Medical Association. The symposium was attended by numerous representatives of human rights organizations, international NGOs, UN affiliates, and people affected by leprosy.

The second symposium took place in New Delhi, India, in October 2012. Among the participants on this occasion were the chair of India's National Human Rights Commission and several members of the Indian Parliament. A highlight was their formation of a cross-party MP forum tasked with combating leprosy.

The third symposium took place in Addis Ababa, Ethiopia, and was attended by that country's prime minister, Hailemariam Desalegn. It provided an important opportunity to make an appeal concerning leprosy and human rights to all the member nations of the African Union.

Rabat, the capital of Morocco, was the site of the fourth symposium. The event was held with the full cooperation of the Moroccan government. Participating on behalf of that country's people affected by leprosy was Naima Azzouzi. Ms. Azzouzi had been diagnosed with leprosy at the age of nine and had been placed in a facility where she remained shut off from outside contact. She spoke of the newly formed association of people affected by leprosy in her country, Morocco's first such organization, in which she was serving as president. The passion with which she spoke left me in no doubt that she was going to make some good things happen in Morocco and other countries in North Africa.

The fifth and final symposium in the series took place in Geneva in June 2015. Here too, a good number of people affected by leprosy participated, including individuals from Brazil, China, Colombia, Ethiopia, Ghana, India, Indonesia, Morocco, and the Philippines.

The second initiative I set up was the international working group. Two individuals would play a central role in this group: Professor Yozo Yokota of Chuo University, who had made selfless efforts as a former member of the UN Sub-Commission on the Promotion and Protection of Human Rights; and Professor Shigeki Sakamoto of Kobe University, who had drafted the "Principles and Guidelines." Its members also included human rights experts and legal scholars from around the world and persons affected by leprosy.

The group had two main tasks: to devise measures for protecting people affected by leprosy, as well as their family members, and to draft an action plan for achieving broad social recognition and realization of the Principles and Guidelines. In all, the working group met on four occasions, between 2012 and 2014, and it compiled a report of its investigations and deliberations, which it relayed to the final symposium in Geneva, and then subsequently the UN.

The report recommended that addressing leprosy-related issues should be a responsibility undertaken at the national level, and that all discriminatory legislation should be abolished. In every country, government agencies at both the national and local levels—judiciary, legislature, and executive—should act in accordance with what was laid out in the Principles and Guidelines, and an action plan matched to the situation of each country should be drawn up and implemented. In addition, the report urged strongly that the principal roles in these matters should be played by people affected by leprosy themselves.

The report also made a strong case for involving religious leaders of all persuasions in the battle to eliminate discrimination. Religious leaders were encouraged to use the power and influence of religion to help bring an end to the common use of the discriminatory word "leper" when referring to people affected by the disease.

One of the most important recommendations issued by the international working group to the United Nations Human Rights Council was its suggestion as to how these issues should be dealt with going forward. The report recommended that the UN Human Rights Council request its Advisory Committee to study and recommend the creation of an appropriate follow-up mechanism at the international level that would have the authority to monitor the actions of member states. In response to this call, under a proposal drafted by the Japanese government, in 2015 the Human Rights Council adopted a resolution tasking the Advisory Committee to conduct surveys over a period of two years regarding the implementation of the Principles and Guidelines, together with any obstacles in their implementation and to submit a report.

The Advisory Committee established a drafting group, and appointed one of its experts, Mr. Imeru Tamrat Yigezu, from Ethiopia, as the rapporteur charged with examining the progress made and reporting back with recommendations. Mr. Yigezu was an international law specialist by training, a reputed academician, and had published numerous papers related to water and the environment, and he was well acquainted with the issues faced by persons affected by leprosy in his country. He showed a high degree of commitment to this task. Professor Kaoru Obata of Nagoya University, Japan's member of the Advisory Committee, became the chairperson of the drafting group.

The report submitted by Mr. Yigezu after two years of investigation showed that on the whole few steps had been taken in setting up any measures or action plans in countries where leprosy was endemic, and there was little sign of recognition in broader society of the existence of the Principles and Guidelines. In many countries, discriminatory prohibitions and practices remained in place, exactly as they had always been. The report stressed that in order to put the principles and guidelines into practice, it was necessary to establish a mechanism with a global mandate for monitoring and reporting.

After Mr. Yigezu's report was submitted to the UN Human Rights Council in June 2017, the Japanese government moved without delay to secure as many nations as possible to support a formal proposal for a resolution on the appointment of a Special Rapporteur.

To be frank, I had not expected the UN Human Rights Council or the Office of the UN High Commissioner to move so quickly toward the appointment of a Special Rapporteur. The speed with which events developed was entirely due to the strong commitment and magnificent diplomatic efforts of everyone at the Human Rights and Humanitarian Affairs Division of the Ministry of Foreign Affairs, and at the Permanent Mission of Japan (to the United Nations and Other International Organizations) in Geneva. Special mention must be made of Ms. Mitsuko Shino, who in 2008, in her position at the time as director of the Japanese Ministry of Foreign Affairs' Human Rights and Humanitarian Affairs Division succeeding her predecessor Ms. Misako

Kaji, had contributed greatly to the adoption of the UN resolution. After serving for several years as Japan's ambassador to Iceland, Ms. Shino had become ambassador of the Human Rights and Humanitarian Affairs Division in Geneva, and thanks to her unmatched powers of persuasion and her tireless diplomatic efforts, again in 2017 we managed to get no fewer than forty-three nations, including Brazil, Ethiopia, Vietnam, Ghana, and Egypt, to agree to be co-sponsors for a joint proposal on the appointment of a Special Rapporteur.

These efforts paid off, and on 22 June 2017 the draft resolution put forward at the initiative of the Japanese government with the co-sponsorship of other nations was passed unanimously at the thirty-fifth session of the United Nations Human Rights Council, paving the way for the appointment of a UN Special Rapporteur on the elimination of discrimination toward persons affected by leprosy and their family members.

The next step was to find a suitable person to take up the post. A great number of people applied from all over the world, but in September 2017 Dr. Alice Cruz, a Portuguese national, was appointed Special Rapporteur by the Human Rights Council. For me, this was a truly excellent outcome, as she was a person I respected and trusted. At the time of her appointment, she was an external professor at the law school of University Andina Simón Bolívar, in Ecuador, but she had obtained her PhD in medical anthropology and had worked with the Brazilian non-profit organization MORHAN. A specialist who participated in the elaboration of the WHO Guidelines for Strengthening the Participation of Persons Affected by Leprosy in Leprosy Services, and who had researched and written on the psycho-social aspects of leprosy and conducted fieldwork in a number of different countries, there was no better person for the job. When asked why she wanted to become a Special Rapporteur, she replied: "It was something I felt I had to do, following years of personal, academic and activist engagement with persons affected by leprosy. Over that time, I have come to know the structural barriers they still face to a full life … However, for vulnerable persons who face multiple discriminations in their daily lives, there is no time to lose."

I was thrilled that such a passionate and dedicated person would be lending her energy to the fight to eradicate leprosy-related discrimination. I wholeheartedly agree with her that there is no time to lose. People affected by leprosy have suffered too long, and they are aging. We have to take steps, tackle the barriers, and bring about changes in society during their lifetimes. I myself am getting on in years: I want to see the changes within my lifetime. It's a fight not only against the disease, but also against time.

2

REACHING THE UNREACHABLE

2001–5

A target that half the world had yet to attain

In May 1991, the forty-fourth World Health Assembly passed a resolution to eliminate leprosy as a public health problem globally by the year 2000. The idea was that once this official target (less than one case per 10,000 population) was reached, infections would cease, and the regular healthcare system in each country would be able to cope. Setting a numerical target was seen as an essential first step. Notwithstanding the significant progress that had been made, however, to most people the idea of trying to control leprosy, let alone eliminate it, seemed like an impossible dream. In 1990, there were still eighty-nine nations with a population of more than 1 million where leprosy was endemic. This was nearly half the nations in the world.

In July 1994, the Sasakawa Health Foundation and the World Health Organization (WHO) held an International Conference on the Elimination of Leprosy, in Hanoi, Vietnam, bringing together representatives from twenty-eight countries that had yet to meet the WHO target of leprosy elimination, along with health experts and NGOs. The principal purpose of the conference, the first of its kind, was to show solidarity with the twenty-eight countries and stiffen their resolve. In my address, I offered to provide WHO with US$10 million per year to fund the free provision of multidrug therapy (MDT) worldwide for a period of five years—a total of US$50 million. The free distribution of MDT is important not only because it cures people of the disease; it also frees governments from the financial burden of purchasing drugs so that they can allocate money for other things—to pay health workers and social workers to find and treat people, or to pay for information and awareness campaigns. It also allows NGOs to redirect funds toward paying for other needs of people affected by leprosy, like reconstructive surgery, artificial limbs, and so on.

In November 1999, we held the third International Conference on the Elimination of Leprosy in Abidjan, Côte d'Ivoire, where we reaffirmed our commitment, identified the countries where it was going to be difficult to eliminate leprosy by the year 2000, and discussed what ought to be done. At this meeting, a new Global Alliance for the Elimination of Leprosy (GAEL) was formed. The members included governments of the countries that had yet to reach the elimination target, as well as members of WHO, the International Federation of Anti-Leprosy Associations (ILEP), the Nippon Foundation, and others. I announced a further pledge from the Nippon Foundation of 24 million dollars based on a new timeframe of 2000 to 2005. After this date, the Novartis Foundation would take over paying for MDT.

GAEL's first international conference was held in New Delhi, India, in January 2001, where we announced what was called the Delhi Declaration, setting a new target of eliminating leprosy in all countries of the world by 2005.

Here is a list of the major countries that went on, one by one, to achieve the elimination target after the Hanoi Declaration of 1994. There are thirty-three of them:

Egypt, Mexico (1994)

Thailand, Sri Lanka (1995)

Colombia (1996)

Togo, Benin, Venezuela, Chad (1997)

Ghana, Nigeria, Bangladesh, Cambodia, the Philippines (1998)

REACHING THE UNREACHABLE

Sudan (1999)

Ethiopia, China, Malaysia, Indonesia, Papua New Guinea (2000)

Mali, Côte d'Ivoire (2001)

Niger (2002)

Myanmar (2003)

Angola, India (2005)

Tanzania, Madagascar, Guinea (2006)

Democratic Republic of the Congo (DRC), Mozambique (2007)

Nepal (2009)

Timor-Leste (2010)

In 1985, there were 122 nations where leprosy was a national health problem. By 1995, the figure was down to sixty-eight. By 2000, the number was eleven. And since 2010, there has only been one country where leprosy remains endemic, and that is the nation of Brazil.

Countries visited in 2001	
January	• India
April	Austria (Nippon Foundation-sponsored Salzburg Music Festival)
May	• Switzerland
	Russia (Moscow; Chernobyl Sasakawa Medical Cooperation conference)
	Serbia (University of Belgrade; SYLFF-related events and refugee issues)
June	• Ghana
	• Uganda
	Tanzania (SG2000 field survey)
August	Malaysia (Meetings)
September	Indonesia
	Finland (Scandinavia–Japan Sasakawa Foundation board meeting)

October	• Czech Republic (Forum 2000 Conference)
	Switzerland (Meetings)
	Finland (Helsinki University; tenth anniversary SYLFF program)
November	Myanmar (Interaction with Myanmar military: visit to a leprosy facility)
	China (Japan–China Sasakawa Medical Fellowship meeting)

• Indicates a trip that features in this section.

SYLFF: Sasakawa Young Leaders Fellowship Fund program.

SG2000: Sasakawa Global 2000 program. An agricultural project supporting farmers in need in Africa.

Forum 2000: An annual international conference launched in 1997 when Václav Havel, Elie Wiesel, and the author invited world leaders to Prague for open debate on the major issues and challenges of the new millennium.

The first GAEL meeting—Republic of India, January 2001

In January 2001, the members of GAEL held their first meeting in New Delhi, India. I attended this meeting. GAEL was a new alliance that had been formed in November 1999 at the Third International Conference on Leprosy, held in Abidjan, Côte d'Ivoire. It was now clear that a number of countries would not be able to meet the target that WHO had announced in May 1991 of eliminating leprosy as a public health problem (defining elimination as a level of prevalence of less than one case per 10,000 population) by the year 2000. The purpose of the meeting was to reaffirm our commitment and set a new deadline of 2005. Those attending included representatives of governments of the countries that had yet to reach the elimination target, WHO regional directors and advisors, ILEP, the Nippon Foundation, the Sasakawa Health Foundation, Novartis and the Novartis Foundation, as well as Danish International Development Assistance (DANIDA), the World Bank, and others. There were ministers of health and representatives from Angola, Brazil, the Central African Republic, the DRC, Guinea, India, Indonesia, Madagascar, Mozambique, Myanmar, Nepal, and Niger.

REACHING THE UNREACHABLE

In my opening address, I reminded participants that we were now walking the final mile of a 100-mile journey, but that the final mile was likely to be the longest—in other words, we could not consider ourselves finished until we had reached the finish line. This announcement seemed to strike a chord, and quite a few people chose to refer to it in their speeches. In his inaugural address, the minister of state for health and family welfare of India, representing the host country, spoke of leprosy as one of the three principal diseases in India that must be eliminated, the other two being poliomyelitis and filariasis. He announced a stepping-up of the distribution system for MDT blister packs and declared that the government would be putting in place a national program and making every effort to decentralize leprosy elimination control activities, bringing diagnoses and treatments to provincial populations.

The declaration adopted at this meeting—later dubbed the Delhi Declaration—recommended collaboration between GAEL members in order to eliminate leprosy as a public health problem by the year 2005. It acknowledged that despite significant progress, access to diagnosis and treatment of leprosy in many endemic countries remained unacceptably low. It expressed concern that other more pressing public health priorities might push some authorities to ignore leprosy and lose this window of opportunity. It supported the strategy of a "final push" to eliminate leprosy in all endemic countries and emphasized the need for leprosy to be integrated within the general health services. It urged all concerned to ensure the uninterrupted availability of free MDT treatment at all health centers, to dispel the negative image of leprosy, and improve community awareness of the availability of treatment.

On the second day, a roundtable discussion with a number of key participants took place on each nation's plans and the kind of overall coordination necessary for effective implementation. It was during these discussions that certain statements were uttered that led to a cooling of trust between WHO and ILEP representatives, and a clear difference of opinion emerged regarding approach. Toward the end of the conference, a proposal came from the delegate from the WHO Office for the Americas that I be appointed Special Ambassador to the alliance, in recognition of my contribution to the cause of leprosy and my success in mobilizing the high level of commitment required in endemic countries; the proposal was adopted with a rising vote, which was followed by a round of applause. The role of Special Ambassador involved me being the "face" of GAEL to the world, strengthening the commitment of governments to get on board with GAEL's principles, and playing the role of intermediary between stakeholders within GAEL. This appointment lasted until 2002, when GAEL was dissolved due to internal disagreements. In 2003, I was appointed WHO's Goodwill Ambassador for the Elimination of Leprosy, a position I still hold today.

A special event at the World Health Assembly on leprosy elimination—Swiss Confederation, May 2001

On 22 May 2001, I visited Geneva to attend the fifty-fourth World Health Assembly at the Palais des Nations.

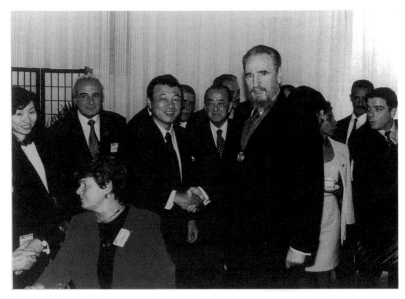

8. At the 1998 WHO Health for All Awards with President Fidel Castro of Cuba (Geneva, May 1998)

During my stay, there was a special event on leprosy elimination, where I was one of the invited speakers. With me on the podium were prominent figures in the field of public health, including WHO Director-General Gro Harlem Brundtland; India's Minister of Health and Family Welfare Dr. Chandreshwar Prasad Thakur; Brazil's Minister of Health José Serra; Madagascar's Minister of Health Rahantalalao Henriette Ratsimbazafimahefa; Mr. Terry Vasey, president of ILEP; and Klaus Leisinger, CEO of the Novartis Foundation.

In her opening address at this special event, Dr. Brundtland described the Nippon Foundation and the Sasakawa Health Foundation as significant partners for WHO and praised the critically important contributions and activities of both organizations toward the elimination of leprosy over the past twenty years. She also made the announcement that I was being appointed GAEL Special Ambassador. "I welcome this appointment with all my heart," she added. "Mr. Sasakawa's devoted effort and his strong sense of commitment to this cause are an inspiration to us all."

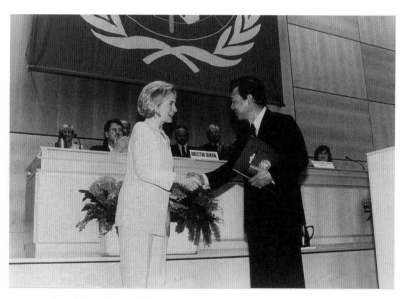

9. At the 1998 WHO Health for All Awards with Mrs. Hilary Rodham Clinton (Geneva, May 1998)

During the plenary meetings of the fifty-fourth World Health Assembly, I was able to have discussions with the health ministers of Myanmar, Nepal, Angola, Mozambique, and Ghana, among other nations. In one of the meetings devoted to presentations of awards, I presented the WHO Sasakawa Health Prize, which this year went to Dr. João Aprigio Guerra de Almeida, who runs a breast milk bank for infants of poor families in Brazil. This is a prize awarded to individuals or institutions, including NGOs, that have accomplished innovative or outstanding work in health development.

Time with two presidents—Republic of Ghana, June 2001

In June, I went to Africa, and my first stop was Ghana. As a former British colony, Ghana is a member of the Commonwealth of Nations. Its first president, Kwame Nkrumah (1909–72), is famous for being an advocate of Pan-Africanism. The country is known for its production of coffee beans. Ghana reached the WHO target for elimination of leprosy in 1998.

I had several objectives during this visit. I wanted to take a general look at the efforts being made toward control and elimination of leprosy. I wanted to hear about an ongoing project researching skin transplants in the treatment of Buruli ulcer, a chronic debilitating disease associated with leprosy that affects the skin and leads to the formation of large ulcers. I also intended to make an on-site inspection of the ongoing operations of the SG2000 project that was spearheading the increase of foodstuff production for impoverished farmers in Africa.

While in Ghana, I paid a courtesy call on President John Kufuor at his elegant private residence (it was a Sunday, so I was invited to his home). President Kufuor stated that his government was getting to grips with eradicating leprosy-related discrimination, which he admitted was still a problem. They were taking measures for the rehabilitation of former patients and extending a helping hand to people who suffered discrimination. He affirmed his government's commitment to step up efforts and extend every support to all initiatives working toward leprosy elimination.

I also paid a call on Jerry Rawlings, president of Ghana from 1993 to 2001, who had been a personal friend for several years. He stated his appreciation of both my father and myself for our efforts in two critical areas of African life, leprosy elimination and agriculture, noting in particular the contributions made by the Sasakawa Africa Association to improving crop food technology and the development of "quality protein maize." Good nutrition, he said, is essential for good health. He had recently been appointed to serve as the first international Year of Volunteers 2001 Eminent Person by UN Secretary-General Kofi Annan. Volunteer work cannot be done without a conscience, he told me. He would do his best to promote volunteerism around the world.

A president under a misapprehension—Republic of Uganda, June 2001

From Ghana, I went straight on to Uganda to attend a Sasakawa Global 2000 (SG2000) workshop. Former President of the United States Jimmy Carter was also one of the participants. The SG2000 project was one that my father established in 1986 in response to the 1984 famine in Ethiopia, with the idea of showing poor farmers in Africa how they could increase their yield, with the cooperation of Jimmy Carter and the American agronomist and Nobel Peace Prize laureate Dr. Norman Borlaug. During my talks with Ugandan President Yoweri Museveni, he told me leprosy was unheard of in his country, though he did know that in the past an island in Lake Victoria was used to isolate leprosy patients. But of course, he said, if Uganda did have leprosy, he would do everything in his power to help eliminate it and likewise the social discrimination attached to it. His words suggested to me the possibility that some leaders in Africa were not being kept up to date with the current situation regarding leprosy in their own countries.

In a briefing I had after that in the Ministry of Health, I was told that 35 percent of the children in Uganda are malnourished. Nevertheless, the government was doing its best to incorporate leprosy treatment in its general health care services, to do away with segregated settlements, and to step up its monitoring of the disease. Uganda had reached the WHO elimination target three years before, in 1998, but armed conflict in five of the northern provinces had

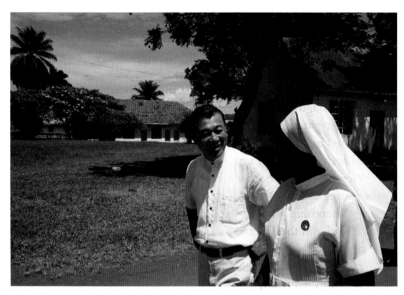

10. With a nurse at the St. Francis Leprosy Center (Uganda, June 2001)

made proper investigation of the leprosy situation impossible. Surveys of these regions were definitely on the agenda. When the political situation stabilized, elimination would be possible. Meanwhile, it was essential to ensure access to medication even in the villages. After this meeting, I went to St. Francis Leprosy Center situated 70 miles from the capital. This was a facility set up as a leprosarium in 1923, originally a Catholic mission run by nuns. Now it served outpatients with tuberculosis as well as leprosy. Every year, fifty or sixty newly discovered individuals with leprosy were being brought in to be cared for.

My first presentation on leprosy and human rights on the world stage—Czech Republic, October 2001

In October 2001, I made my annual trip to Prague, to attend the Forum 2000 Conference. This is an event that happens every year using Prague Castle as its backdrop, gathering together leading politicians, people in the business world and the world of journalism, academics, philosophers, writers, representatives from labor unions, NGOs and non-governmental foundations, religious leaders, and leading intellectuals from all manner of spheres to discuss world issues— ethnic conflicts in a globalizing world, religious conflict, population problems, environmental issues, and other topics—and to reach for solutions through dialogue. This conference was the brainchild of the poet, playwright, freedom fighter, world intellectual, and first president of the Czech Republic Václav Havel, and the writer, professor, political activist, and Holocaust survivor Nobel Peace Prize laureate Elie Wiesel. They asked me whether I would like to lend my efforts to the cause, and together we put this grand undertaking into operation. My friendship with His Holiness the Fourteenth Dalai Lama, the spiritual leader of the Tibetan people and a Nobel Peace Prize laureate, stemmed from this endeavor.

The people attending the conference in 2001 included former US President Bill Clinton; former South African President Nelson Mandela; Israel elder statesman Shimon Peres; former GDR and German President Richard von Weizsäcker; South African statesman and Nobel Peace Prize laureate F. W. de Klerk; Prince Hassan of Jordan; US statesman Henry Kissinger; former President of Ireland Mary Robinson; Indian politician Sonia Gandhi; Costa Rica activist and Nobel Peace Prize laureate Óscar Arias Sánchez; activist, former president of Poland, and Nobel Peace Prize laureate Lech Wałęsa; US political scientist and academic Francis Fukuyama; UK musician Peter Gabriel; notable US economist Jeffrey Sachs; His Holiness the Dalai Lama; South African Archbishop Desmond Tutu; and many other leaders, illustrious personalities, and courageous individuals. Since I was one of the people, along with Václav Havel and Elie Wiesel, on whose initiative the annual conference was founded, I made a point of attending every year for the fifteen years from 1997 to 2011. The conference in 2011 ended up being the last one attended by Václav Havel, who died later that year.

The theme of the conference was "Human Rights—Search for Global Responsibility," which was discussed over the three days from a variety of different perspectives. On the second day of the conference, 15 October, in a special session featuring a panel discussion on "The Human Right to Health," I opened the discussion with remarks on "Leprosy and Human Rights," in which I explained that leprosy had a medical side and a social side, and with a brief history and a few key examples highlighted the human rights dimension of this disease. We were now in the process of eliminating leprosy as a disease, I explained, but a host of problems remain—related to prejudice and discrimination. For years, the prejudice felt toward people who are affected by leprosy and their family members has been a hidden problem; but in many countries it means that people with this disease, and those who have recovered from it, have to live lives blighted by stigma, with curtailed opportunities, often in appalling conditions. The plight of these people amounts to a human rights violation. A panel discussion followed, with, among others, the Somali supermodel and human rights activist in the fight against female genital mutilation (FGM) (1997–2003 UN Special Ambassador against FGM) Waris Dirie, as well as Anwei Law, filmmaker and chronicler of the leprosy-affected community in Hawaii, who is an advocate for those with leprosy in her position of international coordinator for the non-profit International Association for Integration, Dignity and Economic Advancement (IDEA).

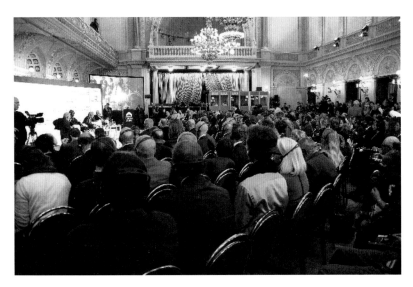

11. The annual venue for Forum 2000, the Zorfin Palace Hall (Czech Republic, October 2001)

REACHING THE UNREACHABLE

This presentation, the first I had ever made on the world stage regarding the issue of human rights and leprosy, clearly made an impression on the conference participants. Afterwards, the Nobel Peace Prize laureate José Ramos-Horta, then foreign minister of Timor-Leste, told me that up till then he had been completely unaware of the existence of this crucial human rights issue in his country, and he vowed to investigate the matter as soon as he returned home. Since then, the issue of leprosy and human rights has been taken up any number of times in sessions in the annual Forum 2000 conference. As I will show in the course of this book, many people present at the discussions, including His Holiness the Dalai Lama, expressed their support and gave us their word that they would do their utmost to disseminate the message of ridding the world of the discrimination shown toward people affected by leprosy and their family members.

Here is the text of the speech I delivered:

Leprosy and Human Rights

By Yohei Sasakawa

President of the Nippon Foundation

Forum 2000, Prague

15 October 2001

Ladies and Gentlemen,

Before I begin, I would like to thank the organizers of the conference for this opportunity to speak to you on the subject, "Leprosy and Human Rights."

I have worked toward the elimination of leprosy for more than thirty years.

To many, leprosy is a disease of a former age, and I am sure that many of you are puzzled as to why I bring it up as a problem for this contemporary age.

But it is still a very big issue. It consists of two aspects. First, it is a medical problem to be tackled. Second, and more important, is its social aspect: discrimination based on the prejudice that it generates.

Leprosy is a chronic bacterial disease that affects the skin and nerves.

In the past, the disease would deform the limbs and disfigure the faces of sufferers. It seemed to strike haphazardly and selectively, and once it struck, it ran an unstoppable course but was not fatal. As a result of these and other characteristics, a tremendous stigma became attached to leprosy, and it became a symbol for that which was most feared. The people it touched were forced to live lingering lives that were worse than death.

We who are working for the elimination of the disease, together with WHO, have set elimination by the year 2005 as our target. We are putting all of our effort into this final push in order to draw the curtain on the long history of leprosy. The leprosy of today can be cured within a year with a highly effective multidrug therapy, known as MDT. For the past five years, my foundation has provided free worldwide distribution of MDT. According to WHO, elimination is defined as a prevalence of less than one person in 10,000. Since 1985, 116 countries have achieved this goal and only six remain: India, Brazil, Myanmar, Nepal, Mozambique, and Madagascar. In my capacity as WHO's Special Ambassador for the Elimination of Leprosy, I am working with the governments of these remaining countries and with international NGOs to further strengthen their activities to achieve this goal as quickly and effectively as possible.

The goal of eliminating leprosy as a public health problem is clearly in sight. Now, however, it is time to seriously consider how we are going to tackle the difficult social issue associated with leprosy: the discrimination that arises from prejudice. Let me give you a picture of how society has reacted to this disease so that you can see the relationship between leprosy and human rights.

History has revealed this relationship very clearly. Since the dawn of recorded history, there have been numerous references to leprosy. Accounts of it can be found in the Old and New Testaments, the ancient documents of China, and Indian classics from the sixth century BC. There are also numerous works of art depicting people who had leprosy. All of these show that, from time immemorial, the individual with leprosy has been treated with all of the fear that dwells deep within the hearts of people: the fear toward that which is different. What is startling is that we find this strong sense of exclusion around the world, regardless of country, religion, or culture. Everywhere, leprosy has been the most feared of diseases and its victims the ultimate outcasts of society, forced to lead lives that denied their very humanity.

From ancient times, and even by family members, sufferers of leprosy were branded as unclean people, as people who had committed transgressions in previous lives. They were ostracized from society and isolated. The Kalaupapa Sanitorium in Hawaii, where Father Damien served in the middle of the nineteenth century, is one example where, out of a sense of crisis about the spread of leprosy, sufferers were sent away to a remote island. Robben Island of South Africa is known as the island where former President Nelson Mandela was exiled, but in fact, the entire island used to be a place to confine people with leprosy. There are countless islands like that in the Aegean Sea, in Asia, and elsewhere, where sufferers lived, completely stripped of their rights as humans.

When people contracted leprosy, their families drove them out, and even stripped their names from them to protect the honor of the family. They thus became people who had no social existence. In this way, they were deprived of a voice with which to speak out against the society. Even their families abandoned them. They lost all identity but the identification numbers forced on them. It is a shock to realize that until the latter half of the 1940s, sufferers confined in the National Leprosarium in the United States were even denied the right to vote.

When I visited a leprosy colony in Indonesia, I had a chance to meet a former patient. She was eighty-five years old but had been living there since she was twelve. I asked, "Since your sickness is completely healed, why don't you go back to your home and family?" She replied, "I cannot because it would only bring trouble and unhappiness to my family. I will be finishing my life here at the colony, quiet and alone." The same kind of story can be found all over the world. Even after death, former patients are not allowed to go back to their families. Families deny the relationship and even refuse to accept their ashes.

Though sufferers have been allotted a fate in which their very families deny their existence, for the most part their plight has not been included on the list of human rights violations.

The countless tragedies associated with leprosy are a terrible and continuing legacy of man's inhumanity to man. They are not something that should be buried in the distant past. Even today in the twenty-first century, we are faced by very real, ongoing challenges. I am specifically thinking of the following two issues:

First, leprosy continues to be a health problem, especially in the developing countries of Asia and Africa. Every year 700,000 new individuals are diagnosed with leprosy. Since there is now an effective cure, it is a global responsibility to help provide treatment in a timely enough manner that deformity and disability do not occur. Then, we will be able to separate ourselves from the long history of discrimination and exclusion.

MAKING THE IMPOSSIBLE POSSIBLE

The second issue is that of just how seriously we all take the question of the dignity and social recognition of former patients. In my own country of Japan, there existed a law justifying the segregation of sufferers until five years ago. Recently, however, those who had been expelled from society sought compensation from the government for the loss of their rights, and in May 2001, they won their case. The fact that these individuals won the court case and that the government admitted its mistake made headlines worldwide. In describing how he felt immediately after this victory, one of the plaintiffs said, "Human rights are like air. I feel that today is the first time that I can breathe freely." This court decision was the first step in returning to former patients the dignity which is every human being's right.

In the dark ages of the 1920s, when leprosy was yet incurable and greatly feared, a Japanese poet named Akashi Kaijin contracted the disease. He nevertheless upheld himself with dignity and pride and left us the following words: "Unless I illuminate myself like a deep-sea fish, nowhere will I find even a glimmer of light." Now, more than ever, a place is needed for those who have been denied their existence by society, to illuminate themselves and raise their voices.

In response to this, for the first time in history, an international support network has been established, whose leadership is primarily made up of individuals who have personally faced the challenges of leprosy. Known as the International Association for Integration, Dignity and Economic Advancement, or IDEA, this organization provides opportunities for individuals to empower and support each other while promoting a positive image of leprosy that is based on ability, achievement, and the wisdom that comes from experience. The organization may yet be small, but its message is immense. Since the message is a vital one, our foundation is providing its wholehearted support to IDEA. The treatment of sufferers of leprosy has been a negative legacy of the human community. We must learn from this mistake and, through education and the media, lead the public down a path of enlightenment to the truth about leprosy and the social issues it has raised.

A minute ago, I told the sad story of a former patient in Indonesia. Those who have been exiled because of leprosy often echo her feelings when they say, "We will only be able to go home when we leave the crematory chimney as smoke."

The history of leprosy is the history of men, women, and families whose lives have been completely determined by this particular disease.

REACHING THE UNREACHABLE

In the twenty-first century, science and technology are making tremendous strides. The danger that this presents us with is that, in the shadow of this extraordinary progress, human dignity and the rights of individuals may be overlooked. We need to fix our gaze on those who are being left behind and are suffering from unreasonable inhumanity. We need to focus on all moving forward together. Then, we will be able to say that humanity is truly progressing.

Thank you.

Countries visited in 2002	
January	Mexico (El Colegio de México SYLFF events)
	Honduras (Zamorano Pan-American Agricultural School)
	• Brazil
February	China (Japan–China security relations)
May	Republic of Korea (Visit to Sorokdo leprosy facility)
	• Latvia
	• Switzerland
June	Singapore (Meeting on the safety and security of the Strait of Malacca)
	• Malaysia
July	United Kingdom (Great Britain Sasakawa Foundation annual general meeting)
September	• Mozambique
October	• The Vatican
	China (Nippon Music Foundation concert)
	Czech Republic (Forum 2000 Conference)
November	• Papua New Guinea
	• Philippines

December	● Bangladesh
	● India (SYLFF award ceremony)

● Indicates a trip that features in this section.

SYLFF: The Sasakawa Young Leaders Fellowship Fund program. A funding program.

Forum 2000: An annual international conference launched in 1997 when Václav Havel, Elie Wiesel, and the author invited world leaders to Prague for open debate on the major issues and challenges of the new millennium.

The second GAEL meeting—Federative Republic of Brazil, January 2002

My first leprosy-related activity of 2002 took place in Brazil, where I participated in the second GAEL meeting, held in the city of Brasília on 29–31 January. It will be remembered that at the first GAEL meeting, held in India, I was appointed Special Ambassador to GAEL, and my express purpose for this trip was to take part in this meeting.

At this second GAEL meeting, Professor Kenzo Kiikuni, chair of the Sasakawa Health Foundation, and Dr. Yo Yuasa, executive and medical director of the Sasakawa Health Foundation (later president of the International Leprosy Association (ILA)), were also attending, and former WHO Director-General (1988–98) Hiroshi Nakajima was also present. The first GAEL meeting had been held in India, the nation with the largest number of people affected by leprosy. This second GAEL meeting in Brazil was being held in the country with the second highest number and was co-hosted by WHO, the Pan American Health Organization, and Brazil's Ministry of Health.

The objective of this meeting was to have delegates from the health ministries of the principal GAEL members where leprosy was still endemic, and delegates from the Nippon Foundation, the Sasakawa Health Foundation, Novartis, WHO, and others, report on the activities they had undertaken over the last year toward the elimination of leprosy and to re-commit to push on with ongoing efforts in the years ahead.

In 2001, as well as delegates from the bodies listed above, we had delegates from the World Bank, DANIDA, and ILEP. In 2002, however, ILEP declined to attend, and the number of NGOs attending was rather small. I will not go into the full story of ILEP's withdrawal from GAEL. Suffice to say, some deep differences had emerged. WHO seemed to want to exclude ILEP from the alliance because it felt that its presence undermined the smooth operation of GAEL's efforts.

The meeting began with a formal address from a delegate of Brazil's Ministry of Health, an address from the delegate of the Ministry of Health of India (who had hosted the meeting the year before), followed by speeches from Dr. Maria P. Neira, director of WHO's Department of Infection Control, Prevention, and Eradication, and myself. This was followed in the sessions by presentations on the activities being undertaken in each nation, a report on the control efforts taking place in Brazil, a statement of Brazil's political commitment to the cause, and a frank exchange of views on future directions.

During this meeting, the deputy health minister of Myanmar suggested that I visit Myanmar in January 2003. I was also asked to suggest to the various members of GAEL that we hold the alliance's third meeting in Myanmar.

Dr. Denis Daumerie, WHO's Group Leader for Leprosy, gave a presentation on the need in the final push for coordinated efforts, free provision of medication, ownership and equality, a policy of complete integration, and a commitment to make leprosy a matter of public health. The elimination of leprosy as a public health problem was well within reach: MDT blister packs were widely available, 11 million people had been treated, 40 million people had been saved from permanent disability, and leprosy was beginning to lose the negative associations that had surrounded it. The main focus for 2002, Mr. Daumerie proposed, should be to get renewed commitments from governments, wider partnerships, full integration of leprosy-control efforts, and up-to-date record-keeping for registered cases.

The meeting was held in Brasília, a planned city that became the capital in 1960. To me, the city seemed bland, arid, and characterless. Almost no one seemed to go anywhere on foot, with the result that the streets were deserted; and building restrictions limited buildings to no more than six floors. The city's design means that it is divided into numbered blocks, and sectors for specified activities, and the only tall buildings are hotels, office blocks, and government buildings. The architecture is modernist, evoking the early 1960s. Legend had it that the city was inspired by a saint's dream of a utopian metropolis. Some intellectuals bewailed the enormous sums of money required to build the city, which left the nation with a huge gap between rich and poor, and a great deficit in human resources because of wholly inadequate public education.

Oscar Niemeyer, the Brazilian architect who designed the UN headquarters in New York, was the designer of Brasília's civic buildings, which received the status of World Heritage Site back in 1987. However, the efforts made by President Juscelino Kubitschek to procure money for the building of Brasília and other industrial projects eventually led to spiraling inflation. After that, there was an army coup, followed by a period of military rule that lasted until 1985. Even after a democratically elected government returned to power, the economy still didn't improve. When the sociologist and political scientist Fernando Henrique Cardoso took the reins as president in 1995, he pegged the Brazilian real to the American dollar, and this finally stabilized the currency and brought inflation under control. President Cardoso remains a popular figure in Brazil, but he was due to leave his post in 2002, and the contest for who would succeed him had already begun (I was told several influential senators had been assassinated in the run-up). Populism seemed to have made a comeback, especially among the poorer members of society, but there were worries that if the labor opposition parties took power, the economy would simply continue to deteriorate.

I had a meeting with President Cardoso during this trip. His first words to me were: "I've heard about what the Nippon Foundation does. I also fully understand the importance of leprosy elimination. I wholeheartedly hope that the elimination targets can be met by the year 2005. In this kind of endeavor, arrangements like GAEL, with collaborative alliances between NGOs, governments, and ordinary people, are by far the most effective in the fight for public health. NGOs play a very important part in Brazil, particularly on the issue of HIV/AIDS, helping patients get treatment." He then added: "Brazil is a wealthy country with many millions of impoverished people. We must help people in many more areas of their lives, outside of making money, and we are currently putting together measures that will make it easier for ordinary people to access what they need in the spheres of education and public health. For example, in the sphere of health, we have started a 'community health agent' program, in which people who are resident in communities and who have a certain level of education are paid to keep an eye on their communities and help households get access to health. Following the example of Cuba, we've also instituted a system that involves teams of people in which family doctors work with these community health agents. Brazil's population is over 90 million, but every single person will be able to get access to proper health care." And, he added, "Leprosy elimination activities will be an integral part of the health service."

I also had the opportunity to visit Manaus, the capital of the state of Amazonas, and the nearby town of Manacapuru, both of which have a high incidence of leprosy. Manaus became a wealthy city in the late 1800s due to the rubber trade, which was monopolized by 100 families of Italian heritage, who became very rich as a result. The city was dubbed the Paris of the Tropics, with an opera house built with bricks brought from Europe, French glass, and Italian marble. One story has it that the wife of a priest secretly took a rubber tree seedling with her and planted it in Malaysia, initiating the rubber industry there.

The Health Bureau of Manaus kindly arranged for us to visit clinics and nearby villages where people affected by leprosy lived. We traveled with local paramedics to small villages on the banks of the Amazon River and visited the homes of leprosy-affected people undergoing treatment. Getting to Manacapuru involved leaving my hotel at 7 a.m., crossing the Amazon River by motorboat, and taking a one-hour car journey to the jungle town. In this town, I was told, there were sixty-two people affected by leprosy, with 500 people who had been cured. Last year, eighteen new cases had been detected, but 65 percent of them had already finished their MDT treatment.

Here, I met with a number of people involved in public health—health workers caring for HIV/AIDS patients, paramedics, the head of the unit in charge of sexually transmitted diseases in the Amazon, the head of the tropical skin disease unit—to find out all I could about the health issues of the district. I was impressed with the health workers' dedication to detection, medical care, record-keeping, and their skilled operational management.

The following morning, I traveled with local paramedics to visit small villages on the banks of the Amazon River, first by a mid-sized riverboat, then by four-passenger motorboat. The first village we visited was called Costa da Pesquidro. Here I visited a forty-eight-year-old man who was affected by leprosy. His three-member family lived in a tiny shack on stilts. Their belongings comprised a mirror, a radio, a portable stove, and three steel saucepans, all scrubbed quite clean. Despite such poverty, the family seemed in good cheer, and both mother and father were clearly doing their best. The next house I went to was also a house on stilts, but this family had a sofa, a small TV, and a generator. The son of the family was bringing home money from a job in Manaus. His wife was the person affected by leprosy. She held a two-month-old baby in her arms. I was deeply touched by the warmth and concern extended to her by family members. In this region, people with leprosy did not seem to be cast out, but rather protected and cared for by their loved ones.

The city of Manaus, with its numerous modern housing complexes and the ambiance of wealth that pervaded the streets, made a stark contrast to this impoverished village, well off the beaten track and with no access to electricity. This is one of the contradictions of Brazil—the huge gap between its rich and poor. It is a rich nation, but millions of its people are still living in poverty, with 10 percent of the country's population holding 50 percent of its wealth.

GAEL conference and exchanges with ministers of health—Republic of Latvia, May 2002, and the Swiss Confederation

In May 2002, I went to Latvia, one of the three sovereign states on the east coast of the Baltic Sea. I also visited Geneva.

I was in Latvia from 12 to 14 May. My purpose was to attend the award ceremony of the Sasakawa Young Leaders Fellowship Fund at the University of Latvia, in the national capital Riga. (The SYLFF is a fellowship program initiated in 1987 to help students pursue studies in social sciences and humanities.) The award ceremony took place on 13 May, with speeches from the rector of the University, Ivars Lacis, the vice minister of the Latvian Ministry of Education and Science, and the Japanese Ambassador to Latvia (and Sweden) Tomio Uchida. This was followed by a concert given by the students.

The University of Latvia was founded in 1919 and has a total student population of 33,000, with thirteen faculties. It originally specialized in the natural sciences, but with Latvian independence in 1990, it has been replenishing its social sciences and humanities faculties.

During my stay in Riga, I paid a courtesy call to President of Latvia Vaira Vīķe-Freiberga (1999–2007) and Prime Minister Andris Bērziņš, and I learned a lot about Latvia: how the cities of Riga and Kobe had been sister cities since 1974; how Riga Zoo sent one of its captive-born elephants to Kobe Zoo in 1996 (at the time of the Kobe Earthquake); how Latvia had applied to join the EU; how the country was concentrating on measures to upgrade the professionalization of its workforce and particularly on training up technicians in IT; and all about the establishment of the Freeport of Riga. This is a major port of international importance with a unique heritage as a trading center and its own highly sophisticated system of operation and governance.

From Latvia, I proceeded to Geneva, to attend a GAEL meeting, a World Health Assembly, and an award ceremony for the Sasakawa Health Prize.

The GAEL meeting was attended by WHO, Novartis, ILEP, delegates from nations, the Nippon Foundation, and the Sasakawa Health Foundation, but this time we also opened the doors to NGOs who were involved in leprosy control or care of people affected by leprosy. So various national NGOs, including Handicap International, Brazil's MORHAN (Movement for the Reintegration of Persons Affected by Hansen's Disease), the International Federation of the Red Cross and the Red Crescent, and the Japan International Cooperation Agency, were there. Sadly, however, members of ILEP chose not to attend. After an address given by Claudio Duarte, a delegate from Brazil's Ministry of Health, the deputy minister at Myanmar's Ministry of Health, Maun Maun Moon, gave a speech in which he announced that the host country for the next GAEL meeting to be held in 2003 would be Myanmar. This was followed by discussion of what kinds of campaigns might be held to remove the stigma surrounding leprosy, with examples of an education and awareness campaign run by the BBC World Service in India, and the educational advertisements that were about to be put out in Brazil. It was agreed that in any campaign it is most important to have the active participation of local political leaders. In Madagascar the previous year, there had been a successful campaign run with funding from Novartis with local programs run at the community level. Opinions were voiced: it was essential to avoid any media campaign that ended up showing leprosy in a negative light. Unless concerted efforts were made to give employment opportunities to people affected by leprosy, efforts toward rehabilitation would be meaningless. Without any specific topic, and without any important resolutions, this was more of an informal gathering and an opportunity to exchange the latest updates.

The Sasakawa Health Prize award ceremony was held on the evening of 16 June, at the Palais des Nations, site of the World Health Assembly. The Sasakawa Health Prize is awarded to an individual or group who has made a unique and significant contribution to health care, and one condition of the prize money ($40,000 for a group; $30,000 for an individual) is that it is used for efforts toward public health. This year, the prize-winner was a group that was providing free dental treatment for women in need in Chile (Programa Nacional de Atención Odontológica Integral para Mujeres Travbajadoras de Escasos Recursos). Miriam Sanchez of Chile's Ministry of Health received the prize on their behalf. In Chile, many women have poor dental health—due to poor water quality and malnourishment. Such women also tend to be very poor. A definite relationship has been shown to exist between oral hygiene, self-esteem, and improved employment prospects. The group gives free dental treatment every year to 14,000 women and thus supports their independence—helping them escape the cycle of poverty.

The objectives of my trip to Geneva were mostly WHO-related, but I was also keen to meet with individuals important to the causes of the Nippon Foundation. First, I visited Ruud Lubbers, who succeeded Sadako Ogata as the United Nations High Commissioner for Refugees. I also visited the office of the UN International Strategy for Disaster Reduction, which runs the United Nations Sasakawa Award for Disaster Risk Management that we award every year to individuals or organizations that contribute to reducing disaster risk, and met with the director of the Secretariat Sálvano Briceño. He gave me a report about the latest activities of the agency and updated me on news about the award.

I also had useful exchanges of information with health ministers from different nations who are working toward leprosy control, something I do every year. In my meeting with the health minister of Myanmar, Major General Ket Sein, I asked him for his cooperation with the GAEL conference scheduled in Myanmar in January 2003, which he confirmed. He was convinced that Myanmar would meet the WHO target for leprosy elimination by that very year. In a meeting with his Brazilian counterpart, Vice Minister of Health Octavio Azevedo Mercadante, I told him that the Sasakawa Health Foundation was arranging for the translation into Portuguese of the *Atlas of Leprosy*, a pictorial manual first published in 1981 and revised in 2002, to assist frontline workers and volunteers in the detection, diagnosis, and treatment of leprosy. It would not be long before we sent copies to Brazil. The Health Minister of Nepal Bhandari told me all about the problems the government was having with the Maoist Communist Party of Nepal, a designated terrorist organization. However, Kathmandu was safe, he told me. The government was determined to rebuild the shattered economy and reestablish security. There was an urgent necessity for international aid, he said, and he was hoping for help from Japan, in particular for funding for a public health center.

In my meeting with the health minister of India, C. P. Thakur, I received confirmation that he would attend the meeting that the Nippon Foundation and the Sasakawa Health Foundation were hosting on leprosy elimination in India, due to be held in Tokyo on 3 June with representatives from the Union Ministry of Health and Family Welfare and ministers from the seven state ministries of health in northern India and several NGOs and charity foundations.

I also held a meeting with Mozambican Health Minister Dr. Francisco Songane, who invited me to visit Mozambique in September that year, and I happily accepted.

I discussed related issues in my meeting with the health minister of Ghana, Kwaku Afriyie, and Dr. Kingsley Asiedu, the WHO medical officer dealing with Buruli ulcers, an infectious disease that mainly affects the skin and sometimes the bone. They expressed their appreciation to the Nippon Foundation for the support we continue to give toward medical personnel capacity building in Ghana.

Visit to Sungai Buloh—Malaysia, June 2002

Route: Narita, Japan → Singapore (flight time: 6h 50m)—one night—(tour of inspection of Malacca Straits)—Singapore → Kuala Lumpur, Malaysia (4h 30m bus transfer)—two nights—Kuala Lumpur → Narita (flight time: 7h)

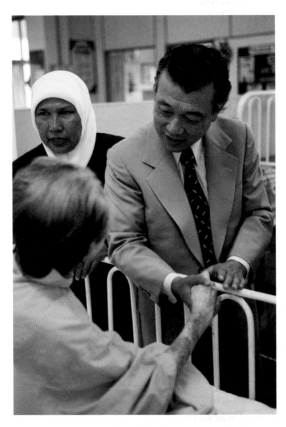

12. Chatting with a person affected by leprosy in the hospital in Sungai Buloh (Malaysia, June 2002)

REACHING THE UNREACHABLE

In June 2002, I visited Malaysia. Leprosy had been eliminated as a public health problem (according to the WHO definition) in Malaysia in 1994. The leprosy colony in Malaysia for which records exist is the one on Pulau Sarimbun (also spelled Serimban, or Srinbun), a small island in the Strait of Malacca, which started in 1850 with twenty-one patients. In 1874, the British imposed segregation policies, with leprosy "centers" built in every state. Each center could only take in about twenty patients, even though around 100 cases were detected annually; most were sent to Pulau Jerejak, to a secondary facility built off the coast of Penang, where the first leprosy patients were brought in 1871. With the enactment under British rule of the Leprosy Act in 1926, all persons affected by leprosy on the Malayan Peninsula were sent to Sungai Buloh (a name that translates as "Valley of Hope"), a settlement built 25.6 kilometers away from the capital Kuala Lumpur. The Sungai Buloh Hospital opened in 1930.

The Second World War utterly destroyed many of the services offered to people affected by leprosy. The number of hospitals dwindled, and many patients were simply told to go home. People who remained at the hospitals despite the lack of care managed to avoid starvation by eating tapioca and snails. The mortality rate reached 30 percent, and ultimately, as records show, only 640 people affected by leprosy remained at Sungai Buloh and 360 at Jerejak (records show 1,200 in 1939). In 1969, six years after the country gained its independence, the National Leprosy Control Program was launched, with an emphasis on early case detection and decentralization of treatment. The Sungai Buloh settlement was officially named the National Leprosy Control Centre, and other clinics and leprosaria around the country closed.

My visit to Malaysia this time involved a trip to Sungai Buloh. There is now a large settlement for people formerly affected by leprosy, home to more than 200 families. There, they grow plants and vegetables and are now completely self-sufficient. The settlement is situated about 25 kilometers from the city of Kuala Lumpur, and people flock there from the city and surrounding towns in order to buy its produce. I was so impressed. It seemed to me to be a wonderful example of reintegration from both sides, and proof that the stigma once associated with leprosy can dissipate completely.

MAKING THE IMPOSSIBLE POSSIBLE

A country with regions where one in three people examined are affected—Republic of Mozambique, September 2002

Route: Narita, Japan → Singapore (flight time: 7h 30m; 3h stopover) → Johannesburg, South Africa (flight time: 10h; 7h stopover) → Maputo, Mozambique (flight time: 1h)—two nights—Maputo → Nampula (flight time: 3h)—one night—Nampula → Pemba city (flight time: 1h)—one night—Pemba → Maputo (flight time: 3h 30m)—one night—Maputo → Johannesburg (flight time: 1h; 2.5h stopover) → London, United Kingdom (flight time: 13h; 5h stopover) → Narita, Japan (flight time: 12h)

In September 2002, I visited Mozambique. By this time, it was one of the six remaining nations that had still to reach the WHO elimination target. Three of these six were in Africa. Mozambique lies in southeastern Africa, bordered by the Indian Ocean. It is roughly twice the size of Japan, though as of 2002 it had a population of almost 20 million. To get to the capital Maputo via South Africa required an airplane trip that lasted a total of thirty hours. Few people know all that much about Mozambique, but in 1992 the civil war that had raged for fifteen years finally ended, the political situation stabilized, and some semblance of peace returned to society. Nevertheless, Mozambique remains one of the poorest nations on earth. A Portuguese colony, then overseas province of Portugal, and then member state of Portugal until 1975 when it gained independence, there is a discernible Portuguese feel to the music you hear on the radio and to the ambiance in the streets. Being there reminded me a little of Brazil, which was also once a colony of Portugal.

At this point, Mozambique was the third most endemic country in the WHO Africa Region. The prevalence rate at the end of 2002 was 3.63 per 10,000. However, there is a large imbalance between provinces, with a few areas in the north reaching numbers as high as ten per 10,000.

My schedule on this trip was a busy one: face-to-face talks with government figures whose support I would need in the fight against leprosy, including Prime Minister Pascoal Mocumbi and Health Minister Francisco Songane, and several other local government officials; a seminar on leprosy elimination hosted by ILEP; a launch ceremony for an anti-leprosy campaign in the northern province of

Nampula, which is one of the worst affected by leprosy; visits to several leprosy facilities; face-to-face talks with key government officials on the latest developments of the SG2000 agricultural assistance program operating in Mozambique since the mid-1990s; and an on-site visit to the plots and fields. I also attended a three-day national conference for extension workers, government representatives, agricultural scientists, and related NGOs hosted by the Ministry of Agriculture.

I also met Minister of Agricultural and Rural Development Helder Muteia, the governor of Nampula province Abdul Razak Noormahomed, the governor of Cabo Delgado province José Condungua Pacheco, and others. I then proceeded to the northern provinces to meet with local political leaders and visit hospitals and health centers. I was accompanied by the Ministry of Health Director of the Department of Health and Sanitation Avertino Barreto, and WHO country office in Mozambique Chief Beatrice Kao Epa.

At the ILEP seminar, titled "Leprosy in Mozambique: Current Conditions and Outlook for the Future," we learned that the incidence of leprosy was high in one central region (Zambezia) and four northern provinces. In the province of Nampula, the prevalence was particularly high—12.9 persons per 10,000 (the national average was 3.9 persons). Here, less than 30 percent of the population had access to medical services; there was a severe dearth of medical personnel and paramedics capable of leprosy examinations; and most villages were at least 5 kilometers away from MDT distribution points, leading to people abandoning treatment midway; the case detection rate was one in three people examined. Concerted efforts were being made to integrate leprosy in the general medical treatment services, to increase the number of volunteers distributing MDT, and to have education and awareness campaigns encouraging detection at the community level—but still, the situation was dire. This became the first of many visits I made to Mozambique, which I regarded as needing particular attention.

While in Maputo, I was shown several self-help projects put together with the aim of helping people who had recovered from leprosy rehabilitate themselves. These included one in which people managed a well and sold water. As Health Minister Songane explained:

"It is in the Mozambique spirit to offer a constructive role in society to physically disabled people." There were all kinds of networks for people with disabilities, I was told. In Nampula, the Mozambican Association of Disabled People ran a factory making shoes, including shoes for people affected by leprosy.

On the second day of my stay, we took a three-hour trip by plane to visit Nampula. The day after that, the health minister and I traveled with several local officials by car, leaving early in the morning, to a small village some 40 miles out of Maputo called Namaíta. Here we took part in the launch of the Communication for Behavioral Impact (COMBI) program, part of a WHO-initiated effort to educate people about leprosy. Health workers sporting yellow T-shirts bearing the logo CYSA ("Check Your Skin Always") would travel from village to village on their bicycles, promoting self-check activities among children and their family members for the early detection of leprosy. Early detection through skin checks was going to be incorporated into the school curriculum, and the most assiduous students would be awarded with a ballpoint pen. Six thousand volunteers had been enlisted. The plan was to carry out a huge campaign involving the media—especially radio. The target was to identify 200,000 new cases.

Several hundred villagers had turned out for the launch ceremony. It began with tribal dances, then a concert given by the military, after which the governor, the chief of the WHO country office in Mozambique, and the health minister gave speeches, followed by little theatrical skits put on by the children. My chief memory is that the health minister gave a long speech, lasting close to forty minutes, using a mixture of Portuguese and the native language. I was quite unable to follow it. When he introduced me, I asked the children whether they knew anything about Japan. The villagers all got lively, asking questions. In my speech, I emphasized how important it was to look out for early signs of leprosy and told them of my hope that Nampula would provide a model for the entire nation. I ended my speech saying "Hurrah for Nampula! Hurrah for Mozambique!!"

Immediately after this, I boarded the airplane for the thirty-minute flight to the port city of Pemba in Cabo Delgado. As soon as we got there, I went to meet with Governor José Pacheco. Governor Pacheco had recently attended an SG2000 conference held in Washington, so he was very clued up and aware of the urgency of capacity training, infrastructure improvement, attracting investments, and so on. He struck me as a politician of considerable energy and vision, although as he admitted to me, he knew little about leprosy. After our talks, we went to the governor's residence, a beautiful place overlooking the Indian Ocean, for dinner accompanied by the Health Bureau chief, the chief of the WHO country office in Mozambique, and a representative of the UN Food and Agriculture Organization.

The return journey involved a four-hour flight from Pemba Airport to Maputo by twenty-five-passenger propeller plane. However, we almost didn't make it. Nobody had told us we had to confirm our reservations, and we had discovered that morning that they had been cancelled. Having put our names on a waiting list, we decided to go to the airport early and negotiate at the checking-in counter. In the end, we managed to get our entire party on board with the exception of one local official. If we had missed that flight, it would have meant a wait of two more days, since our onward flight from Maputo was fully booked.

A second meeting with Pope John Paul II—Vatican City, October 2002

In October 2002, I had the honor of an audience with His Holiness Pope John Paul II. This was an exceedingly moving experience for me. It was in fact the second time I had been in the presence of Pope John Paul, the first being in 1983 when I had accompanied my late father Ryoichi Sasakawa when he had been invited for a private audience.

On that day in 1983, my father and I had met with the pope in his private office in the Vatican. The pope had uttered some words of encouragement and given my father a medal for his efforts to vanquish leprosy. He then enfolded my father in his arms and told him: "You have made great contributions to humankind with your endeavors toward world peace, and also especially toward the eradication of smallpox. You are also doing everything you can to eradicate leprosy.

I am grateful for all that you do to drive out the suffering due to illness and inequality from humankind. I hope that you will continue with your work in the years to come."

Later, when recalling the meeting, my father said he felt as if he was being embraced by his own father.

On the day I had my audience, it was exactly twenty-five years since Pope John Paul had been elected, and a special mass was being held to celebrate. St. Peter's Square was overflowing with more than 15,000 devoted followers who had gathered there from the four corners of the earth. Though I was not one of the Christian faithful, I was led up to the podium for a few brief minutes with His Holiness, and I was able to deliver the message I had prepared—informing him that we were fulfilling the promise my father had made to him all those

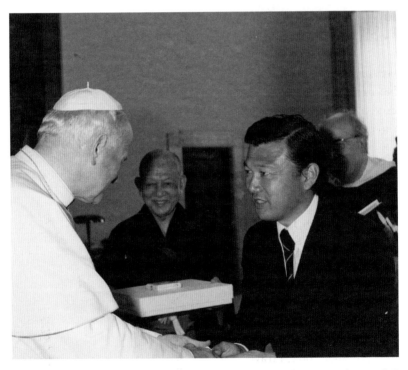

13. The author and his father Ryoichi Sasakawa with Pope John Paul II (Vatican, May 1983)

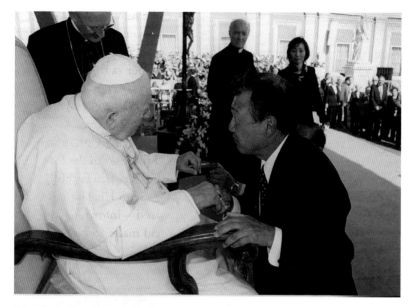

14. The author delivering his message to the pope (Vatican, October 2002)

years ago about eradicating leprosy. I had asked one of the papal aides beforehand to hand the pope a letter with more details. After I delivered my words, the pope nodded, without speaking, and then gently took my hand, covering it in his.

The need for vigilance after elimination—Republic of the Philippines, November 2002

> Route: Narita, Japan → Port Moresby, New Guinea (flight time: 8h)—three nights—Port Moresby, New Guinea → Manila, Philippines (flight time: 5h)—three nights—Manila, Philippines → Culion Island (1h flight from Manila to Busuanga Island; 1h car journey to Coron Port, followed by 1h boat ride to Culion Island)—one night—Culion Island → Manila—one night—Manila → Cebu Island (flight time: 1h)—three nights—Cebu Island → Narita, Japan (flight time: 5h)

In November 2002, I traveled to Papua New Guinea and had my first meeting in several years with Prime Minister Michael Somare. He had started out as a teacher, joined the civil service, and from there entered politics, becoming the South Pacific island's first prime minister after independence from Australia in 1975. He helped my father in his efforts to have the remains returned of the many Japanese soldiers who had fallen in Papua New Guinea during the war in the South Pacific, and he had great respect for him, even going so far as to name his eldest son Ryoichi. Papua New Guinea is an important tuna fishing zone, and the prime minister had enjoyed some wonderful meals of tuna sashimi—in Papua New Guinea and in Tokyo. He liked to call sashimi "sushimi," I remember.

Papua New Guinea is a sovereign state comprising the eastern half of the island of New Guinea and a number of offshore islands of Melanesia, a region in the South Pacific north of Australia. Since 1976, the nation has been an "observer state" in the Association of Southeast Asian Nations, though it belongs to the geographic region of Oceania (which comprises Australasia, Melanesia, Micronesia, and Polynesia). Somare played a pivotal role in securing peaceful independence from Australia: he is often referred to as the "chief" and the "father of the nation." He was a much beloved leader.

While in the Philippines, I visited the Dr. Jose N. Rodriguez Memorial Hospital and Sanitarium in Manila. The hospital, formerly known as Tala Leprosarium, was built in 1940 to accommodate persons affected by leprosy in the entire Luzon region and currently serves as the principal referral hospital for leprosy patients and the premier training and research center for leprosy care and management in the Philippines. It also serves the public health needs of community members of Tala and nearby areas. In a factory attached to the hospital, people affected by leprosy who had completed treatment and had recovered were making high-quality dolls for export abroad. I was happy to observe people who were clearly intent on gaining a level of financial independence.

I also made an excursion to Culion Island, a place that occupies a unique place in the history of leprosy. The island once hosted the world's largest leprosarium, sometimes housing 7,000 people affected by the disease, first established in 1906 under the administration of the United States. From 1907 to 1964, close to 50,000 people affected by leprosy were apprehended and isolated on this island. Today, it is a municipality with a population of 16,000 people, comprising people currently affected by leprosy and people who have been treated and are completely cured, medical staff, and the descendants of both.

The last place I went in the Philippines was the island of Cebu, where I visited the leprosy research laboratory set up in 1928 by the Leonard Wood Memorial for the Eradication of Leprosy, and the Eversley Childs Sanitarium, both important places in the history of leprosy treatment, the first for coordinating important leprosy-related research and the latter for follow-up studies lasting fifteen years. The Eversley Childs Sanitarium was a 52-hectare complex of clinics, dormitories, residences, churches, and a cemetery built in 1982 with funds from the US philanthropist Eversley Childs on a site that was originally a leprosarium as a permanent home to thousands of people affected by leprosy. Only 3 percent of the total number of individuals who were given MDT went on to have further outbreaks of leprosy. It is a sad fact that the leprosy bacillus responsible for leprosy will develop resistance to current MDT therapy, which makes further research into other therapies essential, and I have every reason to believe that the Leonard Wood Memorial research facility will continue to play a key role.

Leprosy, arsenic, and vaccines—India and the People's Republic of Bangladesh, December 2002

In December 2002, I made two trips to the Indian continent, visiting several areas in India and Bangladesh.

First trip to India (5–9 December)

(Visit to a leprosy colony in Lucknow, the capital city of Uttar Pradesh; and others)

Route: Narita, Japan → Delhi (flight time: 8.5h)—one night—Delhi → Lucknow, Uttar Pradesh (flight time: 1h)—one night—Lucknow, Uttar Pradesh → Delhi (flight time: 1h)—Delhi → Narita, Japan (flight time: 8h)

Second trip to India (21–5 December)

Route: Narita, Japan → Singapore (flight time: 6h; 2h stopover) → Dhaka, Bangladesh (flight time: 4h)—two nights—Dhaka → Kolkata,

West Bengal, India (flight time: 1h)—one night—Kolkata → Patna, Bihar state (due to mist, the plane had to go via Lucknow, and the scheduled 1h flight became a 4h one)—two nights—Patna → Delhi (flight time: 1.5h) → Singapore (flight time: 4.5h; 4h stopover) → Narita (flight time: 6h)

At the time of my visit, Bangladesh was the seventh most populous nation in the world, with over 150 million inhabitants. Yet its total land area is only around 40 percent of that of Japan. After India gained independence in 1947, the northern regions became West Pakistan and East Pakistan, in an event that is referred to as "Partition." In 1971, the mainly Bengali-speaking East Pakistan seceded from Urdu-speaking West Pakistan and became Bangladesh, while West Pakistan became Pakistan. People in Bangladesh speak Bengali, and they share this language with their neighbor, the Indian state of West Bengal. Ninety percent of Bangladeshi people are Muslim. Recent years have seen economic development chiefly centering on its textile industry. Agriculture employs close to half the workforce. The country produces many crops, the main one being rice, benefiting from the so-called "green revolution" implemented during the 1950 and 1960s aimed at the development of agriculture in nations of the world and led by the late eminent agronomist Norman Borlaug, who was a Nobel Peace Prize laureate. Bangladesh eliminated leprosy as a public health problem in 1998.

In Dhaka, I met with Minister of Health Khandaker Hossain—at his home, since it was a Friday, a day of prayer in the Islamic faith—and we had wide-ranging discussions. We agreed that notwithstanding Bangladesh's success in meeting the leprosy elimination target, population density and widespread poverty meant that there could be no let-up in vigilance. International cooperation would continue to be vital. Discrimination was less of a scourge, Mr. Hossain told me, because more people now knew that leprosy was treatable. Still, more work had to be done in educating the populace, and for this people with lived experience of leprosy could play a key role. He hoped to see such people organizing themselves. Even so, the amount of governmental public health spending in Bangladesh amounted to a mere 6 dollars per person per annum—13 dollars, if one counted the amount spent by charities and NGOs. A wide array of community programs existed promoting healthy behavior, and education on leprosy had been incorporated into the school curriculum. One major problem in Bangladesh is the arsenic contamination in the shallow and underground water systems of the country—an issue shared by many of the world's delta regions. We discussed the problems around immunization. Bangladesh had long been engaged in polio eradication efforts, with "national immunization days" instituted in 1995; the minister informed me that the country was finally getting close to reaching the official WHO target for eradication, with no new cases detected in the last two years. The Hepatitis B vaccination was also being rolled out in urban areas, with support from the Global Alliance for Vaccines and Immunizations (GAVI), an alliance of public and private sector organizations dedicated to "immunization for all." Tuberculosis is a major health problem in Bangladesh, the minister informed me, with the fifth highest incidence in the world. I assured him of the Nippon Foundation and the Sasakawa Health Foundation's continuing support through WHO, and thanking him for his time, took my leave.

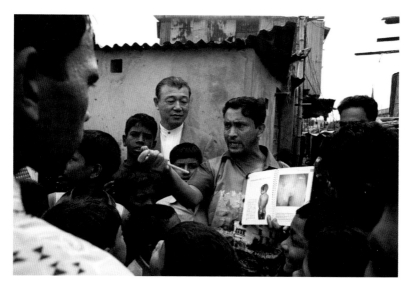

15. A man trying to raise leprosy awareness in the slum community (Bangladesh, December 2002)

During my trip to Dhaka, I visited the Al-Falah Model Clinic in Mohammadpur, one of the smaller clinics that The Leprosy Mission (TLM) has set up. Run jointly by the government and TLM, the clinic concentrates particularly on early detection of leprosy in women and children, providing free services. The narrow corridors were thronging not only with people with leprosy but also outpatients with other illnesses. The clinic uses a combined approach, focusing on treatment, socio-economic development activities and empowerment, and validation of human rights. One of the services being offered (chiefly to women) was access to small-scale ("micro-credit") loans. After my visit, I walked through a nearby slum area. This was an area where refugees originally from East Pakistan (probably originally Muslims from Bihar state in India, with more affiliation to West Pakistan) had settled and formed their own community. People with leprosy were living cheek by jowl with people unaffected by the disease. Despite the terrible living conditions in the slums, the children seemed cheerful. They told me that they went to school outside the slums every day, and one of the girls told me about her ambition of becoming a doctor. I did not see a single beggar.

I then visited the International Centre for Diarrhoeal Disease Research, also in Dhaka. This is a research center that has contributed significantly to reducing infant, maternal, and child mortality, and the Nippon Foundation has provided it with three grants amounting to a total equivalent to US$900,000 to refit its research facilities and other related expenses. I was given an update on the kind of research being undertaken, and I toured other facilities, including the Sasakawa Training Hall.

I then headed to the venue for the Bangladesh Scholarship Council (BSC) award ceremony. The BSC is an NGO that aims to rebuild the nation through educational schemes and issues scholarships to poor students to go to educational institutions in the country. The Nippon Foundation provided grants for its scholarship program from 1995 to 2010. The minister of foreign affairs, Chief Justice Reaz Rahman, was present at the ceremony. On this day, I handed a check for 8,000 taka (then equivalent to 24,000 yen, or US$200) to every one of the 300 awardees. Tuition fees at university range from 200 to 300 taka, so the scholarship money helps them meet these basic costs. I was very happy to see our grant money being used for a brighter future for Bangladesh's youth.

Lagging elimination activities in Bihar—Republic of India (West Bengal and Bihar), December 2002

From Dhaka, after a three-hour delay to our 8.15 a.m. flight due to mist, I went straight on to Kolkata in West Bengal, India. Here, I attended a briefing with several people who had been present at the Tokyo meeting in June 2002, including the principal secretary of West Bengal state, Mr. Ashim Kumar Barman. Mr. Barman delivered a report on the latest developments. He said that the state leprosy officer and his team at the Ministry of Health were putting devoted efforts into working with WHO for leprosy elimination. After the Tokyo meeting, he had been able to get commitment from all sorts of quarters to move things along with speed. The mayors of Kolkata and Howrah had committed to elimination activities. Such statewide effort, involving the national government, local authorities, and NGOs, would be the first of its kind in the world. Education and awareness campaigns were already reducing prejudice and discrimination. NGO interventions had led to detection rates of multibacillary cases (MB; cases with a high bacillary load) dropping by 90 percent; most cases were now paucibacillary (PB; cases with a low bacillary load). Hidden cases had also dropped by 90 percent (i.e. only 10 percent were now hidden in the provinces as opposed to 100 percent), thanks to the awareness-raising campaigns. The media campaigns had been especially effective. He was reporting nothing but successes. This is a phenomenon we frequently encounter. I listened carefully to everything he said, but that didn't mean I believed everything entirely.

At the press conference that followed, with twenty or so journalists present, I explained the current state of leprosy elimination around the world and then in India and West Bengal. An official from the state leprosy office mentioned that cases of leprosy among women in the state of Bengal were on the increase. This was because more young women are now turning up at health clinics and hospitals for examinations. For the real eradication of leprosy, I stressed, we needed much more help and collaboration from the media. We deplored the fact that most of the media's interest seemed only to be in funding and finances—the size of my donations, how much I had given so far, and so on. Despite being so forthright, I was left with the overall impression of how much there was left to do in terms of educating the media on the problem of leprosy.

On the morning of 22 December, we were suddenly told at Kolkata airport that our flight booked to Patna had been cancelled due to mist. In a panic, we started investigating overland routes, but then we were informed that the plane would be departing. We were thus slightly delayed. We arrived in Patna at 1 o'clock and went straight to the State Health Ministry for a briefing. The state of Bihar has 17 percent of the people with leprosy in India. Figures in 2002, however, showed a slight decrease in the prevalence on 2001. In 2000, there were four districts with five or fewer cases per 10,000 population; fifteen districts with from five to ten cases; twelve regions with ten to fifteen cases; and sixteen districts with fifteen or more cases. As of November 2002, there were eight districts with five cases or fewer per 10,000 population; twenty-six districts with five to ten cases; three districts

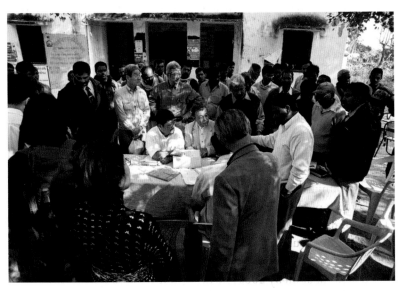

16. On-site visit to the health sub center (Bihar, India, December 2002)

with ten to fifteen cases; and no districts where there were fifteen or more. However, the figures for women had increased by 38.5 percent and for children by 16.13 percent. The main problem was that there were insufficient health sub-centers in each district. Even with 9,000 at the present time, a further 6,000 were needed. The mid-size general health centers in the city were also severely understaffed. The media (TV and newspapers) could only play a limited role in getting messages out about leprosy, since only just over half (52.5 percent) of the population could read and write.

I next went on to the district of Jehanabad, where I had a meeting with an all-female group of social workers known as Anganwadi Workers. ("Anganwadi" is Hindi for "courtyard shelter.") The Anganwadi scheme was started by the government in the 1970s as a way to combat child hunger and malnutrition, and there are about 5,000 of these women in the state of Bihar. They have made the eradication of leprosy part of their work, doing as much as they can to promote awareness at the local levels and participating in the COMBI program—more particularly in the "Check Your Skin" drive. About 400,000 children, ranging from nine to fourteen years of age, participate in this drive. Each child takes three worksheets home: they keep one for their family, and the other two they distribute to any neighboring houses that don't have children their age. The worksheet is designed to help them check up on any abnormalities on their skin. The drive covers 1.2 million families, with nearly 6 million people participating. The drive was showing results, with case detection rates up in every district. Such methods of detection, involving skin checks carried out by children, are used in the state of Uttar Pradesh as well (and Mozambique in Africa) and have been shown to be effective.

The state leprosy officer and WHO state coordinator told me that leprosy elimination efforts had a late start in Bihar (1996), as had the distribution of MDT (1997), but everyone was trying their very best. The overall number of people affected by leprosy was much reduced (from twenty-four per 10,000 population to 6.6 in 2001). However, he added that even though India was aiming to reach the target of leprosy elimination by 2005, he thought it was going to be difficult for Bihar. I found his reasoning for this unclear and unconvincing. I asked him to tell us specifically what we could do to help. If Bihar didn't reach the target, that would mean that India wouldn't reach the target, I told him, and I urged him to do his very best, along with everyone else, to make sure that Bihar state did reach the targets by 2005.

On 23 December, we held a news conference attended by about forty reporters from the local media. The health minister was also present. During this press conference, it became evident that almost none of the reporters knew how serious a problem leprosy was in Bihar state. When I told them that India's leprosy was among the worst in the world, and the prevalence of leprosy in Bihar among the worst in India, they were shocked, and they all started asking the health minister the reason for this and the policies he was instituting to tackle the situation. The exchange was widely reported in the newspapers the next day, and the Patna edition of *The Times of India* featured an article written in English on how more than 4.4 of the 5.5 million persons affected by leprosy worldwide live on the Indian continent and that the state of Bihar has the highest leprosy prevalence in the entire nation. The health minister's statement that he was going to step up anti-leprosy measures was also reported. I also saw the same sort of thing being reported in several Hindi-language newspapers.

Before I departed from Patna, I went to meet the chief minister of Bihar state, Rabri Devi Yadav. She was the first woman to have held this position. Originally a traditional housewife, with no experience in politics, she came to power in 1997 after her husband Lalu Prasad Yadav, the former chief minister, had to resign due to allegations of corruption. She struck me as a taciturn individual. She had come under severe criticism because of her illiteracy and inexperience, but her husband was popular, particularly among people of the lower castes. Our meeting was held in the official residence, and the minister of health and many other government officials were also present. However, the only person who actually spoke was Rabri Devi's husband, apparently the mouthpiece for his wife. He promised to create a "mass movement"—to have huge gatherings of 200,000 people and to tell everybody who had gathered that leprosy was curable and treatment available to them at no cost. But when NGOs were mentioned, he became critical: "Oh, NGOs serve no purpose. They're in it only for themselves. All they want is your money." The fight against leprosy was the concern of the government, he asserted, and if a "mass movement" was created, it would be possible to eradicate it entirely. He then showed me cheerfully around the official residence. In the center of the grounds was a lotus pond, symbolizing India. Pointing to the lotus, he told me "lotuses are a sacred flower that blooms in the mud." And then he said, "I want to become like the lotus flower, blooming in the turbulence and murk of India." He also showed me his stables of white horses. As I looked round, I thought about the rows and rows of shanties, just beyond the residence's walls, inhabited by people who had to live in poverty. On the one hand, wealth, opulence, and power; on the other, poverty, disease, and powerlessness. Would it be this way in India forever?

Countries visited in 2003	
January	China (Japan–China Medical Association Fellows meeting)
February	● Myanmar (GAEL annual meeting)
	United States (The Carter Center, Atlanta)
	Honduras (Sasakawa Zamorano Pan-American Agricultural School)
	Nicaragua (SG2000)
	China (Beijing: Japan–China Field Officer Exchange Program)
March	● India
April	Myanmar (Meeting with government officials)
June	United States (University of Rochester)
	Portugal (Visit to Sasakawa fellows at Coimbra University; visit to leprosy health facility)
	Sweden (Twentieth anniversary of founding of World Maritime University)

July	Switzerland (UN Sub-Commission on Human Rights meeting)
	● India
	● Angola
August	United Kingdom (University of Essex)
	Switzerland (UN Sub-Commission on Human Rights meeting)
	United Kingdom (University of Essex, LEPRA Conference)
September	● Madagascar
October	China (Sasakawa Japan–China Friendship Fund)
	Mongolia (Mongol Business Academy)
	Czech Republic (Forum 2000 meeting)
	United States (United States–Japan Foundation board meeting)
	France (Sasakawa Japan–France Foundation board meeting)
November	● India
December	Cambodia (Celebration of the completion of 100 primary schools)
	Indonesia (Asian Public Intellectuals (Fellowship Program) workshop)

● Indicates a trip that features in this section.

SG2000: Sasakawa Global program. An agricultural project supporting farmers in need in Africa.

WMU: World Maritime University.

Forum 2000: An annual international conference launched after a meeting in 1997 when Nobel Peace Prize laureate Václav Havel, Elie Wiesel, and the author invited world leaders to Prague for open debate on the major issues and challenges of the new millennium.

REACHING THE UNREACHABLE

The third GAEL meeting—Republic of the Union of Myanmar, February 2003

> Route: Narita, Japan → Bangkok, Thailand (flight time: 6h; 3h stop-over) → Yangon, Myanmar (flight time: 1h)—five nights—Yangon → Heho, Shan state, Myanmar (flight time: 1h 20m)—one night—Heho → Yangon (flight time: 1h 20m; 1h 30m stopover) → Bangkok (flight time: 1h; 2h stopover) → Narita (flight time: 6h)

In January 2003, I visited Myanmar to attend the third meeting of GAEL and the opening ceremony for 100 primary schools the Nippon Foundation had founded in Shan state. Leprosy in Myanmar had for a long time been a major health problem in both the rural and urban communities, but in recent months I had received indications that the WHO target was about to be reached.

The third annual meeting of GAEL, which took place on 6–8 February, was held on a grand scale in the Sedona Hotel in Yangon. The meeting began with a speech by General Khin Nyunt, Secretary-1 of the State Peace and Development Council, Government of the Union of Myanmar. He astounded the assembly with an announcement that Myanmar had reached the WHO elimination target—in January 2003. The newly appointed minister of health, Professor Kyaw Myint, then offered a warm welcome to the participants, and this was followed by statements delivered by Dr. Uton Muchtar Rafei, director of WHO Regional Office for Southeast Asia (SAERO), a speech from me as GAEL Special Ambassador, and a speech from David Heymann, executive director for communicable diseases at the WHO, Geneva. The chair of GAEL was then passed formally from Brazil to Myanmar.

In the following sessions, reports were delivered by WHO regional directors and other representatives from the Regional Offices for Africa, the Americas, the Eastern Mediterranean, and the Pacific. After numerous presentations delivered by health ministers of GAEL member countries on the state of affairs in their nations, including challenges and activities underway to further progress toward elimination, a special session was held in view of Myanmar's achievement. A number of debates were also held by working groups involving health workers at various levels.

The GAEL meeting concluded with a meeting to deliberate the contents of a document that came to be called the Yangon Declaration. An agreement was eventually reached but only after a certain amount of wrangling, arising out of the fact that the text originally listed by name countries that looked unlikely to meet the targets by 2005. Brazil and India objected, and the offending sentences were erased from the final text. The Yangon Declaration had a number of points that can be summarized as follows. It endorsed GAEL's original strategic plan to try to reach the deadlines for elimination of leprosy by 2005. It noted that whereas in 1985, the number of leprosy-endemic countries was 122, this figure had now declined to twelve. It noted that a small number of countries looked as if they would not be able to meet the elimination target by 2005, but it encouraged all the member nations of GAEL to make a special effort to help them reach the deadline. It affirmed that Myanmar's achievement of reaching the deadline ahead of time is a cause for celebration. It expressed thanks to the Special Ambassador for his work to accelerate eradication in GAEL's "final push." And it called on all the member nations of GAEL

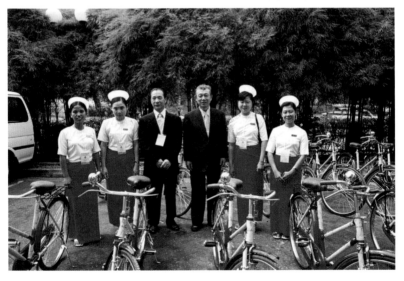

17. The "Red Angels" of Myanmar, with their red bicycles gifted by the Sasakawa Health Foundation (Myanmar, February 2003)

to recommit to doing everything possible to meet the elimination targets by the deadline of 2005.

Sadly, due to contrasts in approach that had emerged over the three years, this was to be the last meeting that the GAEL nations ever had.

Decisions in West Bengal and Jharkhand—Republic of India, March 2003

> Route: Narita, Japan → Bangkok, Thailand (flight time: 6h; 4h stop-over) → Kolkata, West Bengal, India (flight time: 2h 30m)—three nights—Kolkata → Jharkhand state (Ranchi) (flight time: 50m)—two nights—Ranchi → Delhi (flight time: 2h 3m)—one night—Delhi → Bangkok (flight time: 4h; 2h stopover) → Narita (flight time: 6h)

West Bengal had a population of roughly 88 million. In 1994, the leprosy prevalence rate in West Bengal had been 16.98 per 10,000. As of January 2003, the time of my visit, prevalence was 3.06 per 10,000 population, with a total of 24,965 individuals affected by leprosy. This was slightly below the national average; in March 2002, the number of new cases of leprosy in the entire nation of India was 440,000, making an average of 4.2 per 10,000. Jharkhand was the state with the highest prevalence in India, with 12.95 per 10,000, followed by Bihar, with 11.03 per 10,000. The third highest was Chhattisgarh, with 10.85 per 10,000.

I arrived in Kolkata late at night on 6 March and first thing next morning boarded a train from a station in Howrah to travel to the western part of the state. By 9 o'clock, I was visiting a primary health center, the Dhenua Primary Health Center, in Asansol, the second largest urban conglomeration in West Bengal after Kolkata, and, importantly, part of a major coal mining area. This health center had to serve an area of 18,000 square kilometers, a population of 12,270, thirteen villages and hamlets, and eleven primary schools. I met with thirteen people with leprosy, both adults and children, all with relatively light cases. The total was thirty-six, I was told. One thirty-five-year-old woman informed me that she was about to be divorced by her husband. One six-year-old boy whose case was clearly very light told me that his leprosy had been detected by an examination at school.

At the next primary health center, I met with various officials directing leprosy elimination activities in the area, including from the Mines Board and the Department of Health. The Mines Board informed me they now had two clinics, and a health worker network was being put into place. The Department of Health and volunteers were going to take on the responsibility of leprosy care in the districts where the miners lived. I gave a talk on the figures for the present state of leprosy in India and told them what I thought about elimination activities in the seven states of the north. I emphasized the importance of education and awareness campaigns by political leaders and the media and also noted my approval that in West Bengal the detection rate of women affected by leprosy was improving. I stressed the importance of early detection before the disease became so bad that it left people with permanent physical impairments.

After that, I dropped by a hospital. I noticed that people affected by leprosy were now being integrated with patients suffering from other diseases and being treated in the same wards. On my return, some health visitors came to see me, and I heard reports on six more districts. In many districts, there was still a strong stigma about leprosy. Incidence of the disease was affected by migration from other areas. Prevalence in certain districts was thirteen per 10,000. Medical infrastructure in some urban areas was so lacking that local authorities had to depend entirely on NGOs. Particular efforts should be made in slum areas.

On 8 March, I returned to Howrah, where I visited a state-run clinic that was looking after seven outpatients with leprosy. One man had come in for an examination. Right next to the clinic was a row of houses for people with leprosy, and when I dropped by to visit them the residents greeted me with a song composed by the deputy mayor of Howrah to educate people about aspects of leprosy.

On my return from Howrah, I had a meeting with Mr. Subrata Mukherjee, the mayor of Kolkata. I told him about my visit with Mother Teresa in 1980. It was my impression, I told him, that conditions in India were even worse than she had imagined. I asked for his strong leadership in the final stages of our program to finally eradicate the disease. During the train journey from Howrah Station to Asansol, I noticed that there were armed railway police in the carriage. The train ran along the tracks at a leisurely pace and slowed down whenever the tracks curved, giving thieves and pickpockets ample opportunity to board the train. The armed police were there to protect passengers from train thieves.

In Jharkhand, where I visited next, which had a population of 2.75 million, I learned that the total number of registered cases in 2002 was 35,587, making for a prevalence rate of thirteen. Now, it was reportedly 10.5, though there were claims of 8.91. The second figure seemed to have more credence.

Having arrived in the capital city Ranchi, I was given a briefing at the hotel on the latest developments regarding leprosy control in Jharkhand, followed by a meeting with State Health Minister Dinesh Sarangi. He expressed his appreciation for this visit from the Nippon Foundation and the Sasakawa Health Foundation, which he saw as a moment of historic importance. When Jharkhand state was established, separating off from Bihar state in 2000, the prevalence rate was eighteen per 10,000. It was now 10.5 per 10,000 population. He assured me that every official in the state government from the chief minister on down would do their utmost to meet the WHO target of elimination by 2005. He described the efforts that were being put into place—the expansion of the health services and screenings on a daily basis at the clinics. I told him I was glad to be able to act so soon upon the kind invitation he had given me when I met him at Myanmar to visit him in Jharkhand state, and how happy I was to hear him reaffirm his commitment as a politician to helping with our efforts to eradicate leprosy.

He informed me that the clinic I would visit tomorrow, the Barangi Clinic, had been made over into a rehabilitation clinic, and he requested financial assistance in order to sustain its activities going forward. There was a need, he said, for more thoroughgoing education and awareness campaigns. In this region, there was still the strong notion that leprosy was visited upon people as a punishment for sins in a former life. They were going to have to train people up who were capable of dispelling such traditional thinking for good.

At the time, Jharkhand had 6.2 percent of the total number of registered people affected by leprosy in India. There are twenty-four districts in the state, and the average of all the districts was 8.91. The lowest prevalence rate was 3.12 and the highest twenty. Leprosy was being incorporated into the general health service, and general health personnel were getting from three to four hours' training a day in how to deal with the disease. Jharkhand is primarily rural, with many tribal villages, most of which are illiterate or semiliterate, making dissemination of information via print media (newspapers, billboards, handbills, banners, or advertisements) almost impossible. The situation of women in rural areas was of particular concern. In addition to suffering social restrictions, the health of women in the family was disregarded, with the result that there was an alarmingly high percentage of women with sight disabilities. Early detection of disease in children was also dire. Thirty percent of the population in this state were tribal, living in mountainous regions, making it difficult to access them to detect cases and offer treatment. Black magic still held sway, and people relied overwhelmingly on traditional healers. I told the health minister:

"The current approach is clearly ineffective if you want to reach elimination. If you simply wait passively for patients to come to you, by the time they get up the resolve in most cases the disease will have progressed. I think you should conduct an all-out social campaign with a view to controlling the disease. Short, easy-to-understand messages about leprosy detection and diagnosis are what you need. I don't believe that you can't convey appropriate information just because women are unable to read. If there's a clear message, it'll get to them, wherever they live. If you think they're hard to reach, it's up to you to make every effort to reach them. You have to reach the unreachable."

At this, the health minister's eyes widened. "Reach the unreachable," he said. "I think we will use that as our slogan."

That night, we held a news conference, and I asked for the cooperation of the media in our fight to eradicate leprosy. Health Minister Sarangi explained that the movement now had a brand-new slogan: Reaching the Unreachable. The journalists asked how leprosy figures and the measures being taken in Jharkhand compared with those in other states. They also wanted to know the figures for rates of elimination; whether Jharkhand would reach the WHO target by 2005; what was the best way to increase awareness of leprosy in the home and at school; whether Jharkhand had suitable infrastructure to tackle the problem; and exactly how much financial assistance the Nippon Foundation would offer.

Later that same night, I met with Jharkhand's first chief minister, Babulal Marandi. He reaffirmed his commitment to the elimination target of 2005 and told me he had decided to propose a resolution at the next budgetary meeting stating that the government and public sector would put every effort into the elimination of leprosy.

In June, I traveled to Portugal and visited Rovisco Pais, the former national leprosarium. Established in 1947 for the study, treatment, and eradication of leprosy, it officially closed its doors as a leprosarium in 1996, but at this point thirty-five residents remained. Rovisco Pais has now taken on a new role as a medical rehabilitation center plus hospital for people with leprosy. I had a pleasant chat with the last person affected by leprosy to enter the leprosarium, a forty-four-year-old man who was working in the vegetable plot. He was a lovely man, with a charming smile.

A state with the second highest prevalence rate—Republic of India (Odisha state), July 2003

Route: Narita → Delhi (flight time: 8h 30m)—one night—Delhi → Odisha (state capital Bhubaneswar) (flight time: 2h)—three nights—Odisha (Bhubaneswar) → Delhi (flight time: 2h; 6h stopover) → Narita (flight time: 7h 30m)

In July 2003, I visited Odisha, in the northeast of India. This was a state with the second highest leprosy prevalence in India (after Bihar), with 7.3 persons per 10,000 population. Nine of the thirty administrative districts in the state had a prevalence rate of ten per 10,000 or higher. The governor, the chief minister, and the health minister all assured me that they were conscious of the problem and were committed to elimination. Leprosy treatment was part of the general health services, and MDT blister packs were widely available. The reason the figures had remained the same for the last decade or so related first to the poverty and density of population in urban areas, second to the migration in border regions, and third to inaccessible tribal areas. Faced with these adverse conditions, the state governor M. M. Rajendran told me he had drawn up a four-step plan to elimi-

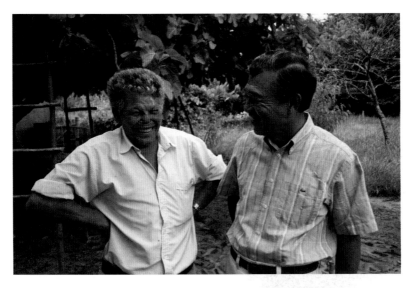

18. Chatting with a man said to be the last person affected by leprosy admitted to the Rovisco Pais leprosarium (Portugal, June 2003)

nate leprosy district by district before the end of 2005. I got a strong sense of his commitment. I was used to getting well-meaning assurances from officials, but here, I thought, was someone who was going to put his intentions into action.

In Odisha, I visited the Cuttack Leprosy Home and Hospital, which had about 200 residents. This is a place of historical significance in that Mahatma Gandhi visited it twice, in 1925 and 1927, on one of his eight visits to the state. I noticed among the residents some young women and children who had clearly once had the disease. That they were still living in isolation despite being cured seemed to me proof of the persistent social stigma attached to having once had the disease. Efforts focused on medicine and healthcare are of course vital for leprosy elimination, but so are separate efforts focusing on ensuring that people who have once had the disease can be fully reintegrated into society.

In the aftermath of conflict—Republic of Angola, July 2003

Route: Narita, Japan → Paris, France (flight time: 12h; 6h stopover) → Luanda, Angola (flight time: 8h 30m)—four nights—Luanda,

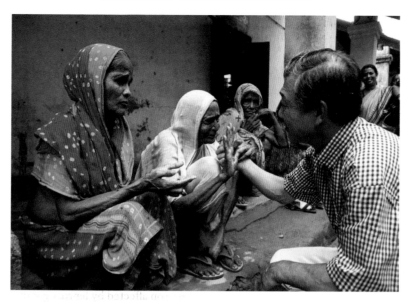

19. Offering encouragement to a person affected by leprosy, cured but still living in a colony (Odisha, India, July 2003)

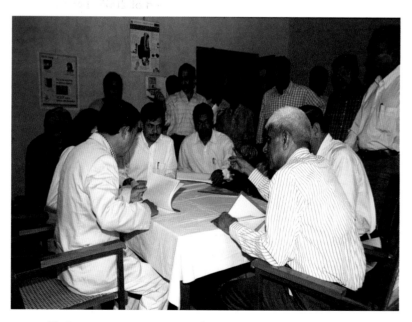

20. Listening to reports at a clinic (Odisha, India, July 2003)

Angola → London, United Kingdom (flight time: 9h; 2h 20m stop-over) → Geneva, Switzerland (flight time: 2h)—two nights (UN Sub-Convention on Human Rights briefing; meeting with Acting High Commissioner for Human Rights Bertrand Ramcharan)—Geneva, Switzerland → London, United Kingdom (flight time: 2h)—one night (meeting to discuss views on leprosy with University of Essex Professor Paul Hunt, UN Special Rapporteur for the UN Human Rights Commission)—London → Narita, Japan (flight time: 11h 30m)

The Republic of Angola, on the west coast of southern Africa, gained independence from Portugal in 1975 after a protracted anti-colonial struggle that started in 1961. But in the same year, the country descended into a civil war, which again lasted many decades, finally ending only in 2002. More than 10 million landmines remain buried in the earth. With the end of the civil war, economic development started to take place, based on the rich resources with which the country is blessed, which include oil and diamonds. The cost of living in Luanda is now said to be the highest in the world.

I flew from Narita to Paris, and then, after a six-hour wait in the airport, took an eight-and-a-half-hour night flight to Luanda, the capital city of Angola. Since the country had recently been at war, the only foreign people on the streets were UN peacekeeping forces. As the only East Asians in the city, we stood out. The Angolan government provided us with bodyguards, since security in the city was still an issue. Once, we got into the car to go somewhere, but one of our staff didn't show up. When he finally arrived, he told us that he had been taking video footage of the town on a small video camera but had been stopped by a man who appeared to be a police officer furious at being filmed. He had passed over a small amount of money, and the man went on his way.

The aim of my visit this time was to go to Bié province, around 600 kilometers from Luanda, which necessitated a one-and-a-half-hour onward flight once we had arrived. We traveled on a fourteen-passenger light aircraft. This was an area that had been the site of ferocious battles, with 20 percent of the population killed in the civil war that had only just ended the previous year. It was also a region with a high prevalence of leprosy, reported to be 5.83 persons per 10,000 population as of the end of 2002. The colonial-style public buildings in Cuíto, the old capital city of the province, were now nothing more than hollow shells. I visited a hospital in a city that was a further 80 kilometers out of Cuíto, called Kamakupa, and everywhere on the unpaved roads we saw bomb craters. The car trip, which lasted three hours, was the bumpiest I have ever experienced. One or two of the people traveling with me were knocked about so much that they got whiplash. Everywhere in the wilderness we saw the burnt-out husks of tanks, left where they were. The mayor of Cuíto informed me with a sad look in his eyes that it was still too dangerous to enter the area of the city on the other side of the river, even though the civil war had ended the previous year, and a huge number of landmines remained in the nearby cultivable fields, making it too dangerous to farm. Anti-leprosy measures were far from adequate, and there was a dearth of MDT blister packs. Despite these adverse conditions, medical staff were doing all they could, together with young volunteers from international NGOs, and he was profoundly grateful to them.

While I was in Luanda, and timed in order to coincide with my visit, there was a conference with key partners that was also attended by the Angolan government's health minister. It was the first of its kind to take place in Angola since the country began its anti-leprosy measures. At this conference, leprosy patients who had been treated and had now fully recovered took part on an equal level with government officials, WHO representatives, and NGOs. I considered this a hopeful reflection of the stance being taken by the Angolan government, which was clearly committed to getting to grips with leprosy from a medical perspective and combating the stigma often associated with the disease. The same sort of thing is being seen in other countries around the world—people affected by leprosy gradually taking their rightful place at the same table as health officials and government administrators.

Salvation in the midst of suffering—Republic of Madagascar, September 2003

Route: Narita, Japan → Paris, France (flight time: 13h; 6h stopover) → Antananarivo, Madagascar (flight time: 10h)—two nights—Antananarivo, Madagascar → Toamasina (flight time: 50m)—one night—Toamasina → Antananarivo → (flight time: 45m)—two nights—Antananarivo → Paris, France (flight time: 10h; 5h stopover) → Beijing, China (flight time: 10h 50m)—one night—(Sasakawa Japan–China Friendship Fund meeting)—Beijing, China → Narita, Japan (flight time: 3h 30m)

In September 2003, I visited the Republic of Madagascar, an island nation in the Indian Ocean 400 kilometers off the coast of East Africa. With a land area of 587,000 square kilometers (over one-and-a-half times the size of Japan), the country's population was 16 million. Following the prehistoric breakup of the supercontinent Gondwana, Madagascar split from the Indian subcontinent around 88 million years ago, allowing native plants and animals to evolve in relative isolation: consequently, over 90 percent of its wildlife is found nowhere else on earth. Among the Madagascan people's ancestors are people from Asia (Indonesia and Malaysia) who traveled across the Indian Ocean 2,000 years ago. This gives the people of Madagascar a somewhat Asian mien. Rice is cultivated on roughly half the agricultural land—it is a staple of the diet. The rice paddies in the country, too, were reminiscent of East Asia.

Madagascar is difficult to access from Japan. My journey involved a thirteen-hour flight from Narita to Paris, a six-hour wait at the airport, and then a ten-hour flight from Paris to Antananarivo.

Meals in Madagascar, by the way, usually involve rice or cassava, along with grain cereals and beans, and perhaps a small amount of meat, and lots of fresh vegetables. However, the restaurants serve excellent French cuisine, due to the French colonial past. Foie gras has become a specialty of Madagascar, and I was amazed by the size of the foie gras that came to me when I ordered it in a restaurant.

In 1997, the leprosy prevalence was high—8.31 per 10,000 population. But this visit I was told it had improved and was now four persons per 10,000. There were certain pockets where eradication efforts were being stymied that had high prevalence, as many as eight or even ten persons.

When I asked what was holding back elimination efforts, I was told it was the fear of leprosy and the social stigma attached to the disease; the lack of sufficiently trained peripheral health workers able to diagnose and treat leprosy cases correctly or use national leprosy program supports; and the fact that a quarter of the nation's population resided more than 10 kilometers from the nearest basic health center in each region, making access to medical treatment difficult. President Marc Ravalomanana had come into politics having risen to prominence as the founder and CEO of a dairy conglomerate, and he was famed for starting his work extremely early in the morning, well before anyone else. His confidant, the chief cabinet secretary, had graduated from the University of Kobe and spoke fluent Japanese, and the president himself was a keen Japanophile.

The aim of my visit this time was of course to hold meetings with government leaders, including the president, the prime minister, the foreign minister, and the health minister. I was impressed that everyone was so well informed about leprosy, and they all showed a strong political will to meet the elimination target. When I met with the president, he told me: "Madagascar is one of the poorest countries in the world, and we have all sorts of public health problems to contend with—malaria, tuberculosis, and others. But leprosy is a huge problem, so I really want to eliminate it by next year. To that end, I plan to put together campaigns to make the people as aware of the disease. It's important to get the people involved. I want to show everyone that people affected by leprosy are as human as the next person, so I will start going out and meeting them myself. And I will tell my health minister to conduct thoroughgoing campaigns urging everyone that hidden patients can come out and get treatment."

I was pleased to see how the issue of leprosy was also getting good coverage on the television and in newspapers. All of this convinced me that the government was doing its best.

I have always argued that strong political will is vital for the eradication of leprosy, and I was very pleased to see how it was more than evident in Madagascar and that the basic policies and strategies were in place. I truly felt that this country would meet its elimination target by 2005. With such political will and determination, I was sure they would succeed.

A place with links to the life of Gandhi—Republic of India, November 2003

Route: Narita, Japan → Singapore (flight time: 6h; 3h stopover) → Kolkata, West Bengal state, India (flight time: 2h 30m)—two nights—

Kolkata → Delhi (flight time: 2h)—two nights—Delhi → Nagpur, Maharashtra state (flight time: 3h)—one night—Nagpur, Maharashtra state → Mumbai (flight time: 1h)—three nights—Mumbai → Singapore (flight time: 6h; 1h 30m stopover) → Narita, Japan

The battle waged by Mahatma Gandhi against the inherent discrimination of the caste system, in support of the so-called "untouchables" at the bottom of society, which he dealt with explicitly in Article 17 of the Constitution, is well known. Perhaps less well known is that he also concerned himself with restoring the dignity of another kind of untouchability—that of people with leprosy. For many centuries, India was famous for being a country where leprosy was endemic, and in fact India still has the highest number of people affected by leprosy globally.

Eradicating leprosy in India has always been my greatest dream. That is why I visit the country as often as I can, usually several times in the course of a single year (and sometimes as many as seven times a year). Ultimately, also, it is my fervent hope and desire to see an end to the stigma and discrimination attached to people affected by leprosy, so that no more of them have to resort to begging in order to survive.

In 2003, I made three visits to India—in March, July, and November. In November, I visited Kolkata, Delhi, Wardha, and Mumbai.

In Kolkata, I visited Garden Reach, an urban slum of 300,000 people with a population density of 30,000 people per square kilometer. In the slum clinic, I found neatly organized records going back twenty-six years for as many as 8,000 people affected by leprosy who had been treated there. I have nothing but admiration for the dedicated efforts of the staff over such a long period. The clinic also has an NGO office and was providing micro-financing for people with leprosy to help them start their own small businesses—evidence that the clinic wasn't only focusing on treating patients but also helping them become self-reliant once they were cured. A good example of how to encourage social rehabilitation.

Elimination activities in West Bengal generally seemed to be proceeding well, although a few problems were pointed out. First, there were flaws in the management of MDT. Availability of drug supplies at the primary health centers was inconsistent. There were insufficient stocks of children's dosages—a point I was asked to convey to the relevant authorities in Delhi. Second was the problem of default-ers—patients failing to complete treatment. With the integration of leprosy services into the general healthcare system in Kolkata, responsibility for case-holding had passed to local government, which was still in the throes of adapting to the changeover. As a result, many patients found that they had been inadvertently dropped from the treatment list or were listed with a different clinic: a good number of examinations had to be undertaken all over again.

In India, 30 January is designated as Mahatma Gandhi Day. Considered the father of the nation, Gandhi was assassinated in New Delhi by a Hindu fundamentalist on 30 January 1948. This day is now also designated as Anti-Leprosy Day to keep alive the memory of Gandhi's selfless efforts to care for people affected by leprosy. He once declared that if India has the breath of life in it, it must stop turning its back on people with leprosy.

As someone who was deeply involved in the fight against leprosy, there was one place I had long wanted to visit and see for myself. This was the Sevagram Ashram in the Wardha district of Maharashtra state. In November 2003, at long last, I was able to do so.

Gandhi stayed in this ashram on several occasions, beginning in 1936, using it as a residence and a place of meditation, and trying out many of his social experiments. It is preserved in its original state as a historical monument. The Sevagram Ashram site consists of a group of huts of modest construction with earthen tiled roofs capping mud walls. Gandhi's room is bare, save for his bedding and his charkha, or spinning wheel, which he used daily and that we often see in photo-graphs of him at the time. Somewhat incongruously, there is also an "office hut," with a telephone, apparently instituted so that the British colonial authorities could check on Gandhi's movements. The tele-phone was also apparently used by Gandhi to keep in contact with the various campaigns taking place around the country aimed at Indian independence. It was in this ashram that Gandhi set about his project of achieving freedom for India from the yoke of British rule through non-violent resistance, relying on mass protest and non-cooperation. Here he chose to live among the people who were traditionally seen as the lowest in society precisely in order to challenge orthodox caste-based social hierarchy, a living source of comfort and inspiration for them. It was also here that he developed his ideas about mental resilience, and his philosophy regarding means and ends in politics ("As the means, so the end"; "There is no wall of separation between means and ends") and expounded his philosophy of universal peace; and cultivated workers who would devote themselves to serving society. Gandhi's *Constructive Programme*, first printed in 1941, was a manifesto aimed at India's independence, a result of the many discussions he had with others in his group in the Sevagram Ashram. The manifesto argues for obtaining self-rule through methods relying on non-violence and non-cooperation. The text comprises eighteen points, with titles such as "Communal Unity," "Removal of Untouchability," "Basic Education." The seventeenth point was titled "People Suffering from Leprosy." Gandhi was clearly positioning the provision of succor to people affected by leprosy, people who heretofore had been completely ignored and left to fend completely for themselves, as one of the major tasks involved in nation-building.

The Sevagram Ashram is also home to the Mahatma Gandhi Memorial Leprosy Foundation. Established in 1951, the foundation mainly carries out education and health training programs in areas where leprosy prevalence is particularly high. When the foundation began its work, the prevalence in Wardha district was unbelievably high: 233 people per 10,000 population. Since the introduction of MTD, it has dropped to 3.4 people per 10,000.

In 1978, the celebrated philosopher and social critic Ivan Illich, a man who was originally from Austria but who had made his home in Mexico, stayed in this ashram: his experience provided the inspiration for his later thesis that autonomy and self-sufficiency are essential for basic human dignity. More specifically, Illich argued that human happiness comes not with material satisfaction and convenience but rather with life characterized by simplicity and earning enough simply to survive. The key to human happiness lies here, much more than in wealth or attributes like beauty, which do not in fact produce happiness in and of themselves. What is needed, Illich argued, is a radical change in people's values, so that rather than acquiring endless amounts of material possessions they gain satisfaction from meeting basic needs. He was the person who started the self-sufficiency movement.

REACHING THE UNREACHABLE

The Sevagram Ashram was swept immaculately clean and was a haven of tranquility. A huge sal tree provided a welcome cover of shade. But one step through the ashram gate took the visitor immediately back to the crowds and hubbub that is so characteristic of India. A cacophony of vehicles streamed by, the destitute of all ages flocked around, and the city streets, filled with noise, extended to the horizon.

Maharashtra state has a population of over 100 million, 42 percent of whom live in urban areas, while the rest live in more than 40,000 hamlets and villages, with many difficulties in access for the provision of medical care. The average prevalence in Maharashtra in 1981 was 62.4 cases per 10,000 population, but by 2003 this had declined to 2.75. The main issues seem to be the difficulties involved in the provision of medical services to tribal districts, the fact that many villages are situated far away from civilization, and that cross-border migration makes it quite hard to keep track of the numbers.

Mumbai is home to the Dharavi, Asia's biggest slum. Some 600,000 people from all over India live here, and the population density is as high as 60,000 per square kilometer. Everyone lives as best they can, despite the lack of running water and unsanitary conditions. Since 1975, the Bombay Leprosy Project has led a campaign to control leprosy in this slum. In 1983, the prevalence rate in the slums was 22.4 per 10,000 population, but by August 2002 it had dropped to 0.7 per 10,000, a dramatic decrease that had occurred due to the devoted efforts of the Bombay Leprosy Project. This NGO not only seeks out and treats patients but helps in the socio-economic rehabilitation of people affected by leprosy who have made a complete recovery, with support from local companies.

I was amazed at how the workers of this organization managed to find their way through the maze of narrow passages pressed together so tightly in the slum, all thronging with people, to lead me to the shanties of people I wanted to visit. Many of these people were Dalit and extremely poor, but I saw no one begging: they were all busily doing work and trying to get ahead, whether it was in the cheap garment industry or in food processing or in cleaning and recycling. At first glance, life for the slum dwellers seemed chaotic, but the postal system worked perfectly, and the crime rate was low.

MAKING THE IMPOSSIBLE POSSIBLE

Reconstructive surgery and socio-economic rehabilitation—Kingdom of Cambodia, December 2003

> Route: Narita, Japan → Bangkok, Thailand (flight time: 6h; 1.5h stop-over) → Phnom Penh, Cambodia (flight time: 2h)—three nights—Phnom Penh → Singapore (flight time: 4h; 3h stopover) → Denpasar, Bali, Indonesia (flight time: 2h 20m)—three nights—Denpasar, Bali → Jakarta, Indonesia (flight time: 1h 45m; 2h stopover) → Narita, Japan (flight time: 7h 30m)

In December, I had a meeting with the Cambodian health minister Dr. Mam Bun Heng in Phnom Penh, Cambodia. Cambodia reached the WHO-defined threshold of leprosy elimination (less than one person per 10,000 population) in 1998, and its current prevalence was 0.47 persons per 10,000 population. Nevertheless, the minister told me, there were still certain areas in the country, particularly in mountainous areas far away from the cities, where access was compromised and amenities, hygiene, and education were less than ideal. Efforts had still to be made to strengthen the systems for identifying cases, registering them, tracing and screening contacts, and monitoring the disease.

During my trip, I paid a visit to the Kien Khleang Center in Phnom Penh. This is a rehabilitation center set up in 2000 by CIOMAL (Campagne Internationale de l'Ordre de Malte contre la Lèpre), a Swiss-registered NGO that provides free medical and surgical rehabilitation for people affected by leprosy and also serves as a training center for patients suffering from the complications associated with the disease. I chatted with about forty inpatients, most of whom had severe long-term sequalae that required surgery. All of them were in the care of Dr. Stephen Griffiths, a medical coordinator for CIOMAL. They looked forward to resuming healthy productive lives in society once their surgery was over. It is important to provide as much care and assistance as possible to people who have been affected by leprosy, even after they are completely cured of the disease itself, and this would be just as important after 2005 when we were hoping that all countries were going to reach the WHO-defined threshold of leprosy elimination.

REACHING THE UNREACHABLE

Countries visited in 2004	
January	• India
March	China (Japan–China Field Officer Exchange Program)
	• Malta
	• Switzerland (Oral statement at the UN Sub-Commission on the Promotion and Protection of Human Rights)
	France (Sasakawa Japan–France Foundation)
April	• Nepal
May	Jordan (University of Jordan, SYLFF)
	Switzerland (United Nations Commission on Human Rights, WHO World Health Assembly)
June	Indonesia (Gadjah Mada University, SYLFF)
	China (Beijing University)
	United States (Meetings at the US–Japan Foundation in New York)
	• India
	• Bhutan
	• Chile (University of Chile, SYLFF)
	• Brazil (University of São Paulo, SYLFF)
July	Switzerland (UN Sub-Commission on the Promotion and Protection of Human Rights)
August	• India
September	Russia (Donation ceremony of the book, Saint Nicholas's Diary to Patriarch Alexy II)
	China (Book donation ceremony)
	• India
October	Sweden (Malmö, World Maritime University)
	United Kingdom (Cardiff University)

November	China (Meeting with World Maritime University fellows; Shanghai forum)
	Mongolia (National Academy of Governance, ceremony commemorating the twentieth anniversary of the SYLFF program)
December	● Philippines
	● India

● Indicates a trip that features in this section.

SYLFF: The Sasakawa Young Leaders Fellowship Fund program. A funding program.

WMU: World Maritime University.

A disease that can make anyone a social outcast—Republic of India (Chhattisgarh state), January 2004

Route: Narita → Singapore (flight time: 6h 30m; 2h 30m stopover) → Mumbai, Maharashtra state, India (flight time: 5h 30m; one-night stopover) → Raipur, Chhattisgarh state (flight time: 1h 30m)—three nights—Raipur → Delhi (flight time: 1h 30m; 7h stopover) → Taipei, Taiwan (flight time: 5h 30m; 2h stopover) → Narita

My first trip in 2004, in January, was to India. The main reason for my trip was to take part in the National Conference on the Elimination of Leprosy in Raipur, the capital of Chhattisgarh. It was organized by the national government and the government of Chhattisgarh, ILEP, and our own Sasakawa Health Foundation and supported by many other bodies and associations.

The leprosy prevalence in Chhattisgarh was 5.08 people per 10,000 population, the third highest in India. More than 34 percent of people affected by leprosy were tribal peoples, with the majority living in places that were geographically cut off from the cities and extremely impoverished. India accounts for more than two-thirds of the world's leprosy cases (and nine-tenths of Southeast Asia's), and this conference lasting three days (27–30 January) focused attention on where the most work remained to be done.

There were more than 500 people attending, including the president of India, Dr. A. P. J. Abdul Kalam, and it was taken up by a great many news sources. In his keynote address, the president made a fervent plea to take concerted steps and devise more effective strategies to reduce leprosy prevalence to less than one case per 10,000 population, within the prescribed time frame. He also emphasized the need for "rehabilitation with compassion" so that all treated patients were helped gently and with understanding to resume lives and work in their communities.

As the Ambassador for Leprosy Elimination, I gave a keynote speech in which I outlined to leading politicians and experts from different parts of India the kinds of things—commitment, awareness-raising, and social support to leprosy-affected persons—that need to take place for the eradication of leprosy to be achieved, giving examples.

The following day, I visited a village roughly 30 kilometers from the city of Raipur, where I accompanied twenty or so female community health workers as they paid home visits. These women are a unique group who go from house to house involving themselves in a wide range of health issues in addition to leprosy, including maternity

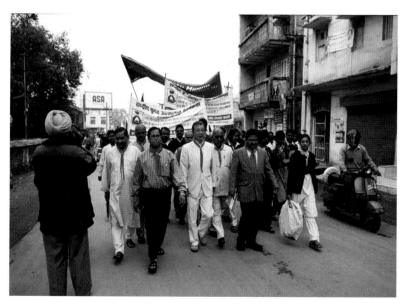

21. The author in a leprosy elimination campaign parade, with the health minister and other officials (Chhattisgarh, India, January 2004)

care, child care, and tuberculosis prevention. In India, they are referred to as Accredited Social Health Activists, or ASHA. On the day I visited, they had gathered to prepare for the leprosy elimination campaign due to start the day after. I was told that these health workers are each responsible for about 5,000 people and do their rounds by bicycle. Many of the homes they visit are far apart, and some can only be reached by foot. I felt humbled and grateful for their dedication. These women were passionately devoted to their cause, the determination clearly showing in their faces. One woman told me with obvious pride how someone from the Brahmin caste had thanked her from the bottom of his heart for making sure he could complete his course of treatment. Ostracization from communities can happen to everyone—high or low in the caste system.

On the morning of 30 January—the day when the entire nation commemorates the life of Mahatma Gandhi, which is also Anti-Leprosy Day in India—several thousand young men and women gathered in a square in the center of Raipur to rally for leprosy elimination. I marched alongside the state health ministers at the head of a long procession of political leaders, government workers, and youngsters as it passed through the center of the city, where the marchers handed out pamphlets promoting leprosy elimination.

Preserving the history of leprosy in a small island in the Mediterranean Sea—Republic of Malta, March 2004

> Route: Narita → London/Heathrow, UK (flight time: 12h; 2h stopover) → Malta (flight time: 3h)—two nights—Malta → Zurich, Switzerland (flight time: 2h; 1h 30m stopover) → Geneva (flight time: 45m)—five nights (meeting with the Sub-Commission on the Promotion and Protection of Human Rights; face-to-face meeting with Acting High Commissioner Ramcharan)—Geneva → Paris (flight time: 1h; 2h stopover) → Narita (flight time: 12h)

In late March, I traveled to the Republic of Malta in the company of Kazuko Yamaguchi, executive director of the Sasakawa Health Foundation and an expert on all matters to do with leprosy. The temperature was 10 degrees C, on the cool side. An island (or archipelago) just off the coast of Sicily, which itself lies off Italy,

Malta has a population of just over 500,000, with a total land area about two-thirds the size of Awajishima. Over the course of 7,000 years, Malta has been a stopping point for people from all over Europe and beyond and witness to the rise and fall of civilizations all around the Mediterranean.

Malta is a fascinating country, home today to three World Heritage Sites. It consists of three islands: Malta, Gozo, and Comino. Malta island in particular is blessed with a complexly formed shoreline along its southeastern coast that historically provided an ideal setting for a natural fortress. Traces remain of civilizations spanning the period from antiquity to the present.

A great stronghold was built on Malta by the Knights of the Order of St. John (originally the Knights Hospitaller, an order that cared for pilgrims of any faith or order; later renamed the Knights of Malta), who were given the islands in 1530. They engaged in heroic battles to defend the island against the Ottoman Empire. In 1798, the Knights were forced to flee after losing to invading forces under Napoleon's command. Just two years later, however, the Napoleonic victors were sent packing by the British, and for the next 160 years Malta remained a British possession, and as such participated in two world wars. Finally, in 1964 Malta won its independence from the British. In 1974, as the Republic of Malta it became a member of the British Commonwealth.

Given its strategically important location in the Mediterranean, Malta has since antiquity been visited by passing ships that carried people, goods, animals, and, not infrequently, pestilent diseases. Particularly in the Middle Ages, Europe was repeatedly racked by plague, and Malta, already the seat of the Knights of the Order of St. John, set up a quarantine station on an island called Manoel away from the main island as a self-defense measure. Called Lazaretto from the generic name given to such isolation facilities, the term can be traced linguistically to the parable of Lazarus the beggar in the Gospel of St. Luke.

Malta's medical history contains reports of leprosy patients throughout the seventeenth and eighteenth centuries. The number of patients increased in the second half of the nineteenth century, a trend largely attributed to the fact that some 6,000 Indian soldiers were sent there by Britain at the time of the Russo-Turkish War of 1877–8. This coincided with a period when increasing numbers of leprosy patients were beginning to become a matter of concern all across the globe, particularly in areas under colonial rule. The British authorities in Malta believed it was necessary, as in other territories in their empire, to isolate and confine the archipelago's leprosy patients. In 1893, they issued an ordinance requiring isolation and set out to establish appropriate facilities. In 1899, a facility for men was created at the Asylum for the Aged and Incurable (commonly referred to as a "poor house") located at Mgieret on the mainland. This was followed in 1912 by a facility for women. According to statistics for the year 1918, the number of leprosy patients then stood at 4.72 per 10,000 population—nearly five times the contemporary WHO-defined threshold.

Malta's history is extremely interesting and complex, and I was interested particularly in the way the island coped with leprosy in modern times. I knew Malta was the first country in the world, in the early 1970s, to institute a leprosy eradication program. All patients given this treatment were reported to be cured. I was eager to know what the situation was of the people who had recovered from the disease. Fortunately, in my quest I was able to avail myself of the help of Professor Victor Griffiths, Professor Emeritus at the University of Malta, who had been on the national committee in charge of forming policies to deal with leprosy. He was able to fill me in from his own recollections and by showing me some important documents.

According to Professor Griffiths, in addition to the pair of isolation centers on the main island already noted, an isolation facility had also been created on the island of Gozo, to the north, in 1937. The isolation facility on the main island (mentioned above) became St. Bartholomew Hospital, while that on Gozo evolved into the Sacred Heart Hospital. Following the development of drug treatments in the 1940s, and in line with the general global trend, the laws mandating compulsory isolation ended in 1953. After that, leprosy came to be treated primarily on an outpatient basis, and all of Malta's leprosaria were closed in the 1970s. The earliest leprosarium later became part of St. Vincent de Paul Residence, a care facility for the elderly, with 1,000 residents at the time of my visit. The isolation wards for leprosy patients that once existed had been removed without a trace.

Statistics for the year 1957 list the number of leprosy patients on Malta at 152, out of a total population of 314,369. The only drug treatment available at this time was dapsone, which required months to take effect. Over time, though, cases of resistance to dapsone were reported, and research began into a new method of chemotherapy. One such program was the Malta Leprosy Eradication Project (MLEP). This was launched in 1972 under the leadership of Malta's health authority with support from the Sovereign Military Order of Malta, the German Leprosy Relief Association, and the Research Center Borstel, also from Germany. It called for the treatment of leprosy using isoprodian—which combined the three anti-tuberculosis agents isoniazid, prothionamide, and dapsone, in combination with rifampicins. A total of 261 individuals, including 201 registered cases of leprosy reported by the health authority of Malta at the time plus patients diagnosed subsequently, proceeded to receive this treatment for periods from six months to seven years. All patients were reported to have been cured. A follow-up study was carried out during the twenty-seven years from the MLEP's start, ending in December 1999. From the Maltese side, the project had been led by Dr. George Depasquale, who had studied under Professor Griffiths, and prior to our meeting Professor Griffiths had confirmed with him what had subsequently transpired. According to Dr. Depasquale's information, around 100 people were still alive who had been treated and cured of leprosy; moreover, no new cases had been reported in the previous six years. However, no one knew who they were, or what their situation now was.

I had heard that when the isolation facilities at St. Bartholomew Hospital and on Gozo were closed in 1974, the twenty-two inmates who had no homes to return to had been relocated to the site of a former army barracks on Malta called Hal-Ferha Estate, where they were provided with places to live and some land to cultivate. They were also said to be receiving pensions and had access to medical care. But when I made inquiries of the health ministry and the Knights of Malta about this prior to my visit, I was unable to receive a definitive answer. When I asked Professor Griffiths about this, he kindly agreed to accompany me to the site. "Thirty years have already passed, so I don't know what condition it's in," he cautioned me. "But years ago, I went there on several occasions, so let's go and take a look."

We drove for about twenty minutes through a number of small towns until we came upon a road sign that said "Hal-Ferha." Proceeding further, we reached a sector where brown stone walls lined both sides of a narrow, twisting lane. There were no homes to be seen. All we found were broken stones and scraps of wood; the whole area was overgrown with weeds and bushes. It was then that we noticed a stone in the lower portion of a corner wall painted with the faded words "Hal-Ferha." And so it was that I confirmed that the Hal-Ferha Estate no longer existed—just as Professor Griffiths had in fact feared. That Malta had managed to eliminate leprosy at such an early point, and through treatment that had been developed on these islands, was a remarkable achievement. And yet, looking at this site, it was clear to me that the history of this remarkable achievement had all but faded away.

As I pondered this situation, I felt rather mournful. I wanted to do something to ensure this important history would not be forgotten. Even if the day comes when leprosy is completely eradicated from the world, its history should never be forgotten. We have a duty to acknowledge both the mistakes that were made in ostracizing people with the disease and to laud the courage of those who endured this treatment.

My first visit to a place with deep associations with my father—Nepal, April 2004

> Route: Narita → Bangkok, Thailand (flight time: 6h 30m; one-night stopover) → Kathmandu (flight time: 3h 30m)—three nights—Kathmandu → Bangkok (flight time: 3h 30m; 5h 30m stopover) → Narita (flight time: 6h)

The other country I visited in March was Nepal, where I spent four days in Kathmandu and its immediate environs. This was one of the six major leprosy-endemic countries. With this trip, I had visited all six in my capacity as WHO Ambassador.

A country known in Japan chiefly for being the gateway to the Himalayan Mountain range, Nepal has only recently attained a degree of political stability. Even after the kingdom was unified in the eighteenth century by the Gorkha Kingdom, political instability continued. The so-called Panchayat partyless system was devised, but Nepalese communism and Maoism gained sway in the 1990s and a civil war raged. In the first decade of the twenty-first century, following a peaceful democratic revolution, the country became a secular state and a federal republic, ending its time-honored status as a Hindu kingdom. However, infighting and strife continued, and it was only in 2015 that the country gained a constitution.

For me, Nepal was a country that had deep personal significance. In 1983, my father visited Nepal's Khokana State Leprosarium and on meeting an elderly woman resident there took her two paralyzed hands in his own, and with tears flowing from his eyes bewailed her fate. The Grammy Award-winning photographer Richard Young captured the encounter in a documentary film and broadcast it all over the world. I was not with my father on that particular visit—I only saw a photograph of the encounter. But the incident made a great impression on me. In all the years that I knew my father, he had always been the picture of forbearance and control. This sudden flood of emotion brought home to me what a hugely compassionate and deeply emotional man my father was. To me, he was a true hero.

Nepal now had a population of well over 24 million. According to health ministry figures, the leprosy prevalence was 2.4 per 10,000 population. Given that the rate was seventy per 10,000 fifteen years prior, in the late 1980s, steady progress was being made toward elimination. MDT had been introduced in 1982, and leprosy had been included in general health service treatment in 1987, with distribution covering all seventy-five of the nation's districts in 1996. However, even though thirty-one of these districts had achieved the WHO elimination target, in the mountainous west and in the southeastern lowlands bordering on India there were pockets where the prevalence rate exceeded five per 10,000, so more effort was needed to reach the official elimination target by 2005.

I met with Prime Minister Surya Bahadur Thapa and Foreign Health Minister Bhekh Bahadur Thapa. I requested that the government lend particular efforts to raising awareness of leprosy. They replied that the government had made elimination a high priority in policy and in practice and were working toward elimination by the end of 2005. Leprosy education was now part of the school curriculum, and the government was determined to spread information about the disease throughout the country by making greater use of the media. For my part, I said that in order to turn leprosy elimination into a major social movement we had to involve a broad spectrum of NGOs concerned with leprosy, making sure to forge even closer ties with them. Both men agreed with me about this. I was very heartened to meet Dr. Rita Thapa, wife of Health Minister Bhekh Bahadur Thapa. Dr. Rita Thapa was a feminist educator and community activist with extensive experience in building links between community, non-governmental, and academic institutions who was working as an advisor to the health ministry on health policy. She clearly understood the need to place leprosy elimination at the top of the list of health priorities and how important it was to eradicate prejudice. She would be a highly effective advisor.

I also had discussions with Health Secretary Lokman Singh Karki and Director-General of the Department of Health Services Dr. B. D. Chataut. I mentioned the example of Uttar Pradesh, where they were achieving education and awareness in families by having the schools incorporate skin checks as part of pupils' homework. They assured me that they were working toward the elimination target by involving government, NGOs, and the private sector in activities at every level, training human resources and fostering a social movement all over the country from village to national level. Dr. Bimala Ojha, director of the Leprosy Control Division, said they were forging ahead with information, education, and communication programs, and that leprosy featured in elementary school textbooks. I wasn't able to see any such textbooks to confirm this, but if true, this would be the second such instance, after Vietnam.

Aware of the key role played by NGOs in the drive to eliminate leprosy, I visited the Social Welfare Council, the government agency that coordinates the work of NGOs, and requested that it help spread my three key messages.

When we held a conference on publicity campaigns and awareness-raising drives for leprosy in Kathmandu, I was very pleased to see officials from the health ministry, various figures from the Social Welfare Council and NGOs that involved themselves in anti-leprosy drives, as well as officers working for WHO and various officials from the media taking part. It is my belief that an important part of my activities lies in associating with people in as many areas related to leprosy as possible. The flame of a single match is only a single flame, but if you light matches in many places, eventually their flames join and give rise to a significant fire.

Because this was a short trip, and also because of the increased security risk due to the continuing demonstrations being organized by rebel Maoist forces, I wasn't able to travel as widely as I would have liked, and I had no choice but to restrict my activities to the city of Kathmandu and its environs. One was the Khokana State Leprosarium operated by the Nepal Leprosy Relief Association (NELRA), and the other was the Anandaban Hospital, operated by TLM. I was delighted to visit these facilities, which were well maintained and being used for their original purposes.

Khokana settlement is located in the village of Khokana along the Bagmati River. On the premises are a clinic, the original leprosarium, new nursing homes, and a job training center. I had the chance to visit with the 200 or so recovered individuals and their families and saw people being taught how to make furniture at the training center.

I also paid a short visit to one of two hostels on the outskirts of Kathmandu operated by NELRA for children of rural families affected by leprosy, which enable them to commute to schools in Kathmandu.

The Anandaban Hospital, established by TLM in 1957, is Nepal's biggest leprosy hospital. It is located 16 kilometers south of Kathmandu in the Lalitpur district, in a valley setting around an hour by car from the capital. It has a total of 121 staff and 115 beds. As a hospital, it undertakes a broad range of activities, including early detection and treatment, prevention of disability, reconstructive surgery, rehabilitation, and elimination campaigns. Dr. Yo Yuasa, executive and medical director of the Sasakawa Memorial Health Foundation (and later president of the ILA), served as medical superintendent at the hospital in the 1970s when he worked for TLM.

Among the hospital's patients were people who had traveled all the way from India because of the hospital's excellent reputation. These people were treated with exactly the same care and attention extended to Nepalese patients, leaving me in no doubt about the devotion and sense of duty of the doctors and other medical staff.

119

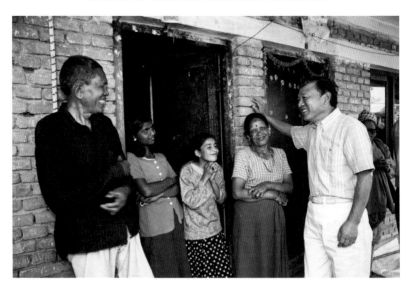

22. In cheerful conversation with residents who have recovered from leprosy in the Khokana settlement (Nepal, April 2004)

The issues affecting leprosy elimination in Nepal seemed to come down to the continuing political unrest arising from the activities of Maoist elements in government, which meant that leprosy campaigns had to be limited to just twenty-five of the country's seventy-five districts; and as yet inadequate human resources that would enable NGOs, which were traditionally at the heart of such activities, and their counterparts in government to work together effectively.

In May, I also visited Geneva to attend the sixtieth session of the United Nations Human Rights Commission and the WHO Assembly.

The role of the media and the important role of people who have lived experience of leprosy—Republic of India, June 2004

> Route: Narita → Jakarta, Indonesia (flight time: 7h 30m)—two nights (Sasakawa Young Leader Prize-Giving Ceremony at Gadjah Mada University—Jakarta → Bangkok (flight time: 3h 30m; 30m stopover) → New Delhi (flight time: 4h 30m)—two nights

On 4 and 5 June 2004, I was in New Delhi to attend a National Consultation Workshop on Advocacy Strategies for the Elimination of Leprosy. Held under the auspices of the India-headquartered International Leprosy Union (ILU), this two-day event brought together government, NGOs, and media representatives, as well as people who had once had leprosy but had been treated and were fully recovered. In my opening speech, I urged that we make every use of the media in disseminating positive, hopeful messages that would capture people's interest; that we create opportunities for people who had experience of the disease to assume positions of responsibility in elimination activities; and that we conduct education and awareness campaigns and integrate leprosy care within the general healthcare system. From now on, I said, leprosy-related discrimination was going to be viewed in the framework of human rights.

After the main session, there were smaller group sessions, and opinions were exchanged about the role of NGOs, how best to involve the media, and the roles that people with lived experience of the disease could play in encouraging others toward self-reliance. Everyone agreed that leprosy elimination and the eradication of leprosy-related discrimination requires transforming a government-led program into a people's movement, and that would involve governmental organizations, but also NGOs, corporations, labor unions, educational institutions, and other groups working in social activism. In order to get the message out to the poorest sections of society who mostly lived on the margins and were in many cases ill-educated, the use of traditional performing arts, such as songs, puppet shows, and dancing, was especially effective. People with lived experience of leprosy could also play an important part as role models. Anybody who had achieved a certain degree of success in self-sufficiency and employment should be encouraged to identify themselves and be made spokespersons.

The workshop ended with the host pledging three follow-up actions. The first was to identify spokespersons from government, media, and people affected by leprosy in the five hyper-endemic districts and to raise their awareness of leprosy control. The second was to look into the creation of a specialized leprosy resource center that could offer information useful to the media when making programs about leprosy (and also allow journalists to learn more about the disease). The third was to find ways in which to involve people

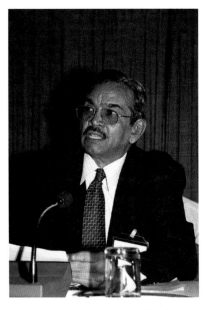

23. Dr. Gopal, representing people affected by leprosy, giving an impassioned speech at the workshop (Delhi, India, June 2004)

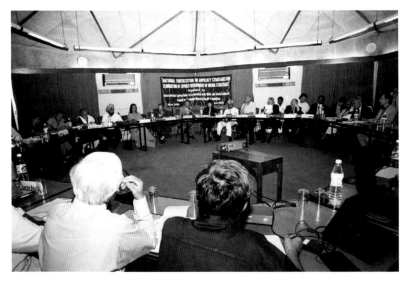

24. The National Consultation Workshop on Advocacy Strategies for the Elimination of Leprosy (Delhi, India, June 2004)

affected by leprosy who had achieved a certain degree of self-sufficiency to play a role in activities such as early diagnosis and the restoration of dignity.

It was a lively workshop, with participants who were highly articulate and passionate—full of ideas. Indeed, they were so eager to contribute to the discussion that not infrequently two people would spring up and hold forth at the same time. This was very much the kind of animated discussion that I was accustomed to seeing in India.

The happiest country—Kingdom of Bhutan, June 2004

Route: New Delhi → West Bengal state (flight time: 2h; one-night stopover) → Bhutan (flight time: 1h 30m)—two nights—Bhutan → Bangkok (flight time: 4h; 10h stopover) → Narita (flight time: 6h)

From India, I traveled straight on to the Kingdom of Bhutan. A tiny nation deep in the mountains of the Himalayas, with a population of about 700,000 at the time of my visit, Bhutan is known for its stunning landscapes and its strong national traditions. It reached the WHO-defined target of leprosy elimination as a public health problem in 1997.

The sole gateway to Bhutan via the air is a narrow landing strip in among several valleys deep in the mountains situated at 2,300 meters above sea level. Taking off and landing at Paro airport is challenging, and only a few pilots are certified to land here because the flight path approaching the airport involves sharp twists and turns. After landing, we drove for almost an hour to the nation's capital, Thimphu, along a narrow twisting mountain road with steep drops, fearing for our lives whenever we had to negotiate space with oncoming traffic. In the square in front of our hotel, we were accosted by a group of about twenty or thirty wild dogs, and the thought of rabies briefly crossed my mind. Everyone I met was wearing the national dress, partly due to a national policy requiring the people to do as much as they could to preserve their traditions. I did not see a single young person wearing jeans. In something of a contrast to this orthodox observation of formality, wherever I went in the town I noticed ornate paintings of penises flanking doorways and the outside walls of homes—I never got the chance to inquire into the background to this. We were now at an extremely high altitude: some members of the team started experiencing headaches, nausea, and shortness of breath. Every room in our hotel, we noticed, was equipped with emergency oxygen cylinders, so we assumed altitude sickness was quite a common occurrence.

The national hospital at Gidakom, built in 1966 originally as a leprosy hospital and until 1981 the main locus of elimination activities, is now a general hospital, one of three in the nation. Nearby is a small settlement for people affected by leprosy, with living space and workshops, which receives funding from the government. Here I met two married couples who were living under one roof, and who had set up a little handicraft business. They were the picture of serenity.

Bhutan began leprosy elimination in earnest in the 1960s. In 1962, the royal family invited TLM to Bhutan, after which the government and various NGOs joined forces to tackle the disease. Before that, people living with leprosy would just form small colonies where they lived out the rest of their days. The only way of getting proper treatment in those days was to trek over to West Bengal, in India, or to await visits from doctors in that country. Thanks to the effectiveness of MDT, which was introduced to Bhutan in 1982, the country achieved elimination in 1997. By 2003, the number of registered cases had dropped from 4,000 in 1966 to eighteen. Currently, about ten designated staff dealt specifically with leprosy, but government policy, as the goal shifted from elimination toward eradication, was now to integrate leprosy treatment into the general healthcare system. The challenge would be to sustain this success, and there was now an emphasis on awareness-raising activities to encourage the social rehabilitation of people affected by leprosy and quash any return of an increase in the numbers of new cases.

The driving force behind Bhutan's success was the powerful political commitment of King Jigme Singye Wangchuck and other members of the royal family. Their involvement in efforts toward leprosy control began in the 1950s. Bhutan at this time was ruled by the king as head of state with a national assembly, a cabinet, and a royal advisory council. (It later became a constitutional monarchy, with a constitution promulgated in 2008.) The king seemed to be ruling with the concerns of his people uppermost in his mind, and as a result he was a trusted leader.

Despite the country's success in achieving the WHO elimination targets, the situation in Bhutan was still fraught with problems. A high proportion of people seemed to be left with injuries or conditions due to late detection of the disease, which of course had to do with the unimaginable difficulties that people living in villages deep in the Himalayan Mountains had to go through simply to access the hospitals. In this kingdom, too, there was still the fear of stigma and what leprosy would mean to individuals and families. People affected by leprosy tended to be kept hidden, with the result that by the time they were discovered, the disease had already wrought its work.

With a national policy of free universal healthcare and education since 1961, and free healthcare services (including emergency services), Bhutan established hospitals and dispensaries throughout the kingdom to provide services to everyone regardless of their locality. Of note is the system of regional healthcare units ("basic health units") with a catchment of 45,000. However, in certain regions people still have to walk for a week to see a doctor. There were still only about 100 Bhutanese doctors, supplemented by thirty overseas doctors, so the resources and infrastructure are far from adequate. Recent diseases on the rise included heart disease, diabetes, high blood pressure, and a range of mental illnesses. Despite the urgent need for MRI and CT scans, the only way of getting tested was to travel to hospitals in India. There was also an extremely high maternity mortality rate.

Bhutan is a country where traditional medicine still holds considerable sway, and it is in fact officially protected by the constitution. The minister of health took me on a tour of the National Institute of Traditional Medicine. The institute collects various medicinal plants, as well as insects and minerals, from around the kingdom to produce pills and ointments and medicinal teas on site, which are then distributed to medical facilities around the country. Traditional medicine, including medicaments but also practices, is an integral part of the medical system and is offered alongside modern medicine: patients are offered the choice of which they prefer. Both are free. Some of the medications include ingredients that would fetch quite a bit of money if they were exported. Officials were considering further R&D and looking into the marketing aspects of some of these ingredients for exports in aromatherapy and cosmetics. I suggested looking into selling some of their ingredients for nutritional supplements, which would enable them to widen their export markets to places like Japan. Bhutan was awarded the Sasakawa Health Prize in 1997 for the success of one of its pilot projects for primary healthcare.

Bhutan has a national policy that the king once expressed as Gross National Happiness (GNH), which takes pride of place over what is generally used by nations as an indicator for their advancement, Gross National Product. Admittedly, GNH is something that is difficult to measure. But it stems from the belief that the collective happiness of the people involves more than material wealth and also includes preserving the country's traditions, the provision of public social services for the assistance of individuals and families in need, and the creation of an environment in which people have the best chance of finding happiness and wellbeing. GNH is based on a set of four basic tenets: equitable and sustainable economic development; conserving the fragile Himalayan environment essential to Bhutan's survival; preserving the best aspects of its culture while carefully choosing what to bring in from the outside; and carefully creating good governance, step by step working toward a constitutional democracy. As ministers explained to me, the hope is that the focus on GNH as an indicator leads to economic development with a human dimension, with a balance between the material and the spiritual. In a world where economic differences between segments of society seem only to be getting wider, I could only feel admiration for such a policy.

On my last night in Bhutan, I attended a party, held outside under the light of the moon, hosted by the ministers of finance and health. At one point in the evening, the ministers performed a traditional dance for us. Singing and dancing, they moved around in a circle to the music. It reminded me of the *bon-odori* dance that communities often perform in Obon summer festivals in Japan. In return, I sang the "Tanko-bushi," a song about coal mining often sung for people in *bon-odori*, and danced.

In Bhutan, everyone wears national dress, even when going about their daily lives. The houses too were all of traditional construction. To some, this might have seemed like a sign of backwardness. However, the truth is that people here were extremely proud of their way of life. Of course, even here TVs and mobile phones were starting to make an appearance, and I was pretty sure that some of the youngsters were going to start to want all the accouterments of modern living. Nevertheless, I could only hope that the people were going to stick by this idea of GNH. My visit this time brought home to me how important it is for a country to have political stability as a basis for economic growth, and how important it is for a people to feel assured that their government was working on their behalf. The same is true of leprosy elimination.

Two nations with vastly different experiences—Republic of Chile and Federative Republic of Brazil, June and July 2004

> Route: Narita, Japan → Los Angeles (flight time: 12h; 3h stopover) → Santiago, Chile (flight time: 11h)—three nights—Santiago → Bueno Aires, Argentina (flight time: 4h; 1h 30m stopover) → Brasília, Brazil (flight time: 5h 30m)—two nights—Brasília → Rio de Janeiro (flight time: 1h 30m)—one night—Rio de Janeiro → Brasília (flight time: 1h 30m)—one night—Brasília → São Paulo (flight time: 1h 30m)—one night—São Paulo → New York, United States (flight time: 9h 30m)—one night—New York → Narita (flight time: 14h)

In late June and early July, my travels took me to South America—to the two nations of Chile and Brazil. I flew from Narita to Santiago, the capital of Chile, via Los Angeles. The weather in Santiago was cool, ranging from 8 degrees to 15 degrees C, but the sun's rays were strong, making sunglasses a necessity.

These two nations have vastly different experiences of leprosy. In mainland Chile, there are almost no records of leprosy patients having existed. The only known cases were 4,000 kilometers away on Easter Island, better known for its monumental statues, or *moai*. Until fairly recently, there was a leprosy hospital on this territory and a small number of patients. Five years before our visit, a survey of the island's 3,000 inhabitants turned up three patients—of Polynesian extraction, leading officials to conclude that the disease had been brought in from neighboring countries. Apparently, leprosy was rarely found in the indigenous population. According to the Chilean dermatologist Juan Honeyman, the reasons for this included the temperate climate, Chile's distinctive topography—a long, narrow country bordered on

127

one side by the Pacific and on the other by the Andes, effectively turning it into an island—and an immunity built up through the BCG tuberculosis and other vaccination programs. I didn't find any of these reasons particularly convincing, still less the proposition that there was something about Chilean DNA that meant they were unaffected by the disease. For now, the reason Chile has had almost no cases of leprosy remains something of a mystery.

Brazil, on the other hand, is a leprosy-endemic country that, after India, has the highest number of registered cases in the world. In 2002, of the country's 5,500 municipalities, 3,521, or 60 percent, have registered leprosy cases, and the prevalence rate stands at 4.52 per 10,000 (roughly 80,000 registered cases in all). There is a particularly high incidence in the Amazon basin and other rural areas where access to healthcare is limited.

In the 1930s, a national crusade to control leprosy was initiated requiring the compulsory isolation of anyone affected by leprosy, even those with less advanced symptoms, in leprosaria. This was followed in 1949 by a policy that required children of parents with leprosy to be placed in orphanages, stripped of the liberty to ever see their parents again, in an effort to impede the ever-rising incidence of the disease. The measures were abolished in 1962 (though not every state followed through), but de facto the practice of requiring people affected with leprosy to live in isolation continued in a number of places until 1980.

The 1980s in Brazil saw an explosion of social movements fighting for democracy and human rights, and one organization that arose out of this was MORHAN. From the start, MORHAN made one of its aims to pressure the government to fulfill its social and public obligations with regard to the inhumane way people affected by leprosy had been treated in the past, which meant monetary compensation and a concerted effort at improvement in their care. Due to MORHAN's efforts, in 2007 President Luiz Inácio "Lula" da Silva signed a bill agreeing to provide monetary compensation to people affected by leprosy who had suffered compulsory segregation. While late, this was at least an acknowledgment of the appalling treatment people had been forced to suffer, and Brazil is one of the few countries in the world that has issued a formal apology and provided compensation to those affected.

At the time of my visit, President Lula had come to power the previous year, in 2003, with a revolutionary government and a raft of policies aimed at social reform and the eradication of unfair economic distribution. He was also keen to make progress with leprosy elimination activities, and immediately after taking office he visited leprosy sanatoria, the first time in nearly a century that a sitting head of state had done so. He expressed his shock that it had taken so long to solve the issues related to leprosy, and his strong determination to make up for lost time. In my face-to-face meeting with him, when I explained only fourteen months were left till the WHO deadline, and that much more effort was necessary, he left me in no doubt that he understood how far behind Brazil had fallen in its measures to deal with the hardships people with leprosy still have to endure and immediately announced a stepping-up of activities.

During my visit, I discovered from talking with many of the program coordinators that leprosy elimination activities in the previous administration had made almost no progress. Officials frankly admitted that health ministry figures published between 1998 and 2003, showing the prevalence rate unchanged, were flawed—not collected according to international guidelines. If the statistics published by the government fail to reflect reality, this posed a real obstacle to implementing an effective elimination strategy. The new administration had recognized this and carried out a root-and-branch reform of the personnel, involving the replacement of about thirty leprosy specialists who had occupied their posts for twenty-two years and done nothing. "We were asleep," a senior health ministry official admitted. Under President Lula and the new health minister, however, a new strategy seemed to be taking shape. Elimination at the national level was targeted for 2005 and at the municipal level for 2010, and there was reason for optimism.

In contrast, the work accomplished by the NGOs and volunteers during that time was nothing short of remarkable. Most notable among these was MORHAN. Established in 1981 by a group led by Franciso Nunes, a leprosy-affected advocate known affectionately as "Bacurau" ("Nighthawk"), MORHAN had around 100 offices all over the nation and with the support of the Nippon Foundation had set up a nationwide toll-free leprosy helpline called Telehansen, which received roughly 10,000 calls a year, 47 percent of which were inquiries about how to diagnose leprosy or how to get hold of MDT blister packs. Health centers in Brazil's outlying regions only rarely had resident doctors, and people were forced to rely on routine visits. As a result, even when patients appeared at such centers, all too often they could not be diagnosed or treated because no doctor was on hand. Hence the reason for the huge number of such inquiries on the helpline. The calls not only concerned diagnosis and treatment; people also wanted to talk about the stigma and discrimination they were forced to endure. One person called in asking what to do about his son, who had developed leprosy for a second time due to inadequate care by a clinic, and who'd had his government support unfairly withdrawn. Another person called in with a story about her mother-in-law who wanted to strip her of her parental rights since she now had leprosy. Often people would call in apparently on behalf of a friend or a distant acquaintance, and then once they discovered the confidentiality of Telehansen admitted that they were really the person who needed help and consultation.

MORHAN now wields considerable influence over government policy toward leprosy and was able to pressure the authorities to fulfill their obligations with regard to the treatment of leprosy. It played a crucial role in replacing the thirty incompetent government officials mentioned earlier.

Another interesting aspect of MORHAN is the way well-known celebrities—singers and actors—work with it, spending time with people affected by leprosy and their families and taking part in nationwide leprosy elimination campaigns. I met two of these people on my visit. Actress Elke Maravilha had been meeting with residents of hospital colonies for fifteen years. Born in the Soviet Union to a Russian father and a German mother, and with a Mongolian grandmother and Azerbaijanian grandfather, Elke went to Brazil right after the Second World War. Never forgetting the hardships she experienced early on in life, Elke now made a practice of visiting individuals with leprosy in hospital, as well as prison inmates and prostitutes, sharing their pain and encouraging them to have hope for the future—and they for their part looked up to her like a godmother. "My former husband asked me if I kissed leprosy patients," the actress told me. "I said 'Yes' and suddenly he decided that he didn't like me. So I divorced him." She said this with a laugh. Ney Matogrosso, one of Brazil's most popular singers, is another celebrity who has been lending his energy to revitalizing the nationwide leprosy campaigns via TV and other media.

The women who play key roles—Republic of India (Bihar state), August 2004

> Route: Narita → Singapore (flight time: 6h 30m; 1h 20m stopover) → New Delhi, India (flight time: 6h)—one night—New Delhi → Patna city, Bihar state (flight time: 2h 30m)—three nights—Patna → New Delhi (flight time: 2h 30m; 4h stopover) → Narita (flight time: 7h 30m)

At the end of August, I visited northeast India—more specifically, the state of Bihar. It was my second visit to this populous state, one of several in India where much work remained to be done if the country was to reach the WHO-defined target of leprosy elimination by 2005. I had recently decided to focus my main attention on eight states in particular: Uttar Pradesh, Uttarakhand, Madhya Pradesh, Chhattisgarh, Jharkhand, Odisha, West Bengal, and Bihar. My first visit had been in December 2002: at that time, the prevalence rate was eleven per 10,000 population. Now, according to the health ministry, it was down to 4.97. The downward trend was encouraging, but Bihar still had 17 percent of the total number of people with leprosy in the entire nation.

In Patna, the capital, I attended two meetings. The first was a workshop to discuss the role of medical professionals, the media, and NGOs in leprosy elimination. The second was a symposium on education and information campaigns, specifically on how to achieve the participation of non-leprosy-related NGOs and other organizations.

Dr. S. D. Gokhale, chairman of the ILU, had organized the workshop. The ILU is an organization headquartered in Pune that was carrying out vigorous awareness-raising activities nationwide on behalf of people with leprosy. I had made a point of participating in all its workshops and symposiums and becoming acquainted with its leaders and members. The aim of the workshop was to explore ways to enable people who once had leprosy but had been treated and fully recovered to lead education and awareness activities. This is by far

131

the best way to neutralize misconceptions and inspire people to come forward for treatment. This workshop was held over three days, looking first at the state and then the district level. On the first day, which was chaired by Dr. P. K. Gopal, president of IDEA India, about thirty people with lived experience of the disease each gave a self-introduction and told us about their aspirations. They included a young MBA student, a housewife, a construction worker, a barber, a stationer, a shopkeeper, a milk-seller, a bicycle repair man, a computer technician, and a preacher. The student announced that after getting his degree he wanted to marry and work in a corporation. The preacher related how he incorporated information about leprosy into his sermons.

The second meeting, a symposium on the role of social organizations in awareness building, was attended by about sixty representatives of companies, banks, industry organizations, and NGOs. Representing the Bihar government was Health Commissioner Dr. A. K. Choudhary; attending from WHO were Dr. S. J. Habayeb and Dr. Derek Lobo (of the Southeast Asia Regional Office); and from the government of India Dr. G. P. S. Dhillon, deputy director general (leprosy). Dr. Lobo made the case for moving beyond the current situation of finding jobs for people affected by leprosy within the leprosy-affected community and argued that it was important instead to help them find jobs in the outside world.

While in Patna, I also gave a speech at Patna Women's College. This college, built in 1940, was the first institution for higher education specifically for women and has about 3,000 students. It is my belief that young women hold the key to raising awareness of leprosy in households. I told my audience of 500 students that leprosy wasn't just a medical disease but a social problem with a long history of humans discriminating against their fellow humans. Each student, I said, should consider leprosy elimination and the restoration of the human rights of those affected by the disease as a problem that they had the power to resolve. I urged them to put Bihar at the head of the movement to eliminate leprosy from India. The students all listened attentively to what was probably the first talk about leprosy they had ever heard. When I told them that leprosy was curable, and that discrimination had no place in the world, they all gave that special Indian head wobble that signifies vigorous agreement.

For the second half of my stay, I visited Patna district. My first call was at the Masaurhi primary health center, which serves a population of 200,000. Under it are two more health centers and twenty-six sub-centers. Health workers and community health workers (known as Anganwadi workers) who discover new patients bring them to the primary health center. Each sub-center sees about ten to fifteen new patients a week. Thanks to early diagnosis and prompt commencement of treatment, there were hardly any cases of lasting disability.

Next, I went by car to Gaya to visit the regional hospital. This journey, however, was far from easy due to the horrendous traffic conditions—something India is famous for. On the roads, I saw trucks, automobiles, carts, and bicycles heading in both directions on the same part of the road, with much tooting of horns. The situation was not helped by cows, sacred animals in India, wandering slowly anywhere they liked through the mêlée. From time to time, we would find ourselves stuck behind a huge truck that was lumbering along, but it was useless to overtake because oncoming traffic would not give way and would come straight toward us. Every time we overtook a vehicle, I felt as if I was putting my life on the line. At the regional hospital in Gaya, I met the district magistrate, the head of the hospital, and about thirty front-line health personnel. There are about twenty-one sub-centers and a total of ninety-five leprosy patients registered. Here, too, thanks to early diagnosis and the effective treatment offered by MDT, I was told there were no cases of lasting disability. (Of course, the wish to present the situation in the best possible light is the same the world over, and I was aware I should not discount the possibility that things were not quite so wonderful as they might seem.)

I concluded my stay in Bihar by calling on Chief Minister Rabri Devi and her husband Lalu Prasad, the former chief minister and now Union railway minister, at their home. This was my second visit to this couple.

When I arrived, officials were already seated on chairs arranged in the garden, waiting for me. I asked whether the large-scale gathering of 200,000 people that had been talked of the last time I visited had materialized. Lalu Prasad now proposed having two gatherings in Bihar state, one of people currently receiving treatment for leprosy and the other of those who had received treatment and recovered. Each gathering would involve several tens of thousands of people, with the purpose of considering ways to work for leprosy elimination and for the social rehabilitation of people affected by leprosy. This would be the start of a movement, he said, that would radiate out from Bihar state to the entire nation. It was proposed that a meeting on awareness and education with people affected by leprosy from Bihar state should be held on 2 October, Gandhi's birthday. I immediately said I would be sure to attend, even if that meant not being able to attend any scheduled international meetings. Unfortunately, however, these mass meetings ended up having to be abandoned for logistical reasons. This was a pity, as such monumentally large events might have been inspiring for the rest of the nation.

That autumn, I had to go to Russia and the People's Republic of China. In Russia, I attended a luncheon and the dedication ceremony for *The Diaries* of Father Nicolas, archbishop of Japan, with Alexy II, the patriarch of the Russian Orthodox Church. In the People's Republic of China, I attended a symposium held in Beijing by the United Nations Environmental Programme (UNEP) in collaboration with the State Environmental Protection Administration of China to commemorate the twentieth anniversary of the UNEP Sasakawa Environment Prize.

After that, I took another trip to India.

Visits to several leprosaria in Goa—Republic of India, September 2004

Route: Beijing → Singapore (flight time: 6h; 4h stopover) → New Delhi (flight time: 5h 30m)—one night—New Delhi → Panaji, Goa (flight time: 2h)—three nights—Panaji → Mumbai, Maharashtra (flight time: 1h; 7h stopover) → Singapore (flight time: 6h; 1h 20m stopover) → Narita (flight time: 7h)

At the end of September, after my visit to China, I traveled to the Indian state of Goa to attend a two-day India Health Secretaries Meeting for Leprosy Elimination sponsored by WHO. The discussion centered on how to achieve elimination by the end of 2005, and the meeting was attended by officials from eleven out of fifteen high endemic regions.

The occasion was significant because of the high level of the Indian government representatives attending—including Secretary of Health J. V. R. Prasada Rao from the Ministry of Health and Family Welfare. With just over a year to go before the elimination deadline, it was important to have these top officials convey the government's determination in front of the representatives of the endemic states and for government and state officials to spend time together, learn about the different strategies each has chosen to follow for reference, and affirm their common resolve.

While in Goa, I visited two teenage boys currently being treated with MDT. One was diagnosed early because his mother had knowledge of leprosy symptoms and had him checked when she discovered a white patch on his skin so that treatment started forthwith. Later, apparently, his cousin was also found to have leprosy. One boy didn't mind receiving MDT treatment, but the other was reluctant, fearful that it would make his skin turn dark. I assured him that any discoloration would only be temporary and encouraged him to take his MDT like his cousin. The conversation brought home to me how important

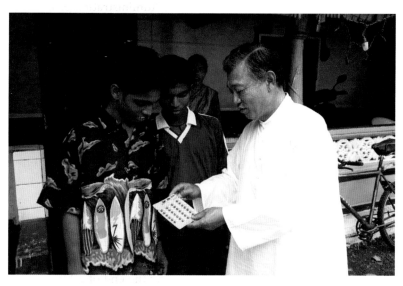

25. Explaining MDT to a young man affected by leprosy (Goa, India, September 2004)

it is to explain everything about the treatment, including the possibilities for leprosy reactions, to people affected by the condition.

I also visited the Goa Central Leprosarium. According to Dr. Froilano de Mello, it was built in 1934 when Goa was a Portuguese colony. Located on high ground in some 60 acres amid coconut palms, jackfruit and mango trees, it is a beautiful place. At one time, it had as many as 280 occupants but today has only eighteen—eleven women and seven men. Their average age was between seventy and eighty. The leprosarium had stopped accepting patients two years before, and there was talk of turning the complex into a hospital for HIV/AIDS or other diseases. The wards appeared spick and span and were run by a staff of seven nurses. The residents all wore uniforms and engaged in a variety of pursuits including electrical repairs, carpentry, and painting. Though every attempt was made to present the facility as a place of peace and comfort, I could not help but see in the expressions in their faces sadness in their isolated existence. One elderly lady told me she had been living there since the age of twelve. In such beautiful surroundings, it was painful to encounter people who had long recovered from the illness but were still required to live separated from society, and I felt even more resolve to end the discrimination that necessitated this state of affairs.

In October that year, I visited Sweden (World Maritime University in Malmö) and then in November the Republic of China (Shanghai Maritime University- and Sasakawa Japan–China Friendship Fund-supported visit of Self-Defense Forces China).

Discussions on post-elimination strategy—Republic of the Philippines, December 2004

> Route: Narita, Japan → Fukuoka (Asian Public Intellectuals fellowships workshop) → Taipei, Taiwan (flight time: 2h 30m; 1h 30m stopover) → Manila (flight time: 2h)—two nights

My last trip in 2004 was to the Philippines. The country had met the WHO-defined target in 1998, but according to reports dating from 2018, rates were once again rising. (Figures for 2018 show 2,178 newly diagnosed persons with leprosy, making the Philippines the second highest country in Southeast Asia after Indonesia.)

REACHING THE UNREACHABLE

The Philippines is home to the largest leprosy settlement in the world, Culion Island, which at one time housed as many as 7,000 people affected by leprosy. Culion also had a major impact on the policies toward leprosy adopted by other countries all over the world. It is situated in the north of the Philippines' Palawan province, around 320 kilometers southwest of the country's main island Luzon. It has a population of around 20,000 people.

The first contingent of leprosy patients, 370 in all, were brought to Culion from Cebu Island on 27 May 1906, under the direction of a Board of Health established by the US authorities (the Philippines was then an American dependency), and they were put in the care of a handful of medical staff, a Jesuit priest, and four French sisters of the Order of St. Paul of Chartres. The number of inhabitants grew steadily at a pace of between 500 and 1,500 patients per year, brought from all regions of the country. With staff and pharmaceuticals in short supply, records indicate that up to 1,221 residents died at Culion Island every year from malaria and other diseases. The island became feared by Filipinos as an island of despair—a land of the living dead. Eventually, the mortality rate declined, and after 1910 inmates were allowed to marry, with childcare facilities created in 1916. After the country gained its independence in 1946, the leprosarium came under the aegis of the new nation's health ministry. It wasn't until 1995 that the history of the Culion leprosarium finally drew to a close. The island was granted regional autonomy.

During my visit, I attended a bi-regional meeting in Manila for WHO's Southeast Asia Regional Office and Western Pacific Regional Office on post-elimination strategies in Southeast Asia and the Western Pacific. It was the typhoon season, and during my stay we were visited by a typhoon that was so strong that the schools had to be closed to brace for the storm. My face-to-face talk with President Gloria Macapagal Arroyo had to be cancelled as she was too busy presiding over the relief efforts. Fortunately, however, the bi-regional meeting with WHO officials was able to go ahead as scheduled.

In my talk, I made a strong argument for sustained vigilance toward leprosy even after elimination and the importance of combining medical treatment with neutralizing the psychosocial aspects of the disease—the stigma and discrimination that blight people's lives even after full recovery. The focus of the conference was on building systems for monitoring, integrating treatment of leprosy into the general health services, and ensuring early detection and treatment.

Transforming personal ambition into selfless service—Republic of India (Madhya Pradesh state and Andhra Pradesh state), December 2004

> Route: Manila, the Philippines → Bangkok, Thailand (flight time: 3h; 1h 20m stopover) → Delhi, India (flight time: 4h 30m)—one night—Delhi → Bhopal, Madhya Pradesh (flight time: 3h)—two nights—Bhopal → Mumbai (flight time: 2h; one-night stopover) → Hyderabad, Andhra Pradesh (flight time: 1h 10m)—two nights—Hyderabad → Delhi (flight time: 2h) → Narita (flight time: 8h)

After Manila, I went straight to India, where I visited the states of Madhya Pradesh and Andhra Pradesh. Both states were working slowly toward the elimination goal. As of October 2004, Madhya Pradesh had a prevalence rate of 1.28 per 10,000, and Andhra Pradesh 1.73 per 10,000. Elimination was close. I had recently been visiting India repeatedly. Of all the countries that have yet to achieve elimination, India has the most cases (266,000 at the end of March 2004).

I landed first in New Delhi, and early the next morning the team boarded a light propeller aircraft departing at 5 a.m. to go to Bhopal, the capital of Madhya Pradesh. (This involved getting up at 3 a.m.) Once we were all aboard, I happened to glance out of the window and saw our baggage left lying on the runway! Quickly, one of my team went to inquire, to be told that the bags exceeded the weight restrictions and would have to be left behind. There was nothing we could do about it. We took off with only one of our ten pieces of baggage. We soon realized we were among the lucky ones: some passengers got turfed off the plane—due to overbooking. Such occurrences are par for the course if you travel as much as I do. I take them all in my stride.

Madhya Pradesh is right in the center of India ("Madhya" is the Sanskrit word for "middle"), and territorially it is one of the largest states in India. Bhopal was once an Islamic principality, and it has 200 mosques, including one said to be the largest in the country. One of the reasons we were visiting this state was to see an example of the so-called "Care and Concern Camps" that take place here from time to time. At these camps, usually held in the open air, people affected by leprosy gather to participate in open-air activities designed to offer a holistic healing approach.

As soon as we got to Bhopal, we went to a small village called Sanchi, 50 kilometers northeast of the city, famous for its Buddhist stupas and other monuments dating from the third century BCE. Here, amid blaring horns of traffic and crowded streets, with due care given not to get in the way of the freely wandering sacred cows, was one such Care and Concern Camp. About fifty people who had recovered from leprosy from the neighboring villages were participating in group activities over a five-day period under the guidance of health workers in marquees erected in front of the local school. Some were washing people's feet in wooden basins, while others were doing simple stretching exercises in groups. Still others were binding the wounds of their companions. The school classrooms had been made over into dormitories for the participants' use. Such camps were apparently excellent at cutting through people's shyness and lack of confidence. On the first day, they were all quite stiff and unfriendly, but on the last they were all shedding tears as they bid each other farewell. I washed the dirty, scarred feet of several of the participants, who smiled at me gratefully to convey their appreciation. (Their feet were pretty filthy.) People from the community— schoolchildren and residents—were encouraged to take part, the idea being to rid them of any misconceptions of risk in contact with people who had recovered from the disease. Within a day or two, schoolchildren who had been looking on with suspicion and hanging back were happily taking part in the activities.

Of all the people I met on this visit, I shall not forget Mr. Malak Singh Shrivastav. A fifty-six-year-old farmer from the village of Malah Pipariya, Narsinghpur district, he had been diagnosed with leprosy two years before. In his region, leprosy symptoms were traditionally seen as one variety of skin disease (leukoderma; vitiligo) and referred to as "kod," which in the *Mahabharata*, one of the two major Sanskrit epics of ancient India, is described as arising out of the curse of a god on a warrior for killing his son. The warrior had to live a life full of sorrows and miseries. At first, Mr. Shrivastav

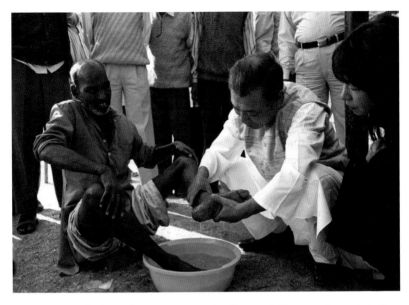

26. Washing the feet of participants in the Care and Concern Camp (Madhya Pradesh, India, December 2004)

assumed that his disease would result in him being cast out of his community. For two days after being diagnosed, he told me, he couldn't eat and began to think about killing himself. He told a close friend, and as soon as his family and fellow villagers got to hear of it, they watched over him twenty-four hours a day for over two weeks to ensure he didn't follow through on his plan. His wife meanwhile visited the regional leprosy officer, who assured her that the disease was easily treatable, that medicine was available at the primary health center, there was no need for him to be segregated, and he would most definitely not be cast out. She went back to her husband and told him this. He began receiving treatment and ended up being completely cured.

As a result of his experiences, Mr. Shrivastav was moved to fund a Care and Concern Camp in his district. Since 2003, he has organized three such camps from his own home, at which those who have lost feeling in their hands and feet receive treatment for injuries and are given a warm welcome by the local community. He also made regular appearances before the media to tell his story.

Looking at Mr. Shrivastav, now working with all his heart to encourage others with the example of his own success, I felt truly humbled. I have always believed that the most effective way to rid society of the stigma and prejudice associated with leprosy is for people affected by leprosy to take a central role. Every word uttered by a person who has been treated and is now recovered has ten times the weight of anything I might say. I was reminded of some famous words of Mahatma Gandhi: "Leprosy work is not merely medical relief, it is transforming the frustration in life into the joy of dedication, [and] personal ambition into selfless service."

We then moved on to Hyderabad, on the outskirts of Andhra Pradesh in central southern India. Here, I visited the Uppal Public Health Center in Ranga Reddy district, where I met about twenty people with leprosy and some forty student nurses from the Yashoda School of Nursing and the Kamineni School of Nursing. As the student nurses and Public Health Center workers looked on, I handed out MDT to the twenty or so people affected by leprosy and told them how to take the medication. Most of these individuals had little or no experience of taking pills: they had quite a bit of difficulty swallowing the medicine, even though they placed the pills right in the back of their throat. I asked the student nurses to remember what they had learned this day whenever they encountered people with leprosy in future.

I also visited the Sivananda Rehabilitation Home, also in Ranga Reddy district. It was established in 1958. At present, it is home to some 500 people affected by leprosy, men and women, including some with families. The facility has a hospital for basic reconstructive surgery and workshops for spinning and weaving. Most of the residents seemed to be in their seventies, with one person who was eighty. The sight of them all spinning away in the workshops made me think of Mahatma Gandhi. I thought of the difficult lives all these people must have led in one way or another, and I was thankful that at least now in their old age, they were living a life where they were secure and safe.

Countries visited in 2005	
January	● India
	● South Africa
February	● Madagascar
	● Brazil
March	● India
	● Cambodia
April	● Mozambique
	● Tanzania
May	● India
	Switzerland (World Health Assembly)
June	China (Japan–China Military Exchange Program)
	United Kingdom (International Maritime Organization visit)
August	Norway (Scandinavia–Japan Sasakawa Foundation board meeting)
	Switzerland (UN Commission on Human Rights)
	● DRC
September	● South Timor
	● India
October	● Czech Republic (Forum 2000)
	China (Sasakawa Japan–China Friendship Fund meeting)
	● India
	United Kingdom (Sasakawa Africa Association board meeting)
November	China (Book dedication ceremony)
	● Malaysia

December	● Indonesia
	● India
	India (Leprosy symposium)
	● Myanmar (Meeting with Ministry of Border Affairs and people affected by leprosy)

● Indicates a trip that features in this section.

Forum 2000: An annual international conference launched after a meeting in 1997 when Václav Havel, Nobel Peace Prize laureate, Holocaust survivor Elie Wiesel, and the author invited world leaders to Prague for open debate on the major issues and challenges of the new millennium.

The power of magic shows—Republic of India (New Delhi), January 2005

Route: Narita, Japan → Bangkok, Thailand (flight time: 6h 30m; 1h 30m stopover) → New Delhi (flight time: 4h 30m)—three nights

Toward the end of January, I was in Delhi to attend a one-day conference on leprosy elimination organized by the chairman of the ILU, Dr. S. D. Gokhale. This conference was designed to forge a sense of solidarity and encourage people affected by leprosy to join our efforts. It was held with the support of the ILU, IDEA, WHO, and related NGOs. The timing and location of the 27 January conference had special significance. January 30 marks the anniversary of Gandhi's assassination. Given Gandhi's long-cherished wish to see leprosy eliminated from India, leprosy-related events often take place around this time of year. It is also commemorated in India as Anti-Leprosy Day. The conference venue was the garden of Gandhi Smriti, a museum dedicated to Gandhi, formerly Birla House, a large mansion in central New Delhi where Gandhi spent his last days, and indeed was assassinated in 1948. There is a well-known anecdote about Gandhi. Invited to formally open a leprosy hospital, he refused. He said he was looking forward to attending on the day that the hospital was closed, when there were no more people affected by leprosy.

Among those attending were the former president of India, Hon. Shri R. Venkataraman; WHO representative to India Dr. S. J. Habayeb;

ILA President Dr. S K. Noordeen; K. D. Gangred, director of the National Gandhi Museum; and the psychologist and actor Dr. Mohan Agashe. Each of these people addressed those attending with words of encouragement and their own declarations of resolve.

The most important achievement of this conference was that we managed to secure the participation and collaboration of people affected by leprosy from all over India. Of the roughly 200 people in attendance, 134 had been treated for leprosy and were now fully cured, from nine of India's states. In India, it still took a great deal of courage for anyone affected by the disease to come forward and declare themselves, but the large majority of these people had reintegrated themselves into society and were playing an active role in their respective fields. Of the 134 people, we selected thirty-two as "Lokdoots" or "special communicators," whose mission it would be to tell their fellow Indians the true facts about leprosy.

The prevalence rate in New Delhi was high: 3.92 at the time of my visit, which was worse than poor Indian states such as Tamil Nadu, Kerala, and Bihar. Migratory and floating populations from other states posed a particular challenge. Often, new cases would be discovered among migratory populations who had come in from the countryside and were living in slum areas, where all too often they escaped official notice. The lifestyles of these floating populations made it extremely difficult for health authorities to register and monitor them, but despite all these challenges, Delhi National Capital Territory Health Secretary S. P. Aggarwal assured me that New Delhi was committed to achieving elimination.

Before leaving New Delhi, I made a brief visit to the Flame of Fire Leprosy Center, a settlement hoping to initiate a rehabilitation program. It had been arranged for me to see a magic show, which was being used to communicate basic information about leprosy and how it could easily be cured. The skit involved a bag that represented a hospital, and a handkerchief with a polka-dot pattern on it, which represented a person affected by leprosy. The magician placed the handkerchief into the bag, along with some MDT, waited, and reaching into the bag, he somehow managed to pull out a handkerchief that was pure white. The message—that the person affected by leprosy had been cured—was unmistakable. The skit was easy to understand

and fun to watch. I thought it a perfect way to get our message across to people living away from the cities in hard-to-reach areas deep in the mountains. Such people often didn't speak Hindi and had little by way of entertainment. I was reminded of how songs and little skits have been found to be effective in Timor-Leste and Nepal.

A leprosy conference and the history of Robben Island—Republic of South Africa, January 2005

Route: New Delhi → London (flight time: 9h; 3h stopover) → Johannesburg, South Africa (flight time: 11h)—three nights— Johannesburg → Cape Town—two nights on Robben Island—Cape Town → Johannesburg—one night

From India, I traveled straight on to South Africa via London. South Africa was in fact the fourth country I visited in January, because before my trip to India I'd had a transit in Thailand.

South Africa is still associated with apartheid, the system of insti-tutionalized racial segregation that existed in the country from 1948 until the start of the last decade of the twentieth century and that drew on the centuries of racist colonial rule that preceded it. But the country is also now famous for the anti-apartheid activist Nelson Mandela, who became the country's first black head of state. Not many people know that Robben Island, where Mandela was impris-oned, was originally an island where people affected by leprosy were forced to live in isolation.

South Africa had met the leprosy elimination target defined by WHO at a country level, but here too, as in so many other countries, there was still prejudice toward people affected by leprosy, and little had been done to enable their social reintegration. Racism is still present in the country, making itself felt in various ways.

I had come to South Africa, hot-footing it from India, principally to attend a four-day conference, the African Leprosy Congress, held just outside Johannesburg from 31 January to 3 February, where I gave an address. This was a conference organized by ILA with the support of the South African government, WHO, ILEP, and others. The ILA, founded in 1931, is a professional society of physicians, scientists, and individuals and organizations in related areas working to understand and relieve the problems associated with leprosy. One of the major ways it does this is by holding congresses on leprosy at approximately five-year intervals. The last such congress, the six-teenth, had been held in Brazil in 2002. This one was the first to be held in Africa and would concentrate on specifically African leprosy issues. In a first for an ILA event of this kind, the opening day was to include a special session devoted to human rights.

South Africa's health minister Dr. Manto Tshabalala-Msimang began the congress with an opening address. In a smaller meeting immediately before the conference, she had announced publicly that for the six years she had been in office, she had not received a single report related to leprosy. She wondered whether the Health Ministry even had a leprosy policy. The prevalence rate in South Africa was presently 0.03 persons per 10,000 population, she explained, but stigma and prejudice remained huge problems, and the rehabilitation of people who had recovered from the disease was an issue that still needed to be tackled. Media involvement to spread awareness of such problems was essential, she said. She then asked who among the audience were from the media. When the answer came back that nobody from the media was there, she announced that she wouldn't allow the conference to start until some media representatives were present. The conference was delayed by an hour, but her admirable stance managed to get the conference excellent media coverage.

In my address, I said I believed this meeting was a truly momentous occasion in the long history of leprosy. For the first time, there was to be a session in an ILA congress devoted to the theme of leprosy and human rights. Of the 273 registered conference participants, twenty-nine were people affected by leprosy who were attending as part of a forty-strong delegation from IDEA. This showed that the conference would concern itself not only with the medical aspects of the disease but also with its social dimensions. In that sense, the congress acted as a clarion call for ending discrimination. Human rights were often discussed in the United Nations, I argued, but until I raised the matter of the human rights of people affected by leprosy, which I had done in March 2004 by presenting an oral statement at the sixtieth session of the UN Commission on Human Rights, the issue had been completely overlooked. In the session on human rights, a number of people affected by leprosy, including Dr. P. K. Gopal, chairman of IDEA, gave presentations on the difficult circumstances that characterize the lives of most people who have recovered from the disease.

During the conference, I had several private meetings with health officials coordinating programs in the six African countries yet to achieve elimination—Angola, Central African Republic, DRC, Madagascar, Mozambique, and Tanzania. Listening to the accounts each gave of their countries, it became apparent that in addition to operational factors common to many endemic countries such as the need to sort out issues of duplicate registration and misdiagnosis, in Africa there are often additional issues—such as regional conflict, refugees, and government corruption. Frankly, I was sure that the state of elimination efforts in each of their countries was worse than their reports were suggesting. I realized that I was going to have to make even more visits to those in power in these countries, to impress upon them in person just how important it was to keep the focus squarely on the goal of leprosy elimination.

On 2 February, I traveled to Cape Town and then took the ferry over to Robben Island. I could not believe how hot it was: the rays of the sun were so strong I could feel myself getting sunburned by the minute. This island, a mere 3.3 kilometers long and 1.9 kilometers wide, once had a maximum-security prison holding 100 or so people—convicted criminals and people who had committed the crime of political activism against the state-sanctioned system of apartheid. The man who eventually became the nation's first black president, Nelson Mandela, was held in solitary confinement here for eighteen years of his twenty-seven-year sentence, until the fall of apartheid and the introduction of full, multi-racial democracy. Visiting the cell in which Mandela was held, I lost myself for a few moments in deep thought. I would never be able to spend that much time in a cell. I lack the strength of will. I was overcome by the thoughts of how fortunate I was to be free. I told myself that I should make the best use possible of my freedom, and that I had to redouble my commitment and my efforts.

There is now a sizeable colony of penguins on this island, which makes for a strange sight. In 1997, the entire island became a museum, called the Robben Island Museum; and every year about 300,000 tourists come across for tours of the island and the prison, one of the sacred places of the anti-apartheid movement. In 1999, it was designated a UNESCO World Heritage Site.

Robben Island was fortified by early Dutch settlers and started being used as a prison in the seventeenth century. This was chiefly for the incarceration of political prisoners, but for a period of eighty-five years, from 1846 to 1931, the island was also used to isolate people with leprosy. The first group of inmates of the leprosy asylum, about sixty or so individuals, were originally living on the mainland, farming their own crops and keeping animals before being forcibly moved to Robben Island. This started a trend. In addition to people with leprosy, the island was also used to hold mental patients. In 1891, with the enactment of the Leprosy Suppression Act, hospitalization became compulsory and more than 800 inmates were brought here, and throughout that decade the number of residents was always more than 500. The residents were segregated not only by sex but also by race, and anyone who showed any sign of not sticking to such racial segregation was punished severely. Any protests against the system, too, would be punished by even stricter enforcement by the British Crown authorities. From 1921, fewer people with leprosy were sent to the island, and in 1931 the Robben Island Leprosy Asylum was closed down. The remaining 108 residents were sent to three other sanatoria on the mainland. The authorities on Robben Island, fearful of infection, destroyed all the buildings, leaving only the church. So while the prison used for prisoners of apartheid remains, the only trace of the history of leprosy on the island is this single church and a small graveyard.

One of the places that the Robben Island inmates were sent to was Westfort, just west of the capital, Pretoria. It opened in 1898 and was one of only two multiracial leprosaria in South Africa. I was shown around by Dr. Okkie Kruger, African director of TLM. In the nineteenth century, the capital city Pretoria had such "forts" placed at strategic positions on its environs, and it was at the west fort that the Westfort Leprosy Hospital was built, executed in a design consistent with that of the hospital on Robben Island. When it opened, Westfort housed 1,450 individuals, but by the early years of the twentieth century it was home to an average of 250 to 300 individuals. It was run like a small town and had a post office, clinic, churches, pharmacy, and shops. However, two guards were posted at the entrance, monitoring all those who came and went; and visits from family members were restricted to once every two weeks, with people affected by leprosy forced to sit behind a glass screen in a prison-like atmosphere when they received visits.

From 1948, under South Africa's apartheid system, patients who were already segregated from society by their disease were subject to further segregation within the hospital on the basis of their race. Inmates were divided into three racial groups—whites, blacks, and "coloreds" (people from the Indian continent and Southeast Asia)— who had separate wards, giving a special character to the leprosy experience in South Africa. The law requiring hospitalization for leprosy treatment remained in effect in South Africa until the 1980s, though a certain loosening of restrictions did start to make an appear-

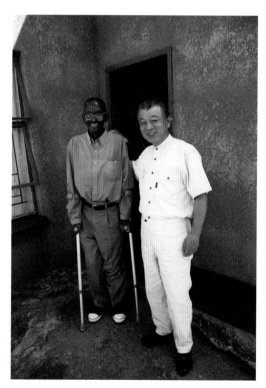

27. The author with Johann, a person affected by leprosy who now lives in the suburbs of Johannesburg (South Africa, February 2005)

ance in the 1970s. After this, specialized institutions for leprosy began to shut down. In the 1990s, only forty or so inmates remained in hospital, and these soon dwindled to fewer than twenty. Westfort was the last of the leprosy hospitals to close, in 1998, thus also bringing to an end the policy of segregating people with leprosy.

Now all that is left of the Westfort Leprosy Hospital compound is rows of small houses lived in by the inmates, the clinic, the church, and a block of offices. TLM was making plans to have the compound designated as a site of historical interest, especially bearing in mind the sites of indigenous peoples that lay dotted about the place. Dr. Kruger told me, however, that the plans were somewhat stymied: the government didn't seem to be interested, and they were having difficulty getting the funding.

After Westfort, I dropped in on the house of a man called Johann, a fifty-five-year-old who had recovered from leprosy and who was living with his wife, daughter, and two granddaughters in a neat little brick house in the suburbs of Johannesburg. He welcomed me into his home and told me a little of his story. Before being sent to Westfort after being diagnosed with leprosy, he was a steel worker. Unfortunately, his MDT treatment was interrupted, leaving him with permanent sight impairment and disability in his limbs. Without regular work, he received a disability allowance from the South African government, equivalent to 15,000 yen (about US$115) a month. His wife, who had waited patiently for him while he was hospitalized at Westfort, managing the family on her own, talked lovingly about her husband. Although he had the support of his wife and family, he had no contact with his neighbors, and on his monthly visits to hospital for a check-up, he was seen separately from other patients. Troublingly, Johann told me he felt he had no place in society, and that sometimes he wondered whether he was better off back in Westfort. The family seemed happy despite everything, but I could tell that Johann had a deeply internalized sense of isolation.

Huge achievements and unresolved issues—Republic of Madagascar, February 2005

Route: Johannesburg, South Africa → Antananarivo, Madagascar (flight time: 3h)—one night—Antananarivo → Toliara (formerly

Tuléar) (flight time: 1h)—one night—Toliara → Antananarivo (flight time: 1h)—one night—Antananarivo → Mananjary (flight time: 1h)—one night—Mananjary → Farafangana → Antananarivo (flight time: 2h; 7h stopover) → Paris (flight time: 10h; 3h stopover) → Narita (flight time: 12h)

From South Africa, I proceeded directly to Madagascar. It was now February. My route took me from Cape Town via Johannesburg and thence to Antananarivo, Madagascar's capital. The last time I had been here was in September 2003, and I wanted to visit to see for myself what changes had occurred and to express my encouragement to people involved in the anti-leprosy activities. In September 2003, the prevalence rate stood at four persons per 10,000 population. In 2004, it had come down to 2.93. The terrain of this country presented some severe logistical challenges to leprosy control: during the cyclone season, heavy rains can cut off communities, many roads and bridges in the country were in a very poor state of repair, and more than 60 percent of the land is difficult to access.

In Madagascar, I attended a World Leprosy Day event held in Toliara, a city situated in the southwest of the country. The temperature was much hotter here than Antananarivo, well over 35 degrees C, and the sun was exceedingly bright. Held in a carnival-like atmosphere, the day-long event included music, dance, puppetry, and film, all of which constituted an excellent platform from which to deliver important messages about the disease. Both the prime minister and the health minister of the country were present at the event.

After Toliara, I visited three towns on the southeast coast of the island, Mananjary, Manakara, and Farafangana, all with high prevalence rates, where I met with health workers and visited local hospitals and health facilities. Basic health centers are at the frontline of the health care system, and each sees to an average of 5,000 to 6,000 people. All told, there are around 2,500 such centers in the country, and the people who work there play a vital role in educating communities and spotting new cases and ensuring follow-up treatment. In this country, unlike India, the system for health visits by mobile peripheral health workers to conduct skin checks did not seem to be systematized. In certain rural areas where people with leprosy are still treated like outcasts, they still often self-segregate at home: when visits from medical staff were not possible, this meant that people with leprosy were left undiagnosed and untreated. The work of peripheral health workers is absolutely vital to leprosy elimination, and the key to improvement lies in a system that supports them and pays them well.

Unfortunately, I also found that not every health center kept strict records of patients—or, for that matter, good stocks of MDT blister packs. In certain remote health centers, they didn't even seem to know the state of their inventory, nor indeed how much they had distributed to various areas. There seemed to be no rhyme or reason to the set-up. In some places, MDT wasn't getting from the regional hospital to the basic health center, while in others there was a surplus. Getting the distribution of blister packs right is essential to the elimination strategy, and I realized that I had to convey this to the prime minister and the health minister and encourage them to spearhead efforts for improvement.

Wherever I travel, I like to talk with as many people affected by leprosy as I can, and this time I was able to chat directly with people at several locations, including the Marovhay Leprosy and Tuberculosis Center in Toliara, the Ambatoabo Community Leprosy and Tuberculosis Center, and the St. Vincent Hospital in Farafangana. All of these hospitals had wards devoted to leprosy patients. Now, however, people with leprosy tend not to be hospitalized (except for the most severe cases) but rather come in as outpatients, basically to collect their medicine. Nevertheless, as I spoke with them, I was struck by their solemn expressions. Their weary, sad demeanor told me right away that they had been through a lot of sadness and struggle. I surmised that they had yet to be cured emotionally and mentally. As always, I felt very sad for them, but at the same time I became ever more determined to do something about their plight.

Malaria is another disease that is endemic in Madagascar, and I was quite apprehensive that the screens in the windows of the places where I stayed were full of holes, with the mosquitoes flying in and out at will—despite attempts to bung the holes up with newspaper. All I could do was plaster myself with anti-mosquito cream and go to bed with mosquito-repellent coils placed all around my bed. As for food, I always like to eat the local fare—this is an essential way of finding out about the culture. In Johannesburg, I enjoyed South African wine, which was cheap and delicious. In Madagascar, it was the foie gras, or stuffed goose liver. The foie gras in Madagascar struck me as markedly heftier than that I had tried in France. Here it was so big, indeed, that it could be eaten as an entrée, whereas in France it is eaten as an appetizer. I remember one time in Tanzania I saw an enormous caterpillar in my salad, and thinking it might be a local delicacy, I was quite alarmed. I am not at all fussy about my food, and I like to think that I can happily eat food from any country around the world. Quite often the food has been prepared or stored in unhygienic conditions, especially in places that are off the beaten track. Nevertheless, in all the years I have been coming here for my

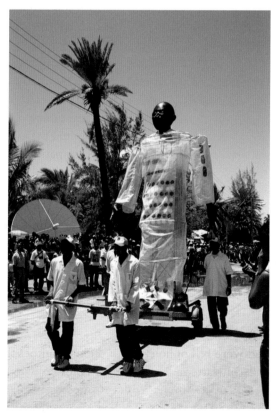

28. A World Leprosy Day event (Madagascar, February 2005)

work, never once have I had to endure an upset stomach. I have very fond memories of the time when I was traveling from India to Chernobyl in the old Soviet Union in order to help out after the nuclear reactor disaster there and had to survive for eleven days on nothing but soup.

Motorcycle Diaries and a conference in Rio de Janeiro—Federative Republic of Brazil, February 2005

> Route: Narita, Japan → Frankfurt (flight time: 12h; 2h 40m stopover) → Rio de Janeiro, Brazil (flight time: 11h 40m)—two nights—Rio de Janeiro → New York (flight time: 9h 30m; 5h stopover) → Narita (flight time: 12h 45m)

After a short time in Tokyo, it wasn't long before I was off again, this time to Rio de Janeiro, Brazil, for a conference the Nippon Foundation was holding there on human rights and leprosy. The trip first involved going to Frankfurt and then straight on to Rio, in effect spending two nights on the plane. On my arrival, I went straight to the venue, where I attended the conference and the dinner, by which time it was close to midnight. It was well after 1 a.m. that I finally got to bed—sleeping in between sheets for the first time in four days.

When I travel by air, I tend to spend the hours reading or sleeping rather than watching inflight movies. I have never worked out how to manage the seat-back video equipment. (I also don't wear a wristwatch, and I don't have a driving license. Nor do I have a smartphone. I don't watch TV. I'm also terrible at shopping. What a hopelessly impractical fellow I am!) But on this flight, the Nippon Foundation's official photographer Natsuko Tominaga twiddled the right buttons and kindly enabled me to watch a movie—the 2004 *Motorcycle Diaries*. This is a movie based on the memoir of the trip across South America taken in 1952 by the Argentina-born Ernesto "Che" Guevara with his friend Alberto Granado. During the trip, the motorcycle broke down, and the two of them had to hitch rides from Argentina through Chile, Peru, and Colombia to Venezuela. Remarkably, the purpose of the journey for these two men, both medical students, was to spend time at the leprosy settlements they would encounter along the way. They stopped off at a number of leprosy settlements and sometimes stayed a few nights, observing the inhabitants and listening to their stories. At the end of the trip, Alberto decided to stay on in a leprosy settlement in Caracas, while Guevara returned to Argentina and graduated from medical school. Though his intention was to re-join Alberto, in the end, as we know, he became involved in a revolutionary movement. It was this movie that gave me the idea of using a motorbike as a metaphor for how we should approach leprosy elimination. It became one of my stock explanations:

> If you want to ride a motorbike, you have to have two wheels. A front wheel and a back wheel. The front wheel is tackling the disease from a medical point of view. The back wheel is destigmatizing the disease. Both wheels have to be moving forward at the same pace, or we make no progress.

In August 2004 in the fifty-sixth session of the UN Sub-Commission for the Promotion and Protection of Human Rights, members had agreed to look at discrimination against people affected by leprosy, and Professor Yozo Yokota, then a professor of international law at Chuo University, Tokyo, and member for Japan of the UN Sub-Commission, had been appointed as a Special Rapporteur to look into this issue. Professor Yokota was due to present his findings at the Sub-Commission's fifty-seventh session in August 2005. This conference in Brazil had been arranged by the Nippon Foundation in order to provide Professor Yokota and other members of the Sub-Commission with the opportunity to conduct interviews and to help him prepare his report. He would be able to hear directly from people affected by leprosy and to visit leprosy settlements and hospitals and find out what people needed. Professor Yokota had attended the African Leprosy Congress held in January, where he collected the testimonies of people affected by leprosy. He was planning to present some of his materials at a conference due to be held in India and collect testimonies and conduct fact-finding surveys there, with a view to using them in his final report to the Sub-Commission.

The Brazil seminar was held in Rio de Janeiro with the cooperation of São Paulo University, the health ministry, and MORHAN. Professor Paulo Pinheiro, a fellow member of the UN Sub-Commission, had set up an administrative hub to coordinate arrangements for the workshop in the Centre for the Study of Violence at the University. (Readers may remember from my account in Chapter 1 that I met Professor Pinheiro during my work in Geneva in 2004, where he had told me about having been transferred to hospital in Myanmar during his activities as a UN Special Rapporteur—he had had a health emergency—and the staff just managed to save his life. The ambulance had been one of the vehicles supplied to Myanmar by the Nippon Foundation.) In addition to Professor Yokota, fellow Sub-Commission members José Bengoa (Chile), Iulia Motoc (Romania), and El-Hadji Guissé (Senegal) also attended. From Brazil, there were participants from the health ministry, the government special secretariat on human rights, legal circles, and NGOs as well as people affected by leprosy.

Professor Bengoa opened the meeting, and I followed with a summary of the steps I had made to get the issue of the human rights aspect of leprosy taken up formally by a body of the UN (the Sub-Commission), and my hopes for events after the next session where Professor Yokota would present his findings. Professor Yokota said that it was shameful that the human rights dimension of leprosy hadn't been raised at the United Nations until now, mentioning testimonies by recovered persons in South Africa. Dr. Rosa Castalia, leprosy program coordinator at Brazil's Ministry of Health, reported that, after my visit in June last year, the ministry had decided to make leprosy a top public health priority. Claiming that important strides had been made for improving the conditions for people affected by leprosy, she outlined the resolve of the government to achieve elimination at the country level by the end of the year in line with the WHO target. Mario Mamede, head of Brazil's Bureau of Human Rights, told the audience, without mincing words, that the way Brazil, which is still a developing country, treated the members of its population who were affected by leprosy was 200 years behind that of most other countries. For too long, the nation had simply chosen to turn a blind eye, he said, to the appalling conditions in which the vast majority of people affected by leprosy, even when cured, have to live their lives. It was essential that the nation get to grips with this problem and work to improve things, not only from the medical point of view but the social one as well. Brazil should involve the whole of society in its anti-leprosy measures. The country's leprosy colonies, he said, are an ongoing stain upon the nation.

Among those who spoke, Cristiano Torres left the deepest impression on me. Now recovered from leprosy, and the head of a leprosy colony committee and the chairman of a leprosy soccer association, he was selected to be one of the Olympic torch bearers when the Olympic flame passed through Brazil in 2004. In his speech, Mr. Torres talked about why the term "Hansen's disease" is a much kinder and more respectful name than the older name of "leprosy." In Brazil, it is now mandatory to use the term Hansen's disease. As Mr. Torres saw it, leprosy is synonymous with suffering, while Hansen's disease is not.

In his speech, Sub-Commission member Professor Guissé stated that "the problems of leprosy have been ignored, and prejudice has arisen, due to ignorance and fear. We see exactly the same sort of situation in countries in Africa," he said. "I hope that we can hold a seminar like this one there as well." He also touched on the possibility of an effective leprosy vaccine. As I wrote before, I sometimes compare myself to a single match that can nevertheless give rise to a large flame. I like to think that my work traveling around the world can light a big fire in people's hearts—one that will dispel fear and ignorance, and prejudice too. If we inspire enough people, we will one day fully tackle leprosy in all its dimensions.

This was followed by a session in which people with lived experience of leprosy gave their testimonies. Artur Custodio Moreira de Sousa, who heads MORHAN, spoke about how leprosy relates to economic circumstances and quality of life and culture. In Brazil, the prevalence rates are highest among the very poorest segments of the population, he said. Leprosy has always been a disease of those who have no political voice, which is why those who have recovered from the disease must take center stage and advocate loudly on their behalf. At one time, he said, the cars used to transport people affected by leprosy would be painted black. People brought to colonies would be told to abandon hope—and that here they would be taught to simply accept their disease. At the entrance to one of the oldest colonies, built by Christians, the residents were exhorted to "renounce all hope so that hope could be reborn."

According to Torres, who lived forty-eight of his sixty-five years in a leprosy colony, such places are treated like dumps where society simply discards those affected by leprosy. It was impossible for people to live with any dignity there. If leprosy colonies could be turned into places of safety, people affected by the disease would be able to recover their pride, providing them with rehabilitative support that would give them the training and support to return to the outside world.

Another individual, Terejina, told us of how she had to leave her young daughter behind when, having caught the disease, she entered a leprosy colony. When she was allowed out, she found her child living on the streets. Yet another tragic story concerned an old man who had been living in a care home with his wife, and who had been taken away and put into a colony when he caught the disease. Left on her own, his wife was subjected to discrimination, and in the end both died of loneliness and depression. As if the floodgates had been lifted, out came all sorts of sad stories about people's experiences. One man became subject to discrimination because it was noted on his ID card that he'd had leprosy; another had caught leprosy in prison and had simply been left to survive on his own. Many others told of the suffering they had to go through when they had to deal with the side-effects of the treatment.

Professor Eleonora Menicucci de Oliveira opened the next session. Professor Menicucci is an expert on public health policy, concerned mainly with the ways in which people get access to health care. She bewailed how people affected by leprosy were treated in Brazil, where for decades they were denied beds in the general hospitals and had to be forcibly segregated in leprosy hospitals. She demanded increased transparency in government health policy, arguing for the importance of greater disclosure of information.

Professor Yokota stressed the importance of including leprosy as a subject in the school curriculum. Leprosy ought to be a theme taken up in school teaching materials and in classrooms. The timing could not be more appropriate, he argued. The world had just seen out the end of the United Nations Decade for Human Rights Education (1995–2004), and the World Programme for Human Rights Education was about to be launched.

The second day of the conference featured presentations of a fact-finding survey the Ministry of Health had conducted in Brazil's thirty-three leprosy colonies in November 2004 with the help of MORHAN.

When I visited Brazil in June 2004, a health ministry spokesman had admitted that government officials had simply let things slip. In relation to leprosy strategy, he had told me frankly, that they had been "asleep." Since then, we were told, the ministry was taking swift steps for improvement. Dr. Rosa Castalia, leprosy program coordinator for the Ministry of Health, told us how the database had been cleaned up, and their statistical methods overhauled. As a result, she said, the discovery had been made that they had 30,000 patients on MDT, not 70,000 as previously thought. As of January 2005, the prevalence rate had drastically decreased, from 4.5 people per 10,000 to 1.7.

This survey looked at a broad range of issues in the colonies that included the number and quality of health personnel, the state of the buildings and facilities, the proprietorship of the land and the buildings, and tax payments, relying on interviews and questionnaires taken of people affected by leprosy, as well as people involved in local government. The results showed that the buildings of most of these colonies were in a terrible state of repair, some places more or less abandoned; they were also poorly staffed. The health personnel also tended to be inadequately qualified. It wasn't just that they were ignorant of how to treat people affected by leprosy medically. Their treatment of them was often insensitive. In the conference, discussion focused on whether and how to improve the infrastructure of these colonies; whether and how to preserve the medical information stored in them for their historical value; how best to provide the residents with better employment opportunities; and how to provide training with that purpose in mind. The residents of these colonies are often fearful of returning to the outside world, and so they have to fight to get residential, property, and parental rights.

Professor Yokota gave his word that he would reflect these findings in the report he would submit to the Sub-Commission. He also proposed asking the UN Human Rights Commission office to set up funding so that people affected by leprosy could travel to Geneva and give testimony at the United Nations.

At a news conference that same day, we were joined by the actress Elke Maravilha, whom I'd met on my last visit, in 2004, as well as Ney Matogrosso, one of the country's most popular singers, and the well-known actress Solange Couto. I was so heartened to see the willingness of these celebrities to join in our leprosy elimination efforts completely out of the kindness of their hearts. However, they were at pains to stress that the media in Brazil could be doing so much more.

That afternoon, there was a showing of *The Best Years of Our Lives*, a documentary by the Brazilian filmmaker Andrea Pasquini. A one-hour documentary comprising the stories of people affected and those who have recovered, all quite elderly, recalling the days when hospitalization for anyone with leprosy was compulsory, it presented a tale of aching sadness and despair, but also, somehow, a triumph of the human spirit. What a wonderful way of getting across the message we wanted to convey, I thought to myself. I decided then and there that we would have to show it during our meeting with the Sub-Commission for the Promotion and Protection of Human Rights at the United Nations in August.

The day after the conference ended, 1 March, I visited a local health center in the Nova Iguaçu district, and I also visited the Curupaití colony hospital in nearby Jacarepaguá district. Both of these districts are quite close to Rio de Janeiro.

Nova Iguaçu has the highest prevalence rate in Rio state, at five persons per 10,000. The health center was shut down for renovations for a period of two years in 1997, and 40 percent of the people in the area had abandoned their medication regimens. I was told that the newly refurbished center was now making concerted efforts to chase up and re-register former patients, conduct follow-up studies, and provide treatment, paying particular attention to ocular lesions. The chief medical officer informed me he had taken up his post just two months previously—before that, basic public health services had barely been functioning. No MDT blister packs appeared to have been given out for the last two years, and other issues had come to light: some major problems existed in their inventory management. Most of the issues were now resolved, thanks mainly to the strong pressure MORHAN exerted on the government. Some unaccounted-for expenses had come to light, and pilfering had clearly taken place. The chief officer strenuously assured us that every effort was being made to improve things, though he also mentioned that for his pains he was now the object of death threats.

The Curupaití colony hospital was a huge set of buildings spread out like a small town on a mountain top, in a suburb of Rio de Janeiro.

In addition to the hospital, it contained five neat residential blocks, home both to people undergoing treatment for leprosy and those who had finished their treatment and their families—around 1,400 inhabitants in all. The colony's buildings were already more than fifty years old, but the residents seemed to be putting a brave face on things and doing their best to look after themselves, despite the deplorable conditions in which they lived.

My return trip involved a plane journey from Rio to New York, and then, after a five-hour wait in transit, a day-long plane journey back to Narita. Again, I spent two nights in a row on the plane.

Belated awareness on the part of the UN—Republic of India (Maharashtra state, New Delhi), March 2005

Route: Narita, Japan → New Delhi, India (flight time: 8h)—one night—New Delhi, India → Pune, Maharashtra (flight time: 2h)—two nights—Pune → New Delhi (flight time: 2h)—three nights

My visit to India in March was already my second trip to that continent that year. Landing in New Delhi, I immediately transferred to Pune, the second largest city after Mumbai in India's Maharashtra state. It was extremely hot—36 degrees C—and the air extraordinarily dry. In Pune, I participated in a conference that was being held to support Professor Yokota, who had been commissioned by the UN Sub-Commission on the Promotion and Protection of Human Rights to prepare a special report on leprosy and human rights and discrimination. The conference was jointly organized by the Nippon Foundation, the Sasakawa Health Foundation, ILU, and the India chapter of IDEA, an organization of and for people affected by leprosy, with a focus on a broad range of topics from health services, education, residence, marriage, families, inheritance, prevention of disability, social segregation, stigma, and legal matters, as much as possible listening to people affected to learn about their life histories and how discrimination had affected them. In addition to leprosy specialists, the conference was attended by representatives from the legal profession, NGOs, human rights groups, and others as well as people affected by leprosy who had responded to the rallying cry delivered by IDEA. Aware that we were now facing a new issue, the battle against the discrimination that people affected by leprosy face, we were keen to find new ways in which we could draw attention to the human side of the disease.

I'll never forget how, as the conference got underway, one of the participants asked why it had taken so long to start dealing with the issue of human rights. A simple question, but utterly to the point. Professor Yokota replied: "We were ignorant. The United Nations had no awareness that such a huge human rights issue even existed." This admission moved me greatly. I also had some reflecting to do. I had spent so many years focused on elimination, I realized, and yet only recently had I started paying attention to the human rights aspect of the disease.

Dr. Gopal, president of IDEA India, explained in his presentation that in India 10 million people had already been cured thanks to MDT. And yet, even in this day and age, he reported, there were still more than 500 leprosy colonies where people who had recovered from the disease had to live, along with their families, having been moved there from a significant distance away. The presence of these colonies attested to the discrimination, misunderstanding, and prejudice that still exist in Indian society. I suggested to him that there were surely signs of hope. As he himself showed by his inspiring example, an increasing number of people affected by leprosy were breaking their silence, forcefully expressing their views, and becoming effective agents for change. This in itself was a major contribution and would one day cause broader Indian society to revise misconceptions about people who had been affected by the disease.

Following the conference, I visited a colony on the outskirts of Pune. The colony was about 100 meters up a dirt-track off the highway and comprised a group of brick houses with simple corrugated iron roofs, looking rather like barracks. The walls had been painted white and pink, and the compound seemed well maintained. Four women in saris were waiting at the entrance to greet me. Each of them held a silver tray containing a small silver dish. The woman nearest me opened my mouth and filled it with sugar—so much, indeed, that I didn't know what to do. At the sight, they all burst out laughing. I had never had such a welcome before. Maybe this practice was a leftover from a time when sugar was rare and very precious, but I felt touched and grateful at this gesture. Twenty or so children, ranging from four years to ten, all gaily dressed in yellow, pink, and green, then put on a little show of singing and dancing for me. To express my thanks, I gave them some sweets that I'd brought along with me specially for this purpose. They sang out "Thank you!" in English, with great big smiles on their faces.

A five-minute walk from the colony was a hospital. This consisted of a men's ward, a women's ward, workshops, and a surgery. The hospital was home for 150 or so people affected by leprosy who required surgery or care for their ulcers or had nowhere else to go. There was one girl, however, only thirteen years old, who was clearly affected very lightly, and I learned that she was only there because there were no health personnel with knowledge of leprosy at the health post near her village. It pained me greatly to think of the discrimination she might experience even after she was cured as a result of having spent time here in this hospital, ostracized from her community, when it might have been relatively simple for her to get treatment living at home.

From the hospital, I went on to visit the factory. With a workforce that included eighty or so people who had once had leprosy but had been treated and were fully recovered, the factory makes engine parts and bumpers that supplied India's largest motor manufacturer, Tata Motors. In a compound with an area of 2,500 hectares lay neat rows of machinery and tools, used for stamping sheet metal, welding it into the correct shape, and applications of chemicals to protect against corrosion. Each of these relatively simple tasks had teams of fifteen women, who were clearly applying themselves assiduously to their work. The foreman informed me that the factory had been established expressly to offer employment to people cured of leprosy. A labor union had been formed in 1987. Until the factory signed a contract with Tata, I was told, it went through some difficult times, even facing bankruptcy. The employees had raised capital from their own salaries to make sure it survived and were able to turn it into a going concern. Despite the various challenges, the wages it pays superseded those of the average Indian workers. There was nothing inadequate about these people's will to work, or their ability. The only thing they had ever lacked was opportunity. I regard it as part of my mission, part of my duty, to be able to create opportunities for people who are cured of leprosy, so that they don't have to beg but can experience the joy and satisfaction of being able to earn their own living.

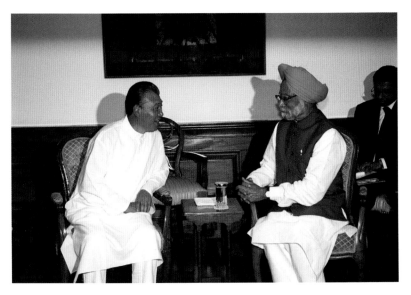

29. With Prime Minister Manmohan Singh (New Delhi, India, March 2005)

On this visit, I had the opportunity to meet Prime Minister Manmohan Singh in New Delhi. The security at his residence struck me as stricter than that of the White House, but his office was surprisingly relaxed. He was well briefed on the leprosy situation in India and our elimination activities. "Mr. Sasakawa," he was gracious enough to say, "you have been an inspiration to India. You are doing noble work." I told the prime minister about our three simple messages—that leprosy is a curable disease, that medicine is available free of charge, and that discrimination against leprosy is unacceptable—and he repeated them several times and then gave me his pledge to do his utmost to eliminate leprosy in India and to redress the human rights problem faced by people affected, and their families.

I also met with Health Minister Dr. Anbumani Ramadoss, who gave me his unequivocal commitment to eliminating leprosy and addressing the human rights issue. He told me: "We have almost achieved elimination. I believe we will be able to make an announcement to the world by the end of this year. We are also doing our utmost on the issue of human rights, because this is a movement begun by Mahatma Gandhi."

REACHING THE UNREACHABLE

The importance of early detection—Kingdom of Cambodia, March 2005

Route: New Delhi → Bangkok, Thailand (flight time: 4h 20m; 2h stopover) → Phnom Penh, Cambodia (flight time: 1h)—four nights—Phnom Penh → Bangkok (flight time: 1h; one-night stopover) → Narita (flight time: 6h 30m)

From India, I traveled straight on to Cambodia. The Nippon Foundation has long made the improvement of the lives of disadvantaged peoples in Southeast Asia an area of concern. In recent years in Cambodia, I had been involved in the establishment of a nationwide organization for the blind. (The prevalence of blindness in Cambodia is relatively high compared to other developing countries—and in large part this has to do with mine explosions. At the time of my visit, there were roughly 140,000 people, 1.2 percent of the population, with blindness and avoidable eye disease.) On this trip, I was due to attend the opening ceremony of the completion of a building that was to be the headquarters of this organization. Another project the Nippon Foundation have been involved with in Cambodia is provision of teacher training (as well as school building construction), and I also attended a ceremony where we awarded 460 young people from rural areas of the country with a monthly stipend for living expenses to help them fulfil their aspirations of becoming teachers.

As always, I was also keen to use my visit to see how the struggle against leprosy in Cambodia was faring. In between my other engagements, I paid a visit to a leprosy colony in the village of Treung in Kampong Cham province. The colony is reached by a tree-lined road and set on beautifully grassy plains. Cambodia reached the WHO-defined leprosy elimination target in 1998. For many decades, people affected by the disease were forced to relocate here—taken away from their villages and their families. Though they are no longer forcibly segregated, it is still a kind of sanctuary for people who are fearful of the prejudice they will meet from the outside world.

The population of this village was 1,107, of whom seven had leprosy and ninety-five were cured. The rest were families of people affected by leprosy—who had been living here for two or even three generations. The ward in the hospital had eight beds. I went inside

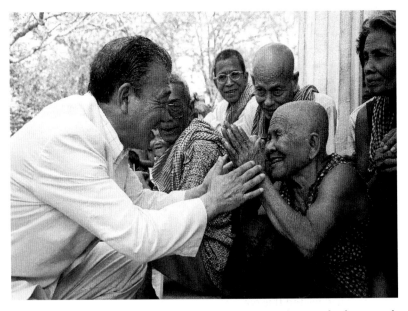

30. The author exchanging a joke with an elderly lady (Cambodia, March 2005)

and shook hands with the residents and asked them to tell me about their lives. They told me how life in the village afforded them a degree of normality: how, even with a certain degree of hardship, they could still marry and have families, without any fear of scorn or discrimination. In my heart, I prayed for a day when the misconceptions about leprosy might be banished, and the people who lived here would feel strong enough to join together and fight for their right to a fair and free existence in the world.

In Cambodia, the fear of discrimination still makes people affected by leprosy reluctant to get themselves checked out at clinics. With little funding, medical personnel rarely travel out to villages to proactively find cases of leprosy and tend to wait passively for patients to report themselves. Information is scant, so most people have no idea that treatment is free. All of which means that the disease is simply left to wreak its damage, with life-changing consequences. In Treung village, I met a young couple who had been treated and had recovered, and who now were now raising pigs for a business. They had made enough profit to buy themselves a motorbike, they told me, proudly, the happiness evident in their sunburnt faces. Listening to them, I felt my sadness and weariness disappear in a trice. Before my return to Japan, I took a brief stop in Laos—to do the same sort of work.

Ingenious ways to deal with elimination—Republic of Mozambique, April 2005

Route: Narita → Hong Kong (flight time: 5h; 45m stopover) → Johannesburg, South Africa (flight time: 12h 30m; 1h 40m stopover) → Maputo, Mozambique (flight time: 1h)—one night—Maputo → Nampula (via Pemba) (flight time: 3h 30m)—two nights—Nampula → Maputo (flight time: 2h)

In April, I went to work in Mozambique, which was one of the nations of Africa that had yet to achieve the WHO-recognized elimination targets. I had visited this country in August 2002, and on that occasion I had meetings with the then Prime Minister Pascoal Mocumbi and Health Minister Francisco Songane, and I had also carried out fact-finding missions in Nampula and Cabo Delgado, two of the regions with the highest prevalence rates in the country. The purpose of my visit this time was to find out if the country had moved forward.

There had been an election in December 2004. A new prime minister and president were now in office, and a completely different line-up of people in positions of government. The new health minister was Dr. Ivo Garrido. Previously head surgeon at Maputo's Central Hospital, I had heard stories that he had flatly refused the official residence and car that came with the office. On my first meeting, I could tell straight off that he was a man of integrity and intelligence, with a deep knowledge of leprosy. He got straight to the heart of the matter. "With leprosy, the issue isn't one of numbers," he told me straight off. "The issue is one of human dignity."

On my arrival in Maputo, I received a briefing from Dr. Bokar Touré, the WHO country representative; Alfredo MacArthur, who was in charge of the health ministry's leprosy and TB countermeasures; and Alcino Ndeve, advisor on leprosy to the health ministry. The recent election meant that they weren't able to give me full

167

details of the new government's public health strategy, which was still being put together. They assured me, however, that leprosy elimination remained a high priority—though they tempered their assurance with the caution that the biggest problems facing the health ministry were Africa's three main scourges, malaria, TB, and AIDS, so there would be resource allocation difficulties.

Sixty percent of the people affected by leprosy live in the north and central provinces of the country (Nampula and Cabo Delgado in the north, and Zambezia, in the center). In these areas, there is only 30 percent health services coverage. Most medical centers are basic and have few staff, who are often over-stretched and in need of training. There was not one ambulance in the entire country.

Figures for leprosy prevalence taken at the end of the previous year showed 2.5 persons per 10,000 population, indicating a steady decrease in the numbers. But even given these hopeful signs it seemed unlikely to me that Mozambique would achieve elimination by the designated date—which was at the end of the current year. I had a consultation with the WHO regional director and other partners to explore ways that would help Mozambique reach its goal as soon as it could. There were several ingenious methods that Mozambique had developed for getting information about leprosy out into communities. One of these was the COMBI project, which involved community volunteers, young men and women, sporting yellow T-shirts who went round villages conducting awareness campaigns, advocating the importance of early diagnosis. Another method involved incorporating the subject of leprosy into what is taught in schools. Pupils were being encouraged to conduct skin tests and then report the results to their schools. This was the kind of campaign I dearly wanted to see in other countries as well, and I often mentioned this as a kind of model for them to emulate.

When I visited Mozambique in 2002, there were parts of Nampula where the prevalence rate was above ten and even as high as twenty. Nearly 70 percent of patients came from four northern states of the country.

From Nampula City, the provincial capital, I drove to the village of Namaita, about 40 kilometers away. Here I attended a festival promoting leprosy awareness, with dancing and theatrical skits and a concert by people affected by leprosy. Addressing an audience of around 3,000 people, I asked whether they had heard of Japan, and only two people raised their hand. (Then again, I had doubts whether many Japanese people would be able to say off the top of their head where Mozambique lay on the map of Africa.) Much of Mozambique's population live in abject poverty, with little or no education, which makes communication through music and theatrical skits the most effective way of getting across our messages, that leprosy is curable, that treatment is free, and that discrimination has no place. Later on that same day, I visited an agricultural workshop and a shoe workshop run by ADEMO (Mozambican Association for People with Disability), an organization for disabled people, and ALEMO (Mozambique Association of Persons with Leprosy), an organization of people affected by leprosy. It cheered me to see them making a living for themselves. These places were exceptional, but they were an inspiring example of what might be done elsewhere.

At the health center in Namaita village, I saw health workers showing people how to take the medicine from their MDT blister packs. In developed countries, people learn how to take medicine as children, either as liquid or as pills; but in developing countries people have no experience of it and have to be instructed in every little thing. Volunteers from the health centers go round from village to village on their bikes teaching people how to take their medicine, diagnosing new cases, and instructing people how to look after one another. I donated funding for 150 bicycles to support them in their work.

I had one more meeting with Health Minister Garrido before I left. After listening to my report of my visit to Nampula, and my doubts that Mozambique would manage to meet the WHO target for elimination this year, he told me he would dispatch health experts to the northern provinces where leprosy was endemic to find out more details, meet with the governors of those provinces to work on strategy after 2005, and ask the president to lend his support. In Mozambique, 10 percent of people who get diagnosed with leprosy on their first visit to a hospital have already developed disability. This is high, and an indication that these visits are being made at too late a stage. Health Minister Garrido admitted that it was going to be impossible to meet the target set in 2005, but he felt sure that the

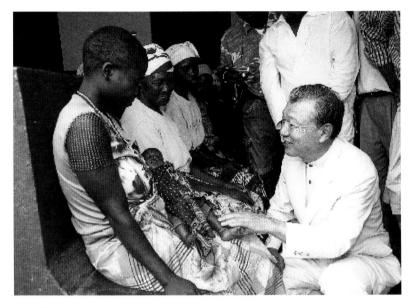

31. The author with a mother with leprosy, and her child (Mozambique, April 2005)

country would meet it within the next few years. He did not look very confident, though, as he said this.

The minister with a father affected by leprosy—United Republic of Tanzania, April 2005

Route: Maputo, Mozambique → Johannesburg, South Africa (flight time: 1h; 1h 30m stopover) → Dar es Salaam, Tanzania (flight time: 3h 20m)—five nights—Dar es Salaam, Tanzania → Johannesburg, South Africa (flight time: 3h 20m; 3h stopover) → Hong Kong (flight time: 12h 30m; 2h 30m stopover) → Narita (flight time: 5h)

From Mozambique, I traveled to Tanzania, another country in Africa where leprosy remains endemic. Located on the east side of the African continent, Tanzania is roughly two and a half times the size of Japan. It has the highest mountain in Africa, Mount Kilimanjaro, and it is also a veritable treasure trove of wildlife. Many years ago, on a safari in this country, I saw twenty-seven species of animals, including a rhinoceros. Even my guide was amazed. It's always been my dream

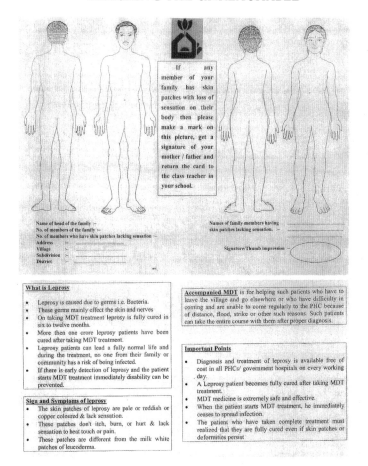

If any member of your family has skin patches with loss of sensation on their body then please make a mark on this picture, get a signature of your mother / father and return the card to the class teacher in your school.

Name of head of the family :-
No. of members of the family :-
No. of members who have skin patches lacking sensation -
Address :-
Village :-
Subdivision :-
District :-

Names of family members having
skin patches lacking sensation. :-

Signature/Thumb Impression -

What is Leprosy

- Leprosy is caused due to germs i.e. Bacteria.
- These germs mainly effect the skin and nerves
- On taking MDT treatment leprosy is fully cured in six to twelve months.
- More then one crore leprosy patients have been cured after taking MDT treatment.
- Leprosy patients can lead a fully normal life and during the treatment, no one from their family or community has a risk of being infected.
- If there is early detection of leprosy and the patient starts MDT treatment immediately disability can be prevented.

Sign and Symptoms of leprosy

- The skin patches of leprosy are pale or reddish or copper coloured & lack sensation.
- These patches don't itch, burn, or hurt & lack sensation to heat touch or pain.
- These patches are different from the milk white patches of leucoderma.

Accompanied MDT is for helping such patients who have to leave the village and go elsewhere or who have difficulty in coming and are unable to come regularly to the PHC because of distance, flood, strike or other such reasons. Such patients can take the entire course with them after proper diagnosis.

Important Points

- Diagnosis and treatment of leprosy is available free of cost in all PHCs/ government hospitals on every working day.
- A Leprosy patient becomes fully cured after taking MDT treatment.
- MDT medicine is extremely safe and effective.
- When the patient starts MDT treatment, he immediately ceases to spread infection.
- The patient who have taken complete treatment must realized that they are fully cured even if skin patches or deformities persist

32. Skin test cards with diagrams of the human body to mark areas affected, a method used in places in India as well as Mozambique

to one day view this country from a hot-air balloon. While the official national capital is now Dodoma, the seat of government is Dar es Salaam, which is situated on the Indian Ocean. Maize (corn) is the main staple grain consumed in Tanzania.

Tanzania had been trying to deal with its leprosy problem since 1977, but its leprosy program is combined with a program for tuberculosis, and since most emphasis has long been given to tuberculosis, which is a major problem in the country, leprosy figures remained high. This time, I got the distinct impression of progress. Government officials were clearly working hard with the German Leprosy and TB Relief Association, as well as NGO workers and WHO health professionals. The day I arrived, 24 April, was a Sunday, but even so, there at the airport was a welcome party, comprising the health minister herself, Anna Abdallah, the director of the WHO office in Tanzania, Dr. Mangane, and other officials. No sooner had I touched down than there was a squall, and the health minister assured me that in Africa rain was seen as a lucky omen—I had obviously brought good fortune with me. I had met Mrs. Abdallah several years before, when she was minister of agriculture. This was when former US President Jimmy Carter and Nobel Prize laureate Norman Borlaug, and the Nippon Foundation set up the Sasakawa Global 2000, a project whose aim was to help farmers in Africa increase their agricultural productivity. She exuded elegance and positivity, and I was happy to learn that she was now health minister.

I was also very impressed with the depth of her knowledge of leprosy. Over a welcome dinner, she mentioned in her speech that her own father had been affected. The people present were amazed. Her father had at one point been a professor at a university, but on being diagnosed with leprosy he had been sent to a clinic far away from where he lived and worked. As a child, the health minister told us, she had never been able to understand why her father had had to go away. "If my father were alive today," she told us, "I'm quite sure he would have done everything in his power to help us in our campaign." She had actually made this fact public on World Leprosy Day in January that year and not long afterwards received a telephone call from her brother who castigated her for talking about it openly. For a health minister to come out with such a thing in a country like Tanzania, where prejudice and misconceptions about leprosy abound, must have required huge resolve and a tremendous amount of courage. But it would also have a positive effect. She wanted of course to eradicate leprosy, but she also intended to eliminate the number-one problem associated with it, which is discrimination. The depth of feeling was evident in her voice.

The next day, I visited the WHO office and the health ministry where I was updated on elimination progress. In 1983, there had been 35,000 cases in Tanzania. In 2004, the number stood at 5,600—

greatly reduced. Over the same period, the prevalence rate had fallen from twelve people per 10,000 to 1.3. This was due particularly to concerted work after 1998. The relationship between the government and NGOs is excellent and is held up by WHO as an example to the whole of Africa. Nevertheless, tasks remain. More than 10 percent of newly detected cases present with substantial disability, indicating that people do not seek treatment early enough—surely out of their fear of prejudice. People cured of the disease continue to live in settlements, the result being that their children are deprived of educational opportunities and grow up to think of themselves as leprosy-affected. The health minister was appealing to these people to let their children go to school rather than hiding them from the outside world.

While in Dar es Salaam, I visited the Mbagala dispensary in the Temeke municipality on the outskirts of the city. Here I met with six people affected by leprosy. A one-hour journey by taxi and ferry took me to Menge, a village for people affected by leprosy, where I gave a talk to an audience of 161 people with disability. This colony had been set up in 1987 in a place called Kipala but had been relocated here in 1970. It now comprised forty-one houses, in which patients and people who had been treated and were fully recovered were living with their families. I learned that most families relied on the government for support.

I then traveled to the capital Dodoma, in the central region of the country, for a meeting with President Benjamin Mkapa. The day I arrived, 26 April, was a public holiday, known as Union Day, commemorating the unification of Tanganyika and the People's Republic of Zanzibar into the United Republic of Tanzania in 1964. I had been invited to the Union Day celebration in Jamhuri Stadium. The marching bands passed solemnly in front of the VIP box, but I couldn't help being privately amused (though I hoped I didn't show it) at some of the marchers who were completely out of step! The president's guest house had barely any security and was a tiny affair, but the building was constructed in a modern style, using huge boulders as part of the construction. The room where I sat for talks with the president had these boulders in it, in between our sofas. No one else was present—it was just the two of us. The first thing the president said to me was that before being briefed ahead of my visit, he had barely even given a thought to the disease. He didn't even know it existed in Tanzania. "In Tanzania," he told me, "there's an expression that equates people who don't work with people who have leprosy. But as of today, I won't ever use it again!" I was reminded of my visit to Uganda in 2001, and President Museveni who had insisted that there were no people affected by leprosy in his country. "As a child, people told me they'd had all moved to an island in Lake Victoria," he had added. In Africa, leprosy strategy tends to be low on the list of priorities in public health policy, and many government officials are either ignorant of it or uninterested. Once I apprised him of the facts, President Mkapa apologized and gave me his word that he would personally convey to his countrymen the three messages that I had brought to Tanzania: that leprosy is curable, that medication is available free of charge, and that discrimination toward people affected by leprosy is unacceptable. In fact, this day I was rather taciturn, which is unusual for me, because I was feeling unwell. I had a fever, and once my meeting with the president was over, I retired to my room and slept.

On the return journey to Dar es Salaam, I stopped off at a care center, formerly a sanatorium, in Chazi, in the Morogoro region. This is an area where the prevalence of malaria is extremely high, with every person said to be bitten by mosquitos a thousand times a year. Here, I found a Japanese doctor who had previously worked in St. Luke's International Hospital in Tokyo. He informed me that his driver had died of malaria just the previous day. My team and I take every precaution to avoid catching malaria in Africa. Fortunately, neither I nor any of the people who accompany me have come down with this illness—so far. There are medications to take to prevent malaria infections, but they have severe side effects, mostly affecting the liver, so I don't take them—and because of this, if I have to attend parties in the evening, which is a time when the malaria-transmitting mosquitoes are out doing their worst, I slather my arms and legs and face with mosquito repellent. Often, the mosquito netting in the doors and windows of the places I stay in is torn, so I have to fill the holes with bits of newspaper, and I sleep with five or six lit mosquito coils all around my bed, with socks on my feet and gloves on my hands and my face covered by the sheet.

About forty people affected by leprosy lived in the care center. The people gathered to see me all looked very downcast, and their rooms were ill-lit, damp, and gloomy. I voiced my usual words of encouragement and hope, telling them that the health minister had told me her own father had been affected by leprosy and had been cured, something that caused some people listening to cry out in shock—as if in astonishment at the thought that a health minister would be able to understand their plight. The drive back from Dodoma to Dar es Salaam took ten hours and was extremely arduous, and though we'd left at dawn the sun was dipping below the horizon when we finally arrived back. As a rule on such trips, we try to avoid activities after sundown. Partly this is just so as to be safe, but we also bear in mind the conditions of the roads, which make for many traffic accidents at night.

I then had a grueling trip back to Japan, first via Johannesburg and then Hong Kong. Eight days of my ten-day trip had involved some sort of journey on an airplane.

A place where God came to see the man—Republic of India, May 2005

Route: Narita, Japan → Itami (1h stopover) → Kansai Airport → Bangkok, Thailand (flight time: 5h 30m; 2h stopover) → Kolkata, West Bengal (flight time: 2h 30m)—two nights—Kolkata → Chennai, Tamil Nadu (flight time: 2h)—three nights—Chennai → Frankfurt, Germany (flight time: 9h 30m; 1h 40m stopover) → Geneva, Switzerland (flight time: 1h)—two nights (Sasakawa Health Prize; meetings with health ministers)—Geneva, Switzerland → Zurich (Visit to CEO of Novartis) (flight time: 1h; 1h 20m stopover) → Narita (flight time: 11h 50m)

In May, I went to Kolkata (formerly Calcutta) and Chennai (formerly Madras). Kolkata is located in West Bengal, a state in India's northeast that borders on Bhutan to the north, Bangladesh to the east, and Nepal to the northwest. The state capital, it is India's third largest city after Mumbai and Delhi, famed as the birthplace of the poet and social reformer Rabindranath Tagore and the Indian nationalist Subhas Chandra Bose, and the home of Mother Teresa's Missionaries of Charity.

An advanced city with skyscrapers and high-speed motorways, Kolkata is like a microcosm of the nation, with extreme differences between rich and poor, who live right next door to each other. On my first visit, I was flabbergasted on the way from the airport to my hotel at the unnerving sight of dozens of homeless people who had staked out places to sleep for the night on the pavement in front of the shuttered shops. But it's a sight I have since discovered is all too common.

I came to Kolkata to attend a conference that had been organized by the ILU, with backing from the Nippon Foundation. Its theme was advocacy strategy and the role of the media in eliminating leprosy. We'd already had similar meetings in Delhi, Bihar, Maharashtra, Odisha, and Uttar Pradesh.

At the conference, a great number of people affected by leprosy made statements about the various ways that discrimination had affected their lives. In my speech, I stated that India has more than 10 million people with lived experience of the disease. Given this situation, we have to think of ways to ensure the reintegration of people affected by leprosy and their families into society. I told the audience that I was making efforts to persuade the UN Commission on Human Rights to require nations to take action to get rid of social discrimination. But the effort requires a social movement, one that makes leprosy everybody's issue, not just that of the specialists and the experts. At every step of the way, the active participation of people affected by leprosy, I said, is essential. I received pledges of solid support from West Bengal's Chief Minister Buddhadeb Bhattacharjee and from its Health and Family Welfare Minister Dr. Surjya Kanta Mishra.

Tangentially, during the conference our driver happened to show his hands to a doctor who was present and straightaway was diagnosed as having leprosy. In India, leprosy is not something that happens to "other" people. It is all around us.

After a quick lunch break of fifteen minutes (we often do not get such breaks, so we were grateful), we headed to the airport to go to Chennai to attend a second conference, the Regional Conference on Leprosy, that was being co-hosted by IDEA India, the Leprosy Elimination Alliance, and the Indian Leprosy Association (Hind Kusht Nivaran Sangh). All three organizations had headquarters in Chennai. This conference was attended by government representatives, people from the medical field, people affected by leprosy, NGO representatives, and members of the legal profession from the four states of southern India where leprosy had formerly been most prevalent: Kerala, Karnataka, Andhra Pradesh, and Tamil Nadu. All four states had succeeded in reaching the elimination target. Opening the conference, Tamil Nadu's health minister, Thiru N. Thalavai Sundaram, told the people present that the number of registered cases in his state had reduced from 800,000 in 1983 to just 5,500 thanks to MDT. However, this was no reason to relax, and it was essential that everyone keep up elimination activities.

Of particular interest at this conference were reports presented by jurists who specialize in human rights issues. They pointed out how many laws in India were still problematic from a human rights perspective, citing provisions such as those restricting people affected by leprosy from accessing public spaces, allowing insurance companies to disqualify people affected by leprosy, and others making leprosy grounds for divorce. Most of these laws are said to date back to when the country was part of the British Empire. One presentation showed how cinema, which is such an influential medium in India, is still being used to propagate false notions, using the example of a film known in English as *Blood Tear*, a 1960s movie that was a huge hit and was re-released in 2004. The main character in the film has dalliances with numerous women, and then as "divine punishment" for his misdeeds he contracts leprosy. The influence of the film industry in fueling unfounded prejudice of this kind needs to be recognized and dealt with.

Thanks to the intervention of leprosy specialists with contacts in the media, we managed to get the media in Kolkata and Chennai to cover our conference quite widely, with articles featuring in about twenty newspapers in each city, including newspapers in the local languages of Bengali and Tamil.

During my stay in Chennai, I traveled to Chengalpattu, home of the Central Leprosy Teaching and Research Institute. When Mahatma Gandhi alighted at Chengalpattu station to visit a nearby temple, leprosy patients streamed to the station to catch a glimpse of him. It happened to be one of the days when he was keeping a "day of silence" (a weekly practice for him), so all he could do was wave and go on his way. He later remarked that he had been going to see God, but instead God had come to him.

The Central Leprosy Teaching and Research Institute, established in 1924, still takes in sixty-two doctors and ninety-two nurses annually for training. However, I was told that its future is now uncertain due to the decrease in leprosy cases. Nearby, an old people's home was being built, started by people affected by leprosy. Construction work was proceeding apace, helped by a grant that Arao Ken and Masako Ken of the National Sanatorium Amami Wakoen, the sanatorium for people affected by leprosy in Amami, in Kagoshima prefecture, Japan, had given to me to pass on. The elderly residents in the home had previously had to sleep on beds made of stone, but soon they would be sleeping in normal beds. I attended the opening ceremony for this home, standing in for Mr. and Mrs. Ken. The home included an art classroom with artworks, mainly centering on the daughter of former President Ramaswamy Venkataraman, many of them excellent. This home has always received funding from the Sasakawa (Memorial) Health Foundation, and it was evident that the funding was being used well.

At this time of year, Chennai was extremely hot. By mid-morning, the temperature was higher than 40 degrees C. The slightest movement brought me out in streams of sweat, and it was utterly exhausting to walk anywhere. Even so, my traveling companions and I made a point of not complaining. We were determined to bear everything—whether it was the heat, jet lag, or unfamiliar food.

The last place I visited was the Villivakkam leprosy colony, located on the outskirts of Chennai. My visit coincided with a monthly meeting of leaders of forty-eight leprosy colonies in Tamil Nadu. At one time, as many as 110 families resided in this colony. In recent years, I was told, many who are not affected by leprosy had moved in to live in the colony. It has long been one of my dreams for the walls between leprosy colonies and society to disappear and for people affected by leprosy to live in their communities, with the recognition that there is no need for segregation.

Inspired by what I saw here, I proposed convening a meeting of leaders from all leprosy colonies throughout India. My proposal was favorably received, and it was decided to hold a meeting that very year, in December 2005. Dr. Gopal of IDEA India said he would undertake an investigation into the current situation of the numerous leprosy colonies said to exist in the country and designate representatives, and use this as an opportunity to create a new network linking people affected by the disease, media, NGOs, and people from business circles. If we could do this, it would be a world-first, I thought, and I was determined to do all I could to support it.

Late that night, or rather in the very wee hours of the following morning, I boarded a plane that took me to Frankfurt and thence to Geneva, where I was to attend a meeting at the WHO General Assembly. I was traveling from a country where the temperature was 40 degrees C to one where the temperature was a mere 8 degrees C. My team and I often find ourselves having to pack for summer and winter on these trips, and this was no exception.

He who imparts light—Democratic Republic of the Congo, August 2005

Route: Narita, Japan → Paris (flight time: 12h; 1h stopover) → Geneva, Switzerland (flight time: 1h)—three nights (attending a meeting with the UN Commission on Human Rights)—Geneva → Paris, France (flight time: 1h; 2h stopover) → Kinshasa, DRC (flight time: 7h 40m)—five nights—Kinshasa → Paris (flight time: 7h 30m; 5h 30m stopover) → Narita (flight time: 12h)

In July 2005, I was promoted to chairman of the Nippon Foundation, having previously been president. Despite the new responsibilities, I was determined to continue with my travels and anti-leprosy work around the globe. In August, after speaking at the Human Rights Commission at the Palais des Nations in Geneva, I traveled to the DRC. This was my first visit to this nation. (My transit via Paris ended up involving a long wait of seven hours in Paris Charles de Gaulle airport.)

I should point out that there are currently two "Congos" in Africa, separated by the Congo River. On the western side is the Republic of Congo; on the eastern side, the DRC. My visit in August 2005 was to the latter. It has about six times the land area of Japan, is rich in mineral resources, and until 1960 was a colony of Belgium. Its colonial history makes it part of the Francophone world. Congo (or "Belgian Congo" as it was once known) achieved independence from Belgium in 1960 under the name Republic of Congo. In 1965, Mobutu Sese Seko came to power in a coup, renamed the country Zaire in 1971, and ran it as a one-party state. For many years, there were ethnic tensions, and by the late 1990s the government began to weaken, and the country was invaded in 1996 by Rwanda. President Seko's long-time opponent Laurent-Désiré Kabila became the new president in 1997 and changed the country's name to the DRC. President Kabila was assassinated in 2001. The DRC shares borders with nine countries: the Republic of Congo, Central African Republic, South Sudan, Uganda, Rwanda, Burundi, Tanzania, Zambia, and Angola. For many years, it was embroiled in warfare with its neighbors and internally as well. Factors including ethnic conflict, dispute over rights to rich material resources, and military intervention by neighboring countries have fueled two "Congo Wars"—occasionally referred to as Africa's world wars since so many nations were involved.

I arrived in the capital Kinshasa on the evening of 6 August. The airport was thronged with people meeting incoming passengers—hugging, or (in the case of men) performing the head knock, in which they touch alternating sides of the forehead, in the traditional greeting. One box in our luggage had not arrived (a common occurrence), the one containing our mosquito nets and mosquito coils. The DRC is a malaria-endemic country, so as a precaution I required everyone on my team to take the anti-Malaria drug Malarone. However, I myself had not been taking it. As mentioned before, this was because—paradoxically—I traveled to Africa so often. I preferred to avoid any risk of the potentially harmful side effects from long-term use of the drug.

I set about my activities early the following morning. To begin with, I traveled to Bas-Congo province to visit the Kivuvu Hospital. My mode of transport was a privately chartered minibus. The DRC has no public transportation system to speak of. People wishing to do long-distance travel have to rely on cars alone. The road conditions were relatively good, and I arrived in four hours.

Kivuvu Hospital is a regional health center that originally functioned as a leprosarium. As illnesses other than leprosy can be readily treated in the nearby city of Kimpese, effectively Kivuvu Hospital was providing necessary treatment only to patients with leprosy, as well as those with leprosy reactions and related afflictions such as neuritis and eye complications. After spending time talking with hospitalized patients, offering them words of encouragement, I proceeded to visit a colony of people affected by leprosy not far away, where I observed how they eked out a modest living from agriculture and needlework. The people looked truly careworn and exhausted, their living quarters barely able to keep out the elements. I was surprised at the lines of drying laundry, and I could only assume that the numbers of children had something to do with it. The children here were like children the world over, friendly and smiling, without any shyness. My heart ached to think of how much they could achieve, how their lives would be bettered, if they could only have just a little schooling.

With its vast land area, the DRC is like a continent in itself. It is also a veritable department store of diseases—not only tuberculosis, malaria, and AIDS but also diseases that are particular to Africa, such as sleeping sickness and Ebola. This posed considerable difficulties for leprosy elimination activities. The situation was exacerbated by poor health services coverage and utilization, few medical personnel, and scant medical supplies, not to mention the fact that in the war zones in the country's northern and eastern sectors, the provisional government exercised no control whatsoever.

Nevertheless, there were reasons to remain hopeful. For example, in recent years a system of trained "community agents" who act as a medium between the local community and the health services had been implemented, leading to greater early detection of leprosy. Further, though I could see that the country was unlikely to meet the WHO's target date for eliminating leprosy, the end of 2005, I sensed a willingness among officials to map out a workable strategy. Rather than bewailing the unlikelihood of meeting the target, it seemed to me more effective to help them work out what kind of approach might lead to definite improvements—with the implication that this would lead to meeting the target sooner rather than later. I told the officials I met that I wanted to do anything I could to make sure that the commitment and passion I saw among medical personnel did not get wasted. Proactive cooperation from the top echelons of government would be indispensable in order to achieve this.

I proceeded to discuss matters with the health minister, the chief cabinet secretary, and with the DRC's vice president, pressing them for a commitment to work for leprosy's elimination and for an end to discrimination against all those affected by the disease. I should add that work in developing countries like the DRC calls for a great deal of sensitivity and tact. I had to choose my words very carefully. If I were too pessimistic and damning in my presentation of the situation, that might be taken as insulting. In the end, the health minister shook my hand and voiced his willingness to hold meetings between government officers and the WHO and NGOs to map out a workable strategy for making effective use of NGO support, which seemed to have been lacking up to that point.

To complement efforts promised by the DRC government, I arranged for a meeting at the WHO office in Kinshasa involving the health minister, officials of the health ministry, NGOs, and members of the media, about 100 people in all. My aim was to enlist everyone's help in spreading accurate knowledge about leprosy to as many people as possible. The meeting was followed by a press conference. Here I outlined our three basic messages—that leprosy is curable, that drugs are available for free, and the social discrimination is unacceptable—and asked that they be disseminated widely. Virtually all the major local media followed up the next day, reporting my visit as the WHO Ambassador for Leprosy Elimination together with the three messages.

After this, I headed to Lubumbashi, the capital city of Katanga province, accompanied by the health minister and a couple of the president's advisors. This entailed a flight in an airplane that seemed alarmingly old and rickety. I had heard a story that the airplane used in an infamous 1970 hijacking incident of Japan Airlines Flight 351 (known as the "Yodo-go hijack") had somehow found its way to the DRC; it had apparently crashed into a mountain sometime before. Throughout the flight, nobody said a word—which was strange for the DRC, where people talk loudly in a lively, animated fashion—until we landed, whereupon they broke out in loud applause.

Lubumbashi, situated some 200 kilometers from the border with Zambia, is the DRC's second largest city. It is also the location of the headquarters of the UN peacekeeping forces in the country. Soldiers in khaki uniforms were a visible presence. Katanga province is rich in deposits of diamonds, copper, cobalt, and uranium, and in former times the uranium produced here was exported via Belgium to the United States, where it was used in the atomic bombs dropped on Hiroshima and Nagasaki.

I began my visit to Lubumbashi with a meeting with Katanga's provincial governor, Dr. Urbain Kisula Ngoy. He told me that the prevalence rate for leprosy in his province was high—3.94 per 10,000 population—and that the measures for combating the disease were far from adequate. He was well aware of the purpose of my visit and was grateful for it.

After our meeting, Nr. Nogy and I, together with the health minister, gave a press conference in a conference room adjacent to the governor's office. Roughly fifty members of the local media were in attendance, and we requested their support and cooperation to help eliminate leprosy in the DRC. The health minister revealed, in front of the cameras, that he'd had two uncles who had leprosy—an admission spoken with a quiet frankness that made a profound impression on me, as well as everyone else present.

For the second half of my stay, I traveled to Katanga province. Here I wanted to pay a visit to Kapolowe, a village 120 kilometers to the northwest. Our group of vehicles traveled at more than 100 kilometers per hour along the roads, and at one point the police car leading the way came to a sudden halt, apparently due to engine trouble, and all the cars behind proceeded to crash into each other, creating a pile-up. But somehow the goddess of fortune must have been looking after us, because the damage to our transport was light: we emerged unscathed. We often have to make long-distance journeys in cars for our leprosy work, and in Africa, despite the fact that the roads are not crowded, there are quite a few traffic accidents. On our journeys, it's not at all uncommon to find ourselves driving past trucks overturned in ditches, or past multiple empty husks of cars. The possibility of a car accident was just one of the many risks we had to be prepared to face during our leprosy-elimination activities around the world.

In Kapolowe, I was welcomed by a throng of people singing and dancing in the main square, located close to the local leprosy hospital

183

and to a small community of people affected by leprosy. There must have been several hundred people, including people affected by leprosy, hospital staff, and villagers. I joined in, dancing with the local children, enjoying myself greatly. The lingua franca of the DRC is French, but in Kapolowe and the area around it the people mainly speak Swahili. Though I always try my best to learn a little of the local language on my travels, and I also adopt the modes of dress, I hadn't learned anything about Swahili, so I used dancing to express my gladness to be there. I then went on a tour of the wards in the hospital, greeting each patient with a shake of the hand or a hug. In the village, the residents were making sandals and weaving baskets. They each make three or four baskets a day, for which they earn the equivalent of $1. Given that the average annual income in the DRC is about $100, this struck me as a decent wage. Nothing brings me greater pleasure than to see people like this eager to be socially rehabilitated, engaging in productive activities. The pride and satisfaction were evident on their faces.

During this visit, I learned that in the DRC the word *sasakawa* often appears in people's names and in place names with the sense of "he who imparts light." I came away with renewed determination to continue my activities here in order to "impart light" to people affected by leprosy and to everyone involved in local elimination activities, so as to live up to the name.

On my return to Japan, once again we spent a long time, five hours, waiting to board the plane in Charles de Gaulle Airport in Paris. My team members stocked up on gifts in the airport shops. Never one for shopping myself, I contented myself, as is my practice, with carrying their baggage.

A land where discrimination does not exist—the Democratic Republic of Timor-Leste, September 2005

Route: Narita, Japan → Denpasar, Bali, Indonesia (flight time: 7h; one-night stopover) → Dili, Timor-Leste (flight time: 1h 50m)—one night—Dili, Timor-Leste → Oecusse (flight time: 45m by helicopter) → Dili (flight time: 45m) → Denpasar (flight time: 1h 50m; 12h stopover) → Narita (flight time: 7h)

At the beginning of September, I made a brief visit to Timor-Leste (sometimes known as East Timor), making my way there via Bali. A tiny country roughly the size of Japan's Nagano prefecture, Timor-Leste had a population of about 1 million people. Timor-Leste occupies half of the island of Timor. The other half is known as West Timor. East Timor was taken over by Portugal (which wanted its sandalwood) in the sixteenth century, and West Timor was colonized by France in the seventeenth century, so the island entered the twentieth century as two countries, occupied by two different colonial powers. The Japanese occupied the island in 1942, and at the end of the Second World War the west half of the island became part of the newly formed nation of Indonesia. The east half remained a colony of Portugal and gained independence only in 1975. But East Timor was then annexed by Indonesia and there followed a prolonged and very violent guerrilla campaign. A referendum in 1999 held in accordance with a UN-sponsored agreement between Indonesia and Portugal showed that the people rejected the offer of autonomy within Indonesia, and Indonesia relinquished control of the territory. For a while, the UN temporarily governed East Timor, until 2002 when the country became independent and officially changed its name to Timor-Leste. The first democratically elected president of the new nation was Xanana Gusmão, a former rebel.

The violent conflict during the Indonesian occupation that had preceded the UN intervention and subsequent independence left a healthcare infrastructure in tatters. Many buildings were just shattered ruins. However, the return of peace saw health services gradually improving. Dr. Alex Andjaparidze, the head of the WHO country office for Timor-Leste, told me that in the last eighteen months or so smiles had returned to people's faces, and the local people were beginning to relax with him. At present, for a population of 1 million people, he told me, there were only about thirty-four doctors. There was a dearth of hospitals and health centers, and very poor sanitation.

Against this backdrop, leprosy elimination had made good progress, due in no small part to the efforts of Dr. Andjaparidze. According to the most up-to-date figures, the current prevalence rate was 3.6 per 10,000 population. However, in a special administrative East Timorese region, an enclave called Oecusse, located in West Timor, the prevalence rate was extremely high: 24.2. The tiny size of Timor-Leste's population, less than 1 million, meant that it could not be included in the WHO list of countries that had yet to reach the target.

In the course of my short stay of four days, I met President Gusmão, Health Minister Dr. Rui Maria de Araújo, Dr. Alex Andjaparidze, and many UN officials, and I asked them, as I always do, to join me in spreading my three main messages. During these meetings, one thing I heard repeatedly was that in Oecusse, people who had been affected by leprosy had long been able to live entirely without discrimination. At first, I thought I had misheard, but it kept being mentioned.

On the second day, traveling by UN helicopter, I flew with UN personnel from the capital Dili to Oecusse. As I stepped out, I was greeted by a band playing "The Rabaul Ditty," a nostalgic wartime song composed by the Japanese composer Shimaguchi Komao. In Oecusse, I took part in a ceremony to congratulate more than 200 people on the successful completion of their treatment. The health minister and the WHO personnel seemed sure that, even if it didn't

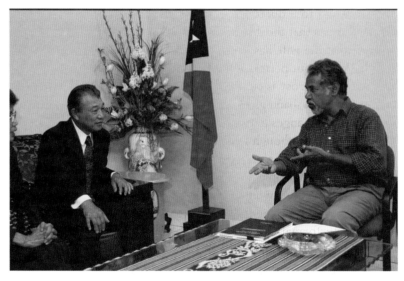

33. In talks with President Gusmão, a man who formerly was imprisoned for a period of 6 years as a rebel (Timor-Leste, September 2005)

meet the 2005 deadline, Timor-Leste would be able to meet the WHO benchmark by the end of 2007, and I promised to visit again to celebrate the achievement.

The ambassadors of the United States, the UK, and Australia were also in attendance at the ceremony. Ambassador Margaret Twomey of Australia told me that her grandfather Patrick Twomey had founded the Pacific Leprosy Foundation, a leprosarium working on behalf of the people affected by leprosy who inhabited Makogai Island in the Fijian Group. She told me how as a child she had helped her grandfather and her father to care for the patients. She thus took a personal interest in leprosy and had found today's ceremony moving.

The event also featured an outdoor play. The people watching it were falling about with laughter, but I couldn't follow it since it was in the local language, and I asked one of the East Timorese officials to tell me what was going on. It was all about a couple of newly-weds. The husband shows symptoms of leprosy and goes to consult a local medicine man, who prepares a concoction for him to drink, instructing him that while taking this medicine he is to refrain from sex with his wife. The husband thinks a little, and then asks if he can wait just a couple of hours before taking the medication. Meanwhile, the wife decides to go to a doctor in a clinic for a screening—though the husband insists that the doctor must not touch her body. The doctor suspects that the wife has leprosy and asks to be allowed to examine her physically, but permission is denied. The doctor explains to the husband that leprosy is curable, and there is no need to be afraid—and finally the husband gives permission for his wife to be examined. Each of the exchanges between the players was very comically performed, and even though I couldn't understand the dialogue I soon found myself laughing along with everyone else. The point of the play was to encourage people not to rely on traditional healers, and to go to clinics: there, they would get medicine free of charge and be sure of getting cured. In regions of low literacy, such methods, involving theatrical performances, dance, and song, even magic shows, are extremely effective in getting the message across.

It was a pleasure to spend time with President Gusmão, whom I had met previously during one of his visits to Japan. A mild-mannered person, it was difficult to imagine that he had once been a warrior who had fought as a leader of the guerrilla forces fighting the Indonesian occupation and had spent six years in prison. He told me of his dreams for Timor-Leste's future, and I promised him that I would do everything within my power to help.

Media Partnership Workshops—Republic of India (West Bengal, Bihar, Assam, and Uttar Pradesh), September and October 2005

> Route: Narita, Japan → Bangkok, Thailand (flight time: 6h; 2h 20m stopover) → Kolkata, West Bengal, India (flight time: 2h 30m)—three nights—Kolkata → Patna, Bihar (flight time: 50m)—one night—Patna → Kolkata (flight time: 50m)—one night—Kolkata → Guwahati, Assam (flight time: 1h)—one night—Guwahati → Kolkata (flight time: 1h; 6h stopover 6h) → Singapore (flight time: 4h; 3h stopover) → Narita, Japan (flight time: 6h 50m) → Beijing, China (flight time: 4h)—two nights (Steering Committee Meeting of Sasakawa Japan–China Friendship Fund)—Beijing → Singapore (flight time: 6h; 4h stopover) → New Delhi, India (flight time: one night) → Lucknow, Uttar Pradesh (flight time: 50m)—one night—Lucknow → New Delhi (flight time: 1h; 6h stopover) (meetings with WHO Southeast Asia Regional Office Director Dr. Samlee Plianbangchang) → Narita (flight time: 7h 20m)

During September and October, I again took trips to India. In 2005, I visited India many times. The trip in September was to Kolkata in West Bengal, Patna in Bihar, and Guwahati in Assam. The trip in October was to Lucknow in Uttar Pradesh. On these trips, I took part in a number of media workshops, in which the aim was to heighten awareness about the important role the media has to play in leprosy elimination work.

The official name of these workshops was Media Partnership Workshops, and they were organized by a communications consultancy, ICONS Media, in association with ILU and IDEA India, and with support from the Sasakawa Memorial Health Foundation and the Nippon Foundation. The workshops had several objectives, the most important being to familiarize the media with leprosy, raise awareness of the movement to ensure the socio-economic integration of people affected by leprosy, discuss ways of fighting the social stigma and discrimination, and discourage sensationalist coverage and the use of derogatory terms such as "leper." Part of the reason the discrimination and social stigma about leprosy remain so deep-rooted in India has to do with the way the disease is often portrayed on television and in newspapers. We wanted journalists and editors to come to the workshops and listen first-hand to what people who had recovered from the disease have to struggle with in their daily lives, so that they could address these issues in their reporting. At the workshops, the journalists and editors were given briefings about leprosy, shown a documentary about leprosy and human rights, and presented with books, written in the Hindi and Bengali language, relating the personal experiences of twelve people affected by leprosy.

No matter how much we strive to reduce the number of people with leprosy, there can be no solution to the problem of social discrimination unless we enlighten the very people who engage in discrimination, so that such views disappear. With this in mind, we planned to hold eight of these Media Partnership Workshops in different parts of the country, out of our strong sense that the media in India tended to perpetuate the problem—often engaging in sensationalist reporting, with incorrect knowledge of the disease and ignoring the privacy and rights of people affected by leprosy. The meetings were attended by state governors, state health ministers, and WHO representatives, who addressed the media on the importance of changing their assumptions and methodology and appealed for their cooperation. In all, around 150 members of the media attended the day-long workshops in the four states in September and October.

As I traveled about the four states where the workshops were held, on some days I was individually interviewed by as many as twelve newspapers and five TV stations. I soon realized that the questions I was being asked were nearly always the same—and most of the questions still had to do with how leprosy was transmitted. I was also disappointed to notice that even after attending our workshop and gaining an understanding of the issues, some members of the media still made unconscious use of the discriminatory term "leper."

One of the most effective ways of ensuring the end of discrimination against leprosy is to get the younger generation on board. I was happy to note that attending each of the workshops were twenty to thirty student journalists in their respective regions. We held contests to create posters on the topic of "leprosy elimination." The call for entries had been issued in advance, and the works submitted were judged during the workshop. The three best teams were presented with awards. Some of the entries depicted people with leprosy in a tragic light, with the aim of eliciting sympathy. I wanted to know whether participation in the workshop had done anything to change their views on people affected with leprosy, so I asked the winners to tell me. They said their notions about people with leprosy had indeed changed, and if another opportunity arose they would concentrate more on positive stories—creating more humanistic portraits, featuring successful outcomes, showing that it was not all doom and gloom. This made me feel as if the project had some effect. All we had to do was give people the right information, while they are still young and with open minds. These young students would go on to become journalists whose work would truly educate and inspire.

Numerous people who had recovered from leprosy participated in the workshops. We wanted to put them up in hotels—and we managed to do this, with the help of the conference coordinating office and the kind cooperation of the hotel staff. For many, this was their first experience in fancy accommodation, and I was happy to see the staff kindly explaining how the buffet worked and how to operate the shower and bath in the rooms.

While in Kolkata, I visited the Premananda Memorial Leprosy Hospital, a facility run by TLM, and spoke with some seventy patients. The hospital was fortunate enough to have a superb plastic surgeon whose sophisticated reconstructive surgery on the damaged hands and limbs of people affected by leprosy (one of the effects of leprosy can be the so-called "clawed hand," and the disease can affect tendons in the feet as well) brought huge benefits to their lives. People affected by leprosy from other states apparently flocked here for operations.

I also gave a special guest lecture at Jadavpur University, at a ceremony marking the tenth anniversary of the founding of the SYLFF, a scholarship for MA students in the humanities and social sciences. I spoke on leprosy and human rights before an audience of roughly 200 faculty and students. The chancellor of the university is West Bengal's governor, Gopalkrishna Gandhi: Mahatma Gandhi's youngest grandson. Like his grandfather, Gopal Gandhi is greatly concerned with leprosy elimination.

Another place I visited was the Gandhiji Prem Nivas Leprosy Centre in Titagarh on the outskirts of Kolkata. Founded by Mother Teresa in 1958 to house an existing community of people with leprosy, it currently sees about 400 patients a month who come for medical attention. I was shown around by the former director, Dr. Chowdry. About 200 people affected by leprosy and their families also live at the center, where there were workshops for spinning and weaving cloth, sandal-making, and carpentry (making artificial limbs). The center stretches across a narrow 10-kilometer strip that runs on either side of the Titagarh–Khardaha railway, donated by the Titagarh municipality, and residents and staff have to step across the railway lines, taking care of passing trains as they go about their daily tasks. With the dedicated care of the Sisters of the Missionaries of Charity, the place seemed to me to be running well. In an ideal world, these people affected by leprosy would be able to gain a living for themselves by returning to their communities. But before that could happen, prejudice against leprosy would have to disappear, and industries in the regions would have to be willing to extend opportunities both in education and in the workplace. I was keen to find philanthropic industrialists who would be able to galvanize local businesses to offer people affected by leprosy jobs and extend funding to provide young people with an education.

My visit to Assam (in northern India; above Bangladesh) was somewhat restricted due to an ongoing insurgency. No sooner had we arrived at the hotel than I was told that as a visitor at the behest of the government, it would be wiser for me not to take one step outside. So there I was, stuck inside the whole time. Members of my team went for strolls in the streets, but I had to wait at the hotel, "on hold," with no option but to read books. Not able to take lunch, I began to feel like a hostage. Several media teams came and interviewed me. The only time I stepped out of the hotel was when representatives of the northeast Chamber of Commerce invited me to dinner—which was, however, only served at 10 o'clock in the evening.

Northeast India is where a famous battle of the Second World War, the Battle of Imphal, took place in 1944. In this battle, Japanese

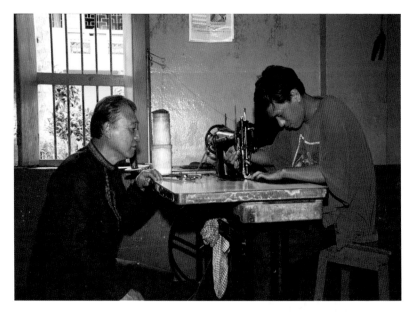

34. A person affected by leprosy at his sewing machine (Bihar, India, September 2005)

armies invaded from Myanmar (or Burma) and attempted to destroy the British forces, which included Indian units, but were driven back into Burma with heavy losses on both sides. In Imphal, there is a museum to Chandra Bose, a man who played a major role in the struggle for Indian independence from Britain, and who also fought in this battle—though he was fighting with the Japanese. In 2019, the Nippon Foundation built the Imphal Peace Museum as a living memorial of that battle. A framed work of calligraphy of the Japanese characters for Heiwa ("peace"), written by Japanese Prime Minister Shinzo Abe and presented to the museum, is on display. As I said at the opening ceremony, India's postwar independence and peace today are the legacy of the ultimate suffering of those who fell in this war. My impression was that there was a lot of interest in strengthening ties with Japan in this area. The opening ceremony, I remember, was attended by the British high commissioner and Japan's ambassador to India.

REACHING THE UNREACHABLE

The Forum 2000 conference and the addition of a new feature—Czech Republic, October 2005

Route: Narita, Japan → Frankfurt, Germany (flight time: 12h; 1h 40m stopover) → Prague, Czech Republic (flight time: 1h)—three nights—Prague → Frankfurt, Germany (flight time: 1h; 2h stopover) → Narita (flight time: 12h)

In October 2005, I visited Prague to participate in the annual Forum 2000 conference. As I have already outlined, this is an international summit that has taken place every year since Václav Havel, Ellie Wiesel, and I started it in 1997, attracting a wide array of illustrious people. In 2001, the fifth Forum 2000 conference, when the theme was "Human Rights—Global Responsibility," I gave the opening remarks in a special session entitled "The Human Right to Health."

In 2005, the theme was "Our Global Co-Existence: Challenges and Hopes for the 21st Century." This time, during the opening ceremony, I talked about the Global Appeal, which I was preparing to launch in January 2006, and I took the opportunity to ask the Nobel laureates and world leaders present at the Forum 2000 in October 2005 whether they would sign it when the time came. Irish President Mary Robinson, Elie Wiesel, Óscar Arias, Václav Havel, His Holiness the Dalai Lama, Archbishop Desmond Tutu, and Prince El Hassan bin Talal of Jordan endorsed the appeal at a later date.

The Forum 2000 had a new feature that had in fact been conceived earlier that year, in April 2005, called the Shared Concern Initiative. It involved giving the option to an open and informal group of personalities present at Forum 2000 of supporting a joint statement with the aim of addressing the major challenges of today's world, "with the understanding that changes towards the better can be effectively promoted with a common voice." Many years later, in 2011, I put together the following joint statement on human rights and leprosy:

STATEMENT: Human Rights and Leprosy

At the end of last year, the United Nations General Assembly unanimously adopted a resolution approving principles and guidelines to end discrimination against people affected by leprosy and their family members.

This resolution marked the culmination of several years of lobbying of UN institutions by groups and individuals devoted to focusing attention on an overlooked human rights issue: the social discrimination suffered by people diagnosed with leprosy. Indeed, the discrimination usually continues even after they are cured, blighting not only their lives, but the lives of other members of their families.

For much of its long history, leprosy was feared as an incurable, disfiguring disease. People who came down with it were ejected from their communities. They often ended up in isolated villages or remote islands, condemned by society to spend the rest of their days as social outcasts.

Today, leprosy is cured by multi-drug therapy (MDT), a course of treatment that kills, after the first dose alone, 99.9 percent of the bacteria that cause leprosy. Since MDT was introduced in the early 1980s, some 16 million people have been cured worldwide. Yet, even after a person is free of the disease, the stigma attached to leprosy has the potential to disrupt people's lives in ways that no drug can cure.

Educational opportunities, job prospects, married life, family relationships, and community participation are all potentially threatened by leprosy. In some countries, discrimination is sanctioned by law, with leprosy treated as legitimate grounds for divorce, for example. Even members of the medical profession have been known to discriminate against patients with leprosy.

Many of the problems faced by people affected by leprosy today stem from society's ignorance about the disease. It is mistakenly assumed to be highly contagious, and therefore sufferers are to be avoided at all costs. Moreover, deeply entrenched notions that leprosy is divine punishment destroy the reputation and self-esteem of those thus diagnosed and cast a shadow over their families.

The principles and guidelines endorsed by the UN resolution go to the heart of the issues. They state that no one should be discriminated against on the grounds of having or having had leprosy. They call on governments to abolish discriminatory legislation and remove discriminatory language from official publications; to provide the same range and quality of health care to persons affected by leprosy as to those with other diseases; and to promote social inclusion.

But the UN resolution is, unfortunately, not a binding document. It can only recommend that states and civil society observe the principles and guidelines that it puts forward. It is very important, therefore, that this resolution is not simply filed away and forgotten. It must be used by states as a roadmap to bring about an end to the unjust and intolerable discrimination that those with leprosy face.

We call on states to use the opportunity afforded by the UN's historic resolution to work toward a world where people affected by leprosy and their family members can live with dignity and play their part in the life of the community. It is time to bring an end to this gross violation of human rights. Such a world is long overdue.

The signatories to the joint statement were His Royal Highness El Hassan Bin Talal, André Glucksmann, Vartan Gregorian, Frederik Willem de Klerk, Václav Havel, Michael Novak, Yohei Sasakawa, Karel Schwarzenberg, Desmond Tutu, and Grigory Yavlinsky.

Jerejak Island, the Valley of Hope—Malaysia, November 2005

Route: Narita, Japan → Kota Kinabalu, Sabah, Malaysia (flight time: 6h)—two nights

In November 2005, I visited Malaysia and Indonesia. Both of these countries had achieved elimination at the national level several years before, but I wanted to observe the current state of leprosy countermeasures and offer my encouragement.

In Malaysia, I visited the province of Sabah, on the north coast of Borneo. Sabah had a population of 2.86 million, or 11 percent of Malaysia's total. Kota Kinabalu is popular with Japanese tourists, famous for its remarkable nature reserve—which has the highest peak in Malaysia, Mount Kinabalu—as well as its forests and amazing wildlife, in particular the orangutan.

For a number of years, the Nippon Foundation has held annual workshops for fifty leading Asian public intellectuals in what we call the Asian Public Intellectual Fellowship program, and one of the purposes of this trip was to deliver the opening speech at the third such workshop. It was sad to think that even in such a tropical paradise leprosy was still to be found in certain places. Nationwide, the leprosy prevalence rate was roughly 0.3 per 10,000, but in Sabah it was rather higher at 0.44, and there were several areas in the province where the rate topped one person per 10,000.

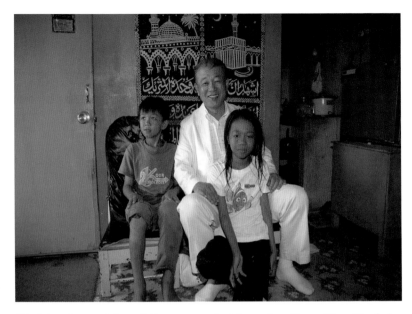

35. A brother and sister fully recovered with no aftereffects (Kota Kinabalu, Malaysia, November 2005)

Local health officials I consulted in Sabah told me that there were plans for concentrated information and education activities about leprosy, with particular focus on five regions that still had high prevalence rates, as well as plans to create a system of home visits. The health ministry was also looking into training up more health personnel. There were programs in place for the distribution and management of MDT supplies, monitoring of people affected by leprosy, and prevention of subsequent complications. All in all, Sabah seemed well clued up about how to deal with the disease. I only hoped that the words I was hearing would be backed up by actions.

During this trip, I visited two families that were living with leprosy. In one family, there was a lively seventy-eight-year-old lady; in the other, a girl of eleven and a boy of ten. In the second family, the girl was the first to be diagnosed with leprosy, then the whole family got themselves checked out—and the boy was found to have it too. The father and the uncle had been affected in the past. Sabah's health services were quick to react, and so the little ones were well on the way to recovery, having been diagnosed and started on a course of treatment at an early stage in the disease. I should mention that I saw a Mercedes-Benz car at the home of the first family. Leprosy is often talked about as a disease of the poor, but it can also strike the wealthiest members of society.

Sabah has a large floating population of migrant workers from Kalimantan, in southern Borneo, which is part of Indonesia, and the Philippines. In fact, some 60 percent of the leprosy cases detected in the province come from abroad—people are either diagnosed while in Sabah or make their way across the border after being diagnosed to benefit from the province's medical services. This poses all sorts of problems, not only in terms of being able to make sure patients complete their treatment but also in that it raises the prevalence figures beyond what they should be. The fact that people prefer to come to Malaysia for treatment also indicates something inadequate in the state of the health services in these other countries.

Giving a boost to the flagging struggle—Republic of Indonesia, December 2005

> Route: Kota Kinabalu, Malaysia → Kuala Lumpur, Malaysia (flight time: 2h 25m; 2h stopover) → Jakarta, Indonesia (flight time: 1h 40m)—one night—Jakarta → Surabaya (flight time: 1h)—one night—Surabaya → Ujung Pandang (flight time: 1h 30m)—one night—Ujung Pandang → Manado (flight time: 1h 30m)—two nights

From Malaysia, I flew straight on to Jakarta, Indonesia. Indonesia achieved elimination nationally in 2000, and the current prevalence rate was just under one per 10,000 population. However, with a total population of 200 million people (at the time of my visit), making it one of the world's most populous nations, Indonesia still had the third highest number of patients in the world, after India and Brazil—with some 20,000 new cases registered every year. (In fact, India, Brazil, and Indonesia have 80 percent of the total number of people with leprosy in the world.) On a national level, the country had achieved elimination, but there were many regions where the target had not been reached. Part of the problem is that this nation consists of numerous far-flung islands, which makes for difficulties in detection.

MAKING THE IMPOSSIBLE POSSIBLE

On my arrival in Jakarta, I went first to a briefing with Health Minister Siti Fadilah Supari and Vice President Jusuf Kalla. I was told that the priority diseases in Indonesia were now malaria, TB, dengue fever, and more recently avian flu. Concern with leprosy at the national level had lapsed. The numbers of registered cases and the prevalence rates had flatlined over the past ten years. Out of thirty regions, twelve had still to achieve elimination, meaning that in those places the prevalence rate was more than one person per 10,000 population. I replied that while I fully understood that the budget was tight, it was still extremely important to keep leprosy high on their list of priorities. I asked that the government issue some stern directives to local authorities to put some fresh energy into their anti-leprosy measures. I also asked that the government disseminate our three important messages pertaining to leprosy.

The main purpose of my trip was to attend a conference on leprosy elimination, where a new objective for leprosy elimination in Indonesia in 2010 was unveiled. The government, local governments, and NGOs all expressed their commitment to working together for this cause. However, I wanted to assess the situation for myself to make sure that this commitment would be backed up by concrete measures, and so I spent the rest of my time visiting two regions where leprosy prevalence rates remain high, the city of Surabaya in East Java and Sulawesi Island, in order to see what the conditions were like with my own eyes. There I took tours of clinics, hospitals, and settlements.

Surabaya is the second-largest city in Indonesia, after Jakarta, and the capital city of the province of East Java. About 30 percent of Indonesia's leprosy cases are to be found in East Java. The prevalence rate is 1.85 persons per 10,000 population. Sulawesi is an island located in the middle of the Indonesian archipelago. Makassar is the capital and the largest city in eastern Indonesia. It is located in the south of the island. Manado is located in the north. Sulawesi has always had a lot of people affected by leprosy. The prevalence rate is 2.27 persons per 10,000 population in the south, and 3.01 persons per 10,000 population in the north.

I visited a number of facilities and clinics, including the Jatinegara Medical Center in Jakarta and the Daya Leprosy Hospital and the

Cendrawasih Medical Center in Makassar. All of them were spick and span, and they had some excellent equipment. But this started to trouble me. The Daya Leprosy Hospital has 200 beds, and 226 members of staff, but I noticed that almost three-quarters of the beds were empty. The state-of-the-art equipment was unused—simply gathering dust. Such large, specialized leprosy hospitals are anyway unnecessary in this day and age now that we have MDT. And nowadays it is generally agreed that people affected by leprosy can be treated in general hospitals, without being segregated in their own wards. And leprosy clinics too are accepting patients with other diseases. Ideally, people affected by leprosy ought not to be admitted to hospital at all but should be able to carry on living in their communities, taking their medicine and having periodic check-ups. This would solve the problem of discrimination and also ease the way for social rehabilitation. The Daya Leprosy Hospital had been built in 1984, I learned, which was after MDT started being distributed free of charge. The fact that it had been built at all was completely out of step with the latest thinking, and pointed to a problem with governance.

In Surabaya, I visited the ninety-three families living in the Babat Jerawat leprosy settlement. Everybody I met seemed in good heart, the women clearly making an effort with their appearance and the children running about happily. The Jongaya leprosy settlement in Makassar had a similarly cheerful atmosphere, and the head of the settlement gave me a loud rendition of a Japanese military song as a welcome. Even if there was discrimination outside the settlement, I thought, within it there was a discernibly positive spirit of self-help and togetherness. Even so, I couldn't help thinking that an effective strategy for information, education, and communication would have taken away any need for a separate village of people affected by leprosy at all. One person asked me why Indonesia was so laggardly in leprosy control. To which I replied: "That's what I've come to find out!"

I was thus heartened by the situation on Bunaken, a beautiful coral island that I reached after a forty-five-minute boat journey from Manado. Here I saw people affected by leprosy living close together with others in the village rather than separately in a settlement. In a population of some 1,500, eleven people were being treated for lep-

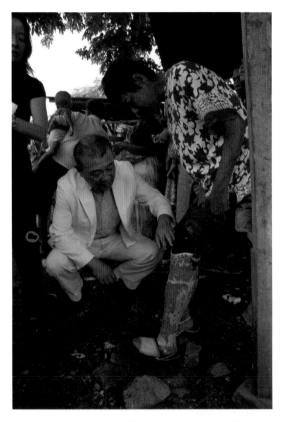

36. How does the prosthetic leg feel? Is it comfortable? (Babat Jerawat leprosy settlement, Indonesia, December 2005)

rosy, and twelve had fully recovered. Eleven new cases had been detected in 2005. Even so, there seemed to be no consciousness of people having the disease, with people socializing freely and wandering in and out of one another's homes without compunction. People being treated for the disease were gainfully employed. Self-help groups had been started by those who had recovered. Admittedly, it was happening on a small scale, but this seemed to me to epitomize what we were working for: people with leprosy living in their communities with joy, pride, and dignity. On Bunaken, I was presented with an example that I hoped very much would be emulated in other parts of Indonesia.

In Makassar, in the south of Sulawesi, I visited the National Leprosy Training Center. Though specialist leprosy hospitals per se are not necessary, this place plays a crucial role both in nurturing human resources and as a resource center for passing on and disseminating leprosy-related information and knowhow. To date, some 3,000 medical officers, 1,500 doctors, and 1,000 medical students had received training here. I had no doubt that it would continue to play a key role in sustaining Indonesia's fight against the disease and in maintaining the quality of the services offered to leprosy patients.

The gifts of dignity and respect—Republic of India (New Delhi, Haryana state, and Rajasthan state), December 2005

Route: Manado, Indonesia → Jakarta (flight time: 2h; 3h stopover) → Singapore (flight time: 3h; 3h stopover) → Delhi (flight time: 5h 30m)—two nights—Delhi → Chennai, Tamil Nadu (flight time: 2h 30m)—one night—Chennai → Singapore (flight time: 4h; 2h stopover) → Narita (flight time: 6h 30m) → Kuala Lumpur, Malaysia (flight time: 7h; 1h 30m stopover) → Delhi, India (flight time: 5h 20m)—two nights—Delhi → Jaipur, Rajasthan (flight time: 1h 40m)—two nights—Jaipur → Delhi (flight time: 1h 40m)—two nights—Delhi → Jaipur, Rajasthan (flight time: 1h 40m)—two nights—Jaipur → Delhi (flight time: 1h 40m)—one night—Delhi → Bangkok, Thailand (flight time: 4h; 2h stopover) → Yangon, Myanmar (flight time: 1h)—one night—Yangon → Bangkok (flight time: 1h; stopover 2h) → Narita (flight time: 6h 30m)

In December 2005, I visited India twice. The first trip to India was simply as an extra leg to the trip I had made to Malaysia and Indonesia in late October. The purpose for that trip was a brief stay to meet with key members in India's business community to ask for their understanding and support principally in raising funds for the establishment of what was to become the Sasakawa India Leprosy Foundation (S-ILF) and go over what needed to be done in preparation. I paid visits to the Confederation of Indian Industry and the India Chamber of Commerce and was able to have constructive meetings with both.

I then returned to Japan, where I had a brief pit-stop of five days, after which I turned right round and set off for India again. This trip would be the seventh trip I made to India in 2005. I would be spending time in Delhi and its environs and a state 250 kilometers to the south, Rajasthan.

On the first day of my trip, I visited a settlement located at Lajpat Nagar in the state of Haryana, thirty minutes' drive out of Delhi. At one time, it had consisted of tents pitched along the side of the road, but now the residents lived in brick buildings. Eighty households, 230 or so people, were housed here. Most survived on begging, but recent years had seen more people making a living by selling water to passersby or working as rickshaw drivers.

It was here that I met a fourteen-year-old girl, called Niram, both of whose parents had once had leprosy. Previously, she had attended a local school, but when her classmates had learned that her parents had recovered from leprosy, she had been bullied and eventually had to leave. She hadn't been to school for more than a year, she told me; she longed fervently to return to her studies. I knew there had to be others in her situation, and I promised her that I would look into setting up a school for the colony's residents. Her eyes filled with tears, and in return she sang me the Indian national anthem. The thought of such sweet, innocent children being bullied by their peers made my heart want to burst. Something had to be done to break the stigma, a thought that accompanies me wherever I go.

The other colony I visited on my trip was the Bharat Mata Kusht Ashram, also in Haryana state. This colony started off as a single hut built in 1973 and is now home to some 300 people. The residents had formed a cooperative association, thus building the foundations of an economically self-reliant community. Over 120 residents were now engaged in weaving and other occupations, and they donated a portion of their profits to the cooperative. This money was used to purchase feed for the chickens and livestock, to pay for doctors to come and visit, and to help support those with severe disabilities. However, the electrically powered looms that the Nippon Foundation had bought for the community after a previous visit were not being put to any use, due to the irregular supply of electrical power. This was our error: we had clearly overlooked the problems with the electricity supply in our original visit to investigate the community's needs. Finding the exact fit to needs and solutions is part of the reason I insist on these visits to the frontlines. Nevertheless, at least we were now acquainted with the problem. If I had not visited, I would have left thinking that the job was done.

The following day, I flew to Jaipur in Rajasthan, in the northwest. From Delhi, it was a roughly forty-minute flight. This is the capital and the largest city in the state and is known as the "Pink City of India" due to the dominant terracotta color scheme in its buildings.

Jaipur is the founding place of the NGO known as the Sarthak Manav Kushthashram, an organization set up by well-to-do ladies some thirty years ago to help people affected by leprosy become self-reliant. The colony that is the focal point of their activities is located near a Hindu temple and is home to thirty-seven families comprising eighty people who once had leprosy and their children. Many colonies in India are located close to temples, and residents look to receive alms from worshippers, though they are not allowed into the temple themselves. (They usually construct their own temples within their colonies.)

At this colony, the residents made a living from weaving and making hand-painted cloths. They also manufactured shoes made to order for people who had recovered from leprosy, which were available free of charge. They had set up a collaborative agreement with a European NGO, direct-selling large quantities of the woven products in an arrangement that allowed the residents to live independently. As with Bharat Mata Kusht Ashram, a portion of the profits went toward food, electricity, medicine, and other necessities for the community and supported those who were unable to work. What was left over counted as each individual's income, and some people were making enough to send money to family members living far away. My guide Suresh Kaul told me that thirty years ago each room would have been home to fifteen or so residents. There were no toilet facilities, and hygiene was extremely poor. It was like a waiting room for death, he said. The head of the colony confessed to me that he had come here in fear for his life: when he contracted the disease, his family had turned him out of the house, and a work colleague fearful of infection had tried to stab him—such was the stigma that surrounded the disease. This was another story that instilled in me the determination to neutralize such fear and discrimination and make the true facts about leprosy known.

MAKING THE IMPOSSIBLE POSSIBLE

The following day, we drove three hours south to Ajmer. This is one of the oldest cities in the state of Rajasthan and an important Islamic and Hindu pilgrimage site.

Along the route, as we were ascending a hill, we passed a conglomeration of simple mud huts, built alongside an Islamic pilgrimage route leading to a sacred shrine. Far away in the distance, we could see the beautiful blue and pink roofs of an ancient city in the sunshine. The mud huts were an impoverished village that had sprung up over the last 100 years. Three thousand people lived here, including 180 children. Two percent of the population, we were told, either have leprosy or once had the disease. The weather that day was extremely hot, but the houses, built of mud, were all cool. There were cooking smells. I learned that, unlike the previous colony, here most of the residents survived by begging—and that many people had moved here specifically in order to do so. A number of projects had been designed to help the villagers become economically dependent but had ended in failure—soliciting people for money had become the only way they could survive. While I had to admire the villagers' tenacity, I could not admire this reliance on begging. It offered the villagers no chance to pull themselves out of poverty or ensure that the next generation have better life chances. It's incumbent on people who have recovered from the disease to make every effort to be self-reliant. I was determined to work, and lend as much support as I could, to help them do so. But any real change would ultimately depend on the efforts and outlook of people affected by leprosy themselves.

On this trip, I was able to find the answer to a mystery that had been bothering me since a visit to India two years before. On that visit, I was walking round a rural village when I was taken short, so I asked if I could use the bathroom in one of the dwellings. I was shown inside to a room with three stones set in the floor. Someone in my party used it ahead of me, and I followed suit. But I always wondered afterwards whether that little space actually was a toilet or simply a space for ablution. The person in my team who had asked to enter the house had mimed washing his hands, but perhaps his full intentions weren't clear. And yet here I could see that, in keeping with every colony I saw in India, every shack had a little space to wash in, separated off with some ragged pieces of material. It occurred to me to ask the person showing us round this time where the toilets were. His reply was that I could choose anywhere I liked—outdoors. It was then that I learned that in places that were rural or cut off, the toilet was anywhere outside. So two years ago, I had indeed relieved myself in the equivalent of the shower room. Oh dear, I thought. What a terrible blunder. The owner of the house could only have concluded that Japanese people have the most appalling manners!

The prevalence rate in Rajasthan was 0.31 per 10,000 population, relatively low for India. But the problem of discrimination toward people who have the disease, or who have had it in the past, remains. Here too, I held one of our Media Partnership Workshops, where we urged governments, medical professionals, the media, and business organizations to join us in our projects to inform, educate, and communicate with people about this disease and provide opportunities for people affected by leprosy. I was pleased to see that our workshop received wide coverage in the local newspapers the next day.

Our work in Rajasthan over, my team and I were waiting in the airport to board our flight back to New Delhi when we saw huge crowds of people all decked out in white robes. We asked them what was going on, and they told us they were all making the pilgrimage to Mecca, in Saudi Arabia. Each one of them looked overjoyed. For a fourteen-day trip, each person had had to pay JPY 280,000. One of the true pleasures of travel is these serendipitous encounters.

On 19 December, we were once again back in New Delhi, for a truly memorable event. This was the establishment of a national organization for individuals who had recovered from leprosy, to be called the Indian National Forum, accompanied by a meeting—the National Conference on Integration and Empowerment of People Affected by Leprosy. It might be remembered that earlier on in 2005 on a visit to Tamil Nadu I had suggested taking a survey of all the leprosy colonies in India with a view to holding a conference specifically for people affected by leprosy, and a team led by IDEA President Dr. P. K. Gopal had undertaken a fact-finding survey with help from the Nippon Foundation. Almost no records exist indicating figures and conditions in these colonies, partly because most of them grew up spontaneously, starting out simply as gatherings of people cast out of their communities trying to survive. According to Dr. Gopal's survey, a total of 630 colonies were confirmed in twenty-three of the country's thirty-five states and territories. (Subsequent surveys confirmed this.) The survey also revealed that all colonies had leaders. A good number of these leaders ended up coming to Delhi to attend this conference.

This was a truly landmark gathering—the first time a national conference specifically for and attended by people affected by leprosy had been held in India. Attending were representatives from the leprosy colonies, as well as senior government ministers, health workers, and activists. The fact that colony representatives from all over India had been able to meet under one roof, and share their knowledge and experience, marked a huge step forward. It was both empowering and inspiring—for them and for us. The representatives proceeded to exchange opinions on a whole variety of topics and formulate ideas about how to move forward on the social front. I had every hope that these delegates, previously scattered all over the country, would now be able to meet regularly, see themselves as part of a network, and become part of a powerful movement for change.

The Federation of Indian Chambers of Commerce and Industry Golden Jubilee Auditorium, where the conference took place, was filled to capacity. Included among the 580 people attending were 450 colony leaders who had gathered from all across India. Most had never traveled by railway or airplane before—indeed, most had never even set foot outside their villages and had certainly never stayed in a hotel. "The bed I slept in was so soft—the sheets so clean and white!" they told me. "For the first time in my life I washed myself with hot water!" I was grateful to the staff in the hotel. For them too this was a new experience, and they extended the most gracious service. I should say that originally the participants had been booked to stay at the YMCA, and a deposit had been paid. But when the YMCA learned that the scheduled guests were people affected by leprosy, the arrangement was cancelled. With trepidation, we tried a hotel run by the state government. Fortunately, someone who had previously worked as a project director for the National Leprosy Elimination Programme in Uttar Pradesh was now working for the National Office of Tourism, and thanks to her help we were able to secure rooms, and our guests were treated like any other.

A key document to emerge from this conference was the Delhi Declaration of Dignity. The declaration was read to the assembled audience by Nevis Mary, an Indian woman, then forty-seven, who had contracted leprosy when she was twenty. When the nature of her illness became known to her family, her father had died from the shock. Nevis herself suffered severe discrimination at school and later at her workplace. Today, she was happily married to a supportive husband, and she had vigorously taken up the cause to help others who had the same sorrowful experience. She was also one of those who delivered statements at the UN Commission on Human Rights meeting we'd held in August 2005.

In one address at the conference, a man called Mr. Sarafudin, speaking of how for many years he had battled vigorously against the authorities to improve the lot of people affected by leprosy, and recalling the discrimination he himself had endured, commented: "I don't think of myself as a weak person. If something needs to be accomplished, then it must be achieved not by others but by one's own hands. For this, it's essential to believe in one's own strength; otherwise, the battle cannot be won." Another man, a leader of a colony in Haryana state close to Delhi, spoke of his own experience. "Twenty or thirty years ago, I was a beggar. I never imagined I would be speaking at a large conference like this," he said with great emotion. "Now that momentum to change things is growing among people with leprosy, we should hold meetings all around the country, even in small villages, to spread the word and change perceptions."

Another participant was Anjan Dey, a man who had overcome leprosy to qualify as a physiotherapist at the hospital near Pune, where he had once swept floors as a patient. "Such an event would have been unthinkable just a few years ago," he told the participants in his address.

Two participants were on hand from the Indian government: Union Minister of Social Justice and Empowerment Meira Kumar, and Union Minister for Statistics and Program Implementation Oscar Fernandes. Ms. Kumar spoke of her involvement in eliminating discrimination by revising her nation's divorce laws and by securing a 3 percent quota for educational and employment opportunities for the disabled, including people affected by leprosy. Mr. Fernandes told us stories of body-building athletes in his state who had come to him with tales of how they had been barred from competing simply because there had been leprosy in their family a couple of generations before; he pledged to listen to the voices of people affected by leprosy, his fellow countrymen and women, and do everything he could to alleviate the prejudice against them, giving them back their dignity as was only right.

As the conference drew to its end, I remember one of the participants, an elderly woman from Haryana, approached me with a look of great joy in her eyes. "I was late in arriving and didn't receive the bag and the shawl that were given to all the delegates," she began. "But what I got here today was two things that I never received in the forty years since I contracted leprosy: Respect and dignity." I felt certain that 19 December 2005 would go down in history as the first time people affected by leprosy had spoken out in public on such a scale, and that the events of that day would mark a new beginning for their activities.

We didn't know it during the conference, but a couple of days later India was to issue its announcement that it had eliminated leprosy as a public health problem. For the country that had the largest number of leprosy patients in the world, it was a momentous achievement and marked an important step forward toward achieving the dream of a leprosy-free India.

Here is the text of the Delhi Declaration of Dignity:

Delhi Declaration of Dignity

New Delhi, India, 19 December 2005

Whereas, the preamble to the Universal Declaration of Human Rights, adopted in 1948, recognizes "the inherent dignity" and "the equal and inalienable rights of all members of the human family" as the foundation for freedom, justice and peace in the world;

We, the participants in the National Conference on Integration and Empowerment of Persons Affected by Leprosy, held in Delhi, India, on December 19, 2005, do hereby join together to affirm our dignity and our right to be involved in decisions that affect our lives and our future.

Therefore, as partners working together to eliminate the stigma associated with leprosy and the destructive effects that it has on people's right to live their lives with dignity, we, the participants in this National Conference, do hereby resolve that the following recommendations be adopted in order to promote quality of life, freedom from degrading treatment, and each individual's most basic human rights.

REACHING THE UNREACHABLE

1. Every effort should be made by government agencies, non-governmental organizations and the people themselves to ensure that individuals affected by leprosy are not discriminated against in any way in their daily life, including the areas of education, employment, housing, public transportation, and the availability of medical services.

2. The government should be encouraged to actively promote the human rights of individuals affected by leprosy, and actively prevent violations of these most basic rights.

3. All discriminatory laws, including the law that facilitates divorce due to leprosy, should be repealed.

4. The use of dignified terminology is essential to eliminating the stigma and appropriate language should be used to address people affected by leprosy. Derogatory terms such as "leper," "maharogi," "kodi," etc., should never be used.

5. Opportunities should be provided for individuals and organizations made up of persons affected by leprosy to work in partnership with government agencies and non-governmental organizations to develop activities and programs.

6. Individuals affected by leprosy should be nominated in the State and National Commissions as members under the Persons with Disabilities Act.

7. Every effort should be made to encourage support and inclusion of the person affected by leprosy within their family.

8. Individuals affected by leprosy and organizations representing these individuals should be supported in efforts to develop productive networks that will ensure that the voice of the persons affected by leprosy continues to be heard.

9. Every effort should be made to ensure that children of persons affected by leprosy receive equal opportunities for education and employment.

10. A national effort should be made to ensure that all types of media, including newspapers, films and television, portray individuals affected by leprosy with dignity. The media should be encouraged to become part of the effort to eliminate the stigma by promoting modern, current information about the disease and those affected by it.

11. Proper housing and care should be given to elderly persons affected by leprosy. A reasonable amount not less than Rs. 500/- as pension should be given to the leprosy-disabled persons.

12. Networks to ensure the prevention and treatment of disabilities should be strengthened, especially among hospitals and private health centers.

13. Sustained training programs for government medical staff should be implemented to ensure the ongoing, comprehensive treatment of persons affected by leprosy.

14. Persons affected by leprosy should be afforded their rightful place in the history of leprosy worldwide. Persons affected by leprosy pledge their support to governments and NGOs to eradicate leprosy from the country and to improve the quality of the lives of the persons affected by leprosy.

In conclusion, we strongly affirm that the final victory in the fight against leprosy should only be declared when there are no more persons to be cured, no more disabilities to treat, no more discrimination and human rights violations to overcome, and when persons once affected by the disease can lead normal, integrated and empowered lives with the same opportunities, rights and duties as their fellow citizens.

Persons affected by leprosy

On 20 December, I left India and headed for Myanmar. The purpose of my visit there was to carry out activities that would help the country move forward. There had been a proposal for a national constitution in preparation for the national election scheduled for 2006, but Aung San Suu Kyi was still under house arrest.

In the 1950s, Myanmar was known to have one of the highest prevalence rates of the disease, with the number of cases in 1951 estimated at fifty per 10,000 population, with 100,000 cases in the country as a whole. However, a concerted effort backed by political will had resulted in the country meeting the WHO target of elimination of the disease as a public health problem by January 2003—well before the deadline. WHO recommended MDT to Myanmar in 1986, but for many years there was only limited coverage. One of the most effective schemes rolled out under the leadership of Prime Minister Khin Nyunt was a national network of health workers, known as the "Red Angels." These were nurses, many of them midwives, who rode bicycles and visited people in their homes. The name derived from the long red skirts that they wore along with white blouses. It was for a celebration marking the twentieth anniversary of the founding of the Red Angels that I went to Myanmar this time.

The Nippon Foundation had chosen to continue its activities in support of Myanmar, specifically for its leprosy elimination activities, despite considerable criticism of its association with the military dictatorship that had ruled the country for decades. The Red Angel network had been able to spread life-saving information to the far reaches of the country in an effective system for combating other public health threats as well. Many of the nurses were midwives who paid monthly visits to patients' homes, monitoring their treatment and detecting new cases. Already an integral part of rural life, they were more trusted than outside specialists by the people living in remote regions. The Nippon Foundation had gifted the Red Angels more than 3,000 bicycles to help them in their work. Many years after this, in 2019, we held a National Leprosy Conference in Myanmar, to which Aung San Suu Kyi came. I remember how fervently she listened to all the speakers. It was clear that Health Minister Dr. Myint Htwe had a deep knowledge of leprosy in Myanmar. I vowed to continue to help Myanmar in its elimination activities.

3

THE DRIVE TO SELF-EMPOWERMENT

2006–9

People affected by leprosy who take on the future of humanity

At the end of January 2006, India announced that it had achieved the World Health Organization (WHO) target of leprosy elimination—meaning that its national leprosy prevalence rate was now less than one person per 10,000 population. In the history of leprosy, this was a triumph on a level with the discovery of a cure. Most experts had considered such a thing impossible: leprosy elimination in India required a miracle. Some specialists in Europe and the United States refused to believe it, and one or two even claimed there must be a mistake in the figures. But it was absolutely true: the result of an incalculable amount of effort put in by people in the field who had never swerved in their belief that they could make elimination a reality.

In June 2002, at a conference in Tokyo hosted by the Nippon Foundation, the Sasakawa Health Foundation and WHO's Southeast Asian Regional Office, the Tokyo Declaration was adopted, aimed at eliminating leprosy in India in 2005. At a National Conference on the Elimination of Leprosy held in Raipur in January 2004, we adopted the Raipur Declaration, outlining the specific strategies to be taken.

213

Needless to say, on the front lines, medical workers, NGO staff, and volunteers kept up the fight on a daily level, believing that elimination was possible. And by 2006, they had brought down the prevalence rate, which at the time of the Tokyo Declaration was 3.8 per 10,000 population, to a figure that was less than one—nearly a quarter of what it had been.

Nevertheless, in India, a country with a vast population (as of 2023, 1.41 billion people), 100,000 new cases were still being detected every year, and numerous areas still had a high prevalence rate. Many people affected by leprosy still had no choice but to beg in order to live, even when cured, due to stigma and discrimination. Of course, our ultimate objective was to wipe out leprosy completely, as had been done with smallpox. But unless stigma too was wiped out, and people who had once had the disease were allowed to lead lives like anyone else, instead of being marked indelibly by the experience, that would be meaningless. Of all the many diseases that exist, it is only leprosy that marks a person forever. We never talk of former tubercular people, or people affected by malaria. In the case of those diseases, once a person has recovered, all talk of their previous condition disappears.

In a conversation I once had with the Dalai Lama, I mentioned that my dream was to eradicate begging. I remember His Holiness turned to me with a big smile on his face: "That," he said, "is going to be an impossible job." I had to reply: "But until we try, we will never know. We will never know what's possible or impossible." "Ah yes," His Holiness replied, "Well, you have a point." Leprosy had been eliminated in India, despite all predictions to the contrary. If people give up on things without having even tried, nothing will ever be achieved. His Holiness graciously agreed that it was a goal worth pursuing and has lent me his support ever since.

Over the course of 2005 and 2006, I created two bases through which to conduct leprosy work in India. In December 2005, we took preliminary steps to establish a nationwide organization of people affected by leprosy, fully funded by the Nippon Foundation, to be called the National Forum. (In 2013, it changed its name to the Association of People Affected by Leprosy, or APAL.) In November 2006, I set up the Sasakawa-India Leprosy Foundation, or S-ILF, an organization to provide support to anybody whose life was impacted by leprosy—either currently living with leprosy or recovered from disease—fostering self-empowerment and economic self-reliance; and to support the children of people affected by leprosy.

I also initiated what I decided to call the Global Appeal, a rallying cry issued every January to the whole world, in which I get individuals, organizations, and foundations to publicly put their name to our cause. The idea is to broadcast to as many people as possible the unendurable circumstances faced by people who have experience of leprosy. My first such Global Appeal took place in January 2006. Ever since then, every year I have been issuing a new Global Appeal on the last Sunday of January, World Leprosy Day.

Countries visited in 2006	
January	● India
	United States (New York, the Juilliard School SYLFF work)
February	● Ethiopia
March	● Vietnam
April	● India
	● Philippines
	● Switzerland
May	Malaysia (Presentation ceremony for training ship for navigational safety to Malaysian Maritime Enforcement Agency)
June	● Brazil
	China (Japan–China Field Officer Exchange Program)
July	● United Kingdom (Great Britain Sasakawa Foundation annual general meeting)
	● India
	● Lesotho

August	● Angola
	● Mozambique
September	China (Sasakawa scholarship student workshop)
	● India
	China (Sasakawa Cup Japanese Knowledge Contest)
October	● India
	Czech Republic (Forum 2000 Conference)
	China (World Maritime University Dalian Branch)
	United States (Sasakawa Peace Foundation USA board meeting)
	Mali (SG2000 twentieth anniversary)
November	● Laos
	Thailand (Asian Public Intellectuals fellowship meeting)
	Nepal

● Indicates a trip that features in this section.

SYLFF: Sasakawa Young Leaders Fellowship Fund program.

SG2000: Sasakawa Global 2000 program. An agricultural project supporting farmers in need in Africa.

Forum 2000: An annual international conference launched in 1997 when Václav Havel, Elie Wiesel, and the author invited world leaders to Prague for open debate on the major issues and challenges of the new millennium.

The first Global Appeal and India's announcement of leprosy elimination—Republic of India (New Delhi, West Bengal, Jharkhand), January 2006

Route: Narita, Japan → Bangkok, Thailand (flight time: 5h 40m; 2h stopover) → New Delhi, India (flight time: 4h)—two nights—New Delhi → Kolkata, West Bengal (flight time: 1h 30m)—one night—Kolkata → Ranchi, Jharkhand (flight time: 1h)—two nights—Ranchi → Delhi (flight time: 1h 3m) → Bangkok, Thailand (flight time: 4h; 3h stopover) → Narita

216

THE DRIVE TO SELF-EMPOWERMENT

On 29 January 2006, World Leprosy Day, we launched the very first Global Appeal, in New Delhi. This Global Appeal was a new initiative designed to draw the world's attention to the barriers faced by people affected by leprosy and their family members, with a public announcement made with much fanfare and endorsed by influential individuals—eleven on this occasion (or twelve, including myself)—who lend their voices to the call for a world free of leprosy and leprosy-related discrimination. The voices of these luminaries carry much more weight than I could hope to have as a mere individual working on my own. The launch received widespread media coverage, and it was also reported by twenty-four media outlets in Japan.

Signatories of the first Global Appeal included five Nobel Peace Prize laureates: former US President Jimmy Carter; former President of Costa Rica Óscar Arias; His Holiness the Dalai Lama; Archbishop Emeritus of Cape Town Desmond Tutu; and Elie Wiesel, president of the Elie Wiesel Foundation for Humanity. Other signatories were Prince of the Jordanian Hashemite Royal Dynasty El-Hassan bin Talal; former President of the Czech Republic Václav Havel; President of the Federative Republic of Brazil Luiz Inácio Lula da Silva; President of the Federal Republic of Nigeria Olusegun Obasanjo; former President of Ireland and former UN High Commissioner for Human Rights Mary Robinson; former President of India R. Venkataraman; and myself.

I firmly believe that the endorsement of such eminent leaders from around the world, and this demonstration of their clear determination to join the fight against prejudice and discrimination toward leprosy, will greatly help to radically change society's perceptions of the disease.

A whole host of other people who had either taken a deep interest in leprosy or served on the front lines were also present that day, including former Chief Justice of India Y. V. Chandrachud; International Leprosy Union (ILU) President Dr. S. D. Gokhale, who had long devoted himself to our activities in India; Chuo University Professor and Special Rapporteur in Leprosy and Human Rights for the UN Sub-Commission on the Promotion and Protection of Human Rights Yozo Yokota; and International Association for Integration, Dignity and Economic Advancement (IDEA) President

Dr. P. K. Gopal. Representatives of people affected by leprosy from Indonesia, the Philippines, and Nepal also participated and gave speeches touching on the social discrimination they and their families had experienced.

At the ceremony, I announced that I was making plans to set up a new organization, using funds raised in Japan and India, that would serve as a foundation and a lending mechanism to support the self-reliance of people affected by leprosy in India and increase their chances for social and economic rehabilitation.

This foundation would have three aims: to create vocational training programs for people affected by leprosy and secure employment opportunities with cooperation from India's business community; to launch a microfinance program under which people affected by leprosy in need—especially women and families—could acquire skills such as embroidery and handiwork to enable them to secure a livelihood; and to create opportunities for education for children from leprosy-affected families through a scholarship program. I saw it as my task to raise the funds to support this new foundation, but it would be up to people affected by leprosy themselves to devise the ways in which they would be used, and to put such plans into action. I hoped they would seek collaboration from experts in public health, law, and social work. This plan eventually materialized in S-ILF, established in November 2006.

I also stated that I was providing guidance and financial resources for the establishment of a national organization for people affected by leprosy, the National Forum India (later renamed the Association of People Affected by Leprosy or APAL).

All over the world, there are people affected by leprosy who play leading roles in the struggle against the disease. One such person is Mr. Hilarion M. Guia, the first elected mayor of Culion Island in the Philippines, which has a long history of segregation, who participated in the ceremony for the first Global Appeal. Now a teacher, he made a strong speech stressing that education was essential to dispel stigma and bring about change in nations and in the wider world. At present on Culion, he explained, the inhabitants depend on support from the Ministry of Health and overseas funding—there is no industry on the island. The question of how the leprosy-affected population will survive as they grow old, and how their second- and third-generation descendants will live, is an urgent one. Oli Parwati, a person affected by leprosy from Nepal, reported on her difficulties in being self-reliant. With support from a leprosy-related NGO, she trained as a nurse and currently teaches trainee nurses herself. It was evident from her speech that women who are affected by leprosy have it especially hard, suffering double barriers.

The following day—30 January, the day that India's leader Mahatma Gandhi was assassinated, which is also Leprosy Day India—we shifted to Kolkata, capital of West Bengal state. Here, in the presence of the city's mayor and the state minister of justice, we again announced the Global Appeal through the local media. Pictures drawn by people affected by leprosy decorated the venue, and we also held an on-the-spot picture-drawing event, in which everybody drew their own pictures on a single integrated painting.

On the third day of my stay, I headed to Jharkhand, a state in northeastern India that would take me forty minutes to get to. Not unusually, I rose at 3 a.m., and got a 6 a.m. flight. Domestic flight services start early in India, making it possible to make effective use of a single day. From the state capital Ranchi, I took a two-and-a half-hour taxi ride to the city of Jamshedpur, where I visited two colonies and attended a human rights seminar. My team and I then turned around and took the same ride back. It was a visit carried out at a rather frenetic pace, since we were aware that the grasslands between Ranchi and Jamshedpur were a place where Maoist-oriented Indian militia, collectively known as Naxalites, operate. We also wanted to avoid being held up and mugged, so the aim was to reach the city before sundown. As a guest of the state, I had been issued with my own personal bodyguard, but as dusk came he insisted we stop the car right there in a spot in the open grasslands for him to answer the call of nature. He seemed quite at ease and able to disregard the fact that he was in an area of high risk.

In Jamshedpur, I visited the Jaiprakash Hindu Mainz colony and the Mahatma Gandhi Ashram. The latter was supported by Bharat Sevashram Sangha, a Hindu charitable organization headquartered there that has worked tirelessly to promote leprosy elimination. The colony comprised roughly ninety households with 400 or so resi-

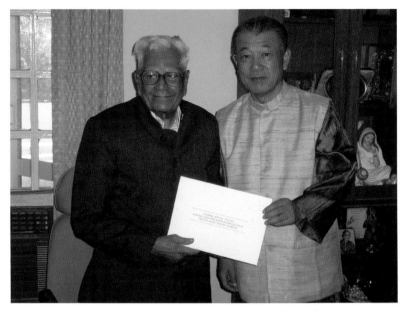

37. Handing the text of the Global Appeal to former President of India Ramaswamy Venkataraman, a longtime keen supporter of the anti-leprosy struggle (New Delhi, India, January 2006)

dents. It was equipped with a care home for the elderly and a hospital, where residents and patients were being well looked after. I was, however, dismayed to see numerous people in the colony begging. During my visit, people came up to me and welcomed me with dancing, even singing, and presented me with garlands of flowers. In January, the mornings and evenings are often chilly in India, so I was wearing a scarf for extra warmth. Thinking it might be rude to keep wearing it, I removed it, only to immediately find my neck festooned with garland upon garland of flowers, some of them drenched in cold water. I felt like a human pole in a fairground game of toss the ring. Thinking it would be rude to immediately take the garlands off, I carried on, my head gradually disappearing amid flowers, which kept on coming. Pretty soon, the drops of water on the flowers made my head feel numb with cold. The next thing I knew, I was having the space between my eyebrows painted with a dot of red paint (known as a "bindi") by one of the women. Normally, red bindi are worn by married women (for widows, the bindi is black), so I imagine that here it was used as a sign of auspicious welcome. I have deep vertical wrinkles in my brow, and I have to scrub when I want to remove the traces of this paint. My visits to India are regularly accompanied by my forehead feeling tender and raw.

A large number of local boy scouts attended the human rights seminar. These members of the national scouting and guiding association of India work with local volunteer groups, going door to door to visit elderly people affected by leprosy in their homes. They also help in mass awareness campaigns, distributing pencils, notebooks, and exercise books printed with our three messages (leprosy is curable; treatment is available; discrimination has no place), and collecting signatures of people on huge pieces of cloth to use as banners in marches, and so on.

The aim of this seminar and the media workshop held the following day was to publicize the Global Appeal and to discuss how we could enlist the state media to raise people's awareness of the human rights dimension of leprosy. Present at the seminar and workshop were numerous people from health-related agencies, the mayor, the health minister, and leprosy program government officials, who discussed strategies for leprosy control in Jharkhand state. On my visit three years before, the prevalence rate was 4.1 persons per 10,000 population, but it was now 1.41 persons—drastically reduced. One state health official noted how the media, always quick off the mark, had already featured stories on the medical and social side of leprosy. Fifteen media companies came to our human rights seminar and nineteen to our media workshop.

Immediately after this, on 30 January, the Indian government announced that the country had reached WHO's official target for leprosy elimination. In a country that had the largest number of people affected by leprosy, this was a historic event. It had been one of Gandhi's dreams. Not long afterwards, we received news that Angola had also achieved the target. Now only seven countries had yet to reach it—Brazil, Madagascar, Mozambique, Tanzania, the Democratic Republic of the Congo (DRC), the Central African Republic, and Nepal.

When news of India's elimination reached me, I ought to have felt elation, but instead I felt an inexplicable sense of physical exhaustion.

I had made eighteen visits to India over the last three years. Maybe only now was I feeling the effects of having made trip after to trip to place after place in that vast nation. Who would have believed, twenty years ago, that a country with more than 11 million individuals affected by the disease would be able to reduce the figure to 100,000? I would like to express my deep sense of gratitude—to the Indian government, to WHO, and to everyone else who worked on this huge effort.

Ethiopian National Association of Persons Affected by Leprosy and a support program for agricultural production—Federal Democratic Republic of Ethiopia, February 2006

> Route: Narita, Japan → Paris, France (flight time: 12h; 4h stopover) → Addis Ababa, Ethiopia (flight time: 7h 20m)—three nights—Addis Ababa → Paris (flight time: 7h 20m; 6h stopover) → Narita (flight time: 12h)

In February, I paid my first visit to Ethiopia in ten years. I went via Paris, and my return trip involved two consecutive nights spent in the airplane. The time I spent in Ethiopia on this seven-day trip was relatively short.

For many Japanese people, mention of Ethiopia immediately brings to mind the Ethiopian marathon runner who won a gold medal in the Tokyo Olympics of 1964, Abebe Bikila. There is also the Ethiopian coffee that Japanese now consume in vast quantities, which is in fact a major Ethiopian export. Ethiopia is one of the oldest nations in Africa, and its civilization emerged thousands of years ago. Christianity is likely to have been introduced here as early as the first century. A missionary converted the king in the fourth century, and 60 percent of Ethiopian people are now of the Christian faith. It is one of the two countries in Africa that were never subject to colonial rule, the other one being Liberia, a nation founded by freed slaves.

The terrible famine suffered by Ethiopia in 1984 was a calamity. Under the direction of my father Ryoichi Sasakawa, the Nippon Foundation contributed emergency relief to the "mercy flights" organized by the UK government. But my father's preferred solution to the problem of famine was, as he explained, not simply to "give people fish" but to "teach people how to catch those fish for them-selves." At his behest, I and former NHK foreign correspondent Itaru Tanaka set out to try to persuade former US President Jimmy Carter and the American agronomist and Nobel Peace Prize laureate Norman E. Borlaug to find a solution. Although Mr. Carter was more than willing to be involved, Dr. Borlaug was somewhat diffident. He had no experience in Africa, he said, and he was now over seventy, of an age to retire. My father back in Tokyo immediately telephoned him. "I am well over eighty," he said, "but that's not going to stop me from doing all I can for the starving people of Africa. Please, Dr. Borlaug, join me!" And Dr. Borlaug consented. This is a story that Dr. Borlaug himself happily recounted on many occasions.

As a result of the consultations, in 1986 the Nippon Foundation initiated, with former President Carter and Dr. Borlaug, an organiza-tion called Sasakawa-Global 2000 (SG2000), whose objective was to help countries in the African region produce quality agricultural goods at a more efficient rate. Thanks to this organization's work, the name Sasakawa is now widely known throughout Africa.

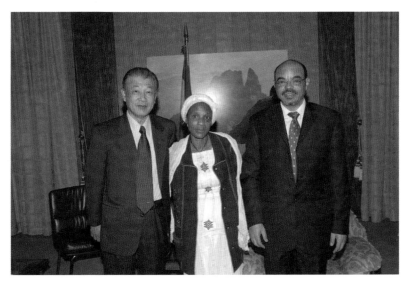

38. With Ms. Birke Negatu, chairperson of ENAPAL, and Prime Minister Meles Zenawi (Ethiopia, February 2006)

At one time, leprosy was a major issue in Ethiopia, but in the 1950s the German Leprosy Relief Association (GLRA) actively addressed it, with some truly astonishing results. By 1999, the number of people affected by leprosy had dropped from close to 81,000 in 1983 to just under 5,000. The country achieved the WHO elimination target in the same year and now registers only about 5,000 new cases annually—amid a growing population—an achievement due to concerted efforts from various quarters, including the health ministry, WHO, and NGOs.

As the staff in the health ministry and WHO confirmed, the Ethiopian government was taking a proactive role in reducing the numbers, creating more "health posts" and training up more health workers. Unfortunately, over 40 percent of the new cases registered involved disabilities. Even if they included people who were relapsed, and who had developed disability before the development of multidrug therapy (MDT), this was too high. I urged the staff to do everything they could to step up early detection measures.

Most of the people affected by the disease in Ethiopia had to live extremely deprived lives—they were often very poor and ostracized from their own communities. I could imagine that many people would be hesitant to go to hospital to get treated out of the fear of being shunned once their illness became known. To improve the situation, it was essential that people with lived experience of the disease take center stage and advocate against stigma and discrimination. At present in Ethiopia, the most active organization in this regard is the Ethiopian National Association of Persons Affected by Leprosy (ENAPAL). First proposed in 1992 and established in 1996, it now had fifty-four branches around the country. Currently, in addition to promoting accurate information about leprosy, it runs a number of programs that include providing small-scale loans for individual businesses and fostering professional embroidery groups.

Birke Nigatu, ENAPAL's chairperson, told me about her experience with the disease. She developed symptoms at the age of six, and after being shown to a number of traditional faith healers, she was taken to the All Africa Leprosy, Tuberculosis and Rehabilitation Training Centre (ALERT), where leprosy was diagnosed. ALERT is a hospital and rehabilitation center built in 1961 on the site of the

Princess Zänäbä Wärq Leprosy Sanatorium. It remains the pre-eminent facility for leprosy treatment, rehabilitation, and training programs. But Birke Nigatu's mother refused to let her daughter go to the hospital for treatment for fear that the diagnosis would become known in her community. At the age of ten, Ms. Nigatu borrowed money for the bus fare from a family friend and went straight to the hospital. She was completely cured, but the delay in treatment meant she was left with slight disability in her fingers and toes. Knowing that her family and community would shun her, she never returned to her village but lived close to the medical facility, making a living through embroidery. She founded a group of professional embroiderers that now has close to thirty members who make clothes, bags, and other accessories to sell. "Getting back into the workforce," she said, "is the one sure way for a person who has had the disease, particularly if that person is a woman, to reclaim her dignity."

Ms. Nigatu took me to the Saint Gebrechristos Church, located on the same site as ENAPAL. It was a Sunday, so the church was thronging with worshippers. Ethiopian Orthodox Christianity is the main religion in Ethiopia. The church had long offered alms to people affected by leprosy, so quite a few colonies had sprung up all around it. As we walked around the church, and through the colonies, I saw many young boys and girls. Ms. Nigatu informed me these were children of people who had recovered from leprosy but who were unable to go to school; their families lived well below the poverty line. Even the lucky ones who, perhaps with financial assistance from the church or an NGO, were gaining an education, would find it hard to find work when they were adults because of the social stigma.

A rather pleasing event happened on this trip. Ethiopia had managed to emerge from the famine with the help of the SG2000 projects and the effort of Prime Minister Meles Zenawi, and it was now one of the most agriculturally productive nations in Africa, even exporting grain to Kenya. The prime minister had sent me a book about how all this had been achieved, which I was very happy to receive. Despite his many prime ministerial duties, he always accompanied us on our tours of the villages in the countryside and made sure to attend the harvest festivals. I brought Ms. Nigatu with me on my courtesy call on the prime minister—without telling his office beforehand. I limited my own remarks to allow her time to speak, and they had a long conversation in Amharic, widely reported in the newspapers the next day. The headlines of the *Ethiopian Herald* ran: "Prime Minister Zenawi Expresses His Strong Intention to Eradicate Leprosy in Ethiopia."

On my final day, we drove to Shashamane, about 250 kilometers south of Addis Ababa. The roads were paved, but the journey was about four hours' drive amid unending grass plains. Shashamane comprises about fifteen villages totaling 60,000 people, some of which are communities of Rastafarians (the Rastafarian religion venerates Ethiopian King Haile Selassie as a god). The word Rastafarian is now known all over the world for its associations with the reggae music of Jamaica, including the most famous reggae musician of all, Bob Marley.

About 12 kilometers from the center of Shashamane is a general hospital. Established as a leprosy hospital in 1951 but today treating TB, AIDS, and other illnesses, it cares for the large number of leprosy-affected people living nearby. Near the leprosy ward is a workshop manufacturing prosthetic limbs, funded by GLRA and the Ethiopian government. As well as prosthetic limbs, people were making made-to-order protective footwear and comfortable rubber sandals. On offer for persons with relatively light disabilities were deck shoes with rubber insoles. Little different from ordinary shoes, these were apparently highly popular and selling well.

For lunch, we stopped at one of the famously beautiful lakes in the Great Rift Valley of Ethiopia. The landscape was breathtaking, but the strength of the sun's rays was too much for me.

One of the villages I stopped at was Kuyera, home to about 7,000 people affected by leprosy and their families. In a joint ENAPAL and GLRA initiative, self-help groups of ten to fifteen people meet once a week and inspect each other's injuries, looking over each other's hands and feet. Those whose hands and feet were well looked after are rewarded with applause, while those found to be neglected and dirty or to have ulcers were told to be careful, and some even fined for not taking better care of themselves. There were about fifty such groups in Kuyera.

Some 60 percent of those affected by leprosy in Shashamane were said to have serious disability, and 99 percent live in penury. Despite

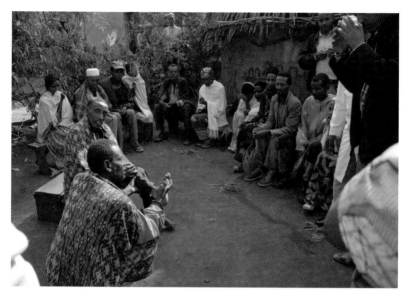

39. With the self-help group members, who meet regularly to check sores on feet (Ethiopia, February 2006)

the large number of people affected by the disease, social stigma was rife, making work difficult to obtain. Many resorted to begging to make a living. A few were apparently involved in agriculture, but yields were poor, and they were hard-pressed to grow enough to meet their own needs.

On the way back to Addis Ababa, I stopped to inspect an initiative of the Sasakawa Global 2000 Agricultural Program. In this particular one, a farm was trying out a new type of irrigation system. Ethiopians are normally only able to work the land for a couple of months of the year—during the rainy season. However, by installing this simple system, the farm had extended the cultivation period by two months, enabling it to grow better-quality vegetables and raise dairy cows. The farmer's wife Beretsu told me proudly that they had been able to make enough money to have their own bank account.

I also visited a chicken farm run by people affected by leprosy, who sold the chickens they raised in the market. However, on this day not a single chicken was to be seen. I was told that they were all being vaccinated as a precaution against avian flu.

The people running the SG2000 mentioned that it had been possible, by using quality protein maize in the chickens' feed, to significantly improve the nutritional value of the eggs the hens laid. This set me thinking. It occurred to me that we might teach some of the agricultural innovations being developed under this program to people affected by leprosy living in the rural settlements. Giving them access to innovative agricultural techniques would greatly improve their lives but also encourage neighboring farmers to come and learn, and so break down the barriers of discrimination. I immediately told my idea to an official from the Sasakawa Global 2000 Agricultural Program and directed him to put it into action.

Full of life and free from stigma—Socialist Republic of Vietnam, March 2006

> Route: Narita, Japan → Hong Kong (flight time: 5h; 1h 30m stopover) → Hanoi, Vietnam (flight time: 1h 45m)—three nights—Hanoi → Kansai Airport, Osaka, Japan (flight time: 4h 25m)—one night— Osaka Itami Airport → Haneda (flight time: 1h)

March 2006 found me in Vietnam to mark the fiftieth anniversary of the founding of Vietnam Maritime University. My last visit had been in 1994, when I attended the first International Conference on the Elimination of Leprosy as a Public Health Problem, held in Hanoi (later called the Hanoi Conference). I had announced my intention for the Nippon Foundation to fund the distribution of MDT globally for the next five years, to energize anti-leprosy activities. Vietnam had achieved elimination in 1995, but even now more than 400 new cases were still being detected each year.

During my stay, I used the opportunity to visit a leprosy treatment center in Qua Cam, about ninety minutes by car from the capital Hanoi. I had last visited Qua Cam in 1994. The center had been established in 1913. Alongside the center is a settlement that is home to around 200 people who have recovered from leprosy and about 100 children. There is also a residential section for the elderly, where I met a seventy-six-year-old woman who had lived there for fifty-two years, as well as another elderly woman of ninety-six. About fifty residents gathered in a hall to greet me. I was struck by how full of life they were, and the general atmosphere of wellbeing.

The reason for this lively, comfortable atmosphere was, they all told me, the absence of stigma, which had existed in the past, but today was as good as gone. The elementary school within the leprosy treatment center was the local village school, with about 300 pupils. The center also functioned as a dermatological clinic, with beds for general patients and twenty beds for people affected by leprosy. I was told there are about twenty such leprosy settlements in Vietnam, operated by the government and the National Hospital of Dermatology.

While in Vietnam, I also met with Le Tien Thanh, vice minister of social affairs. He thanked me for the support the Nippon Foundation had offered over the years—for leprosy control measures, for the provision of prosthetic limbs for the 70,000 people who had been injured in the war, and for our support for people with hearing disability. And he also stated that the five-year free supply of MDT all over the world that I had proposed during my last visit to Vietnam in 1994 had played a huge part in changing people's perceptions of leprosy by helping to dispel the stigma toward people affected by the disease.

Establishing a new foundation for the social rehabilitation of people affected by leprosy—Republic of India, April 2006

Route: Narita, Japan → New Delhi, India (flight time: 10h)—three nights—New Delhi → Narita, Japan (flight time: 7h 30m)

The purpose of my visit to India in April was twofold: I wanted to lay the groundwork for establishing a foundation for the social rehabilitation of people affected by leprosy and to meet with senior figures in the Indian business world to explain the foundation's objectives—in short, to raise funds. I also wanted to deliver a message of congratulations to the Indian government and WHO for achieving the elimination goal at the end of the previous year. Officials at the health ministry told me that they did not consider the fight to be over, and that India's next goal was eliminating leprosy on the state level. The previous year's achievement had clearly raised their confidence and sense of commitment.

In the run-up to the conference in December 2005 for representatives of all the colonies in India, we had conducted surveys and learned that nearly 800 colonies existed, and that most of the residents of these colonies lived in penury, many forced to rely on begging for a living. The motivation for my decision to establish a completely new foundation in India was to alleviate the need for people affected by leprosy and their families to beg. To discuss the proposed foundation, I made visits to both the Confederation of Indian Industries (CII) and the Progress Harmony and Development Chamber of Commerce and Industry. I met up with leading figures in the worlds of business, academia, the media, and other fields.

As we pondered a possible name for the foundation that would be easy to understand, I posited one that implied eradicating the practice of begging once and for all. How about "No to Beggary?" I suggested. This, however, only drew laughter from the others in attendance. "In India," I was told, "being a beggar is a recognized profession. Beggars even have unions. Such a name will only fill beggars with fear and outrage that you intend to take their jobs away. You're liable to get a full-scale uprising on your hands."

The 100-year history of Culion, Island of Despair—Republic of the Philippines, May 2006

> Route: Narita, Japan → Manila, the Philippines (flight time: 4h)—one night—Manila → Busuanga (flight time: 1h) → Culion Island (by car and boat)—one night—Busuanga municipality → Manila (flight time: 1h) → Narita (flight time: 4h)

For thousands of years, until the development of an effective cure, the history of leprosy has involved people affected by leprosy being cast out of their communities and having to live in segregation. All over the world are islands where people affected by leprosy have had to live separated from the outside world: Molokai Island in Hawaii, Nagashima Island (Okayama prefecture) and Oshima Island (Kagawa prefecture) in Japan, Sorokdo Island off the southwestern coast of South Korea, Robben Island in South Africa, Jerejak Island off the eastern coast of Penang in Malaysia, the Fijian island of Makogai, and several islands in the Aegean Sea. The island of Culion in the Philippines, which I visited in May 2006, was a prime example of just such an island.

THE DRIVE TO SELF-EMPOWERMENT

In the first decade of the twentieth century, the American colonial authorities decided that segregation was the answer to the Philippines' leprosy problem. The island of Culion, which is about half the size of Sado Island off the north coast of Japan's main island Honshu, was designated as a leprosy colony. The first arrivals were brought ashore in May 1906. The purpose of my visit in May 2006 was to attend a ceremony commemorating the centennial anniversary of this event.

The Nippon Foundation had conducted a number of aid activities on Culion since 2004 through the Sasakawa Health Foundation: providing small-scale business loans, supplying schools with educational equipment, and so on. A number of sanatoria around Japan continue to support the island, and the marker unveiled at the centennial celebration was built with help from Nagashima Aiseien Sanatorium. There was also a musical connection. Culion has a band made up of people affected by leprosy, and Nagashima Aiseien has a similar music group called the Bluebird Band. Koichi Kondo, one of the core members of the Bluebirds, gifted their counterparts in Culion with new instruments and uniforms. On my arrival at the port, the Culion band were there to meet me, decked out in their new uniforms and playing their new instruments.

Getting to Culion from Manila involved a plane trip to Busuanga Island, a car trip, and then a trip by boat. (The plane was a small propeller aircraft, with tight weight restrictions: at Manila airport, my luggage was weighed, and so was I.) From the airport, we traveled for about an hour along a dirt road, reached the coast, then boarded a boat for an hour's ride to finally reach Culion. A half-day's journey. The broad open space where the commemorative marker was to be unveiled was already a scene of bustling excitement when I arrived. The tiny island's infrastructure was strained to capacity, as many former residents who had relocated to other islands or provinces or even overseas had returned for this special occasion. Over the past few days, there had been chaos—with the water supply suddenly running dry and unexpected power cuts.

The ceremony began with a re-enactment of the arrival of the first leprosy patients to the island 100 years before. Watching with me was Miyoji Morimoto, the chairman of the advocacy group IDEA Japan, and his wife. As we observed scenes depicting how individuals with leprosy were parted from their families, or of the Catholic sisters and priests receiving people affected by leprosy as they were carried in on stretchers, many in the audience were in tears.

Following the unveiling, the venue shifted to the Culion Museum and Archives for a ribbon-cutting ceremony to mark the opening of this new facility—funded by the Sasakawa Memorial Health Foundation—in which Culion's history as a leprosy colony is laid out. The ground floor is dedicated to showing how the leprosarium looked in its earliest days, with exhibits of early medical instruments and photographs of individuals with leprosy and their treatments. The upper floor is home to the Culion Archives. On this visit, it was stacked high with assorted boxes of materials, patient medical records, and the like, all awaiting proper archiving on microfilm. (This archiving work was subsequently undertaken by experts who volunteered to help.) The bulk of the items on display were collected by Dr. Arturo Cunanan Jr., who had played a central role in establishing the museum and the archives. Dr. Cunanan's grandparents were among the first individuals with leprosy to be sent to Culion, and he grew up on the island. He later won a scholarship to study medicine

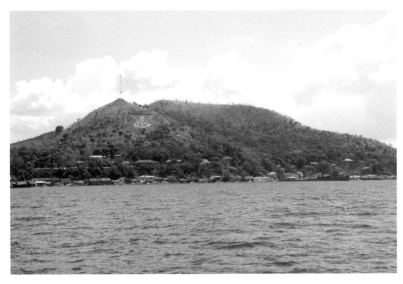

40. Culion Island (The Philippines, May 2006)

in a university in Manila. Although he could have easily made a life for himself in Manila, he chose to return to Culion in order to help the island's residents. In addition to serving as the chief physician at the sanatorium, Dr. Cunanan is a leading force in the drive to revitalize the island. To preserve Culion's heritage, he personally searched for, collected, and preserved materials that might have otherwise been thrown away as detritus. With the completion of the new archives, these precious materials can now be passed on safely to future generations.

In my speech marking Culion's centennial anniversary, I spoke of how, along with brilliant advances, the history of humankind had also been marked by numerous mistakes, among the gravest being the way that people with leprosy were stripped of their dignity and fundamental human rights by being forced to live in isolation. And tragically, the stigma and discrimination attendant on leprosy continues to exist all around the world. So many hundreds and thousands—no, millions—of people had been forced to live subjected to untold emotional pain simply because they had contracted this disease, which in reality ought to be treated no differently from any other. I explained that as the WHO Ambassador for the Elimination of Leprosy I was going around the world, visiting all the countries that had yet to reach the target of eliminating the disease as a public health problem and doing all I could to support the fight to eliminate the disease. And we had made huge progress. The Philippines had reached the WHO target on a national level. And recently so had India.

Leprosy had also been eliminated on Culion Island, where we were today. Here, thanks to the efforts of Dr. Cunanan and his team, the target had been reached. Only six nations in the world had still to achieve it, and eliminating the disease medically was only a matter of time. Nevertheless, it was important to be aware that the struggle against leprosy involved other dimensions apart from the medical one. There were also the psychosocial aspects of the disease. True eradication of and liberation from leprosy would only be achieved once we had rid the whole world of the stigma and prejudice that were sadly linked to the disease. The history of Culion Island provided a demonstration of the truth of this fact.

I told the audience about the Global Appeal launched in January of this year, with the endorsements of Jimmy Carter and His Holiness the Dalai Lama. With this Global Appeal, I wanted to cast a light on the stigma and prejudice due to the ignorance and misperceptions that have become ingrained in people's hearts and minds and effect a complete and radical transformation, fostering an environment in which people affected by leprosy, either currently or in the past, as well as their family members, could be allowed to live ordinary human lives.

In the light of the 100 years of pain endured by the residents of Culion, this development had of course come far too late. I asked for my audience's forgiveness. Today, I said, I wanted to dedicate this Global Appeal, with the endorsements of the twelve luminaries who had signed it, to the people of Culion Island and to all those who had lived and died here.

I assured them they would never be forgotten. There were now people around the world who would be taking a personal interest in their fate. The leaders who had signed the Global Appeal would be standing with them, and I would never give up in my struggle and

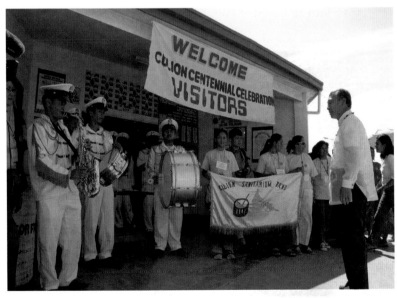

41. With the Culion Band, decked out in their blue tasseled uniforms, a gift from the Nagashima Aiseien sanatorium in Japan (The Philippines, May 2006)

would devote the rest of my life to fighting leprosy and bringing about a world in which discrimination would have no place.

The Global Appeal would provide the momentum to rid the world of the problem of leprosy once and for all. And the help of all of the people affected by leprosy would continue to be essential in that project.

At one time, I had heard, there had been a movement to do away with the name Culion, but the people on the island had resolved, bravely and proudly, to keep it—a decision I heartily applauded. As the residents of Culion thus set out to begin the next 100 years of their history, I voiced my hope that the first 100 years would be duly recorded and preserved. And to that end I hoped that the museum would be further improved. The history of this island, I felt, was an important legacy for all humankind.

In Culion, a place where people had overcome the stigma and discrimination associated with their disease and were creating a community based on solidarity and mutual support, I wished the residents the very best in their efforts to turn the place from an erstwhile Island of Despair into an Island of Hope.

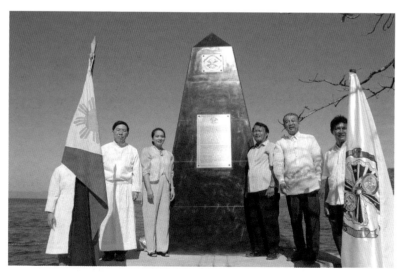

42. By the commemorative marker on the centennial anniversary of Culion Island (The Philippines, May 2006)

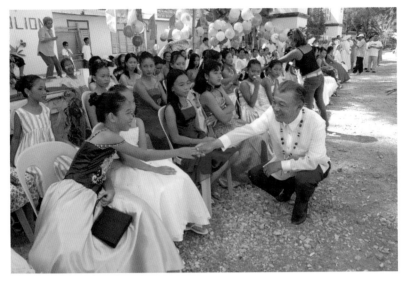

43. Children of persons affected by leprosy participating in a "Beauty Contest" (The Philippines, May 2006)

Talks with world health ministers—Swiss Confederation, May 2006

Toward the end of May 2006, I was in Geneva for the World Health Assembly. I like to attend this every year, since it allows me to be present at the award-giving ceremony of the Sasakawa Health Prize and also to meet and have talks with health ministers from around the world.

This year, the Sasakawa Health Prize was awarded to two organizations. The first was the Agape Rural Health Program, a non-profit NGO that seeks to address the needs of vulnerable and marginalized populations in the Philippines. This organization had been carrying out philanthropic work in communities for more than twenty years. It had trained 4,000 volunteers and provided care to 57,000 people. The other recipient of the award was ILU India, with which I had a long association, for its services to leprosy work. The prize was received by its president, Dr. S. D. Gokhale. The ILU had been working for more than twenty years, engaging in various activities for the social rehabilitation of individuals affected by leprosy and their family members. One of its prime objectives was to rid society of the ingrained stigma and prejudice associated with the disease. India had eliminated leprosy as a public health problem (per the WHO definition) at the end of 2005, but stigma and prejudice remained a huge issue, making the ILU's work ever more important. The ILU was chosen according to objective criteria, but I couldn't help feeling a sense of personal joy.

On this trip, I attended the first ever global leprosy forum, which took place as a special session during the fifty-ninth World Health Assembly. It was attended by health ministers and top officials from India, Angola, Brazil, Myanmar, and Tanzania, among other places, as well as the Novartis Foundation, the International Federation of Anti-Leprosy Associations (ILEP), and many other leprosy-related NGOs.

The opening remarks were delivered by Margaret Chan, assistant director-general for communicable diseases as well as the director-general's representative for pandemic influenza. Speaking on behalf of the late Director-General Dr. Jong-Wook Lee, who had died suddenly the month before, Dr. Chan commended the Nippon Foundation and the Novartis Foundation and noted the success achieved by the elimination strategy. However, this was not the time to relax or be complacent: there were still pockets where the disease remained endemic. "As with any control program," she noted, "the final phase is the most difficult phase. We need to put in that extra effort." Some participants suggested setting a target of 2010 for dealing with all the issues attendant on the disease. I stated that I thought it was important to consider elimination as one milestone along the road to eradication. I was aware that some people misunderstand this and feel that once elimination is achieved, the work is done. I, however, was going to continue to visit countries, especially those that have yet to achieve elimination, emphasizing that it is one important step toward eradication. I mentioned that I had been newly reappointed as Goodwill Ambassador and noted that my new mandate included a reference to tackling the social aspects of leprosy. This would serve as a big boost to my efforts to get the UN Commission on Human Rights to adopt a resolution on stigma and discrimination.

India's Health Minister Anbumani Ramadoss then gave a speech. India had indeed reached WHO's target of elimination of leprosy as a national health problem in 2005, he noted. The prevalence rate in

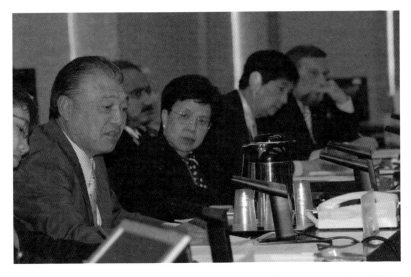

44. In the Leprosy Forum held by the WHO. To the author's left is WHO Assistant Director-General for Communicable Diseases Margaret Chan. To her left is Myanmar Minister of Health Kyaw Myint. (Geneva, May 2006)

December 2012 was 0.95 persons per 10,000, which in March had further reduced to 0.84. He attributed India's success to concerted efforts to detect new cases, thoroughgoing improvements in the training of health service personnel, better dissemination of information about the disease using the help of the mass media, and streamlining the distribution of MDT. He was proud that his country had finally achieved Gandhi's long-held dream, and confident that India could achieve eradication in the next ten to fifteen years.

Dr. Jarbas Barbosa da Silva Jr., director of the National Center for Epidemiology in Brasília, within the Ministry of Health, stated that he thought Brazil was close to elimination, and perhaps able to reach it within the current year. For too long, he said, leprosy had been disregarded. But anti-leprosy programs had been renewed in 2003 and given a high priority. The prevalence rate had fallen to 1.4 per 10,000 population. With a new plan for 2006–10, they would achieve elimination at both the national and sub-national level.

Everybody else present voiced their views and reported on the state of leprosy efforts in their country. Despite some differences,

I felt that the fact we had been able to hold a leprosy forum at the World Health Assembly marked a huge step forward. The forum ended with the chair Dr. S. K. Nordeen of the International Leprosy Association (ILA) paying tribute to the late WHO Director-General Dr. Jong-Wook Lee, who, as Dr. Nordeen said, had devoted his life to public health. "Elimination" had been Dr. Lee's byword since the start of our efforts in 1991. Achieving the elimination of leprosy had been Dr. Lee's dream.

While in Geneva, I also had an opportunity to pay a courtesy call on Ibrahim Wani, who was serving as Chief of the Africa Branch and Director for Research and the Right to Development in the Office of the UN High Commissioner for Human Rights. Born and brought up in Uganda, he was extremely well informed about leprosy. He told me that the UN Commission on Human Rights would be sure to look into the matter of the human rights of individuals affected by leprosy on the basis of the findings of the Special Rapporteur. He did ask me, however, whether it might not be better to ask for the issue of leprosy to be placed in the context of other illnesses and diseases. I insisted that leprosy had to be treated as a single issue.

Mr. Wani advised me in that case to carry out as much lobbying activity as I could over the next few months so that leprosy would remain uppermost in the minds of the Human Rights Council's members. The next session would be held in September, and all sorts of matters would have to be considered between now and then. At present, they had as many as forty items on the agenda that were being looked into by special rapporteurs. However, he assured me, once we managed to get our issue recognized by the national delegates as worthy of consideration, it was sure to go forward for deliberation by the Office of the UN High Commissioner for Human Rights. For me to hear such specific advice from a high-ranking official of that very office was truly inspiring and made me feel much more hopeful about our chances of success.

"Here hope is reborn"—Republic of Brazil, June 2006

Route: Narita, Japan → New York, United States (flight time: 13h; 9h stopover) → Rio de Janeiro, Brazil (flight time: 9h 30m)—two

nights—Rio de Janeiro → Brasília (flight time: 1h 30m)—one night—
Brasília → Fortaleza (flight time: 2h 30m)—two nights—Fortaleza →
Teresina (land trip) → Brasília (flight time: 3h; 4h stopover) → Manaus
(flight time: 2h)—three nights—Manaus → Miami, United States
(flight time: 5h; 2h stopover) → New York (flight time: 2h)—two
nights (visit to United States–Japan Foundation)—New York → Narita
(flight time: 13h 30m)

In July 2006, I made another trip to Brazil, which was now one of a
handful of countries yet to achieve the WHO's goal of eliminating
leprosy as a public health problem. Under the direction of President
Lula, the government, WHO, and various NGOs were getting to
grips with leprosy, and the prevalence rate stood at 1.4. There were
some 18,000 registered cases. The federal government predicted
that Brazil would reach the elimination goal at the national level at
around the end of the current fiscal year or the beginning of the next.
Elimination at the sub-national level would occur within the next
five years.

There are still only a few direct flights from Japan to the countries
of South America (or, for that matter, to Africa). To get to Brazil, I
had to go via New York. My return trip from Manaus had to involve
first Miami, and then, again, New York. On this trip, I was accompanied by Chuo University Professor Yozo Yokota in his capacity as UN
Special Rapporteur.

My first stop in Brazil was Rio de Janeiro, where I visited the
Hospital Frei Antônio, in the city itself, and then a leprosy colony in
Itaboraí, about ninety minutes by car in the suburbs. There are three
government-run leprosy settlements in the environs of Rio.

Hospital Frei Antônio is the oldest leprosy facility in Brazil—well
over two centuries old. The original building belonged to the Society
of Jesus, but after the expulsion of the Jesuits in 1759 the Sisterhood
of the Sacred Sacrament of Our Lady of Candelária installed a leprosy hospital here, and it remained active until the 1980s. At the
time of my visit, there were only four elderly residents. They were
being taken care of and were well dressed and cheerful. Among the
four, I was especially taken with Lydia, a woman of ninety-one who
had been a resident since the age of seven. For a while, she had lived
in the outside world, with her husband, but when he died, she

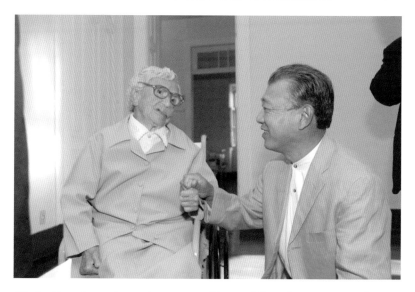

45. Lydia, whom the author met in Hospital Frei Antonio (Brazil, June 2006)

returned to this facility. "What's most precious to me is that pine tree over there," Lydia told me, pointing to the garden. The tree had been planted as a sapling by her father when he left her at the hospital. Now, more than eighty years later, it had grown tall and stood straight in solitude.

The original church had been constructed when Brazil was still a Portuguese colony. The main building, entirely in baroque style, and the chapel—even the dining table—were built in the shape of a cross. The interior, kept immaculately clean, provided a pleasant environment for the residents. On the second floor was a room with a large religiously themed stained-glass window etched with the message "aqui renasce a esperança" (here, hope is reborn). The same message was etched above the huge wooden staircase.

Later that day, I visited the Tavares de Macedo colony in Itaboraí, outside Rio proper. The colony was established by the federal government of Brazil in the 1930s. My arrival was greeted by lively music and people dancing and singing under streamers in Brazil's national colors —yellow and green. The colony had some 2,000 inhabitants,

241

with only 250 people affected by leprosy—the non-leprosy affected population was noticeably larger. One elderly couple made an impression on me. The wife's face was severely disfigured, she was blind, and she used a wheelchair. I wondered how her condition had been allowed to deteriorate so badly in a government-run colony with a hospital and nurses. Despite her multiple disabilities, she seemed eager to talk. She told me she had seven grandchildren, two of whom were living with them and taking care of them.

Tavares de Macedo is a government-built colony, with the government providing everything necessary to support the lives of people affected by leprosy. Families are permitted to reside on the premises together, and utilities are provided free of charge. Apparently, however, this attracts people who are in no way affected by leprosy to settle inside the colony, illegally. And even though the colony is supposed to be a government-operated one, I learned that no support had been forthcoming for the past forty years. No one seemed to know where the money had disappeared. At the time of my visit, subsidies equivalent to upward of JPY 2 million (equivalent to around US$15,000) a year were coming the colony's way but were used for building repairs and the like. Dishonesty and fraud are always unforgiveable but especially in a leprosy facility where people are desperately in need.

Most of the arrangements for my trip were made by the Movement of Reintegration of Persons Afflicted by Hansen's Disease (MORHAN), a grassroots movement headquartered in Rio. I visited their office and received a briefing on the latest developments.

MORHAN is a social movement that operates tirelessly on behalf of people affected by leprosy, working to eliminate leprosy and the stigma associated with it, mostly with the government, but on occasion standing up in opposition against it. Brazil has some active civic movements, and political decisions concerning health issues are made by a forty-eight-member National Health Council. Half of its members are representatives drawn from private and civic groups and organizations, MORHAN among them. The council makes proposals to the health minister based on resolutions that it has passed, and it also has health committees in 5,500 municipalities spanning Brazil's twenty-seven states to deal with local health issues, public hygiene, human rights matters, and the like. This cooperative approach by the private and public sectors toward shared goals has proven highly effective. To illustrate: until a few years ago, Rio had a high leprosy prevalence rate: four per 10,000 population. The head of the municipal health authority concluded an agreement with MORHAN under which the NGO went into areas of the city where the state government was unable to penetrate and carried out an awareness-raising campaign that enabled Rio to achieve elimination at the municipal level.

After Rio, I visited the federal capital, Brasília, where I had meetings with Brazil's health minister, the head of the Special Secretariat for Human Rights, and the senator representing Acre state. While in one sense the meetings were productive, I was distressed by the distractions—not uncommon in Brazil in my experience. Continual replenishment of refreshments (coffee ... water ... much appreciated, to be sure), people whispering while others are talking, people leaving partway through the discussion, mobile phones ringing, or people making calls themselves—the noises and disturbances were endless.

From Brasília, I went to Fortaleza, the capital of Ceará state, some 2,300 kilometers to the northeast. Brazil has an abundance of attractive coasts, but the shoreline around Fortaleza is surely one of the most beautiful. I had a stunning view from my hotel room in the early morning. I saw couples strolling along hand in hand, people taking their dogs for a walk, and several people jogging, working up a sweat.

I first paid a courtesy call on the state health secretary. After that, I was scheduled to visit a leprosy colony outside the city, but that day Brazil was playing its first match in the 2006 FIFA World Cup finals taking place in Germany—an event of such national importance that all government offices and banks were closed. The whole country was swept up, the atmosphere wildly festive, and serious work impossible. In the end, we joined in, and from the local beach we watched Brazil battle against Croatia. Large screens had been set up for people to watch together, and they did so, drinking beer and cheering. We had worried that our schedule for the following day might be affected by the outcome of the match, but to our great relief, the ever-powerful Brazilian team won the game.

The next day, 14 June, I had a formal meeting with the state health secretary, who informed me that the state prevalence rate was 1.76, the state was increasing the number of its health personnel, and steady progress was being made toward the elimination goal. These are assurances that are often made, but I always take them with a grain of salt. I need to see the improved results with my own eyes. Ordinarily, the idea is to think of ways in which to get people affected by leprosy out of the colonies and back into society without delay. In Brazil, they seemed to be doing the opposite of this: encouraging people who were in no way affected by leprosy to settle in leprosy colonies.

I visited two colonies that day. The first was Antônio Diogo, located in the municipality of Redenção. The leprosy hospital here was originally established as a convent in 1927. With their ochre walls and red-brick roofs, the buildings exuded a softness and warmth I associate with southern Europe. The colony, I was told, was home to ninety-two people affected by leprosy and 194 of their family members, and when we arrived we were greeted by a large throng of them singing. The houses surrounding the main convent building were clean, and equipped with the necessary electrical appliances, including a TV and refrigerator. The pots and pans hanging on the walls were also spick and span. The lives of the colony residents seemed comfortable.

The second colony was the Antônio Justa colony in the municipality of Maracanaú. MORHAN had a branch here, and I spoke with its sixty-six-year-old coordinator, who had himself been affected by leprosy. He told me that, unlike Antônio Diogo, Antônio Justa had at one time been in the charge of nuns who ran a brutally strict regime. Leaving the premises without permission after 10 p.m. was forbidden, and if someone broke this rule the nuns would set the colony's watchdogs on them and lock them up in the colony jail. As a consequence, the man said, in an agitated tone, Antônio Justa used to be dubbed the "town of the dead." The colony was surrounded by a tall barbed-wire fence to prevent anyone escaping, and on entering the colony the residents were stripped of their normal civil rights and the word "lepra"—the Portuguese word for "leprosy"—stamped on their identity card.

The difference between the two colonies was like night and day. Unfortunately, the regime at Antônio Justa in earlier days is by no means rare in a global context. Listening to the suffering endured by this man, visibly shaken by his memories as he angrily related them, I felt outrage that one supposedly rational human being could treat another with such cruelty. How frightening ignorance is. And these were nuns. The residents of Antônio Justa were now free to come and go as they wished, and it was a much more lenient regime. The barbed-wire fence around the colony remained in place. Now, however, it was keeping out illegal intruders from the surrounding "favela" (slum), who might take up residence within the colony to enjoy its free housing and land and subsidized utility costs.

The next day, my destination was Manaus, the capital of Amazonas state, located in the middle reaches of the Amazon River. Some technical failure delayed take-off, so we departed six hours late and made a detour via Brasília. A journey that ordinarily took three and half hours took eighteen. When we arrived, there was nowhere open to eat dinner, and we finally went to bed close to midnight, with empty stomachs. Manaus originally thrived on its rubber industry, supported by the labor of Italian immigrants who had traveled to this distant

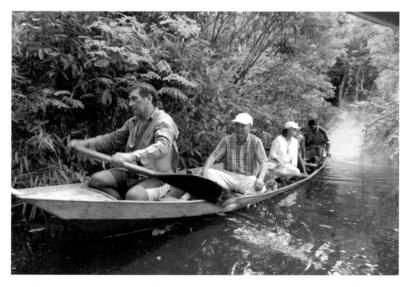

46. The Amazon forest had flooded, so the author visited people affected by leprosy by boat. (Brazil, June 2006)

245

country in response to the Brazilian government's proactive immigration policy. There are some imposing stone buildings left over from this time, and even an opera house of all things. I had come here once before, in January 2002.

It was in Manaus that I met Dr. Maria da Graca Souza Cunha, head of the Alfredo da Matta Foundation, an institution supported by the Brazilian government. She and her staff kindly arranged for me to visit the Paricatuba health center in Iranduba, a jungle town of some 800 inhabitants reached by boat traveling upstream on the Rio Negro ("Black River"), which takes its name from its unusually dark waters that look black from afar.

The people living here each received a monthly stipend of 350 Brazilian reals (about US$70) from the federal government plus a social welfare payment of 175 reals (about US$30) from the Amazonas state government. Altogether this was quite a sum, and the house of the couple I visited had a television and a refrigerator. The husband was clearly a cheerful, sociable person. He made no mention of the tribulations he must have suffered due to his disabilities but animatedly told us how as a young man he had been popular with the ladies, and how blessed he was to have grandchildren and great-grandchildren. I find people who remain cheerful despite the hardships they have suffered in the past a true inspiration—their good spirits are contagious.

The following day, I paid a visit to another family, living on the banks of the Rio Negro. To reach them, we traveled by a small boat for two hours or so, passing by the odd isolated dwelling en route. Every now and then, the river dolphins poked their snouts above the water surface as if in greeting. Midway through our journey, the larger boat accompanying us sprang a leak, and everyone had to get out and stand in the river, legs apart, struggling not to be swept away. Then suddenly the captain shouted that he'd seen a crocodile (was it a joke? we never found out), and panic-stricken everyone clambered back into the boat …

The family was a couple affected with leprosy who were living with their son, daughter-in-law, and grandchildren. When we arrived, we were told they were out gathering fruit. We got back into a small boat and set off to try to find them, but then we ran into them—on their way back. Their hunting dog had been attacked by a jaguar. The dog was lying in the bottom of the boat, covered in blood, trembling with fear. It was the rainy season, when the river floods its banks and animals lose their habitats. At such times, attacks from jaguars and other animals were a frequent occurrence. This was the explanation from the husband, who sat there in the boat, his rifle now at the ready. Lucky for us that we had run into them, I thought. Otherwise, we might have gone deeper into the jungle and ... become a tasty snack for the jaguar.

The small cottage, painted blue, was a single house, located by the riverside, with no others beside it. Inside we saw hammocks, and wood-carved pictures adorned the walls. The kitchen and bedroom areas were kept neat, and all in all, aside from the cracks in the walls, open invitations to mosquitos, it seemed a passable living space. But the shirt the husband was wearing was in tatters, and the wife had only the one dress she was wearing. The couple eked out a living making skewers for cooking from the wood they gathered in the jungle. It took ten seconds to make one skewer, and together they made 4,000 in a day. For every forty skewers, they earned roughly 25 cents, making for a daily income equivalent to about US$25. There was no guarantee of a steady livelihood, but they seemed to be managing, their clothing aside. They had their own generator and some electrical appliances.

Talking with them, however, it was clear that discrimination was having an effect even here. The husband had been the first to develop symptoms of the disease. He received medicine on a regular basis from a visiting nurse. But when the wife came down with the disease, she chose to go a hospital in Manaus, using a pseudonym. Soon their daughter contracted the disease: she also attended the hospital under a pseudonym. This daughter refused to meet us. Even in such a remote and lonely location, it seemed, people felt it necessary to conceal the fact of their disease from others.

Visit to Mother Teresa's clinic—my first for twenty years—Republic of India, July 2006

Route: Narita, Japan → London, UK (flight time: 12h)—two nights (Great Britain Sasakawa Foundation board meeting)—London → New

MAKING THE IMPOSSIBLE POSSIBLE

Delhi, India (flight time: 8h 30m)—four nights—New Delhi → Narita (flight time: 7h 30m)

In July 2006, I paid a visit to India, going via London where I had to attend a Great Britain Sasakawa Foundation board meeting. The objective in India was to make progress with activities preparatory to establishing the Sasakawa-India Leprosy Foundation (S-ILF).

I had visited Mother Teresa's clinic in Kolkata, West Bengal, in 2005. This visit to the New Delhi clinic was my first in twenty years. I remembered when I had visited in 1985 for a tour of the clinic with Mother Teresa, the cars had to progress up a dirt road, the tires flicking up sand. Now we could go along a tarmacked road to the gates of the building. In the operating room, where once there had been nothing but a single barely sufficient table, now there were three—with all the necessary equipment. The scrawny saplings that had lined the road to the main hall had grown into tall trees. I had a clear memory of Mother Teresa, a strong, determined figure despite her tiny frame, showing us round. I had hoped one day to facilitate a tripartite conference between my father, Ryoichi, His Holiness the Pope, and Mother Teresa. Sadly, Mother Teresa subsequently fell ill, so it never came to pass. That was all such a long time ago, I reflected, and so much had happened. The fact that India had achieved elimination of leprosy had to be making Mother Teresa smile from her place up in heaven. At present, this clinic was home to 250 people. Medical personnel apparently visited only once every fifteen days, so it was more like a residential care home.

Setting up a foundation in India first required registering an office there, so after my visit to the clinic I conducted an urgent search for appropriate premises. They were not easy to find. The chief problem seemed to be the sign that we would put up announcing that we were an organization concerned with leprosy. The owners of the first two properties were not keen, but we struck lucky with the third one. "My dear friend's father," he told us, "was a leprosy doctor with a practice in Kolkata. I am someone who understands." I decided immediately that this was the place.

During my trip, I also paid a courtesy call on Delhi Chief Minister Sheila Dikshit. I briefed her on the latest news: I told her that we were putting together a national organization in India for people

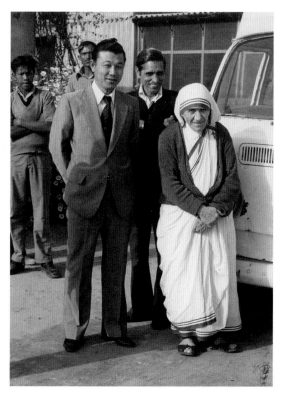

47. With Mother Teresa. (New Delhi, India, 1985)

affected by leprosy, that we were conducting surveys into leprosy colonies, and that we intended to hold a nationwide conference of people affected by leprosy in October in Delhi. She for her part explained that the Delhi government currently provided a monthly stipend of 800 rupees to people affected by leprosy who live within the metropolitan area, but that in common with other urban areas Delhi had to cope with migrants arriving from elsewhere in the country, which kept the prevalence rate high (2.11 persons per 10,000 population). The influx also put pressure on services provided for people affected by leprosy, she told us. "It's a problem," she said. "We would like to offer them more facilities, but the more facilities we provide, the more people come." She expressed an interest in attending the upcoming nationwide conference and offered to help if we required it. (As we will see, Chief Minister Dikshit's administration later agreed to a request put forward to increase the stipend given to leprosy-affected people from 800 to 1,800 rupees.)

The cassava tree myth—Kingdom of Lesotho, July 2006

Route: Narita, Japan → Singapore (flight time: 7h; 8h stopover) → Johannesburg, South Africa (flight time: 10h; 1h 30m stopover) → Maseru, Lesotho (flight time: 1h)—one night

At the end of July, I made my first visit to Lesotho, a landlocked country situated right in the middle of South Africa. I went via Singapore first and from there caught a 2 a.m. flight to Johannesburg, South Africa—where I then had to get on a small light aircraft to the capital Maseru. Trips to Africa often have to go by way of Johannesburg. By now, I knew it was best to leave any non-essential luggage there before going on—traveling lightly was more comfortable and reduced the chances of luggage going astray. I set off, after leaving bags I wanted to take to Angola, the next port of call after Lesotho, to pick up in a hotel near the airport.

Lesotho had a population of 1.8 million at the time of my visit. It is sometimes referred to as a kingdom in the sky, as it lies in a shallow valley in the foothills of mountains. The city of Maseru is on a plateau listed as 1,600 meters above sea level. Summer in Tokyo that year was fiercely hot, but here in the southern hemisphere it was winter. Snow had been forecast, the first time in twenty-five years—we would be carrying out our activities in a snowstorm. Unequipped for such weather, local people went about wearing blankets over their shoulders. I did the same, wearing a blanket that someone gave me wrapped closely about me. As an extra precaution, I also wore pajamas under my trousers.

The WHO representative Dr. Angela Benson took me straight from the airport to the office of the minister of health and social welfare, where I was informed that the country now had only twelve people with leprosy, and official eradication of the disease was close. Admittedly, Lesotho is a small country, but this was a commendable achievement, and a model to hold up for other African countries. The minister put the success down to the way chronic personnel shortages had been dealt with, and good opportunities offered to trained medical staff. Nevertheless, there were still areas of concern on the road toward leprosy elimination, including the high infection rate of AIDS—close to 30 percent. Two hundred thousand orphans had lost both parents to the disease. Average life expectancy in this country was a mere thirty-two years. There was every possibility that in remote regions people affected by leprosy had yet to be detected. Checks and regional monitoring would continue to be necessary.

During my stay, I paid a visit to the Botshabelo Leprosy Hospital. Built in 1914, after the Boer War, this facility had housed people affected by leprosy from northern regions of South Africa and Swaziland. In 1976, there were over 1,000 people hospitalized here. Now there were just seven. At first sight, all seemed well: the place was clean and well-staffed. But I did wonder about the logic of people being hospitalized for six months to a year—when treatment on an outpatient basis would have worked just as well. Most of the people under treatment were suffering from disabilities, suggesting that stigma had inhibited them from seeking treatment sooner. The corridors and rooms of the hospital were jam-packed, but the atmosphere was strangely gloomy, with people looking fearful and waiting in complete silence to be examined by the medical personnel. Nearly all of them were waiting for treatment for HIV/AIDS. Indeed, the place seemed to be fast becoming a relief center for this disease. At one time, I learned, a rumor had gone around that sex with young virgin girls was a cure for HIV/AIDS, resulting in many fatalities. In Africa, superstition still seemed to reign supreme, and with medical services that were rudimentary, many people feel they had no option but to rely on traditional faith healers.

It did seem that Lesotho was well on the way to eradication of leprosy, but stigma and discrimination were clearly an issue, and many new cases already had permanent disabilities. Stigma was clearly making people unwilling to undergo leprosy checks. I decided to convene a press conference, with the health minister alongside me, in which I told journalists about the Global Appeal that I had launched in January, with eleven other signatories endorsing it, and about the three messages that inform my mission. One journalist asked if I knew the popular saying about the cassava tree: "If your cassava tree grows more than

1 meter tall, then you will get leprosy." Superstitions and myths about leprosy abound all over the world. But this only underlines the validity of my mission. The sole way to counter these superstitions and myths was to continue to inform, educate, and communicate.

The day of my flight back to Johannesburg saw another big snowfall. I expected the flight to be cancelled, but the plane ultimately took off on schedule. The airport runway with its white layering of snow reminded me of sherbet. I considered putting off our trip to Angola by a day. Surely the pilot would have little experience of taking off in such conditions. Not wishing to make my traveling companions anxious, I refrained from saying this out loud. It was probably the first time that pilot had ever seen snow—maybe he didn't know how risky it was. To my great relief, the plane left the ground with no mishap. But in all my travels, this was one of the scariest moments.

A theatrical skit in the Funda Community Center—Republic of Angola, August 2006

Route: Maseru, Lesotho → Johannesburg, South Africa (flight time: 1h)—one night—Johannesburg → Luanda, Angola (flight time: 4h)—three nights

From snowy Lesotho, I returned briefly to Johannesburg, South Africa, and went on to Angola. Our Angola Airlines airplane was a rickety old wreck, with mosquitos flying around in the cabin. I later heard that international organizations and people in the diplomatic service make sure never to use this airline. The nature of our activities means that we frequently have no choice but to use airlines and railways that are officially avoided, and to work in areas of high risk. Of course, we make sure to be well informed, and only travel with the country's express permission.

Angola achieved the elimination target at the same time as India, at the end of December 2005. To be honest, this was sooner than I had expected. But good collaboration between the government, WHO, and NGOs had led to this excellent result. The prevalence rate now stood at 0.94 per 10,000 population.

In Angola, I was met by Dr. Luís Gomes Sambo, the WHO's regional director for Africa and a native of Angola, and Health

Minister Sebastião Veloso and numerous reporters. Dr. Sambo had graciously come all the way from the Republic of Congo, and I knew him well, often encountering him during my work at the WHO General Assembly. A specialist in public health, and the author of a huge number of scientific publications, he cut an extremely elegant figure, and I was always struck by his calm, courteous manner. Dr. Sambo was of the view—and I agreed with him—that the government should produce a plan for sub-national-level elimination, with an emphasis on clinical examinations and monitoring.

The health minister and the vice minister accompanied me to most of the places I went to during my trip. The partners' meeting was attended by representatives from The Leprosy Association (TLA), part of ILEP, and the Angolan Association of People Affected by Leprosy (ARPAL) as well as other NGOs. There was lively discussion, covering the need to increase the number of health centers offering proper diagnosis and treatment, since there were still individual provinces where the prevalence rate was in excess of five persons per 10,000 population, and the ways in which we could enlist the help of civic and governmental groups to ensure dissemination of accurate information about the disease.

The next day, I visited Camp Funda, a village 50 kilometers or so outside the capital Luanda. At one time, there were many sanatoria in Angola, but now only six were left, one of them at Funda. The rest have been converted into general hospitals or old people's homes. At the leprosarium, I was told there were just under forty patients, all outpatients. The village had a population of 700, of whom 162 individuals had once had the disease and were now cured. Angola actively encourages the reintegration of people affected by leprosy into the local community, providing housing and assistance so that they can live with their families. Six families from Funda had apparently received assistance and moved to the suburbs of Luanda; another five were to follow. Assimilation, one of the main difficulties in rehabilitation, appeared to be happening relatively smoothly, and there seemed to be little sign of the stigma that is the source of so much distress. At Funda, people made money from manufacturing shoes and wooden mobility vehicles, selling them to the other sanatoria. A little play was put on for me by the village boys and girls about a girl who developed symptoms of leprosy. At first, she is shunned by all her friends. However, once she learns about MDT, all is well, and she is able to live in her community. The health minister and I gave it our hearty applause.

My field visits in Angola were organized with the help of ARPAL, a local NGO formed by people affected by leprosy that currently had a total of about 300 members in four cities. ARPAL carries out a variety of activities, including helping people affected by leprosy build homes and offering them micro-credit and campaigning for their human rights. It receives help from the government for its activities: its headquarters, once a leprosy treatment center, was donated by the health ministry.

Indolent officials—Republic of Mozambique, August 2006

Route: Luanda, Angola → Johannesburg, South Africa (flight time: 4h 45m)—one night—Johannesburg → Maputo, Mozambique (flight time: 1h; 1h 15m stopover) → Beira → Nampula (flight time: 3h)—one night—Nampula → Maputo (flight time: 3h; 2h 45m stopover) → Johannesburg (flight time: 1h; 7h stopover) → Singapore (flight time: 10h; 2h 45m stopover) → Narita (flight time: 7h 20m)

The final stop on my African journey was Mozambique, yet to achieve elimination. I had made two previous visits, in 2002 and 2005. As of 2006, Mozambique had a leprosy prevalence rate of 2.5 per 10,000 population, with most of the cases in the northern provinces. Among these, Nampula province, directly north of the capital Maputo, had a prevalence rate of 6.3. I headed straight there—the flight took a further three hours. A population of 4 million, most of them illiterate, was spread over a wide area. This is a region of the country where there are many anthills, some extremely high—twice my height. It's also not too uncommon to hear of farmers being attacked by crocodiles, and lions making sudden appearances in villages.

A visit to a health post in the town of Murrupula provided a stark picture of the challenges. Queues of people were waiting under the open sky for their medicine. Health personnel were having to give directions on how to take the drugs. In Mozambique, this kind of health post was where most people would be getting their MDT, yet only 25 percent of the population in the region lived within a 5-kilometer radius of such places. The rest lived well beyond that, with no means of transport. I could bet that most people probably didn't even know such health posts existed. Brazil has a similar problem of pockets of the population living in outlying places, but there they have a system of health patrols who go out to these remote settlements. Here there was no health service delivery at all, and information was non-existent. Most shockingly, we discovered that the health post didn't even have any MDT. Deliveries of medications to health posts in such out of the way areas are always cross-checked. I had never heard of such a thing before.

In the square in front of the municipality government building, I addressed a crowd of people: "Who thinks that leprosy is a sign of a divine punishment?" Most people raised their hands.

I found myself unable to identify a single improvement that had been made since my last visit. If anything, things had deteriorated, something that made me feel inwardly very angry. That day, during the official tour, we spent two and a half hours on lunch. Yet the partners' meeting with the Health Ministry, WHO, and NGOs,

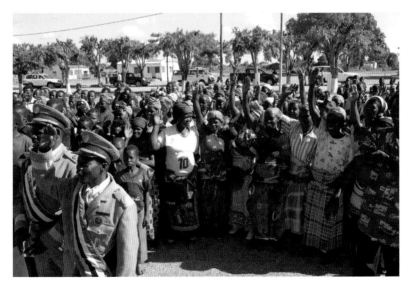

48. "Who thinks that leprosy is a sign of a divine punishment?" A crowd raising their hands in response. (Mozambique, August 2006)

lasted only one and a half hours—and the reports had been short to the point of cursory. Where was the sense of commitment? Two and a half hours on lunch, and one and a half hours on a meeting? When I thought of the long, complicated route we had taken to get here— starting in Tokyo, changing flights at Singapore, going first to Lesotho, then via South Africa, Angola, then going back to South Africa, traveling on to Mozambique, and once we had got to Mozambique getting a further onward flight up here to Nampula, which itself required a further four and a half hours … And all of that for this? Normally, I choose my words carefully so as not to make the officials present feel small, but on this occasion I spoke plainly, raising my voice. I told them I would be coming again in April next year, and I wanted to see much better results. It was essential that drug supplies were maintained, I said, and also that people were clinically examined. It was these things that brought the prevalence rate down. They had only themselves—and their indolence—to blame.

In the capital Maputo, I had meetings with President Armando Guebuza, Health Minister Ivo Garrido, and President of the Assembleia da Republica Dr. Eduardo Mulémbwè. I spoke to them all of my visit to Nampula and stated the need for committed leadership with appropriate countermeasures. "It is our job to help the sick and diseased in our country," the president of the assembly told me. "One possibility would be to create a parliamentary committee on leprosy. Every assembly member should undertake to go back to their constituency and make sure that accurate information is disseminated about the disease."

President Guebuza told me he had given a radio address about leprosy to the nation in January that year, on World Leprosy Day. I thanked him for doing so. Most of Mozambique's problems are caused by poverty, he told me: and poverty was the major obstacle in dealing with them. He thanked me for the efforts being made by the Sasakawa Global 2000 program to increase food supply. The next year would be the thirtieth anniversary of diplomatic relations being established between Mozambique and Japan. He was looking forward to visiting Japan to mark the celebrations. He thanked me for my efforts on behalf of leprosy elimination in Mozambique and assured me that leprosy would remain a public health priority. "We will do our best to show you that it has been worth your while."

THE DRIVE TO SELF-EMPOWERMENT

Burgeoning networks for people affected by leprosy—Republic of India,
September and October 2006

September

Route: Narita, Japan → New Delhi, India (flight time: 8h 40m)—two
nights—New Delhi → Raipur, Chhattisgarh state (flight time: 1h
40m)—one night—Raipur → Bhubaneswar, Odisha state (flight time:
1h)—one night—Bhubaneswar → New Delhi (flight time: 2h)—one
night—New Delhi → Narita (flight time: 8h)

October

Route: Narita, Japan → New Delhi, India (flight time: 8h 30m)—two
nights—New Delhi → London, England (flight time: 11h 50m; 1h
45m stopover) → Prague, Czech Republic (flight time: 2h)—four
nights (attending Forum 2000)—Prague → Frankfurt, Germany (flight
time: 1h; 2h stopover) → Narita (flight time: 11h)

The nature of my work requires that I am constantly traveling to
remote places all over the world. Japan's national holidays are consequently barely on my radar. Nevertheless, my trusty personal assistant Taeko Hoshino tries to arrange my schedule so that I get about
two free weeks in August to use as summer holidays. I usually spend
that time in my retreat in the Mt. Fuji highlands—weeding the garden. Every day, for about six or seven hours, I put everything else out
of my mind, and sitting down on the ground just pull out every single
tiny weed. In Zen terms, it's like a kind of *shugyo*, or mind–body
training. When I need to rest, I simply lie there on my back, listen to
the breeze in the trees and the chirping of birds, and gaze up at the
clouds or the snow on Mt. Fuji's peak. It's my way of reminding
myself of how I am but one part of a natural universe that surrounds
me … And then I get back to work.

In 2006, I followed my summer holidays with two separate trips
to India in September and October. The trip in September was to
Chhattisgarh state, where leprosy remained endemic at the state
level; and where I wanted to push the state government and the media
for concerted efforts toward elimination. I was also going to visit
Odisha, which had achieved elimination this past August, to offer my
congratulations and to give a talk about initiatives for self-empowerment and self-sufficiency. In October, I went to attend a National

Conference on the Integration and Empowerment of People Affected by Leprosy. This was the second conference of this kind, and it was organized by the National Forum of People Affected by Leprosy, an organization that had been put together at my suggestion.

This was my second visit to Chhattisgarh. The first had been in 2004. As of June 2006, Chhattisgarh had 4,612 registered cases of leprosy, and a prevalence rate of 2.3. In India, there are more people affected by leprosy in eastern regions, and on my last visit, the prevalence rate stood at thirteen. This represented a remarkable improvement, the result of much effort by all those involved.

On my arrival in Raipur, the state capital, I went straight to an empowerment workshop. Some eighty people were taking part, including the state governor Dr. Raman Singh, the chief minister, health minister, and health secretary. During the workshop, Health Minister Dr. Kristhanamurty Bandhi argued persuasively that just as regional cooperation and social awareness had helped to defeat polio, the same would be true of leprosy.

After the workshop, I visited a health center in Durg, 30 kilometers from Raipur, where I spent time with about twenty people in a foot-care camp. They were soaking their ulcerated feet in basins of saline wash. Keeping wounds clean is one way of preventing the ulcers from spreading. Among the health workers supporting the camp, however, I noticed women volunteers from the Lions Club charity organization. I immediately detected that the camp was not a regular event but had been put on specially to impress me. Back in Raipur, I called on the office of Chief Minister Dr. Raman Singh. He assured me that my three messages—leprosy is curable, treatment is free, social discrimination has no place—were being taken to every district and street in the state, and that children were being taught about leprosy at school. I pay careful attention to everything I am told by local leaders to see if they are just saying these things to please me, and I try to discern whether their actions bear their words out.

My final appointment of the day was a meeting at the official residence of the health minister Dr. Bandhi, where I had further discussions with him and his health secretary B. L. Agrawal. Mr. Agrawal spoke of the practical difficulties involved in socially and economically rehabilitating his state's nearly 50,000 people affected by leprosy, many of whom lived in colonies. There were limits to what the government could do, he said: NGOs were far better equipped to know the most effective schemes to put in place to help people affected by leprosy, and it was up to them to make proposals. It is always vital for government and NGOs to work together. It made me keenly aware that each state is different, and the ways in which people affected by leprosy can be helped back into society after recovery have to be devised with that in mind.

The following day, I was due to fly to Odisha, but a hastily arranged meeting with Indian President A. P. J. Abdul Kalam meant that I had to quickly return to New Delhi. The president's official residence is a truly magnificent building, a fitting symbol of this 1.3-billion-strong nation, and the huge reception room only seemed to accentuate the delicate-looking president's small frame as he welcomed me with a smile. The president hails from Tamil Nadu state in southern India. Originally from an impoverished family, he paid his own way through education, eventually becoming an authority on astrophysics. He was a true leader of the people, whom the masses rightly adored. We had a productive meeting. I congratulated the president on India's achievement of leprosy elimination, reminded him that elimination was a necessary milestone on the way to our goal of eradication, and asked for continued attention to be paid to leprosy. He assured me that leprosy remained on the agenda. He said he was against the idea of colonies, which only perpetuated the segregation of people affected by leprosy from ordinary citizens and assured me that he understood how important social and economic rehabilitation was for helping people affected by leprosy truly recover from the emotional pain they had experienced.

The following day, I flew to Bhubaneswar, the capital of Odisha. This was my second visit to Odisha since 2004, and I was particularly satisfied that this once highly endemic state had achieved elimination. I attended another workshop dealing with the subject of leprosy elimination and beyond (in states that have achieved elimination, this was now the focus of the workshops). Over 200 people took part, despite the fact that we had the workshop at the weekend (delayed by one day due to my sudden trip back to New Delhi). Participants included Health Minister Duryodhan Majhi, Principal Secretary

Chinmay Basu, and Women and Child Development Minister Pramila Mallik, as well as people from the media and NGOs. A passionate discussion ensued, of the kind I always saw in India, often with two people leaping up out of their seats at the same time to animatedly voice their point of view.

While the slight delay to the start of the workshop made little difference to the number of participants, such sudden changes of schedule demand a lot of my team of staff, who have to deal with a huge number of rearrangements—securing hotel rooms, air tickets, reserving multiple cars for transfers, registering the number plates for entry into the president's official residence, informing the Odisha state government and the chief minister's office of the change in our schedule, and so on. The Indian officials watched in astonishment as my staff dealt efficiently with each problem one by one. It should be obvious to my readers by now how much I rely on the devoted efforts of my staff at the Nippon Foundation and the Sasakawa Health Foundation. Not infrequently, we find ourselves having to check out of hotels at 3 or 4 in the morning and checking in at close to midnight. As soon as we arrive, they have to sit down and book flights, arrange for cars for land travel, confirm appointments, and so on. I think nothing of going to bed on an empty stomach, as I regard it as part of my work. But I am very conscious of the demands I make of my team.

The following month, I was back in India again, this time to attend the Second National Conference on the Integration and Empowerment of People Affected by Leprosy, which was held in New Delhi on 4 October. Close to 700 delegates attended from leprosy colonies all over the world. I had suggested these conferences as a way for people affected by leprosy, both those who have leprosy now and those who have recovered from the disease, to advocate for themselves. The conference was inaugurated by India's Vice President Bhairon Singh Shekhawat and attended by Delhi's Chief Minister Sheila Dikshit as well as many experts in the field of social work and rehabilitation.

The Indian vice president's participation in the conference meant that the event could be held in Vigyan Bhawan, New Delhi's premier conference facility. This was not lost on the delegates. For them, the venue was of enormous symbolic significance as a mark of the progress that their movement was making. One individual remarked, eyes shining: "Previously people like me would not have been allowed anywhere near this building. It's like a dream—us holding our conference here!"

Clearly hugely knowledgeable about leprosy, Vice President Shekhawat acknowledged the importance of India having eliminated leprosy as a nation but also stressed the overwhelming necessity to now make sustained efforts to change the social image of the disease. He mentioned the famous example of "Baba" Amte, who was known for his work in the care, rehabilitation and economic empowerment of people affected by leprosy in Maharashtra state, and the vocational training and small-scale business support being offered to people affected by leprosy in Jaipur, in Rajasthan state.

This was followed by accounts given by around twenty individuals about their struggles and what life was like living in leprosy colonies, and what they had decided to do as members of this organization to work for the rehabilitation of others affected by the disease. I was

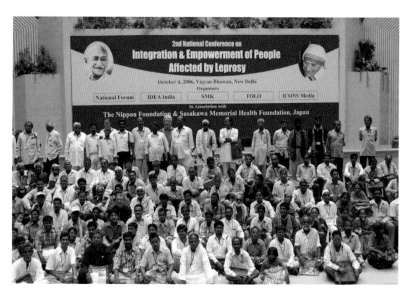

49. A gathering of the colony leaders at the second National Conference on the Integration and Empowerment of People Affected by Leprosy. Note the images of Gandhi and Mother Teresa on the billboard. (New Delhi, October 2006)

particularly struck by the speech of one woman called Maya, who hailed from somewhere near New Delhi. She herself was unaffected by leprosy, but she had chosen to marry a man who had been affected in the past, and together they had two children. Her contentment with her husband was well known to those around her, and she was determined that her story serve as an example that leprosy need make no difference to living a happy married life.

Not a few people demanded an improvement in the meager living allowances given by the government to people with leprosy. Regional inconsistences in public assistance meant that some people received 200 rupees (the equivalent of about US$2) per month. Others, living in Delhi and its environs, received 850 rupees. It was impossible to live on either of these amounts, and the reality was that most people had to beg to survive. Listening to these pleas, I resolved that in every state in India that I went to from now on, I would visit the chief minister, the health minister, and the secretary of health and welfare, in the company of at least one individual who had recovered from leprosy, and vociferously petition for an increase in the amount of financial support given to people affected. In the end, I managed to get several states, including Bihar and Uttar Pradesh, to make big increases in the amount of state support they provided. In this conference, Delhi's Chief Minister Sheila Dikshit committed to increase the amount of support for people affected by leprosy living in Delhi from 850 rupees to 1,800 rupees, an assurance that was greeted by huge applause from everyone present.

A country with a single village for people affected by leprosy—Lao People's Democratic Republic, November 2006

> Route: Narita, Japan → Bangkok, Thailand (flight time: 6h; 3h 30m stopover) → Vientiane, Laos (flight time: 1h)—two nights—Vientiane, Laos → Luang Prabang (flight time: 40m)—one night—Luang Prabang → Vientiane (flight time: 40m)—one night

In November, I visited Laos, the only landlocked country in Southeast Asia, surrounded by Thailand, Vietnam, Cambodia, Myanmar, and China. Though it has 60 percent of the land area of Japan, the topography of Laos is largely mountainous; elevations are typically high. At the time of my visit, its population was a mere 6,900,000. The country had made the transition to a market economy, but it remains a single-party state, run by the Lao People's Revolutionary Party.

The first day, I left my hotel in the capital Vientiane early, skipping breakfast, and traveled for roughly two and a half hours by car to Somsanouk, a village about 130 kilometers north. It is the only village in Laos expressly created for people affected by leprosy. According to the head of the village, the Laos government created the village in 1970, and people affected by leprosy from Vientiane and every area in the country had come here to live. Somsanouk had a population of 1,136, drawn from three ethnic groups (the Laos Thais, the Laos Theung, and the Laos Sung). Forty-one of the families here had been designated as extremely poor. Of the 1,136-strong population, 165 were affected persons, 109 of whom had disabilities. Most of the population eked out a living from subsistence farming. Their life was hard, with inadequate rice supplies for four months of the year.

At first glance, it seemed that the people affected by leprosy were living alongside the other villagers, not in separate areas of their own.

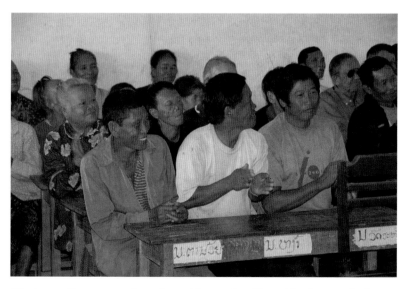

50. A meeting arranged to chat with people affected by leprosy in Luang Prabang (Laos November 2006)

But this didn't mean that there was no stigma. From what I was told, people still thought that leprosy was a form of divine retribution and that the disease originated not from contagion but very much from within. I noticed many who were severely disabled and very much at a disadvantage compared to their able-bodied neighbors. At a gathering held when I arrived, I gave a speech in which I emphasized repeatedly that leprosy is curable—that it is not at all a punishment from the gods. I also told them that discrimination is fundamentally wrong. I told them I wanted them to have confidence and live happy lives.

Very unusually, my team and I had time to spare, so we went to see the city of Luang Prabang, often described as the Kyoto of Laos. It's a beautiful old town with numerous Buddhist temples and monasteries and famous for a daily ceremony whereby every day at first light twenty or thirty Buddhist monks and acolytes form a procession and hold out begging bowls for alms—which take the form of sticky rice. Bright and early in the morning, we duly purchased some sticky rice and waited on the street for the monks to appear and pass by. As soon as they did, we placed rice in each of their begging bowls. But what we'd bought soon disappeared. The procession was never-ending—everywhere we looked, more monks seemed to be coming. Catching on to our dilemma, street sellers rushed over to us and offered us more alms to buy. We ended up using all our money. After this, we visited the beautiful and richly decorated monastery complex Wat Xieng Thong, climbing all the way up the 1,000 steps till we were sweating profusely. But it required money to enter—and we had no money left. All we could do was make our way down again.

On the outskirts of Luang Prabang, we encountered some of the Hmong people, all dressed up in their traditional costumes, celebrating the Hmong New Year. There are nearly 800,000 Hmong people in Laos, who mainly make a living from slash-and-burn farming in mountainous areas. The girls all gathered in a square, accompanied by their parents. There were stalls selling food, and little skits being put on, and all in all it was a wonderful atmosphere. The Hmong people are known for their fierce sense of independence. In years past, they had helped US forces, which means they are looked on askance by the present Laos administration. Such mass gatherings were frowned upon by the government. These New Year's celebra-

tions would go on for two weeks and also offered the younger generation the opportunity to look for suitable marriage partners. Some of
the participants had walked for two or three days to get here, others
from even further afield, requiring seven days of walking. No one
could accuse these people of not taking the search for a life partner
seriously. All about us, we caught sight of boys and girls standing
opposite each other in rows 2 meters apart. They threw oranges at
whoever they wanted to chat with. It was a playful way of signifying
interest. If a person wasn't interested, they would simply fail to catch
the orange.

That night, I went out with my team to enjoy the cool night air in
the famous open market. I have never enjoyed shopping, and in fact
have never bought anything on any of my trips. However, I always
encourage my team to do so—as a way of helping the local economy.
While we were looking around the stalls, I caught sight of a small boy
sleeping by the side of his mother as she sat there selling her wares.
A vision of myself as a six-year-old rose up before my eyes. It would
have been in the 1940s, immediately after Japan's defeat. Our house
had been burned down in the air raids, and my mother and I had to
stay with a succession of friends and acquaintances. (My two brothers
had been evacuated out of the city.) Still a small boy, I had little
understanding of anything that was going on in the wider world, but
we definitely had no money, because I remember one day sitting with
my mother on a mat on a pavement in the Ginza district—she was
selling things on the black market. After introducing herself to every
shopkeeper on the road, she laid out some things with hands that
were obviously quite unused to this line of business. She was trying
to sell calico. All of a sudden, there were shouts and signs of panic.
Arrest warrants had been issued for anybody selling on the black market. Police officers arrived, and we were all told to get into a truck.
I was lifted into the truck with my mother—crammed in among a
whole load of people and their belongings. The next thing I remember is a big room on the second floor of the police station—everyone
had just fallen asleep where they were sitting. I was crying loudly—I
was so scared about what might happen. I remember so clearly—like
it was yesterday—the elderly lady sitting next to me telling me:
"Don't worry, little boy. You'll be able to go home tomorrow ..."

I don't remember what happened after that, but the sight of that small boy sleeping by his mother in her stall in the night market brought back vivid memories of my own experiences at the same tender age.

Progress amid political turmoil—Nepal, November 2006

Route: Vientiane, Laos → Bangkok, Thailand (flight time: 1h; 3h stop-over) → Phuket (flight time: 1h 20m)—one night (participation in Nippon Foundation-founded Asian Public Intellectuals Fellowship meeting)—Phuket → Bangkok (flight time: 1h 20m; 2h stopover) → Kathmandu, Nepal (flight time: 3h 30m)—three nights—Kathmandu → Pokhara (flight time: 25m)—two nights—Pokhara → Kathmandu (flight time: 25m; 4h stopover) → Bangkok (flight time: 3h 30m; 4h stopover) → Narita (flight time: 6h)

From Laos, I went on to Nepal, with a couple of stops along the way in Bangkok and Phuket. There were some momentous political developments happening in Nepal. The previous April, the Seven Party

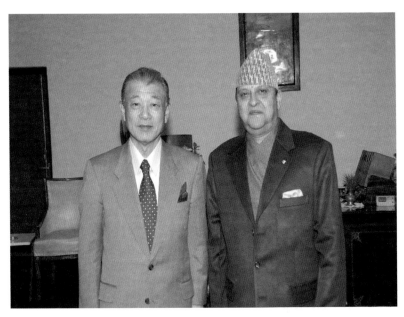

51. The author's audience with King Gyanendra (Nepal, November 2006)

Alliance had joined forces with the Maoist insurgents and held demonstrations—and then staged a general strike. On the direction of King Gyanendra, Prime Minister Girija Prasad Koirala and other leaders had entered into peace talks with the Maoists and preparations moved toward holding elections for a national constituent assembly. There were signs that a decade of conflict was coming to an end.

On 27 November, I had an audience with King Gyanendra. It was dusk, and the sight of countless ravens swooping around the palace gave me a rather odd feeling as I approached the audience chamber. I was shown into a remarkably plain and rather small room, and then the king entered, completely alone. Seated on a chair with the skin of a leopard (head attached) thrown over it, he listened good-naturedly as I explained my role as Goodwill Ambassador and my concerns about tha stigma attached to people with leprosy. Somehow, he exuded a sense of loneliness, no doubt because he was preoccupied by the continuing political uncertainty.

The next day, I traveled south of the capital for yet another visit to Anandaban Leprosy Hospital (this was my third visit). Founded in 1957 by The Leprosy Mission (TLM), it is the biggest leprosy hospital in the country and the main leprosy referral hospital in Lalitpur, Bagmati province. The number of people affected by leprosy had decreased to sixty-nine, and the number of beds had also been reduced. In recent years, the hospital had switched its focus: it was now treating general outpatients—and also looking after people with tuberculosis. I went around every ward and had a chat with as many people as I could. I was slightly disturbed to learn that numerous people were getting leprosy reactions here, as a side-effect of the MDT therapy.

Another reason for visiting Anandaban was to attend a general meeting of the Nepal chapter of IDEA. It was held in a packed meeting hall in the hospital grounds. I gave a speech in which I told the audience that it was up to them, as people with lived experience of the disease, to let the government know about the problems they faced in their lives, and how they wanted them fixed. They couldn't expect the government to know without being told. The government would provide help once it was pointed out where help was needed. I urged them to do all they could to strengthen the Nepal chapter of

IDEA. My hope was that with cooperation from their government, the Nepal chapter of IDEA would become a model for other countries in the world.

The following day, I attended a seminar organized by WHO on leprosy elimination. It was a two-day affair intended to cover a range of topics, including a review of the latest situation in Nepal and identification of issues yet to be dealt with: leprosy detection and treatment in the area along the border between Nepal and India, and the role of the media, social service providers, and other related groups. Specific action plans and proposals were drawn up. Lending their support and experience was a six-person team from India's health ministry, who gave examples of case studies in India, with advice on leprosy cases in their common border areas. The Minister of Health and Population of Nepal Amik Sherchan regretted that Nepal had not achieved the WHO-defined target by the original date of 2000 but affirmed that the country would continue to pursue the aim of eliminating leprosy, using the advice given.

For the last part of my visit, I flew from Kathmandu to Pokhara, located about 200 kilometers west, a trip of about one hour. Many domestic journeys are made by small airplanes in Nepal, with not a few accidents, I'd heard. A storm was brewing when we were due to depart, and I prepared myself for the flight to be cancelled. But in two hours' time, the weather cleared, and all was well. From the airplane windows, we were able to catch a view of the Himalayan mountains, the world's rooftop. It had always been a dream of mine to go trekking in these mountains. But before that, there was something much more pressing to attend to: my dream that we could one day eliminate leprosy in Nepal.

In Pokhara, I was shown around the Green Pastures Hospital and Rehabilitation Centre (GPHRC), a leprosy facility created in 1957 by the International Nepal Fellowship (INF), a British Christian mission. Improvement in leprosy control services and the introduction of MDT had led to a fall in patient numbers, so the GPHRC had broadened its scope to help people with all kinds of disabilities, offering counselling, reconstructive surgery, occupational therapy, and vocational training.

According to Dr. Iain Craighead, the GPHRC superintendent who took me around, the facility currently had seventy-two in-patients,

60 percent of whom were people affected by leprosy. At one time, he told me, the extensive grounds were feared by the locals as a place where "evil spirits" resided—and had been left unused.

Here too, though, disturbingly, I was told that numerous people who were being treated were getting side-effects from MDT in leprosy reactions. This was similar to what I'd been told in Kathmandu. Dr. Craighead expressed his hope that more could be done to develop treatment for these leprosy reactions. Research had shown, he told me, that they were more common in people of Mongolian extraction.

Countries visited in 2007	
January	Denmark (Meeting for twentieth anniversary of SYLFF program at University of Copenhagen)
	Sweden (WMU)
	● Philippines
February	Sri Lanka (Ceremony marking food aid delivery)
	● Timor-Leste
	● Indonesia
	Thailand (Meeting with WMU Fellows)
March	Malaysia (Symposium on the Straits of Malacca and Singapore)
	● India
April	Switzerland (Visit to WHO)
	Philippines (University for Peace opening ceremony)
	● April: India
	France (Fondation Franco-Japonaise Sasakawa board meeting)
May	● Madagascar
	● Mozambique
	● Switzerland

	Myanmar (Negotiations for peace talks; meetings with government officials)
	United States (Received Honorary Doctorate of Humane Letters, with President Clinton, from University of Rochester, New York)
June	Switzerland (UN Commission on Human Rights)
	China (Japan–China Field Officer Exchange Program)
July	United States (Washington, DC, award ceremony for presentation of Congressional Gold Medal to Dr. Norman Borlaug)
August	Mongolia (WHO Interregional Workshop on the Use of Traditional Medicine in Primary Health Care)
	China (Ceremony commemorating twentieth year of Japan–China Sasakawa Medical Fellowships)
September	Switzerland (Visit to WHO; UN Human Rights Council parallel meeting)
	● Vietnam
October	Greece (Meeting on maritime matters)
	● India
	● Nepal
	● Turkey
	Georgia (South Caucasus Conference on Regional Security)
	● Azerbaijan
November	● DRC
	● Tanzania
	Philippines (Asian Public Intellectuals fellowships workshop)
December	United Kingdom (Meeting on Malacca Straits Aid to Navigation Fund)

	Lebanon (WHO Eastern Mediterranean Region Program Managers Meeting on Elimination of Leprosy)
	● Thailand

● Indicates a trip that features in this section.

API: The Nippon Foundation Fellowships for Asian Public Intellectuals, a fellowships program operated by five partner institutions across Asia.

SYLFF: Sasakawa Young Leaders Fellowship Fund program.

WMU: World Maritime University.

A hotel restaurant scene—Republic of the Philippines, January 2007

Route: Narita, Japan → Manila, the Philippines (flight time: 4h 30m)—three nights—Manila, the Philippines → Bangkok, Thailand (flight time: 3h 30m; 5h stopover) → Colombo, Sri Lanka (flight time: 3h)—two nights (launch ceremony for new wing of Sri Lanka School of Prosthetics and Orthotics; food aid)—Colombo, Sri Lanka → Singapore (flight time: 3h 50m; 1h stopover) → Narita (flight time: 7h)

On the morning of 29 January 2007, the restaurant of the Heritage Hotel in Manila was bustling with guests enjoying a buffet-style breakfast. The room echoed with laughter and the clink of china and cutlery. Sipping my coffee, I felt particularly elated as I gazed out over the scene. Among the guests were forty or so people affected by leprosy from various places in the Philippines. The Heritage Hotel was the oldest premiere hotel in the Philippines, with a five-star rating. People affected by leprosy were staying here as registered guests and enjoying their breakfast like everyone else. I had long dreamed that I might see this most ordinary spectacle happening before my eyes. All the long years I had spent working for people affected by leprosy to do this really quite unexceptional kind of thing as if it really was quite unexceptional came back to me.

This was the day when we launched the Global Appeal 2007, in the Philippine International Convention Center in Manila, with people affected by leprosy gathered from all over the globe. This appeal, calling for an end to leprosy-based discrimination, had been signed by sixteen representatives of people affected by leprosy from thirteen countries, and by me as WHO Goodwill Ambassador. From Japan,

Ko Michihiro, president of the National Hansen's Disease Sanatoria Residents' Association, was also a signatory. Over 300 people, including people affected by leprosy and officials from WHO, had been invited from a huge number of countries, and every corner of the Philippines, for a day of speeches, songs, and messages of support. After an opening speech from Health Secretary Francisco Duque III, the noted Filipino film historian Nick Deocampo gave a presentation on representations of people affected by leprosy in movies, and Yokota Yozo, who had served as a member of the UN Sub-Commission for the Promotion and Protection of Human Rights, and professor at Chuo University, gave a talk on leprosy and human rights. After this, with me standing by her side, and with the world's cameras trained on her, ten-year-old Kristina Sacdalan, who once had leprosy but was cured with MDT, read out the manifesto. A huge round of applause followed.

The Philippines was at one time home to the world's largest leprosy colony on Culion Island. This island marked its centennial in 2006. Thanks to the efforts of the former mayor Mr. Hilarion M. Guia, who himself had once had leprosy, the island has transformed itself from an island of despair into an island of hope, full of lush greenery and with a vibrant community—a desirable living spot for anyone, not just people affected by leprosy. It had been during events in 2006 commemorating the island's history that I had got the idea of staging our second Global Appeal, in 2007, in the Philippines, with people affected by leprosy putting their names to the appeal.

Among the people in the restaurant enjoying their breakfast were people affected by leprosy from Culion Island. For most of them, as well as their first experience of staying in a hotel, this was their first trip away from home. Dr. Arturo Cunanan, Medical Center chief of Culion Sanatorium and General Hospital, visited all the rooms making sure they knew how to use the showers and wouldn't burn themselves—people affected by leprosy are prone to injury since they lack sensation in their nerves. I have no doubt that they were all very nervous about a trip away from the island—worried lest other guests at the hotel object to their presence and scared that they may face discrimination. I felt a deep sense of gratitude to the hotel staff who so warmly welcomed them. I knew I had been right to want to hold this Second Global Appeal in Manila.

THE DRIVE TO SELF-EMPOWERMENT

Progress amid political turmoil—Timor-Leste, March 2007

Route: Narita, Japan → Denpasar, Bali Island, Indonesia (flight time: 7h 30m; one-night stopover) → Timor-Leste (flight time: 1h 50m)—one night

In February, I visited Timor-Leste, going via Bali Island, in Indonesia. The political situation in Timor-Leste was still unpredictable. In May 2006, a political crisis began when soldiers from one part of the country went on strike and protested they were being discriminated against in favor of soldiers from another area and were relieved of their duties. The disaffected soldiers protested against the authorities in the streets, and several people were killed—and then things got out of hand, with 2,000 homes in the capital Dili set on fire and 130,000 people made internal refugees. Near the airport, a refugee encampment was established by the UN High Commissioner for Refugees, where 40,000 people had to set up home.

I was met at the airport by the WHO country representative in Timor-Leste, Dr. Alex Andjaparidze, whom I'd met and got on well with on my last visit. Born in Georgia during the Soviet period, he had personal experience of being an internal refugee during the turmoil of Georgia's fight for independence from the Soviet Union. I could see in his eyes that he cared deeply for the plight of internal refugees here. Directly above his desk in the WHO office was a large hole caused by some sort of bomb—thankfully with no casualties. At one time, all UN-related offices had been ordered to leave, but Dr. Andjaparidze told me proudly that he and his wife had insisted they stay. In such dangerous times, no hotel rooms were available for foreign visitors, and I slept on a mat in a temporary lodging put up by the UN. The building had a moat round it and looked a bit like a jail, but I felt lucky to be able to get lodgings with a secure roof over my head.

Due to the political unrest, on my arrival at Dili Airport I had to be escorted to my hotel by armed UN security guards, who accompanied me for the duration of my stay. The leprosy prevalence rate had decreased from 7.5 people per 10,000 population in 2003 to 2.4, a big improvement. Five of the thirteen regions had eliminated leprosy as a public health problem; in the remaining eight regions, con-

273

certed efforts were being made to control it. Between 2003 and 2006, 1,217 new cases had been diagnosed. Of these, 888 individuals (73 percent) had completed treatment, while 222 people were undergoing treatment. The remaining 107 hadn't completed their course of MDT, but this was largely due to the political turmoil, which prevented leprosy work from being carried through. Regarding disability rates, in 2003 15.9 percent of new cases presented with disability, where in 2006 the figure dropped to 8.5 percent, indicating that new cases were being detected earlier. However, on-site screening was considered too risky an undertaking, so for the time being it was suspended.

In addition to leprosy, lymphatic filariasis and other intestinal parasitic diseases remain a huge challenge for public health in Timor-Leste. The Health Ministry and WHO had set up a five-year strategy and by pushing forward integration of their health services—combining health strategy for leprosy with that for each of the other parasitic diseases and incorporating these into general health services—were doing their best to improve the situation. At the WHO office, I was given a briefing on the current situation regarding lymphatic filariasis by Dr. Atsuhide Takesue, who had been seconded to Timor-Leste by the Sasakawa Health Foundation from Aichi Prefectural University. Dr. Takesue had been implementing preparatory investigations with a view to introducing a urine sample method of testing developed at his university to replace the previous method of testing based on taking blood samples. The political turmoil had forced him to abandon this in the May of the previous year and return to Japan, but in November he resumed his investigations. Once urine sample testing becomes a possibility, he told me, testing would be easier and much more economical.

In a salutary reminder of the current security situation in the country, the UN vehicle that came to pick me up the next morning arrived with cracks in the back window. It had apparently been pelted with rocks. My first call was on Vice Prime Minister and Minister for Health Dr. Rui Maria de Araújo, whom I met on my previous visit in 2005. Dr. Andjaparidze advised me, rather white in the face, that I should get to the airport without delay, so I quickly got back in the car, and we hurried to the airport. Only later, once

I'd got to Jakarta, did I learn that all the roads in Dili had been closed, and international flights diverted, shortly after I departed. I had got away in the nick of time.

So-called neglected tropical diseases—Republic of Indonesia, February 2007

> Route: Dili, Timor-Leste → Denpasar, Bali Island (flight time: 1h 55m; 4h stopover) → Jakarta (flight time: 1h 40m)—three nights— Jakarta → Singapore (flight time: 1h 35m; 2h 30m stopover) → Bangkok, Thailand (flight time: 2h 20m; 6h stopover) → Narita (flight time: 5h 45m)

Leaving Timor-Leste on the afternoon of 12 February, we arrived in Jakarta, after a four-hour transit in Bali. In capitals of developing countries, our hosts often give us motorcades of police cars and white-helmeted motorbike riders. On this trip, we were given two motorcycle policemen to precede us. The traffic jams in Jakarta are notorious, and arriving thirty minutes late for appointments is far from unusual. Our two motorcycle policemen at times rode alongside us, at times before us, and at traffic lights and crossroads used hand signals to tell drivers of other cars to slow down or shift over, without making any use of their horns. The skill and coordination they demonstrated as they created space for our car to proceed through the busy streets was impressive. Normally, I expect such policemen to use their authority and arrogantly force drivers over to the side—but this was quite a graceful spectacle. I was thrilled, so I got them to take a photograph as a memento.

On 13 February, I called on Indonesia's health minister Siti Fadilah Supari. Though Indonesia had achieved elimination on a national level in 2000, I urged the minister to continue to make every effort to sustain the achievement, with an explanation of why it was so necessary, choosing my words carefully so as not to offend. I also made the case for more to be done to end discrimination toward people affected by leprosy. Indonesia has its own National Human Rights Commission, which is independent of parliament and government. It has twenty members and concentrates on monitoring, arbitrating, and raising awareness of human rights infringements. No such institution exists in Japan, despite a UN request. When I met with the chair of the Indonesian commission Mr. Abdul Hakim Garuda Nusantara and informed him of the social discrimination faced by people affected by leprosy, he candidly admitted that leprosy had not been one of the concerns of the commission. He promised he would launch an investigation and take steps to improve the situation immediately. We also discussed plans to hold a workshop sponsored by the commission. In the evening, I met with Indonesia's coordinating minister for social welfare Aburizal Bakrie. His position of "coordinating minister" meant that he was in charge of several ministries at once, the Health Ministry, the Social Welfare Ministry, and the Ministry of the Environment, and had to coordinate between them, a rather unique arrangement designed to eliminate the deleterious effects that arise when (as happens all too often, all over the world) government ministries operate entirely separately. He agreed that it was important to have a long-term strategy for education through public awareness campaigns but suggested that poster campaigns would have more immediate impact. He said he would do everything he could to help. It transpired that the minister's son owned a TV station, and the minister urged me to appear on TV and deliver my message.

The following day saw the opening of a two-day Meeting of Partners on Tropical Diseases, organized by the WHO's Regional Office for Southeast Asia. WHO was currently focusing on thirteen so-called neglected tropical diseases (NTD)—including leprosy, lymphatic filariasis, onchocerciasis, Buruli ulcer, and yaws—all of which are characterized in this way because they tend to be overlooked by policymakers relative to diseases like malaria and dengue fever. This was the second such gathering; the first took place in India in 2005. I myself am not too fond of this designation. To my mind, the word "neglected" sounds slightly patronizing. People who are unlucky enough to come down with such diseases have to struggle with them every day, and it ought to be the duty of medical professionals to offer treatment while looking at things from their standpoint. It always strikes me that the word "neglected" does a disservice to what the people suffering from these diseases are actually going through.

I had been invited to deliver the keynote address and discuss lessons to be drawn from the global leprosy elimination program. I stated that I believed that the success of the elimination campaign was due to cooperation between WHO, NGOs, pharmaceutical companies, and donors; to the setting of a numerical target for elimination (less than one case per 10,000 population); and to working to a deadline (the end of 2000, later extended to the end of 2005). I also urged that they should now be looking at the social aspects of leprosy, namely the stigma and discrimination that people experience. Leprosy, I said, should be seen in a human rights context. I used my motorcycle metaphor, comparing the front wheel to medical treatment and the back wheel to eradicating social discrimination and stigma, explaining that both wheels have to rotate at the same speed and be the same size. Our future challenges, I said, were going to involve how to incorporate help from corporations into our efforts. I also emphasized the importance of developing preventative as well as curative medicine.

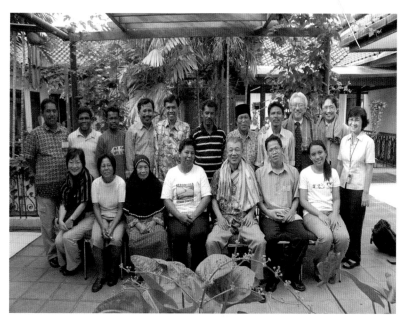

52. With members of the Independent Association of Leprosy (PerMaTa), a national networking organization of persons affected by leprosy in Indonesia—the only association of its kind (Indonesia, February 2007)

In the afternoon, I did the TV interview that had been arranged the previous day, through the coordinating minister for social welfare. ANTV, a nationwide commercial network, sent a camera crew to my hotel. I delivered my three simple but extremely important messages—that leprosy is curable, treatment is free, and social discrimination has no place. I had arranged for Adi Josep, one of the people affected by leprosy who had signed the Global Appeal 2007, to appear with me. He talked about the tough experiences he had been through.

The next day, 15 February, I attended a meeting of a dozen people affected by leprosy, who, along with Adi (the person who had come with me to the TV station), had gathered together in Jakarta from all around the country—for the very first time. They ranged in age from people in their twenties to people in their forties and fifties, and all were determined to make their voices heard and take action to better their position. I was truly impressed and promised that the Sasakawa Health Foundation would support them. Indonesia has the third highest number of people affected by leprosy in the world, and so these people could potentially play a hugely important role in our work. I looked forward to seeing what they would do.

The start of S-ILF—Republic of India, March 2007

Route: Narita, Japan → Delhi, India (flight time: 9h 30m)—two nights—Delhi, India → Narita, Japan (flight time: 7h 30m)

My visit to New Delhi in March 2007 was mainly to attend the first Board of Trustees meeting of S-ILF. This new foundation had been officially inaugurated at my initiative in November 2006, to work to facilitate the empowerment and economic advancement of people affected by leprosy and their families and to promote their integration into mainstream society. I felt some hesitation about using my surname in the foundation's title but ultimately decided to do so. The name "Sasakawa" had achieved considerable recognition, I was told, due to all the work I had undertaken all over India during many years in the fight against leprosy, and this would serve us well in attracting funds. The Nippon Foundation had already committed to a grant of US$10 million. The position of chairman was filled by Dr. S. K. Noordeen, who for many years had been in charge of leprosy-related matters at WHO and who at this time was serving as president of the ILA. We also welcomed on board as trustee Tarun Das, a core member of India's business community. Dr. Vineeta Shanker, a prominent sociologist, was appointed executive director of the foundation.

Discussions centered on the way forward for the new foundation's activities: we agreed on investigating the conditions at leprosy colonies nationwide, creating a database, setting up a website, forming a strategy for fundraising, and establishing an advisory committee. Mr. Tarun Das, who, as director-general of the CII (1967–2004), had long pushed for social contributions from India's corporate sector as part of its commitment to social improvement, explained that the business community was already extending small loans to unskilled laborers who wished to undergo vocational training or to people who aspired to start their own companies. Indian businesses also frequently dispatched advisors to offer advice free of charge. In his view, given the existence of organizations already possessing expertise and a solid

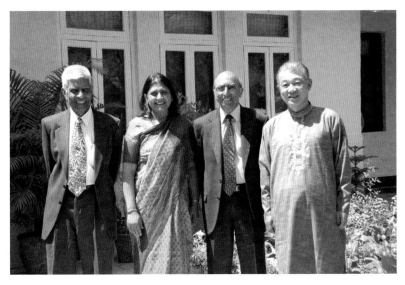

53. From left to right: Dr. S. K. Nordeen, Dr. Vineeta Shankar, and Mr. Tarun Das, former director-general of the Confederation of Indian Industry, with the author (Delhi, India, March 2007)

track record in these areas, S-ILF would best serve as an intermediary—a catalyst—linking organizations possessing information, technology, and resources with India's leprosy colonies. I considered it important, if S-ILF was going to meet its remit, that individuals and groups were able to create "partnerships" in a variety of forms, which would allow for better quality and more efficiency in the work undertaken. The drive toward corporate social responsibility in India is surely due to the country's economic strides in recent years. The focus of India's corporate philanthropy seems to me to be much more practical and sensible than that of Japan—where in the era of the "bubble economy" money seemed to be thrown around indiscriminately at all manner of cultural and artistic pursuits.

One more thing I wanted to do in Delhi was to visit the headquarters of the National Human Rights Commission of India. This commission, which exists independently of the parliament and government, is mainly composed of judges in the Supreme Court or the High Courts of India and spends its time inquiring into human rights violations, as well as protecting and recommending measures relating to and promoting research on human rights. I explained how discrimination and stigma constitute a violation of the human rights of people affected by leprosy and their family members. The acting chair of the commission, Dr. Shivaraj Virupanna Patil, promised he would do his utmost to rectify this situation: he would work on the Indian government to require the commission to look into the matter and make sure it was brought up as a formal topic for discussion. I also suggested that discrimination toward people affected by leprosy might be made part of school education.

On my last day, I went to visit the office of National Forum North, part of the organization set up after the National Conference on Integration and Empowerment of People Affected by Leprosy in New Delhi in 2005 to help to unite people who reside in leprosy colonies nationwide—this chapter covering the ten states of northern India. The office had been set up with help from the Sasakawa Health Foundation in 2006 and though small was equipped with PCs and bright furniture. The representative, Sarat Kumar Dutta, was a ball of energy, clearly on good terms with key people in government and seemed a lovely person—very easy to get along with. He had been one of the signatories to our Global Appeal in Manila in January 2007.

I then went to see the Nava Jeevan leprosy colony in Ghaziabad on the outskirts of New Delhi. Thirty-eight families, comprising around 100 people affected by leprosy and their family members, currently reside in this colony, which was set up with funds from the local Catholic church in 1979. They made a living from growing and selling vegetables (making a profit of about one-third or one-fourth of what they manage to grow above what they need to feed themselves), but they also relied on charity from neighbors and begging. They lived in a constant state of uncertainty, and they worried about how to educate their children. These were just the kind of people whose needs S-ILF must concern itself with, I thought to myself.

The Hindon River flowed just past the colony. On the banks of the river, I saw the little rectangular structures of funeral pyres. Many of these people were too poor to afford to buy kindling to burn the bodies of their loved ones who had died, and I was told it was not uncommon for the bodies to be borne away by the river before being fully burned, or to see wild dogs gnawing on the corpses, scattering their bones on the ground. The riverbed was apparently clogged with the bones of dead people. Meanwhile, there were people swimming in the river and eating the river's fish. As much as I love India, there are some things about it that I find hard to take.

Baba Amte's "Forest of Joy"—Republic of India (Maharashtra state), April 2007

> Route: Narita → Manila, the Philippines (flight time: 4h 30m)—one night (University for Peace graduation ceremony)—Manila → Singapore (flight time: 3h 40m; one-night stopover) → Hyderabad, Andhra Pradesh (flight time: 4h 40m; 3h 30m stopover) → Nagpur, Maharashtra (flight time: 1h)—three nights—Nagpur, Maharashtra → Mumbai (flight time: 1h 15m)—one night—Mumbai → Singapore (flight time: 5h 25m; 3h stopover) → Narita, Japan (flight time: 7h)

In April, I made another trip to India—following on from my trip in March. I stopped first in Manila to attend a graduation ceremony at Ateneo de Manila University's branch of the University for Peace, an intergovernmental organization with its main campus in Costa Rica that trains young Asian professionals to become peacebuilding practitioners. I then went on, via Hyderabad (the capital of Telangana and the de jure capital of Andhra Pradesh), to land in Nagpur, Maharashtra state. In the eastern part of Maharashtra state, in roughly the center of India, is a town called Wardha, with a population of 12,000. It's a special place, known to every Indian alive. In a village called Sevagram, 8 kilometers or so outside Wardha, is the location of the ashram where Mahatma Gandhi lived from 1936 to 1948 (the year when he was assassinated), developing his personal philosophy, nursing people affected by leprosy, and directing the Indian movement for independence. This was the location of the first All-India Leprosy Workers' Conference, held in 1947 at Gandhi's behest.

I first visited the ashram in December 2003, and this time I felt blessed to have the opportunity to visit again. In recognition of my many years of leprosy work, Wardha's Gandhi Memorial Leprosy Foundation had decided to present me with the International Gandhi Award, and accordingly on 12 April I went to receive the award at an official ceremony. Gandhi once stated that leprosy work is not merely medical relief; it is transforming the frustration of life into the joy of dedication, personal ambition into selfless service. This aptly encapsulated my own feelings about leprosy work, and when I received the award from the hands of Vice President Bhairon Singh Shekhawat, chair of the awards committee, Gandhi's words were running through my mind. In my acceptance speech, I spoke of the need to change society, since it is still pervaded by discriminatory attitudes, and quoted Gandhi's famous words: "A disease of the mind is far more dangerous than physical disease. If there is purity of mind, bodily diseases will disappear of their own accord."

After the ceremony, I paid a visit to the ashram. Now preserved as a historical site, this was the place where the famous photograph was taken of Gandhi at his spinning wheel. The temperature in the afternoon was around 40 degrees, and the sun dazzlingly bright. The ashram was still a haven of tranquility, and I paused in the shade created by the huge sal tree looming above me. More than half a century had passed since Gandhi expressed his anguish over the leprosy problem. Yet notwithstanding the tremendous efforts and contributions made by so many people over the decades since, this disease was still causing unspeakable suffering for those it affected and their family mem-

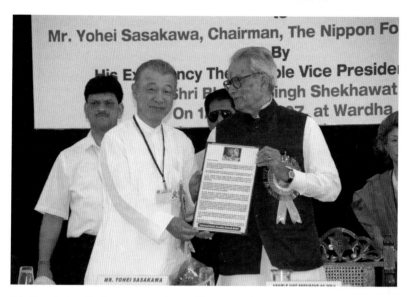

54. Receiving the International Gandhi Award from Vice-President Bhairon Singh Shekhawat (Maharashtra, India, April 2007)

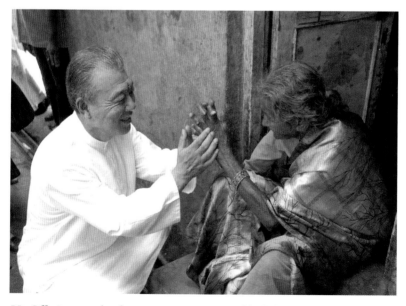

55. Offering words of encouragement to an elderly lady affected by leprosy (Maharashtra, India, April 2007)

bers because of the stigma attached to it. A disease of the mind is indeed not easily cured.

The next day, I took the opportunity to go by car to Warora, a special place several hours' drive out of Wardha, to visit a man called Baba Amte, a legendary social activist who concerned himself with leprosy in India. I first learned of Baba Amte's work from the Dalai Lama. His Holiness had told me that if I intended to carry out my activities in India, I should do all I could to meet this man. He had visited Baba Amte and stayed with him more than once.

Baba Amte had been born in 1914 into a family of considerable wealth, and after receiving an education available only to India's elite, he became a lawyer. One day, he had an experience that changed his life. He passed a person with leprosy on the wayside who was clearly near death and found the scene so frightening that he panicked and fled. After regaining his composure, however, he began to castigate himself. "What if someone in my own family had leprosy? Would I have fled like that, doing nothing to help?" Feeling shame at how he had behaved, he resolved to become involved in supporting the cause of leprosy. This commitment ultimately led in 1949 to his creation in Warora of a community where people affected by leprosy could live peacefully. He named the community Anandwan, meaning "Forest of Joy." A man who has won all sorts of prestigious awards, including the Ramon Magsaysay Award, Asia's premier prize and highest honor, and who counts the Dalai Lama as a close friend, Baba Amte was by now nearly ninety-three, and to get around the facility he used a specially equipped bed-on-wheels, his spine having been injured from the heavy labor he had performed as a young man. As good as bedridden, his speech was at times difficult for me to comprehend, but I was nevertheless able to converse with him, and his words gave me great inspiration and encouragement.

Baba Amte also had another name by which he was known. India's caste system divides Hindus into four main categories with Brahmins at the top, followed by Kshatriyas, Vaishyas, and the Shudras, and outside these categories are the untouchables. Each caste has its own particular hereditary occupation, with sub-castes said to number as many as 3,000. Among the sub-castes, the lowest of the low is populated by those who work collecting night soil. Even today, there are

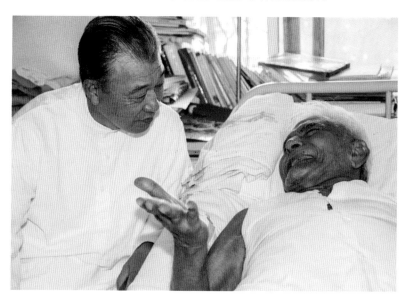

56. Chatting with Baba Amte (Maharashtra, India, April 2007)

many individuals, especially in rural areas, who make their livelihood, as did their forefathers, by collecting human waste. Baba Amte had formed a union of those who belonged to this sub-caste at the nadir of Indian society, and it was in recognition of this that he had won the name King of the Scavengers.

Anandwan is not a charity. Its distinguishing characteristic is that its residents all eke out their livelihoods by engaging in some kind of productive work: it runs as a virtually self-reliant self-sufficient community. Financially, it is completely independent. Amte's son, Dr. Vikas Amte, who had taken over the running of the place, took me on a site visit. It was large—some 176 hectares in all, and some 5,000 inhabitants who had gathered there from all over India (or, more truthfully, who had been turned out of their homes by their families) were hard at work, farming the land, or laboring in any of the various factories on the premises: there was a sewing factory, a printing factory, a carpet factory, a brick factory, a crafts center, metalworks, and factories making plastics and recycling tires. The site was also home to a bank, post offices, shops, and a hospital and a university, both operated by the community itself. Anandwan really was a self-contained town.

For more than half a century since its foundation, Anandwan has functioned as a "shelter" protecting India's most vulnerable citizens, who, even today, face intense public prejudice and discrimination. The significance of the community's existence truly defies description. "Our mission is really to close Anandwan," Dr. Vikas told me. "In other words, to create a society in which Anandwan will no longer be necessary." I found myself in full agreement with those sentiments: the ultimate goal of our activities isn't to protect people affected by leprosy from prejudice and discrimination but rather to see a world in which such prejudice and discrimination will have vanished. To borrow Dr. Vikas's words, our mission is truly to close the Sasakawa-India Leprosy Foundation and create a society in which S-ILF will no longer be needed.

I asked Baba's wife Sadhana Tai, who had been with him all along, what it had been like at Anandwan at the very start. Thinking back, she recounted her memories. For one thing, the area was rife with venomous snakes and not fit for human habitation, she said. "But now," she said, "it's a paradise."

The next day, I flew to Mumbai, the biggest city in Maharashtra, on the west coast of India, and paid a visit to the Sanjay Nagar leprosy colony in Borivali, north of the city. This colony was led by Mr. Bhimrao Madhale, who also represents Maharashtra's thirty-seven self-settled colonies. Located alongside a stench-filled muddy creek about 30 meters wide, it is home to 700 families—some 5,000 people affected by leprosy and their family members. In 2005, thirty homes were destroyed by flooding and hundreds more were damaged. Under Mr. Madhale's leadership, most were rebuilt, though the residents shared communal toilets and sanitary conditions remained far from perfect.

I next visited the Acworth Leprosy Hospital. Founded in 1890, the hospital had established a small museum two years before my visit. With support from the Sasakawa Heath Foundation, it had copied all the historical documents related to leprosy for the past 100 years in the state archives. An initiative that is still rare for India, this will be of great benefit to students and researchers in their study of the history of leprosy in Maharashtra state.

THE DRIVE TO SELF-EMPOWERMENT

The fight continues even after elimination—Republic of Madagascar, May 2007

Route: Narita, Japan → Paris, France (flight time: 12h)—four nights (Fondation Franco-Japonaise Sasakawa board meeting)—Paris, France → Antananarivo, Madagascar (flight time: 10h 30m)—three nights

In May, I made my third visit to Madagascar. After attending a Fondation Franco-Japonaise Sasakawa board meeting in Paris, I flew straight to the capital Antananarivo. On my last visit to Madagascar, in 2005, I had promised I would return to congratulate the country when it officially eliminated leprosy. Finally, less than two years later, that goal had been reached. As well as conveying congratulations, I wanted to discuss the next steps to take to ensure progress was maintained. In three days, I met with president, health minister, foreign minister, and the speakers of the lower and upper chambers of parliament. I also had the honor of addressing the lower chamber. During my stay, I made a five-hour round-trip to visit a hospital outside the capital.

For Madagascar, passing the elimination milestone was a major achievement. When I visited the speaker of the upper chamber at his official residence, and complimented him on his country's success, he told me straight out: "I am happier than I can say. This is the first time we have done something that has received this much world recognition." When I met President Marc Ravalomanana, after thanking him for holding true to the personal promise he'd made to me, I stated that the whole world was impressed with his efforts and those of the people of his country. He replied that he was glad to have been able to fulfil his promise to me. "This is all due to your passion," he told me, "and to the help over so many years from WHO, the Nippon Foundation and the Sasakawa Health Foundation. And now we set our sights on eradication! So please continue to take an interest in us!" He had a huge smile on his face, and his whole body exuded joy. The photograph taken of me and President Ravalomanana holding the commemorative glass shield that I gave him to mark his country's achievement was shown all over the news media in Madagascar.

However, I was a little dismayed to see that the people in the leprosy elimination program—people such as Dr. Marie Monique

Vololoarinosinjatovo—who had fought long and hard at a time when the situation was most dire, were playing a back-seat role in the celebrations. I was surrounded by officials from the Health Ministry whom I barely knew, and they were all acting as if they could be credited for the achievement. Yes, they were all relatively high-ranking, all appointed by the president himself; yet they had not done the heavy lifting. They were simply acting as if they had—and most of them were indifferent. Elimination had been achieved more swiftly than anticipated, and they'd all quickly gathered round and joined in, pretending as if they had been involved all along. Aha, I thought to myself, so this kind of person isn't unique to Japan. Quietly, making sure not to draw attention to myself, I made sure to give the small commemorative glass shields to four people who had put a huge amount of work into the elimination effort. They accepted them with a modest smile and a "Merci beaucoup!" Needless to say, the top officials who had done no real work received no award from me.

During my stay, I had the honor of delivering a speech in the lower house of the Madagascar parliament. There was no fixed topic, so I decided to speak on "Leprosy Elimination in Madagascar and Challenges for the Future." The site for the speech was the lower chamber. The building could not compare with the grandness of the National Diet Building in Japan, but as in the latter, the chairman sits in an elevated seat on a high podium, with a seat for the speaker just below him. Unlike the main chamber in Japan, the seating is not arranged in a fan shape but in a rectangular shape (the "classroom" arrangement).

I began my speech by offering my congratulations to Madagascar for reaching the WHO target, despite forecasts suggesting it would be impossible, under the strong guidance of its president and with the collaboration of parliamentarians. This achievement might seem small against the backdrop of the other challenges the country faces in terms of public health, but I believed that Madagascar's success in solving this very difficult challenge, which involved the Nippon Foundation, the Sasakawa Health Foundation, and various international NGOs all working together in concert, provided an excellent reference model for future challenges that the country would encounter as it grew as a nation. "The nations of the world have observed your success in eliminating leprosy with amazement and huge admiration," I told them. "You can be proud that you have won their trust and esteem. But please bear in mind that elimination is only one step along the way toward eradication of the disease. I ask you now to redouble your efforts in letting all your fellow citizens know of three important messages. First, leprosy is curable. Second, treatment is freely available. And third, leprosy is a condition like any other, and so stigma and discrimination toward people with the lived experience of leprosy have no place."

Most of the parliamentarians were in suits, but one person seemed to be attired in a raincoat, and another in scarlet sweatpants and matching top. Some chatted among themselves, but most were looking at me, listening intently to my words. In the audience, I heard people saying "Arigato!"—clearly speaking in Japanese. I knew that Japanese is taught in ten schools in the country, and quite a few Madagascans have experience of living in Japan in initiatives like the state-supported technical intern training programs and university courses. I had heard that close to 1,000 Madagascans can now speak conversational Japanese. Under-Secretary Ibo working in the Office of the President had graduated from the faculty of economics at Kobe university and had been selected for his post as trusted advisor to the president when he was still only thirty-two.

One reason for the high level of interest in things Japanese was a book titled *Japon sy ny japone* (Japan and the Japanese) written by Pastor Ravelojaona. Set in the period that followed the Russo-Japanese war (1904–1905), when quite a bit of world attention was directed toward Japan, it describes the mind-boggling progress Japan achieved economically and politically and bewailed the way Madagascar was bemired with old-fashioned ways and impotent leaders. I was told that the book, first published in 1913, still sells well in Madagascar and has inspired many youths to know more about Japan and feel positively about the country.

At one point during my stay, I visited a leprosy facility in a town called Moramanga, accompanied by Health Minister Jean-Louis Robinson, to offer encouragement to the residents. Moramanga was the health minister's native village. For nearly two and a half hours, we traveled by car over twisting mountain roads, swaying violently to the right and left—in a journey that if nothing else served perfectly to unblock any intestinal obstructions. The town's mayor came out to welcome us, all smiles. He had the longest name, Ravoloronjatvo George Kurodo, sported a moustache, and was wearing a white uniform like that worn by a ranking officer in the Japanese maritime Self-Defense Forces. He apparently held a third dan black belt in judo, and he told me that he was extremely moved and impressed by the Meiji restoration and Japan's recovery after the Second World War and that his favorite Japanese phrases were *seishinryoku* ("spiritual strength"), *giri ninjō* ("duty and compassion"), and *yūki* ("courage"). He clearly felt a great affinity to Japan.

With the health minister hosting, we enjoyed lunch at a Chinese restaurant with a French name, Au Coq D'or, in a little alley in town. Seemingly impatient for all thirty of his guests to take their seats, the minister called the waiter over and got him to fill his tumbler a quarter full of whisky, diluted it with water, and downed half of it. The mayor, seated opposite him, was visibly shocked. "Erm, this evening, Minister," he ventured, "I understand that you have a meeting with the speaker of the Upper House ..." "Oh, you're telling me we should head home already? Is that what you mean?" the minister retorted. "Not at all, not at all," the mayor replied, in a soothing tone. "Today," the minister told him, "I've come back to my hometown, and I've brought Mr. Sasakawa with me. It's the highest honor. I've never been so happy in my life." And with another gulp he finished off what was left in his glass. "Do you know that yesterday," he went on, "in a press briefing with the president, Mr. Sasakawa said the whole world was amazed by Madagascar's enormous effort in achieving leprosy elimination. I suppose you saw the huge photographs of Mr. Sasakawa and our president in all the newspapers? After that press briefing, the president issued an urgent invitation to all of us in the health ministry to a meeting," the minister said, in the same high spirits. "The president was in an excellent mood. In all the time I've been a minister in his government, I've never seen him so pleased with us all. And Mayor, do you know what the president did next? He said that as a reward he would give each one of us a house!" The mayor's mouth fell open as he listened.

There's a detailed description of a battle between the Japanese navy and Russian Baltic Fleet that ended in Japan's victory in the

Russo-Japanese war in Shiba Ryotaro's historical novel *Clouds Above the Hill*. On 29 December 1904, the Baltic Fleet arrived in Madagascar (having set off from the Baltic and traveled around the Cape of Good Hope in Africa) and requested supplies of coal and food and water provisions from the Merina Kingdom (a pre-colonial state that dominated what is now most of Madagascar) but was given nothing but evasive answers and kept waiting for three months. During that time, some of the soldiers caught malaria and died, and some even committed suicide, and the fleet set sail again on 16 March 1905, bereft of any fighting spirit and utterly demoralized. Two months after that, on 27 May 1905, there was a naval battle in the South China Sea that ended in a decisive victory for Japan. If the Russian Baltic Fleet had been able to set sail on time and fully provisioned, the outcome of that war may have been completely different. My French interpreter Yoshikazu Ozawa told me that the story of how this information was brought back to Japan by a woman called Ito, who had somehow left Japan and worked as a prostitute in a port in Madagascar, features in Nishiki Masaaki's novel *Sun Yat-Sen's Women*. A memoir titled *A Man of the Castle Town*, written by the intelligence officer Ishimitsu Makiyo who was deployed to Russia before the Russo-Japanese War, also describes how Japanese prostitutes working on the borders between Russia and China were sources of important information and intelligence. It seems that even women like this who had landed up in the world of prostitution retained their pride as Japanese citizens.

Confident of elimination—Republic of Mozambique, May 2007

Route: Antananarivo, Madagascar → Johannesburg, South Africa (flight time: 3h 20m; one-night unexpected stopover) → Maputo, Mozambique (flight time: 1h)—three nights—Maputo, Mozambique → Johannesburg, South Africa (flight time: 1h; 5h stopover) → Singapore (flight time: 10h 25m; 4h stopover) → Narita, Japan (flight time: 6h 50m)

From Madagascar, I traveled on to Maputo, the capital city of Mozambique, going via Johannesburg, South Africa, where I was due to wait for four hours in transit. But the onward flight was cancelled. The reason: the lights in the runway of Maputo airport were not functioning, making take-offs and landings impossible. We had no option but to check-in at a hotel, taking all our baggage, only to have to rise at 4 a.m. and go back to the airport. This only happens occasionally, but it means that our stay has to be shortened, which is a pity.

On my last visit to Mozambique, in August 2006, I had heard all sorts of excuses for the delay in elimination. There were budget allocation difficulties, there were no trained personnel in provincial areas, the drugs hadn't reached some places, and in certain areas they were even being sold on the street (when they ought to be free of charge). There was the possibility that activities might have to be suspended. But in the space of nine months, the commitment of President Armando Guebuza had provided the impetus for a turnaround. He had set the government wholeheartedly onto the cause, getting the health minister and other officials in his team to brief the entire Cabinet about leprosy activities. It was now a matter of national policy that Mozambique would reach the WHO target at some point between 2007 and 2008. On my last visit, the leprosy prevalence rate was 2.5 per 10,000 population, but that figure had now come down to 1.3.

The delay in South Africa meant that this time I only had one-and-a-half days to spend in Mozambique, and I had to forego any visits outside the capital. Nevertheless, I was able to meet with the prime minister, the health minister, and influential parliamentarians, as well as local WHO officials, and hold a press briefing. Prime Minister Luísa Dias Diogo, a woman whose eyes missed nothing, told me how much she appreciated my frequent visits and said that Mozambique would continue to work for elimination. She also promised that she would instruct the national assembly to spread my three messages in every sector at the state, city, and township level throughout the northern part of the country where leprosy prevalence figures remained high. They had to bring about a complete change of mindset, she said, involving the entire country. I still had my doubts about this, remembering my experience the previous year. On the other hand, with the permission of the government, WHO had decided to install a leprosy officer in the north. That gave me hope. Health Minister Garrido told me that he felt confident about attaining the WHO elimination target in the next eighteen months. On our previous meeting, he had been much less upbeat. The desire had been there, he said, but no clear idea of how or when. He was happy to be able to give me the good news this time and said he would leave it to WHO to confirm the figures and conduct the proper analysis of the statistics. Though some may wonder whether it was really worth my while to go all that way to Mozambique for such a short stay, meeting with officials in person and talking with them face to face, reminding them of the importance of the task, encouraging the media to get on board, and repeating my encouragement to frontline workers not to give up, is the most effective way of pepping up their activities and making sure they don't kick things into the long grass. There is no such thing as "resignation" in the work I do. I went home the usual way—going back first to South Africa, then to Singapore, and finally arriving back at Narita.

Meetings with health ministers of Brazil, Nepal, and Tanzania—Swiss Confederation, May 2007

In May, I attended the World Health Assembly in Geneva, which had now become an annual practice, and while there I met with several health ministers, who briefed me on the progress of leprosy activities in their countries.

Dr. José Gomes Temporão, Brazil's minister of health, told me that the Brazilian government was strongly behind the fight against leprosy. A recent evaluation had shown good progress. There was an important social movement for the protection of the rights of people affected by leprosy, which the president supported, and the government was working closely with it. The secretary of health happened to be a dermatologist specializing in leprosy, so there was a strong commitment to tackling leprosy in the health ministry. President Lula had initiated a law providing all people affected by leprosy with a pension for life. At present, the number of new cases detected annually was between 40,000 and 50,000; the exact figure would be reported shortly. The situation seemed hopeful, though there was no room for complacency.

The minister of health and population of Nepal, Mr. Giriraj Mani Pokharel, told me that Nepal was in the process of political transition right now and was going to need even more assistance from other countries than before. The new constitution stated that free access to health care services would be available, but resources were limited. This seemed to be a request for financial help in other areas, but I stressed that for us the priority would always be leprosy.

The minister of health and social welfare of Tanzania, Professor David H. Mwakyusa, expressed his relief that his country was close to achieving the WHO benchmark of elimination. Last year, he told me, the prevalence rate was 1.1 individuals per 10,000 population, and they were doing their utmost to get rid of that final 0.1. But a large number of people affected by leprosy had been detected in the border areas between Tanzania and Mozambique. Both countries were now integrating their leprosy and TB programs, and many leprosaria were being closed. He was committed to providing protection for anybody who found themselves with nowhere to go, ensuring that they were not reduced to begging for their livelihood.

I also received reports from the ministers of health of Indonesia, Angola, and the DRC.

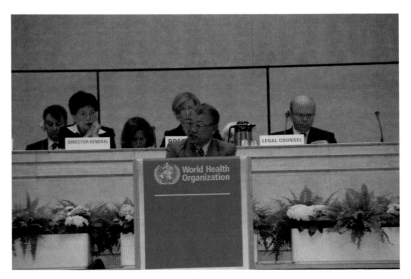

57. The author giving a congratulatory address to that year's recipient of the Sasakawa Health Prize in the World Health Assembly. The Director-General Margaret Chan listened attentively. (Geneva, May 2007)

THE DRIVE TO SELF-EMPOWERMENT

The recipient of the Sasakawa Health Prize this year was Dr. José Antonio Socrates of the Philippines for his pioneering work in the government's delivery of health care services to rural communities, particularly on Palawan Island.

An excellent facility in Quốc Oai—Socialist Republic of Vietnam, September 2007

In September, after participating in a parallel meeting at the UN Human Rights Council in Geneva, I made a brief visit to Vietnam. Vietnam had achieved the WHO target of elimination of leprosy as a public health problem in 1995. At the end of 1996, there were 572 registered cases of leprosy, making for a prevalence rate of 0.1 per 10,000 population. During 2006, 666 new cases of leprosy were recorded. Of these, 5.56 percent were children, and 17.27 percent involved grade 2 (visible) disability. I consider that one reason for the high incidence of disability among new cases is the fact that the correct information about leprosy is not reaching Vietnam's ethnic minorities, of which there are fifty-four. Part of the problem must be related to language. We urgently had to come up with some innovative innovations to reach these communities.

From Hanoi, I traveled to the Quốc Oai Leprosy Treatment Center in Hà Tây province. There is a total of twenty such treatment centers in Vietnam. For the most part, they serve as residential homes for older people affected by leprosy who are suffering from disabilities. Quốc Oai had 125 residents when I visited. They were being looked after by a staff of three doctors and twelve nurses. In Hà Tây province as a whole, there were said to be around 500 people affected by leprosy. Residents of leprosy treatment centers got all medical care free of charge and they were also entitled to a monthly allowance equivalent to US$12. Quốc Oai currently received support from the Netherlands Leprosy Relief (NLR), which was also planning to begin a scholarship program for children of people affected by leprosy. I have been to numerous leprosy facilities on my travels, and Quốc Oai, which I found to be clean and well-run, was definitely one of the best.

MAKING THE IMPOSSIBLE POSSIBLE

Promoting S-ILF—Republic of India (Delhi, Maharashtra state), October 2007

> Route: Narita, Japan → Frankfurt, Germany (flight time: 11h; 1h 30m stopover) → Athens, Greece (flight time: 3h)—two nights—Greece → Dubai (flight time: 4h 15m; 6h stopover) → Delhi, India (flight time: 3h)—two nights—Delhi → Mumbai (flight time: 1h 55m)—four nights—Mumbai → Delhi (flight time: 2h; 2h stopover) → Kathmandu, Nepal (flight time: 1h 45m)—two nights—Kathmandu → Bahrain (flight time: 4h 45m; 4h stopover) → Istanbul, Turkey (flight time: 4h 20m)—two nights—Istanbul → Ankara (flight time: 1h)—one night—Ankara → Istanbul (flight time: 1h; 1h 30m stopover) → Tbilisi, Georgia (flight time: 2h 20m)—two nights—Tbilisi → Baku, Azerbaijan (flight time: 1h)—two nights—Baku → London, UK (flight time: 6h; 6h stopover) → Narita (flight time: 11h 45m)

In October, I made a long trip lasting eighteen days that literally took me traveling around the globe—I went to six countries. My first visit was to Athens, Greece, by way of Frankfurt. In Athens, I had a meeting with the professor in charge of the Sasakawa Young Leaders Fellowship Fund (SYLFF) at the University of Athens. I then went on to India. Here, as well as visiting leprosy colonies, and having meetings with people affected by leprosy, I wanted to explain the workings of the organization I set up at the end of 2006, S-ILF, to various people in business and government. The role of this foundation would be to help people affected by leprosy and their families to gain access to education, skills training, and microfinancing to enable their reintegration into society.

On 9 October, we held the second S-ILF board meeting in Delhi, and a launch ceremony. The chief guest was former president of India, Dr. Abdul Kalam, who admitted that there was no excuse for the leprosy colonies that still existed in India. He knew that it would take time, but he was hopeful that the day would come when such colonies were nowhere to be seen. He delivered a heartfelt speech, gesturing passionately with the full force of his slight frame.

The next day, we traveled on to Mumbai, the financial center of India, where we held a similar reception. Many of India's top industrialists were present, including Mr. Jamshyd Godrej, one of the major figures in the Godrej Group and chairman of Godrej & Boyce, and former president of the CII.

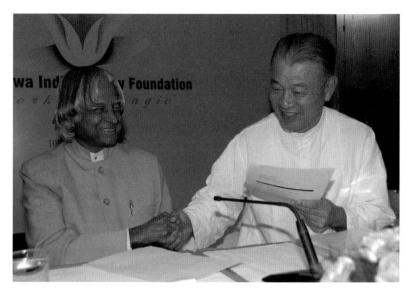

58. With former President of India Dr. Abdul Kalam who came to the launch (Delhi, India, October 2007)

People with lived experience of leprosy were of course invited to both these events, but at the buffet reception after the launch ceremony, I was concerned to see that those present—businessmen, health officials and experts, and people who were affected by leprosy—all seemed to be standing and talking to one another in three separate groups. Since the whole point of what I do is centered on collaborative work, it was disappointing.

On the last day of my stay, I went on a short field visit to Trombay, a colony on Mumbai's outskirts—about one-and-a-half hour's drive away. Founded in 1942, it is home to 3,500 people affected by leprosy and their families, including about 1,040 pre-school children. The colony had its own school, and the sight of these children gathering together and studying in one place soothed my heart. Over half the children in the school came from outside the colony, from poor households in the neighboring villages, to get an education at no cost. I noted that no one was begging in this colony. But self-sufficiency was a concern. City authorities had put a stop to the production of bootleg liquor, which had provided income, and the colony was now

297

looking for another means of subsistence. I hoped that something would present itself.

An encounter with a young man from Japan—Nepal, October 2007

From India, I traveled to Nepal to attend a seminar on leprosy elimination organized by the Nepalese government's Ministry of Health and WHO. Downtown Kathmandu was, as usual, clogged with traffic. The number of cars keeps soaring, and the infrastructure doesn't keep up. At the seminar, held in a hotel in the city center, were forty or so people, including the minister of health and population, WHO representatives, and related NGOs. There were updates on Nepal's progress with the elimination goal and discussion of necessary support strategies. This was followed by a press briefing with about thirty journalists. I got the impression that some advances had been made in people's understanding of the condition.

The next day, there was a meeting in which support groups of various sizes and organizations of people affected by leprosy came together under one roof in a Leprosy Awareness Gathering. The objective of the meeting was to encourage collaboration between government and these various organizations, and between the groups themselves, to work toward a solution to the issues faced by people affected by leprosy. Organizations such as the Nepal Leprosy Relief Association, TLM, INF, and IDEA were there and reported on their activities and challenges.

Unfortunately, with the insurgency being waged by Maoist militia, the political instability in Nepal remained unresolved, and it was too dangerous for us to visit any sites that were remote, but we were able to make a brief visit to the Khokana Leprosy Center on the southern outskirts of Kathmandu. The Sasakawa Health Foundation had been supporting this facility since 2004. There I encountered a young Japanese man, Daisuke Yoshioka, engaged in education- and health-related volunteer work all alone in this land far from home. He belonged to the Cancer Society Nepal, a registered charity, and the Himalaya Ikuei Kai ("Himalayan Association for Youth Development"), and he had helped build a primary school. He told me he sometimes came to the Khokana Leprosy Center for acupuncture and moxibustion treatment, and he was keen to get people affected by leprosy interested in gateball, the croquet-like sport popular in Japan. I did see some people playing a game of gateball in one spot in the leprosy center. These encounters with young men and women from Japan doing good work in far-off corners of the earth greatly move and encourage me.

The innovative approach of Dr. Türkan Saylan—Republic of Turkey, October 2007

After finishing my work in Nepal, I went straight on to Turkey. Leprosy has a long history on the Turkish peninsula, with the disease appearing to date back to the time of Ancient Greece. It is known that leprosaria were built in Roman times both in Istanbul and Anatolia. With the advent of the Turkish Republic in 1923, systematic attempts to screen and record cases began, and at their highest there were around 10,000 cases of people affected by leprosy. As of my visit in 2007, the Turkish government claimed that around 2,500 were affected by leprosy, with most of the cases in the impoverished areas in the south and eastern regions of the country.

In the leprosy hospital I visited on the outskirts of Istanbul, I found twenty-two inpatients with leprosy-related disabilities receiving social support, the youngest of them forty-five years of age. The hospital also had outpatients. A remarkable lady who has played a leading role in fighting leprosy in Turkey is the physician, academic, and activist Dr. Türkan Saylan, whom I had the pleasure of meeting on this visit. Born in 1935, Dr. Saylan had now retired from her work on the front lines, but she still worked periodically for three NGOs and a hospital with German affiliations. She first became involved in leprosy work in 1976: as a medical student, she went on an observation tour of a segregated ward in a leprosy hospital, and what she saw there, she told me, changed her life. Discrimination and prejudice regarding leprosy were rampant, even evident in the doctors charged with providing care. When she qualified, Dr. Saylan did her best to rectify this with the students she was training, and she also encouraged the medical staff in the country's health centers to conduct awareness campaigns, but nothing seemed to change. In the end, she decided to become an agent of change herself. Dr. Saylan had served as the voluntary director of this hospital for twenty-one years, between 1981 and 2002.

From the start, the hospital had adopted a dual approach. With a commitment to providing medical treatment and psychological and social support, it had implemented a social welfare program to everyone, even patients whose needs were relatively mild, offering a full palette of care, including support for the social rehabilitation and self-reliance of patients, but also creating a system of grants for their children and providing prosthetic legs and glasses. The foresight and leadership of Dr. Saylan, who had discerned the value of a holistic approach to people affected by leprosy at a time when it was common even for medical personnel to treat them in a discriminatory way, is admirable indeed.

It is a source of regret to me how late it was that I became aware that liberation from leprosy would never truly be achieved unless we take steps to neutralize the problem of social discrimination. It was only in 2003 that I knocked on the door of the office of the UN Commission on Human Rights to argue for acknowledgment of the human rights dimension of the disease. Dr. Saylan told me that her approach, forming networks between health providers and NGOs, and paying attention to education and training for people affected by leprosy, provides a model for ways to approach other illnesses too. Getting several bodies and organizations to link up and find a collaborative solution to an issue, she said, is one of the most effective ways to approach the many problems that afflict contemporary society. I was deeply impressed by Dr. Saylan and looked forward to working with her again in the future. But tragically, an illness made that impossible, and she died in May 2009.

A life with venomous snakes and frogs—Republic of Azerbaijan, October 2007

From Turkey, I traveled to Georgia, where I attended an informal gathering with Sasakawa scholarship students attending the World Maritime University in Sweden and had talks with Prime Minister Zurab Noghaideli on strengthening relations with Japan. I then headed to Azerbaijan. A country located in the Caucasus, the area to the south of Russia bounded by the Black Sea to the west and the Caspian Sea to the east (and comprising present-day Georgia, Armenia, and Azerbaijan), Azerbaijan gained its independence in 1991 with the breakup of the Soviet Union. In 2007, its population was 8.3 million. Roughly 90 percent were Azerbaijanian, the rest Russian and Armenian. The vast majority of the populace was Muslim. The capital city Baku was the birthplace of Richard Sorge, a famous Soviet spy who was assigned to Tokyo just before the outbreak of the Second World War. There is now a concrete monument to him in one of the city's parks. Leprosy had been eliminated in Azerbaijan, and I was told that the last person to have caught the disease had done so two years previously.

My purpose this time was to go to the Umbaki leprosy sanatorium, located some 70 kilometers from Baku. To get to it, we took a speedway that followed the coastline of the Caspian Sea, and then took a turning at a sign to go inland. From here, it was only 25 kilometers, but we had to go at a crawl along a road whose surface was in desper-

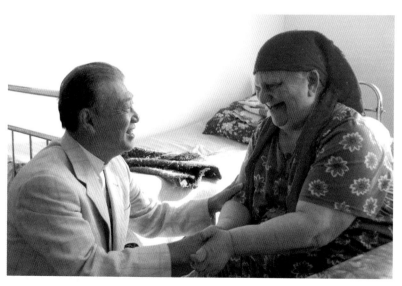

59. Chatting with a person affected by leprosy who had been living in Umbaki leprosy sanatorium for several decades (Azerbaijan, October 2007)

ate need of repair, so this part of the trip took one and a half hours. As we crept along, lurching from side to side, over the barren landscape, the hard-to-reach, isolated location seemed to speak volumes about the prejudice held by society toward people affected by leprosy.

Eventually, just beyond Umbaki village, the sanatorium came into view—a cluster of buildings. In contrast to the stark nature of the surrounding landscape, well-tended gardens dotted the compound, many with trees heavy with pomegranates.

The sanatorium was home to around thirty residents who had either had leprosy in the past or were undergoing treatment for it now, with fifteen staff to see to their care. In the days of the Soviet Union, Umbaki was the only leprosy sanatorium in the southern Caucasus, and at its peak there were roughly 200 residents who had been brought there from various regions.

We were first taken on a tour of an old building in a dreadful state of repair to show us how residents used to live—until (amazingly) just four years previously. Windows were broken or missing, there were holes in the walls and the roof. One of the former occupants, an elderly man, told us: "We shared it with venomous snakes and frogs!" For the fifty years since the sanatorium's establishment in 1953, the buildings of the facility had been left to go to rack and ruin, and so it might have continued if not for the intervention of a group of volunteers who had been assisting the sanatorium for some time and who, led by an English businessman called John Patterson, raised funds and built a new clinic and refurbished the residential buildings. The residents could now live in their own well-lit rooms and apartments, with heating provided by gas stoves. I was struck by how nicely the residents had decorated their rooms, with lace cloths on their beds and other personal effects on the shelves.

I had been told how Azeris like to give a warm welcome to guests, and that was certainly the case here. In each room I visited, the residents greeted me warmly and repeatedly invited me to come back again. I enjoyed a nice slice of cake with sanatorium staff and residents—a very pleasant memory. This facility had started using MDT in 1988, and now every resident here had been treated with it. Nevertheless, mistaken notions about the disease still retained their hold on people's hearts—in larger society and among the residents themselves. We witnessed it for ourselves when one young girl remarked that she had contracted the disease because her parents had been "too closely related"—meaning that she thought her condition was punishment for incest.

A trip to see the pygmy people—DRC, November 2007

Route: Narita, Japan → Paris, France (flight time: 12h 30m; one-night stopover) → Kinshasa, DRC (flight time: 8h)—five nights

In November, I went to do some work in the DRC and Tanzania. The total flight time for this round trip was thirty-nine hours, and including the extended transit time in Paris, it amounted to eighty hours. Just a single outbound trip from Japan to Tanzania via the DRC takes sixty-three hours if one factors in transit time. It was my second trip to the DRC: I had last visited in 2005.

It was 6 p.m. when we touched down in the capital Kinshasa, having flown via Paris. The local media were waiting for us at the airport, and one reporter asked me: "How easy is it to catch leprosy? Can you get it from simply touching someone with the disease?" I thought to myself: If that's the level of knowledge of someone who works in the media, it must be next to nothing among ordinary folk in this country, unless they work in the health services. I could tell we were going to encounter the usual misplaced notions—that leprosy was the result of some sort of divine punishment, or a curse, or could be inherited, and so on.

According to what I was told, in this country even qualified doctors earned about US$50 a month. The level of poverty was striking. Walking through the streets, we were continually followed by people trying to sell us things—a pair of shoes or a SIM card. As in so many countries in Africa, mobile phones seemed to be everywhere, notwithstanding the totally inadequate state of most of the infrastructure.

In my meeting with Health Minister Dr. Victor Makwenge Kaput, he gave me his word that the government considered public health an issue of utmost importance. He indicated his strong determination to implement measures to eliminate leprosy and even to eradicate it. With authorization from the prime minister, Dr. Kaput agreed to take leave from his duties and accompany me for two days on my tour of the DRC.

Prime Minister Antoine Gizenga described to me how many of his country's citizens had been forced to leave their homes during the war, a situation that prevented the DRC from being able to document the numbers of people affected by leprosy. But he assured me that after seeing the work that I, a foreigner, was doing in his country, he would lend his full support to my activities. President of the National Assembly Vital Kamerhe, a dapper figure in a necktie and socks in matching colors, assured me that in the National Assembly the following morning he would drive home my three messages to the parliamentarians—that leprosy is curable, that free treatment is available, and that discrimination has no place. We could be sure that they would take the messages home to their constituencies.

The foremost purpose of this visit to the DRC was to travel to Orientale province, in the country's northeastern sector, to investigate the state of leprosy among the pygmies who resided there. I had long hoped to travel here. The northeastern quarter of the country was still quite dangerous due to lingering skirmishes, I was told, and there were qualms about my safety as well as doubts about whether we would be able to locate the pygmies, who characteristically move continuously about in the forests—but we ultimately succeeded in our mission.

The pygmies are hunter-gatherers who typically live in the tropical rainforests close to the equator. They can be found throughout Central Africa. There are indeed several pygmy groups, all with different names, who speak various languages. They are very short in stature, adults usually being around 1.5 meters tall. The name "pygmy" actually derives from a Greek word and was used by colonists, so really and truly I should avoid use of it and use the names that the people themselves prefer. But I have consciously chosen to use the name used by anthropologists.

From Kinshasa, it was a four-hour flight, across 1,600 kilometers, in a seventeen-seat propeller plane to Kisangani, the capital of the former Orientale province. From Kisangani, our destination—an administrative district called Wamba, in dense rainforest—was another 600 kilometers to the northeast. This time, our mode of transportation was a single-engine Cessna, with seating for nine passengers. After roughly an hour flying above nothing but deep, dark green rainforest, we spotted a small open area of red dirt with a few tall trees still standing at either end that had obviously been cleared in the middle of the jungle. Our pilot, who was an American, started circling a few times, looking down through his window and shaking his head. I could see he was nervous about attempting a landing. Again and again he circled, trying to gauge how he should do it, and then, swiftly and suddenly we found ourselves making a descent into such a tight space that I thought the plane's wings would end up touching the branches of trees. Clouds of dust went up as we landed. Shuddering and jolting violently, the plane came to a stop just before the end of the airstrip.

Our arrival was greeted enthusiastically by hundreds of pygmies, gathered there from a nearby village, the level of their excitement raised all the more by the uncommon sight of the airplane—and the prospect of strange guests from far away. Accompanying them were the military forces on hand to guard us: soldiers, dressed in full combat gear including gas masks, plus a good number of police officers armed with rifles. This was a degree of welcome and security befitting the visit of a president. The air strip was really so in name only: it appeared to be more of a hastily prepared dirt clearing. After the people had sung and danced their welcome, we got into the cars and advanced along the dirt road to the heart of the village. Here and there, we saw traditionally made dwellings, plain mud huts constructed out of earth and woven branches. In honor of my visit, the sides of the roads had been swept clean, and every 40 or 50 meters I saw decorations of flowers placed on wreaths of palms. The village school had declared a holiday in honor of the guest from Japan, and all the inhabitants stood by the sides of the road, waving as we passed by.

Nearly 500 people had gathered in the village from their dwellings in the surrounding rainforest. I was told that skin diseases were rife, since in the forest habitat they generally avoided washing in the rivers, fearing attacks from animals in the jungle. As I walked among them, I noticed a few people whose feet were misshapen or who had permanently bent fingers, but I saw virtually no cases of severe disability. I later learned that only those capable of walking had made the journey from their jungle homes; those with severe disability had remained back in the forest. As I walked along shaking hands with each of them, I paid attention to the state of their skin. Some of them flinched visibly when I touched them. Perhaps they were nervous about being touched by someone from a distant land—I couldn't tell. All of them—men and women—had bare upper torsos, and almost invariably their skin showed signs of a disease of one sort or another: some with the patches characteristic of leprosy, but others with blisters or ulcerations of the kind caused by chicken pox. The sight provided me with ample indication of the harsh lives they endure in their forest habitat.

A young girl emerged from the crowd and with her small hands offered me a bouquet of flowers. By her side stood her mother, pregnant, holding a small infant—the young girl's child, I was told. Pygmies marry and start families early, some at the tender ages of twelve and thirteen.

We were in 30 degrees heat, and the air was drenched with humidity. The Wamba district has a total population of around 100,000, including 30,000 pygmies. I was informed that the district's prevalence rate was fifty-seven cases per 10,000, but I had no way of knowing just how accurate this statistic was. Being hunter-gatherers, pygmies moved from place to place with the changing of the seasons, never settling down in a permanent domicile, which makes keeping track of cases extremely difficult. I was told that doctors and nurses go deep into the forest on a regular basis looking for leprosy patients, and when they discover them they entrust the drugs to the headman of the group, giving him a thorough explanation of how to manage and distribute the drugs. However, a Catholic priest based in the diocese of Wamba told me with wry amusement that pygmy society treats all its members equally, and as a result the headman apparently distributes the drugs he receives equally to everyone: both those who are ill and those who are not.

The same priest also told me that pygmy life has gradually become more settled: over the past five years, schools have been built, and at the time of my visit some 5,000 pygmy children were already attending. The priest informed me, with evident pride, that five teachers had already emerged from among these newly educated pygmy students. To be frank, I felt mixed emotions at hearing this news. Pygmies are people who thrive in the forest. They had a unique way of life, living in the wild, coexisting with forest ecosystems, never causing destruction to the environment, taking what they needed, and then moving on. I couldn't help wondering whether it was truly appropriate and even ethical to encourage them to settle down, to give them a modern education, to draw them into a cash economy and transform them into people intent only on satisfying material desires.

When we left the village, we were offered two parting gifts: a little deer and a mynah bird. We had to refuse them, as politely as we could, and we requested that they be returned to the forest. I was also given a "lucky cane"—a thin, narrow piece of wood, about 40 centimeters long, which I was very happy to receive.

When we returned to the open area that was the airstrip, our pilot had a worried look on his face. Before our departure from Kisangani, he told us, he had been assured that the runway here was at least 1,000 meters long. That was why he had agreed to undertake the flight. But after landing, he had discovered that the airstrip was no more than 650 meters long. We would be taking off into a headwind, he said, and he warned us that if we didn't achieve adequate lift he would have to abort the takeoff. "So don't be too surprised if that happens," he told us. And he peered up several times at the tall trees rising high into the sky at the end of the runway. To achieve adequate power for takeoff, the pilot maneuvered the plane down the entire length of the airstrip and then made a quick U-turn, and he repeated this several times. Finally, it seemed that we were about to take off, and there was a moment of anticipation that seemed unbearably long—the bodies of everybody on board seemed to lift off the seats … As a sense of despair was beginning to spread through the passengers, at the very last possible moment the nose of the Cessna lifted, and we headed upward, just managing to escape the tops of the trees … We all joked that our success was surely due to our having been protected by the newly acquired lucky cane.

Not long after our visit, I received the following email from the priest we had spoken with in the village. He had written it in French:

> The man who brought light to Wamba left with words saying "I will be back."

He was a man who did not give many gifts to the people but he poured out his love to all poor pygmies with his affection and his respect.

He is a very modest and shy man but he hugged and encouraged people affected by leprosy among the pygmies and gently touched the afflicted skin.

With children he bent down to talk at the same height with them.

He danced with pygmies to the Tam Tam rhythm.

We would like to thank him from the bottom of our heart for paying attention to the pygmies who had been abandoned by society.

Conditions in Zanzibar—United Republic of Tanzania, November 2007

Route: Kinshasa, DRC → Johannesburg, South Africa (flight time: 4h; one-night stopover) → Dar es Salaam, Tanzania (flight time: 3h 30m)—two nights—Dar es Salaam, Tanzania → Dubai, United Arab Emirates (flight time: 5h; 4h stopover) → Kansai Airport (flight time: 8h 50m; 2h stopover) → Narita (flight time: 1h)

From the DRC, I went on to Tanzania, making the usual stop in Johannesburg. When I last visited in 2005, I had promised to come back and celebrate when the country passed the elimination milestone, so it was with real pleasure that I returned to mark Tanzania's achievement. Among the guests at the celebratory reception was former Health Minister Ms. Anna Abdallah (whom I mentioned earlier), and we were able to raise a toast and celebrate together. As a woman whose father had been affected by leprosy, she told me it meant a lot to her that the target had been reached.

I also met two people involved in two organizations for the empowerment of people affected by leprosy, Dr. Sira Manboya and Mr. Richard. When I'd last visited, Dr. Sira had been in charge of the leprosy control program in Zanzibar. Now she was working as the general secretary of the Tanzania Leprosy Association, which had reorganized itself in September that year, tackling issues of stigma and discrimination and empowerment. Richard was the representative of the Samaritan branch of the Tanzania Leprosy Association in the capital Dodoma. The Tanzania Leprosy Association was aiming to establish a branch in each of the thirty-nine leprosy settlements in

Tanzania, and I was told that so far they had succeeded in establishing eighteen. Tanzania was now one of those nations seeing the emergence of self-empowerment organizations. The movement was still in its infancy, but, as with self-empowerment in India, the important thing was to take that first step. And as I knew, it was vital that someone took an interest in their cause. I talked to them about what I had learned in India and told them that I would do everything I could to support them.

I also included a visit to Zanzibar on my itinerary. In 1963, the island of Zanzibar gained its independence from Britain, and the next year saw a revolution, known as the Zanzibar revolution, after which the country merged with Tanganyika to create Tanzania. Its two main islands are Unguja and Pemba. It is situated just off the coast of Tanzania in the Indian Sea, and though it is part of Tanzania, it still enjoys a high degree of autonomy.

From Dar es Salaam, we went by plane to Unguja island, where I learned from the health ministry that (despite the country having met the WHO target at the national level) prevalence of newly recorded cases here was high—as much as 1.4 per 10,000 population. President Amani Karume was familiar with my name from our Sasakawa Global 2000 agricultural project in the country. I impressed upon him the need to make sustained efforts, and he promised to see that schools would screen for the disease and that pupils would be taught about leprosy in the classroom.

I then flew on to Pemba. Here too I had been told to expect the number of people affected by leprosy to be high. After a fifty-minute flight in a chartered single-propeller plane, we went by car through the jungle to the village of Makondeni, where I stopped at a kindergarten and the children sang songs and danced to welcome me. Here it seemed that children of people affected by leprosy studied side by side with children of families who had no experience of the disease—suggesting that there was little discrimination, and no exclusion. A gathering was held in my honor in a little square outdoors, and as I sat on the grass watching the dancing, which seemed simple but was performed with great passion, I suddenly heard a great thud next to me. A huge coconut had fallen to the ground. Looking up, I saw clusters of similar coconuts hanging from all too slender-looking trees. A close call. Thank goodness it hadn't fallen right on top of me! What would have happened if it had? Everybody had a good laugh imagining what the papers might have said. "Yohei Sasakawa, WHO Goodwill Ambassador for Leprosy Elimination in Critical Condition in Zanzibar after a Coconut Lands on His Head."

Countries visited in 2008	
January	● United Kingdom
	● India
February	● Nepal
	● Cambodia
	● India
March	United States (Washington, DC: US–Japan Sea Power Dialogue; Gallaudet University)
April	Sweden (Ceremony marking twentieth anniversary of establishment of SYLFF program at Uppsala University)
May	● Switzerland
June	Sweden (Conference at WMU in Malmö on impact of climate change on maritime industry)
	Switzerland (UN Commission on Human Rights)
	United Kingdom (Roundtable of international shipping associations; Great Britain Sasakawa Foundation board meeting)
	● Guinea
	Indonesia (Signing ceremony of Agreement for Association of Southeast Asian Nations (ASEAN) Secretariat and the Nippon Foundation Comprehensive Partnership)
August	● Republic of the Niger
	● DRC
September	Czech Republic (Forum 2000 Conference)

	Jordan (WANA Forum)
	United States (Des Moines SG2000)
	China (Dalian University of Foreign Languages)
	Philippines (University for Peace graduation ceremony)
	● India
October	India (S-ILF board meeting)
November	China (WHO Interregional Workshop of the Use of Traditional Medicine in Primary Health Care)
	United States (Meeting with Dr. Norman Borlaug)
	Costa Rica
	Peru (Visit to incarcerated former President Alberto Fujimori)
	● Brazil
	Malaysia (International symposium on safety of navigation and protection of the environment in the Straits of Malacca and Singapore)
December	● Nepal

● Indicates a trip that features in this section.

WMU: World Maritime University.

SYLFF: Sasakawa Young Leaders Fellowship Fund program.

WANA: West Asia–North Africa, a non-profit think tank based in Amman, Jordan, comprising intellectual leaders in economic, environmental, energy, educational, and social spheres.

SG2000: Sasakawa Global program. An agricultural project supporting farmers in need in Africa.

Forum 2000: An annual international conference launched in 1997 when Václav Havel, Elie Wiesel, and the author invited world leaders to Prague for open debate on the major issues and challenges of the new millennium.

Launch of Global Appeal 2008, endorsed by international NGOs—United Kingdom of Great Britain and Northern Ireland, January 2008

Route: Narita → London, United Kingdom (flight time: 12h 35m)—three nights

In January 2008, I visited London for the launch of the Global Appeal 2008—our third such event, endorsed this year by the Nippon Foundation and nine international organizations, including Amnesty International and Save the Children. We chose London in view of its central importance for global communications and the fact that many international NGOs are headquartered there, the aim being to deepen understanding of leprosy and human rights in as wide an audience as possible, including those whose work is not directly related to leprosy.

The event was held at the Royal Society of Medicine on 28 January. There were 126 people present, including representatives of the signatory NGOs, ambassadors, WHO officials, people from leprosy-related organizations, people affected by leprosy, and medical professionals. Victoria Hislop, author of the best-selling book *The Island*, a story that features the former leprosy colony belonging to Greece on the island of Spinalonga, was also attending.

We began with a ten-minute documentary film on leprosy, made specially for the event, after which I gave a speech. We then listened to messages of support from Barry Clarke, chair of Save the Children Alliance, and Sir Edward Clay, a trustee of the charity Leonard Cheshire Disability. Sir Edward noted that many Leonard Cheshire facilities in Asia and Africa started out as homes and care centers for people affected by leprosy. "Overcoming the stigma and discrimination that people with leprosy have to endure is a major objective for us."

This was followed by speeches from José Ramirez, one of the signatories of the Manila Global Appeal 2007 and a board member of the American Leprosy Mission, and Dr. Sira Mamboya, a doctor tackling leprosy in Tanzania. Mr. Ramirez told the audience about being taken by a hearse from a hospital in his hometown Laredo, Texas, to the Carville leprosy sanatorium in Louisiana. He challenged the audience

312

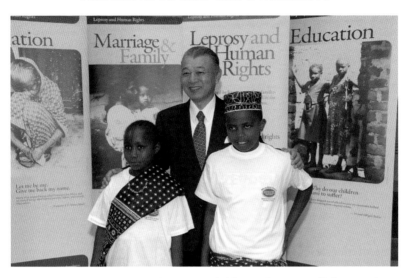

60. Ame (right) and Sahira (left), two children who came all the way from Zanzibar and gave a splendid reading of the Global Appeal text (United Kingdom, January 2008)

to educate others about the true facts about the disease. Dr. Sira talked about the two children she had accompanied to this event to read out the appeal, whom she had treated in Zanzibar. As a doctor, she was delighted they had been cured, but the problem was that "the community does not understand when people have been cured, and still calls them 'patients.'"

Finally, eleven-year-old Sahira Hamadi and twelve-year-old Ame Juma Muhamed from Tanzania (which I had visited at the end of the previous year) read out the text of the Global Appeal. These two children were on their first trip away from their island—their first trip abroad. Doubtless nervous, they nevertheless proudly read out the appeal in English, which they had studied hard to learn.

International Leprosy Conference—Republic of India (Andhra Pradesh state), January 2008

> Route: London, United Kingdom → Dubai, United Arab Emirates (flight time: 7h; 3h stopover) → Hyderabad, Andhra Pradesh, India (flight time: 3h 20m)—two nights

After the Global Appeal in London, I traveled to India via Dubai to attend the opening of the seventeenth International Leprosy Congress in Hyderabad. This congress, which is organized by the ILA, takes place every five years. Ten years previously, it was held in China, and five years previously, Brazil.

Representatives of NGOs, officials from ministries of health from various countries as well as from the WHO, and doctors and scientists working in the field of leprosy had all gathered in the International Conference Center. More than 1,200 participants, in total, with 430 people from overseas and 830 from within India. Most notable of all, 140 people affected by leprosy from twenty-four countries all over the world were attending. A good third of the topics for the conference concerned issues to do with the discrimination and stigma arising from leprosy. The conference took place from 30 January to 4 February and was divided into sessions dealing with elimination activities, human rights, education and awareness-raising, psychological aspects, pathology, and medical aspects. Much lively discussion ensued. There are any number of medical associations in existence, but I am pretty certain that this is the only one in which people affected by leprosy take an active part.

In the special inaugural session on the first day, after speeches given by Rigo Peters, head of ILEP, and Klaus Leisinger, chair of the board of Novartis Foundation, the organization that had taken over free delivery of MDT worldwide from the Nippon Foundation, I gave my address, comparing, as I always do, our work on leprosy with the two wheels of a motorbike—the front wheel dealing with the medical dimension of the disease, the rear wheel the social dimension of the disease. Both wheels have to be the same size and run at the same speed. Later on, I gave a speech titled "Leprosy and Human Rights," in which I touched on the Global Appeal 2008 that we had just launched in London with the endorsement of several international NGOs and organizations and reported on the appeal I was making to the UN Human Rights Council.

In the afternoon of 31 January, I seized some brief moments to visit the Parvath Nagar colony, on the outskirts of Hyderabad. A colony built on a rock-strewn area of land, it has no trees and is the picture of barrenness. This is a colony established by Mr. Mohammed Salahuddin, one of the strongest leaders of all the leprosy colonies in

India. Born into a wealthy family, he was diagnosed with leprosy at the age of sixteen. Although he tried to pursue his original ambition for a professional career, in medicine or in the navy, eventually he had to abandon all his previous aspirations, but his proficiency in English and typewriting skills meant that he could be financially self-reliant. As his illness grew worse, he was hospitalized, but even then, with the endorsement of a doctor, he eventually gained employment as an administrator and provided training to other people affected by leprosy so that they could be similarly employed. After that, he became involved in government-supported leprosy facilities working to support the reintegration of people affected by leprosy into society, helping them into employment. He had established this colony in Parvath Nagar in 1978 on the basis of these experiences with the aim of helping people affected by leprosy gain skills and confidence to go out into the world.

This colony has grown to comprise about 8,000 people, of whom 600 are affected by leprosy. It is an integrated community, with large numbers of people who have no experience of the disease at all. Many of the people affected by leprosy I met had their own businesses, which included little ironing shops, shops selling sweets and puddings, rickshaw businesses, a business loaning telephones, a vegetable shop, and a butcher's. The business owners looked happy and cheerful. However, the elderly people, who had disabilities, told me of their worries for their grandchildren—they would do anything to make sure they got an education. They were like all grandparents the whole world over. Even though their own situations were far from easy, they had more thoughts for their little ones.

Support from the king and the Maoists—Nepal, February 2008

> Route: Hyderabad, Andhra Pradesh, India → Delhi (flight time: 2h; 3h stopover) → Kathmandu, Nepal (flight time: 1h 45m)—one night—Kathmandu → Chitwan (flight time: 30m)—one night—Kathmandu → Bangkok, Thailand (flight time: 3h; 4h stopover) → Narita, Japan (flight time: 5h 45m)

After my trips to London and New Delhi, I traveled on to Nepal (with a three-hour wait at the airport in New Delhi). I had made a previous visit in October 2007. In addition to Kathmandu, I visited Chitwan, a district located in the southwest on the border with India. At this point, Nepal was still one of four countries left in the world that hadn't reached the WHO elimination target (the others being Brazil, the DRC, and Mozambique). The prevalence rate was 1.2 people per 10,000 population, very close to the target.

On my last visit, the unstable political situation and security issues meant that my activities were limited to the environs of the capital Kathmandu, but this time I could go further afield. We traveled by eighteen-seater propeller airplane. Chitwan, just 100 kilometers south, is a low-lying densely forested zone, famous for the Chitwan National Park, a World Heritage Site. We booked accommodation in the Royal Park Hotel, avoiding the riskier city center. The hotel had a grand name but in actuality was a plain wooden building more like a jungle villa. Though we were in a jungle, it was February, and the temperature at night was zero degrees. A cold wind blew in through the cracked windowpanes, the radiators didn't work because of a power cut, and there was no hot water. My room was bone-chillingly cold, and I got into bed wearing gloves and socks, but the bed covers were damp, heavy, and offered little warmth. As accustomed as I am to rough-and-ready places to stay, this had to be one of the worst. I had terrible difficulty getting any rest.

After what turned out to be a sleepless night, I took breakfast dressed in a coat, my breath showing white in the air. When the sun rose, the temperature eased a bit, and we could set about our work. Imagine my surprise when the mode of transport that came to collect me was not a car but an elephant! It seemed well trained and got down on its knees for me to mount it. I enjoyed looking at the scenery from my elevated position on top of its back. I proceeded to form part of a grand parade, accompanied by musicians leading the procession and following behind. The journey could not have been more eventful: at one point, I caught my head on one of the electrical wires hanging down low over the road, and I had to be disentangled by the elephant handler, who used his bamboo rod to move them aside. Then, when I was getting down from the elephant's back, it was in the process of defecating, and if I hadn't moved fast, I would have ended up covered in elephant dung.

Chitwan seemed like a peaceful rural village, inhabited by simple people, but during my stay I was told that there had been bombing and rioting incidents close by. I had thought that the political situation had settled down somewhat, but evidently this was not the case. Such incidents occurred frequently in Tarai. Nepal is a socially complex nation, home to more than thirty different ethnic minorities, including of Indian, Tibetan, and Central Asian extraction. Adding to this complexity has been the presence of the Unified Communist Party of Nepal (Maoist), comprising radical elements opposed to the monarchy that ruled Nepal for 240 years. The party gradually gained strength, allowing it to join a provisional government formed in 2006 ahead of parliamentary elections scheduled for April. In December 2007, a resolution was passed to abolish the monarchy, but the political upheaval was still ongoing. This political turmoil and dire insecurity posed obstacles to our anti-leprosy efforts in Nepal.

Against this backdrop, on this visit to Chitwan and accompanied by an official from the Ministry of Health, I called on a leprosy clinic and paid visits to two health posts in the city of Tandi: the Bakulahar

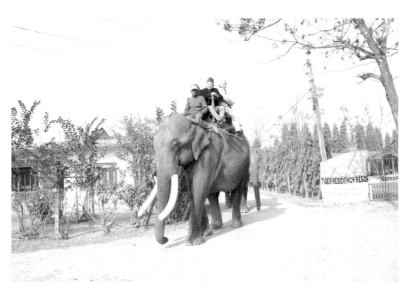

61. The author traveling to a health post by elephant (Chitwan, Nepal, February 2008)

health post and the Bachhauli sub-health post. The staff seemed to be doing their best, despite the political situation and not having received any specific instructions from the government for achieving the elimination target. I was told that the area suffered from a shortage of capable staff due to the frequent changes in personnel. Every year, I make a point of going to the WHO General Assembly in May and receiving briefings on the latest developments relating to leprosy from each country's health ministry, so I know almost every health minister by face, but not so with Nepal, where the health minister is replaced every year, and we have to start the pleasantries of first meeting.

Everywhere I went, I was impressed by the presence of female health workers who were working as volunteers, improving the health of local residents, offering encouragement to people affected by leprosy and their families, and detecting many hitherto undiagnosed cases. It was due to the tireless efforts of such people amid so many challenges to basic health services that leprosy figures had steadily decreased. But the leprosy prevalence in Chitwan was still much higher than it should be—1.9 per 10,000. In some places, the prevalence rate was two or three persons per 10,000, or even more, and a stepping-up of control measures was clearly in order. On this tour, I was accompanied by Dr. Kan Tun, the WHO representative in Nepal. A report of our findings was submitted to the minister of health and population, Giriraj Mani Pokharel.

On 4 February, I met with King Gyanendra. I reported on leprosy elimination efforts in Nepal and the latest efforts to neutralize the social discrimination attached to the disease.

As the leprosy endemic regions are mostly areas under Maoist sway, I decided it would be helpful from a humanitarian standpoint to try and get the cooperation of the Maoists. With the help of an old friend Santa Bir Lama of the Nepal Mountaineering Association, a well-known guide to climbers from Japan, I scoured the streets of Kathmandu for the Maoists' headquarters, and finally after about an hour, we located them—a three-story building in the narrow back lanes of the city. The entrance was adorned with a huge painting with three photographic portraits of Lenin, Stalin, and Mao Zedong. After a few minutes, an old, white-haired gentlemen came into the room.

This was Chandra Prakash Gajurel, the party leader who dealt with the Maoists' external affairs. I told him the reason for my visit. He noted that compared with the former era, when leprosy patients were hidden away in shacks, understanding of the condition now seemed to be making steady progress. And then he said: "Some communities may refuse to admit foreigners out of wariness of their motives. If you need specific support of any kind, at any time, let me know." This seemed to me to be very like a gesture of cooperation.

In effect, I realized, I had succeeded in winning understanding for my leprosy elimination activities from both sides in Nepal—from the king, and from the Maoists. Now we could go with confidence to regions where leprosy efforts lagged and work till we achieved elimination. Exhilarated by this totally unexpected achievement, once we had left the room, in my joy, I couldn't help giving Mr. Santa a hug.

Issues yet to be resolved—landmines and discrimination—Kingdom of Cambodia, February 2008

> Route: Narita, Japan → Bangkok, Thailand (flight time: 7h 20m; one-night stopover) → Phnom Penh (flight time: 1h 15m)—two nights—Phnom Penh → Bangkok (flight time: 1h; 2h stopover) → Narita (flight time: 5h 40m)

In February 2008, I made my first visit in three years to Cambodia. This was a country where even now injuries from landmines and unexploded ordinance continued unabated, despite the civil war having ended over ten years before. According to 2006 figures, every year 440 people were still injured or killed by landmines. I wanted to observe the removal of landmines and unexploded ordnance by the Japan Mine Action Service, a non-profit organization supported by the Nippon Foundation, and show support to the experts—mainly retirees from the Japanese Self-Defense Forces—who undertake this deadly work. Apparently, it will take another 100 years before all landmines and unexploded ordnance in Cambodia are safely removed.

I also paid another visit to Treung township (I previously visited in March 2005). The journey there took two and a half hours, driving along roads clogged with traffic. This is the only leprosy colony in Cambodia, comprising people forcibly sent there during the 1960s and early 1970s to live separately from society. In 1975, the segregation policy was discontinued, and the colony closed, and many residents returned to their native villages, but a lot of them came back, unable to bear the open prejudice and discrimination directed toward them in the outside world. For that reason, Treung is still thought of as a place solely inhabited by people affected by leprosy. Of the 1,243 residents, eighty-seven are completely cured. The number of people who have had leprosy in Cambodia is estimated at 300, which means that roughly 30 percent of them live in this village.

At the village hospital, a nurse, together with two technicians who make protective footwear and prosthetic limbs for people affected by leprosy and who have disabilities in their legs and feet, and one locum doctor—four people in all—were treating patients. Once a month, a person visited from the Omar Foundation, an off-shoot from the leprosy division of the Knights Hospitaller of Malta, to give instruction in the prevention of ulcers. Most of the people here were elderly, with disabilities to their hands or feet. The footwear and prosthetic limbs cost 150 dollars, quite expensive, but I had observed people

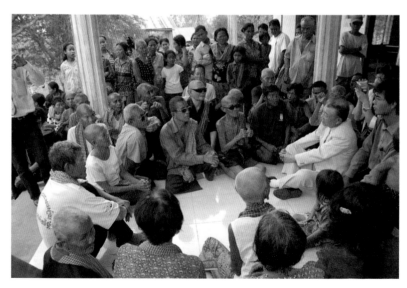

62. A meeting arranged to talk with the villagers of Treung township (Cambodia, February 2008)

affected by leprosy engaged in cutting stone for construction and at work in the rice fields. The average monthly salary in Cambodia was 70 dollars, which meant that the equipment would cost two months' pay. Notwithstanding the high price, such equipment seemed key for anyone with disabilities to gain employment.

In this village, it was not unusual for people affected by leprosy to get married to one another. The local school had 125 pupils, which included the offspring of these marriages. Young men and women with their babies in their arms told me that they wanted cows and pigs so that they could earn a living from them. Cows would produce milk and calves, and pigs would produce piglets. These could be sold for money, which could be reinvested for more money-making opportunities.

One more reason for making this trip was to speak at the opening of an eight-day festival in Phnom Penh for physically challenged performing artists, funded by the Nippon Foundation. In Cambodia, people with disability still face discrimination, and many internalize that discrimination and fear to go out into the wider world. Twelve groups from seven Asian nations were taking part. Nearly 800 people attended the opening night, which was also graced by the presence of Princess Norodom Rattana Devi. I had also invited a group of about forty people affected by leprosy from Treung township who at the time were in a Phnom Penh rehabilitation center. For people who tend to spend the greater part of their time tucked away in care centers and the like, appearing in public would encourage their capacity for self-reliance. Everyone on stage gave bold, confident performances and seemed not to give two hoots to their impediments; they were met with fervent applause from the audience. There were dances in wheelchairs, and pantomimes staged by people with hearing impairments. A strong performance by the world-famous Japanese drumming troupe Koshu Roa Taiko drew particular praise. Other similar festivals followed, held in Vietnam, Laos, Myanmar, and Singapore.

A third S-ILF board meeting—India, March 2008

> Route: Narita → New Delhi (flight time: 10h)—two nights—New Delhi → Chicago, United States (flight time: 15h 50m; 3h stopover)

→ Washington, DC (flight time: 1h 45m)—two nights—Washington, DC → New York (flight time: 1h 25m)—two nights—New York → Narita (flight time: 14h)

After Cambodia, I returned briefly to Japan, and then I was on my way again, this time to New Delhi, in India. From there, I flew on to Washington, DC, where I attended the US–Japan Sea Power Dialogue and also had the opportunity to deliver a lecture on leprosy and human rights at the Woodrow Wilson International Center for Scholars.

In New Delhi, I attended the third board meeting of S-ILF. As already explained, S-ILF aims to enhance the employability and livelihoods of people affected by leprosy and their families through skills training, scholarships, and micro-financing. The meeting was attended by the chair of S-ILF, Dr. S. K. Nordeen; immediate past director-general of the CII Mr. Tarun Das; and S-ILF's director, Dr. Vineeta Shanker, who discussed future financial assistance activities for S-ILF and drew up the following guidelines:

S-ILF Guiding Principles of Financing:

1. SILF's initial target groups are the self-settled colonies.

In order to not spread itself too thin as it begins its work: SILF Board has decided that in the initial years SILF will undertake projects that benefit people in the self-settled colonies.

2. SILF will in the initial years focus exclusively on livelihood creation projects.

The objective of its grants and assistance will be to create and enhance opportunities available to leprosy-affected people and their families living with them in these colonies to undertake sustainable income-generating activities.

3. SILF will give priority to project proposals that are put up by leprosy-affected people themselves.

It believes that its work should respond to the felt needs of the leprosy-affected people as expressed and understood by them.

4. SILF will consider only those proposals that are forwarded by colony associations.

These may be either individual or group projects. SILF believes that this will help to strength the colony associations as well as provide the collective ownership and oversight of the projects.

5. SILF will give greater priority to projects by and/for women.

6. SILF will consider proposals for either an individual or group project.

An individual project is one where a single individual or family is the beneficiary. In a group project, several people/families are participants in the activities and the benefits to accrue to the group.

A meeting of the UN Human Rights Council in Geneva—Swiss Confederation, May 2008

Route: Narita, Japan → Paris, France (flight time: 12h 30m; 2h stopover) → Geneva, Switzerland (flight time: 1h)—three nights—Geneva → Paris (flight time: 1h; 4h stopover) → Narita (flight time: 11h 50m)

There were three items on my agenda when I traveled to Geneva in May 2008. First, to attend the WHO-Sasakawa Health Prize presentation ceremony. Second, to liaise with health ministers at the World Health Assembly to hear the latest on leprosy elimination efforts and post-elimination measures. And third, to meet with and make appeals to numerous ambassadors representing member countries ahead of the meeting of the UN Human Rights Council scheduled for June.

This year, the Sasakawa Health Prize went to MORHAN, a Brazilian NGO dedicated to fighting leprosy and rehabilitating people affected by the disease. I was delighted that the selection committee saw fit to honor a close partner, an organization that had done so much with us for the social rehabilitation of people affected by leprosy and their families in Brazil.

Established twenty-four years prior, in response to the WHO's "Health For All" initiative, the Sasakawa Health Prize recognizes outstanding contributions made by individuals or organizations in the field of primary health care. MORHAN was the second NGO involved in anti-leprosy efforts to be awarded the prize, the first being the ILU. The Brazilian government was delighted, with the Brazilian health minister and the leader to the Brazilian mission at the UN showing as much pleasure as if they were receiving it themselves. Cristiano Torres, chair of MORHAN and once affected by leprosy himself, gave a moving acceptance speech. The regional director and the head of the country office for the Pan-American

Health Organization, the specialized health agency for the Americas in WHO, were also quite evidently delighted.

In my meetings with health ministers, I stressed the importance of continuing to provide leprosy services to control the disease in countries where it had been eliminated as a public health problem. I also urged the ministers of Brazil and Nepal, the two countries yet to reach the goal, to redouble their efforts. Brazil was the birthplace of MORHAN, and both the president and the health minister were determined to reach the elimination targets. All that was needed was to ensure early detection and speedy distribution of medication and they were sure to achieve the target. The Nepalese health minister reported that the Maoists had achieved a victory in the recent election, and democratization was proceeding in his country—it wouldn't be long before the government issued a resolution to eliminate leprosy. Mozambique and the DRC had already achieved the elimination target and were currently only waiting for international recognition of this fact. In fact, every country in Africa had now achieved the elimination target, including Guinea. This was a historic achievement. At one time, Africa had been considered a hopeless case, a continent where elimination was impossible.

The third reason for my presence in Geneva was to seek the understanding and support of ambassadors of members of the UN Human Rights Council for a draft resolution to end discrimination against people affected by leprosy and their families, due to be proposed in June by the Japanese government at the eighth session of the council. I visited delegates from the twenty-seven member states and met with ambassadors and managed to get strong backing from all. Even so, I got the clear impression that many of them lacked knowledge of the extent and depth of the problem. European delegates in particular believed that leprosy was a thing of the past, with no idea that millions of people, along with their family members, still endure prejudice and exclusion because of the disease. Some ambassadors were clearly shocked at the situation as I explained it and agreed there was a definite need for much more awareness-building if the general public was to fully grasp the issues. If things went our way after the Japanese government tabled the resolution, it would be passed on 18 June, the session's final day. Even after the resolution was passed, I was determined to keep making appeals to the government of every nation.

THE DRIVE TO SELF-EMPOWERMENT

At the start of June, I visited Malmö in Sweden to attend a conference at the World Maritime University on the impact of climate change on the maritime industry, and I made another trip to Geneva, Switzerland.

Route: Narita, Japan → Frankfurt, Germany (flight time: 12h; 3h stopover) → Copenhagen, Denmark (flight time: 1h 30m) → Malmö, Sweden (transfer by car)—two nights—Copenhagen → Geneva, Switzerland (flight time: 2h)—two nights—Geneva → Paris, France (flight time: 1h; 2h 30m stopover) → Narita (flight time: 11h 30m)

NGOs that insist on going it alone—Republic of Guinea, June 2008

Route: Narita, Japan → London, UK (flight time: 12h 30m)—three nights—London → Paris, France (flight time: 1h; 3h 30m stopover) → Conakry, Guinea (flight time: 6h 20m)—four nights—Conakry → Paris (flight time: 6h; 6h stopover) → Narita (flight time: 11h 40m)

In June, I visited the Republic of Guinea, first stopping in London to attend the roundtable of international shipping associations and the board meeting of the Great Britain Sasakawa Foundation, and then going on to Guinea via the Charles de Gaulle Airport in France. Guinea is an Islamic country that gained independence from France in 1958. Despite ongoing political uncertainty, it reached the WHO goal of eliminating leprosy as a public health problem in 2006.

Guinea has a reputation for being a country where corruption runs rife. As a country, it lacks basic foodstuffs, and life for the people is precarious. Just two days before I was due to arrive, on 16 June, some policeman went on strike over pay owed to them for several months and barricaded senior officers in a building in the capital Conakry, and the next day there was a shoot-out between the police and the army, which led to the closure of the airport and some of the streets in the city. Seven policemen were killed, and sixty-four people were wounded. The flight I had boarded in Paris was grounded for a while. Worried about security, I quickly sent two female members of my team back to Japan, and after confirming from officials in WHO in Guinea that we would be allowed to land, I decided to go ahead.

On our arrival at Conakry, I stepped out of the aircraft to be enveloped in intense humidity. The temperature was 25 degrees. There to meet me was Health Minister Sangare Hadja Maimouna Bah, who was clad in colorful traditional attire and a striking headwrap. She promised that her ministry would remain committed to fighting leprosy, though the country was currently much preoccupied with other initiatives to tackle diseases like HIV/AIDS and TB. Also present was Dr. Bide Landry, the official in charge of the leprosy program of WHO's African Regional Office, who told me that Guinea's leprosy program was one of the most successful in all of Africa, an example for others to emulate. According to Genji Matsumoto of the Sasakawa Health Foundation, who had arrived ahead of us, only the day before shots had been heard being fired in the city, but today the streets were quiet, and the only sign of the fighting was a single abandoned tank lying by the roadside.

Later in the day, I was briefed by Dr. Fatou Sakho, the coordinator of Guinea's national leprosy program. Like the health minister, she too was clad in colorful traditional attire. In Africa, many extremely able women are in high positions in government.

She told me that in 1990 Guinea had a registered prevalence of 11.9 per 10,000 population. In 2007, the rate had dropped to 0.74. The message that MDT was available free of charge was being broadcast frequently throughout the entire nation, and public awareness was 100 percent (I wanted to see if this was true). Every year on the last Sunday of January, they observed World Leprosy Day with awareness-raising events. In 2002, they had also initiated rehabilitation efforts aimed at supporting the social rehabilitation of people affected by leprosy, with support offered by home visits, skills training, and micro-finance support. In the six provinces where leprosy remained endemic, more work had to be done to reinforce detection to bring down the number of people with disabilities and alleviate the social and economic consequences of the disease.

On the morning of 20 June, I paid a short visit to a health center in Madina, a suburb of Conakry. This was an outpatient facility that saw some eighty patients a day, including those with TB and leprosy. When I arrived, early in the morning, there were already many people present, and I chatted with them. Many had come especially to meet me. Dr. Bide Landry told me that Guinea has a well-developed system of primary health care, which has played its part in early detection and the country achieving the elimination goal.

From there, I went straight to an appointment with Prime Minister Ahmed Tidiane Souaré. He filled me in on the measures being taken in Guinea to control leprosy, and I asked him to pass on the three messages that leprosy is curable, treatment is free, and social discrimination has no place. I also called on the president of the National Assembly, El Hajj Aboubacar Sompare, to deliver a similar request.

That afternoon, I received briefings from the NGOs that support Guinea in its fight against leprosy. The Mission Phil Africaine, from the Netherlands, has the longest presence in Guinea, dating back to 1982, when it opened a center in Forested Guinea and began providing medication. Currently, the center offers microfinance services, employment skills training, and reconstructive surgery. The Raoul Follereau Association, a French NGO, has been in Guinea since 1985, working in Upper and Lower Guinea, supporting the health ministry by supplying medication for people with disabilities, training staff, providing vehicles and fuel, and also conducting awareness campaigns in rural communities. A local version of this association had been established by and for people affected by leprosy in 2005, with the purpose of going into the interior to investigate people's health needs, but the health ministry's leprosy program coordinator Dr. Yakite told me that to date its activities had been constrained due to lack of funds. The Order of Malta had operated in Middle Guinea since 1986, but its leader had just been appointed to the new cabinet and could not be present at our meeting. Dr. Landry told me that relations between the health ministry and the NGOs were not cordial, which was why in six provinces the prevalence rate never got any better. He had lobbied for a scheme that required regular updates and effective coordination between the ministry and the NGOs, but despite all efforts certain individuals in the NGOs seemed to prefer to go it alone, with the result that nothing had got off the ground.

The following day, I visited a health facility in Kindia, an upland city some 135 kilometers east of the capital, in a vehicle that negotiated the paved but narrow road at 100 kilometers per hour. When we arrived, there was a power cut due to heavy rains, and no lights were on inside the buildings. I was greeted in a spot outdoors by the mayor and city officials. I asked the mayor how many people lived in the city, but he looked puzzled and asked the official standing next to

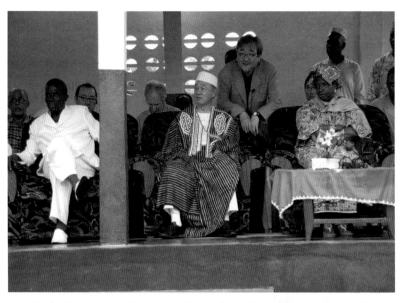

63. With the mayor of Kindia, who had no idea of his city's population (Guinea, June 2008)

him. He didn't know either. Another official answered my question, but I instinctively knew that the figure he gave was inaccurate. The health post at Damakanya is one of twenty in Kindia prefecture and specializes in patients with HIV/AIDS, leprosy, and TB. Originally set up to treat sleeping sickness caused by the tsetse fly (now treated elsewhere), the health post sees an average of twenty patients a day. To welcome me, about twenty people affected by leprosy had come in from the surrounding area (that is, within a radius of 100 kilometers), and among the other events in the welcoming ceremony, they put on a little skit. The story of the skit was as follows. A man visits a health center, where he is diagnosed with leprosy, registered as a patient, and prescribed MDT. On his return home, his wife flees in horror to her parents. But after being given the facts about leprosy by her mother, who is properly informed about the disease, the sobbing wife calms down and goes back to her husband. It was quite a performance, and utterly convincing as the performers had all had experience of the disease.

I stayed a total of four days in Guinea, but the political situation was so unstable that with the exception of the trips I took for visits and face-to-face meetings with officials (with armed vehicles leading the way), I spent the entire time in my hotel room, unable to go out. Unusually, I was not invited to any formal dinners, so apart from a hastily snatched meal on my visit to Kindia, for the four days I spent in the largely empty hotel, I had to take all my meals there. The menu was extremely limited, so every single day I had an omelette for dinner. At my age, I don't particularly need sumptuous meals, and I am happy to take what is on offer wherever I go on my travels. But I feel bad for putting the younger members of my team, who had hearty appetites, under such testing experiences.

In traditional attire—Republic of Niger, August 2008

Route: Narita, Japan → Paris (flight time: 12h; one-night stopover) → Niamey, Niger (flight time: 5h 20m)—three nights

In August, I made my first trip to the Republic of Niger, via Paris. This was the twenty-third African country I had visited. A landlocked nation, Niger shares borders with seven other countries—Libya, Algeria, Mali, Burkina Faso, Benin, Nigeria, and Chad. One-third of the country lies in desert, and it is the hottest country on earth. Niger achieved the WHO's goal of eliminating leprosy as a public health problem in 2002—the leprosy prevalence rate in 2007 stood at 0.39 per 10,000 population. According to the UNDP's Human Development Index rankings, however, it was among the poorest nations in the world. Inflation was rampant, and unemployment high. Ten thousand recent university graduates were without employment.

At the airport, I was met by Minister of Population and Social Reform Zila Manane Bookani, and Minister of Public Health Issa Lamine, the latter one of eight high-ranking female officials in the cabinet, charged with social rehabilitation of people with disabilities, including people affected by leprosy. Minister Issa, a member of the Tuareg ethnic group, wore traditional attire, his entire head and face swathed in a long white head cloth. I make a practice of wearing the clothing of whichever country I am visiting as a way of expressing affinity, and this time was no exception—I asked if a head cloth could be procured for me to wear during my stay. I was given a *cheche* (the head cloth) and the *grand boubou* (the flowing wide-sleeved robe). It was quite a task to wrap the headcloth, which was more than 5 meters long, round my head, and every morning I had to ask for assistance from the hotel staff. Everyone seemed to do it in a different way—or perhaps it was just that there are several different styles. Looking at my reflection in the mirror, I felt like an avenger fighting for justice, or even, I thought, Kurama Tengu. Sadly, the younger members of my team were probably unfamiliar with this legendary Japanese hero with supernatural powers … This is a little off-topic, but once when my father visited the French premier Valéry Giscard d'Estaing in the Palais de l'Élysée in Paris, the premier several times expressed his admiration for the formal Japanese *hakama* and *haori* that my father wore and wanted to know all about them. At the time, the premier was avidly reading *The Book of Five Rings* and wanted to know all about what samurai wore and did.

At the WHO Niger office, I learned that in addition to eliminating leprosy as a public health problem nationally, at the sub-national level the disease prevalence rate had fallen below one in 10,000 in all but two of its forty-two provinces. In the two provinces in question, the nomadic life of the Fulani people who lived there was cited as one difficulty. Also cited were the lack of trust toward the government leprosy control programs, the fact that no new plan for the past three years had been drawn up to sustain progress, the lack of priority given by the government to leprosy, and the lack of cooperation between NGOs and government. The government was not taking advantage of the free MDT available from the WHO, relying instead on one sole NGO to supply the drugs. We could only assume that this had to do with historical connections—perhaps this NGO had been supplying medication to people before WHO became involved in elimination efforts. For the patients, it didn't make much difference, as they were still getting their medication. But if the NGO had availed themselves of the free MDT available from WHO, this would have freed up money to spend on other services. It was incomprehensible.

Health Minister Lamine was surprised and delighted to see me dressed in Tuareg attire. I thanked him for what Niger had achieved so far and urged him to make it the first country in Africa to wipe out leprosy altogether.

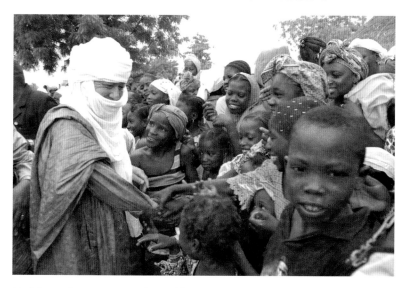

64. The author imagining himself as Kurama Tengu (Niger, August 2008)

My next appointment was with Minister of Population and Social Reform Zila Manane Bookani, to whom I underlined the necessity of ending stigma and discrimination against people affected by leprosy. She assured me the government was working with various NGOs including the Raoul Follereau Niger to address the social rehabilitation of people affected by leprosy and to secure support for self-reliance, housing, and food relief, but something told me that this was not working very well. In the afternoon, I met with a couple of NGOs—Raoul Follereau Niger and Serving in Mission. They were involving themselves in all sorts of efforts for social rehabilitation of people affected by leprosy—offering skills training, literacy programs, agricultural support, and microfinancing. All of this was small-scale, but over the long term these efforts, often carried out against the odds, would all prove important.

On my third day, I visited the National Center for Dermatology and Leprosy. Built in 1981, it initially specialized in leprosy, but it now treats other skin diseases as well. I then went on to Koira Tégui, a village in Niamey of 250 households of people affected by leprosy and other people with disabilities that had grown up on land made available by an NGO. As I arrived, the villagers and their children gave me a wonderful welcome, singing and dancing. Without any hesitation, I joined the rows of children and danced with them. The young men then put on a demonstration of the local form of wrestling, apparently very popular, and carried out with deadly seriousness. I found it fascinating—it seemed that the first to hit the ground with their body was the one to lose. I was pleased to see that these scenes were being recorded by a TV crew. I believe such positive images go a long way to lessening the stigma and discrimination attached to leprosy. There were three such self-settled colonies in Niamey, and about five in each of the other provinces. Organizations of people affected by leprosy were springing up all over the country, and hopefully they would form wider networks that would be able to lend their strength to enabling social rehabilitation.

The same day, I was invited to the private residence of Prime Minister Seyni Oumarou, whom I had met earlier in the year in May at The Fourth Tokyo International Conference on African Development held in Yokohama. On seeing me dressed in traditional Niger attire, he raised his hands in surprise. He told me, "This sends a message that you are thinking about Niger's problems with us."

My visit concluded with a press conference, where I was joined by the health minister and the population minister, to brief those present on the latest efforts in Niger on leprosy elimination.

Toward the end of my stay, I found myself with a few hours to spare before my evening flight, and a liaison officer from the Foreign Office recommended that we go to view the giraffe reserve. We were about an hour's drive along a highway out of Niamey when we saw several giraffes ahead of us gracefully walking across the road. The liaison officer and the WHO official had the cars stop for us to watch and take photographs. This ended up landing us in a spot of bother. Somebody seemed to have reported us to the paying observation platform located about five minutes' drive along on the road. "There is a rule that you are only allowed to take photographs once you have paid the observation fee," an official came and told us. "You have committed an offense. For this, we will have to confiscate your cars and your cameras." Someone in our party went to negotiate. At first, I was confident we would get on our way quickly, aware that in Africa

matters can sometimes be quickly solved by "money under the table."
But I was mistaken—the negotiations took ages. Ever the optimist, I
tried to make a joke of it all, telling my companions that "spending
two or three days in a prison in Niger will make a great story."
Finally, after about an hour and a half, during which we waited while
craning our necks in anticipation till it felt like they were as long as
the necks of the giraffes we had come to observe, the person we had
asked to negotiate came back with a smile on his face. Ultimately, we
paid the goodly sum of $105 for our photographs of the giraffes. And
we were allowed to go on our way.

Issues after elimination is reached—DRC, August 2008

Route: Niamey, Niger → Paris (flight time: 5h; one-night stopover) →
Kinshasa, DRC (flight time: 7h 45m)—four nights—Kinshasa → Paris
(flight time: 7h 45m; 14h stopover) → Narita (flight time: 11h 30m)

From Niger, I made my way to the DRC. This involved traveling back
to Paris, where I stayed overnight in a hotel near the airport before
taking a roughly eight-hour flight to Kinshasa, the capital of the
DRC. This was a visit following up one I'd made the previous year.
The DRC had achieved the WHO's leprosy elimination goal at the
end of 2007. To be frank, I hadn't expected it to do it so soon. Parts
of the country were still at war, its infrastructure needed building up,
and diagnosing and treating the hunter-gatherer tribes that live in the
extensive tropical rain forests of the Congo River basin presented a
real challenge. The fact that the DRC was able to achieve the elimination goal was a credit to all involved. The purpose of my visit was
both to mark the achievement with those responsible—government
officials and people working on the ground—and to see for myself an
area where the prevalence rate remained troublingly high.

The morning after my arrival, I visited the WHO office and met
representative Allarangar Yokoude. "Much leprosy work remains to
be done in the DRC," he told me without hesitancy. "During this visit
we would like you to see not only what progress has been achieved
but also what issues remain to be dealt with." According to Alexandre
Tiendrebeogo of WHO, the results of a survey taken at the end of
2007 for the entire African region had shown a prevalence rate of

0.45, so Africa as a whole had reached the elimination target. Nevertheless, in certain countries there were numerous places where leprosy remained endemic. The prevalence rate in the DRC was high in four provinces, Katanga, Orientale, Équateur, and Bandundu. I opted during this visit to go to Katanga province's Moba district, where the prevalence rate was 2.01.

At the health ministry, I reunited with Minister of Health Makwenge Kaput, who said he would accompany me on my observation trip to the provinces. I also met with Nzanga Mobutu, who as deputy prime minister for basic social needs ranked third in the DRC's political hierarchy. President Joseph Kabila and Prime Minister Antoine Gizenga were out of the country on official visits, so I wasn't able to convey my congratulations directly. Nzanga Mobutu is a son of former President Sese Seko Mobutu, the dictatorial leader who ruled the DRC for thirty-two years, until 1997, when his government was overthrown. I had met President Mobutu once in Tokyo, when he attended the state funeral of Emperor Showa in February 1989. I was still wet behind the ears and perhaps somewhat naively said to the president: "We are grateful that you could come. I hear that the situation in your country is unstable." To which Mr. Mobutu, who was wearing his trademark leopard-skin hat, jokingly responded: "Everything's just fine. I brought the guys mostly likely to rebel against me with me to Japan." The man who overthrew President Mobutu was Laurent-Désiré Kabila, father of Joseph Kabila, the president between 2001 and 2018. So two sons of former political enemies were working side by side in the interests of national unity.

With Health Minister Dr. Victor Makwenge Kaput and the WHO country representative, I set out for Moba district, flying first to the provincial capital Lubumbashi, 2,000 kilometers southeast of Kinshasa. From there, we transferred to a sixteen-seater propeller plane for the 600-kilometer flight north to Moba. When we landed, on a runway that was little more than an open area of red dirt, we were given a rousing greeting with much rhythmical music by a 1,000-strong crowd of local people. Moba is a region where war broke out for a second time in 1997 between government and rebel forces (the former including ex-Rwandan army troops). In 2000, the war became particularly ferocious, with kidnappings and pillaging and acts of arson, along with massacres, and many villagers made their escape by boat across Lake Tanganyika to Tanzania and Zambia. Now that the fighting had ended and peace restored, in the last six months more than 3,000 people had returned to this village. Altogether, about 18,000 people had come back to the country, I was told, though many regarded Rwandan people with fear.

Lake Tanganyika is a vast expanse of water, in all of Africa second only in size to Lake Victoria. It is surrounded by the countries of Tanzania, the DRC, Zambia, and Burundi. The morning after I arrived, we journeyed by boat along the shore of Lake Tanganyika south for about an hour to the village of Mulunguzi, whose population of some 1,900 included many people affected by leprosy. Hundreds of villagers had gathered, eager to meet us, some standing waist-deep in the water. As we jumped ashore, they broke into applause, and women yelped in excitement, their hands over their mouths. We were escorted on foot to the Mulunguzi health center.

Leprosy had been rife in the area around Mulunguzi since the mid-1980s. According to a study of the almost 14,000 people living in the region served by the health center, new cases were being detected at the rate of 110 per year, and the prevalence rate was unusually high, at twenty-five per 10,000. I was told that a plan was underway for a joint investigation of this anomaly to be carried out by the health ministry, NGOs, and a group of American researchers.

As so often happened, before leaving I was invited to join the villagers in dancing and worked up quite a sweat before it was time to take our leave. Our leave-taking was very moving. As I boarded the boat, the villagers—even more numerous than when we had arrived—waded into the lake, yelping excitedly and waving their hands in farewell. They continued doing this until they were but tiny specks far off in the distance—all for this Japanese visitor they might never see again.

After Mulunguzi, I called at the Moba hospital, a large facility with 150 beds. Dr. Kaput's father had once served as a physician here, and Dr. Kaput himself, I was told, had spent part of his childhood in Moba. Here again, I was surrounded by villagers, and again I worked up a sweat dancing with them, this time to loud music blaring from loudspeakers. Several families of people affected by leprosy were living not far from the hospital's main building. I was told that even though they had been cured of their disease, they were unable to return to their villages because of discrimination and had no choice but to settle where they now were.

Since Moba has no facilities for lodging visitors, we put up in a beautiful red-brick church that had been constructed 100 years before by a member of a Belgian mission, situated within a village of thatch-roofed houses. I was given the pastor's room to use. On the wall was a photo of Pope John Paul II, who was deceased; there was no photo of his successor Pope Benedict XVI. I had no way of knowing whether this unusual circumstance was due to the remoteness of the location or to the personal taste of the pastor himself, but either way I felt this was a bit strange.

Dinner was served in the attached convent where the nuns lived. We were all craving a beer, knowing all too well that this was not a

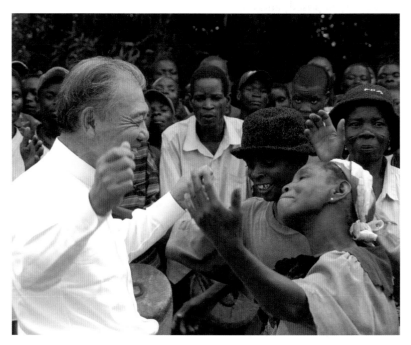

65. One step out of the airport and a warm reception awaits (Democratic Republic of the Congo, August 2008)

place where we would find one, but by a stroke of luck one of the two people serving us, a woman of robust physique, appeared with a bottle for each of us. That beer, drunk in such a remote location, tasted especially good. Watching the efficient manner in which our two servers went about their work, I turned to Dr. Kaput, who was sitting next to me, and asked, "Are those two nuns?" The health minister immediately broke into laughter: "They're members of parliament who hail from here. They came back home a week ago to prepare for your visit." Just at that point, a platter with a big black mound of caterpillars was offered to me, but I could not face it, and I had to decline.

My bed was equipped with a mosquito net, but the toilet was out-doors. The mosquitoes that transmit malaria (genus Anopheles) come out in the morning and evening. As usual, I lavishly sprayed my face, hands, and feet with mosquito repellent, but in the morning when I went to the toilet, it suddenly occurred to me that my rear end was completely exposed, and I had neglected to spray it. I realized that I shouldn't dilly-dally and finished up with all speed.

At 5.30 a.m., the church bells started to ring. Entering the church, I saw that twenty or so worshippers were already quietly at prayer, though the priest had yet to appear.

We returned to Lubumbashi, once again by the propeller plane. At the hotel, we saw European peace-keeping forces in army fatigues who were stationed there, with female soldiers among them.

In the evening, a ceremony was held in Lubumbashi at which the DRC government issued an official declaration that leprosy had been eliminated from the country as a public health problem. It took place in the Katanga governor's mansion, and many members of the press and TV crews were on hand to cover it. Dr. Kaput, as health minister, read out the formal declaration of elimination, and then we had questions from the media. Many of the questions were shockingly basic: "Is leprosy hereditary?" "Is there a risk of 'catching' leprosy?" And so on. I was made painfully aware that the world's media still needed quite a bit of education and awareness-raising about the disease. Only recently, I had seen a major newspaper in the United Kingdom using the discriminatory term "leper," and I'd had to issue letters of complaint.

MAKING THE IMPOSSIBLE POSSIBLE

Like the River Ganges—Republic of India (New Delhi, Uttar Pradesh, West Bengal), September 2008

> Route: Narita, Japan → New Delhi, India (flight time: 8h 35m)—two nights—New Delhi → Varanasi, Uttar Pradesh (flight time: 1h)—two nights—Varanasi → New Delhi (flight time: 1h 20m)—one night—New Delhi → Kolkata, West Bengal (flight time: 2h)—two nights—Kolkata → Bangkok, Thailand (flight time: 2h 40m; 2h stopover)→ Narita (flight time: 6h)

September saw me journey to India, where I went to three cities: New Delhi, Varanasi, and Kolkata. My purpose in visiting India this time was to attend a seminar in New Delhi to brief Indian media and partners on the Human Rights Council resolution in June, to go to the holy city of Varanasi, and to take part in a meeting in Kolkata of the National Forum for People Affected by Leprosy, to which I had been giving my wholehearted support since its founding in 2005.

In New Delhi, I visited the WHO's Southeast Asia Regional Office, which works with us in leprosy control efforts, and the Indian health ministry, and discussed the current state of leprosy elimination efforts both in Asia and in India itself. In Asia, the only two countries left to achieve the WHO target were Nepal and now Timor-Leste. In 2008, the latter had joined the countries covered by the WHO target due to a population increase.

On this day, we held a symposium with the participation of specialists in law, human rights, medicine, and leaders of relevant civic organizations to tell them about recent developments in the UN Human Rights Council. The Japanese government had submitted a resolution to the council in June 2008 calling for an end to discrimination against people affected by leprosy and their families, and it had been passed.

I then went to Varanasi, in Uttar Pradesh state, which has a population of around 190 million people. This town, situated on the banks of the sacred river, the "mother Ganges," is a sacred city for people of Hindu faith and proponents of Buddhism. Bodies are continually being cremated in funeral pyres on the riverbank, and it is believed in the Hindu faith that throwing the ashes into the river will enable the deceased to be released from the wheel of transmigration. As a result, the city is filled with people who are near the end of their lives. I had long been determined to visit this holy city, knowing of its intimate links with the faith of Indian people.

At the Sankata Mochan colony, I was interested to learn that this colony had a policy of having children move out when they marry, to give them a better chance of broadening their opportunities. I was also greatly impressed by the musicians who performed for me—with accordions and drums—sitting on the ground, playing. In this colony, in addition to the psychiatrist, Dr. Tulsi, a number of NGOs offer support, and one of the methods they use to do this involves teaching the residents to play musical instruments. It seemed to be working. The expressions on the players' faces spoke of the healing power of music and its ability to nourish the soul.

The following day, I visited two primary health centers, in Harhua and Pindra. Here, I met a group of women, Accredited Social Health Activists known by their acronym ASHA, who greeted me by intoning a Hindu prayer. These women are not formally employed: their work is undertaken voluntarily, with occasional remuneration. On six days of the week, they head out to villages, going from house to house, examining the inhabitants for signs of leprosy or other diseases. Each activist is responsible for about 1,000 inhabitants. For every person detected with leprosy, an activist receives 100 rupees (roughly equivalent to US$1). They are then charged with making sure that the patient takes MDT for the next six months. At the end of the treatment, the activist receives a further 200 to 400 rupees. Thanks to these workers, early detection rates improved, more people were cured, and fewer people were left with disabilities.

On my last day in Varanasi, I rose at 4 a.m. and boarded a motorboat to go out on the Ganges. The part of the river that runs through the city is not all that wide, but it flows swiftly. In contrast to Japan, where the purest water is used in religious ritual, the water of the Ganges is filthy, with rubbish and plastic bottles, and corpses of cows floating past, and sometimes, so we were told, the dead bodies of children wrapped in cloth. On the banks, people were praying fervently, splashing water over their heads, and assiduously gargling. Not 100 meters away was a crematorium, where the ashes of the dead were tipped into the water. From further upstream came a stream of effluent from the city sewers. Apparently, it is the mark of the highest respect to put the ashes of the deceased into an urn and throw it into the river. However, not everybody gets put into an urn: the ashes of people affected by leprosy, pregnant women, people who died of smallpox, anyone who had died after being bitten by a venomous snake, and children younger than ten years are just thrown in without ado. Gazing out from the boat, everywhere I looked I could see people exposing their rear ends and performing their morning business straight into the river. This was, I thought, a quintessentially Indian experience—where things that I would rather not see forced themselves into my line of vision.

From there, I went to Kolkata, in West Bengal, where a meeting was taking place of the National Forum. An all-India meeting of this organization, founded in 2006, had so far been held twice in New Delhi, with one meeting of the west India chapter in Mumbai in Maharashtra state. This was the first time a meeting had been held in Kolkata, in east India. Nearly 300 people affected with leprosy attended, from West Bengal, Odisha, and Jharkhand, and several states in the northeast. It was essential, if the organization wanted to be taken seriously by the rest of India, for it to keep expanding and enriching its operations and also to foster talented young leaders who would be able to take it forward into the future.

In the final panel of the conference, as I was making my address a vision of the scenes we had witnessed on the River Ganges flitted before my eyes. The river had its source in the Himalayan Mountains, far away in Nepal, and was formed by several tributaries that came together to form a magnificent river, which then flowed all the way out to sea. It seemed like a fitting metaphor for the National Forum, which was also formed from all sorts of small forces coming to it from localities all over India. I told myself that I had to keep up my efforts so that these smaller forces could become a powerful river, eventually large enough to create the changes in society that we wanted to see.

Talks with a president and people affected by leprosy—Republic of Brazil, November 2008

Route: Narita, Japan → Los Angeles, United States (flight time: 9h 40m; one-night stopover) → San José, Costa Rica (flight time: 5h 40m)—two nights—San José → Lima, Peru (flight time: 3h 40m)—one night—Lima → São Paulo, Brazil (flight time: 4h 40m; 7h stopover) → Brasília (flight time: 2h)—two nights—São Paulo → Frankfurt, Germany (flight time: 11h 25m; 3h stopover) → Narita (flight time: 11h)

In November, I visited Brazil, going via Los Angeles for a trip of ten days and nine nights, though five of those nights were actually spent on board an airplane. Along the way, I stopped for an event at the University of Peace in San José, Costa Rica, where I had a meeting with President Arias. I also visited former President Fujimori in prison in Peru.

On my arrival in Brasília, I called on the offices of Grupo de Apoio as Mulheres Atingidas pela Hanseniase (GAMAH), an NGO founded in 2003 by Mrs. Marly Araújo, a woman affected by leprosy. Every day, some two dozen or so people affected by leprosy come to the organization's offices and engage in income-generating activities such as making sandals and drying flowers. Mrs. Araújo originally served as a health worker treating leprosy patients before she herself contracted the disease. She founded GAMAH to fill what she recognized as a need for a place where those affected by leprosy coping with disability and facing discrimination could gather.

That afternoon, I paid calls on the local offices of WHO and the Brazilian health ministry. In my discussion with the official in charge of the government's leprosy program, I was shocked to notice that he did not once mention the word "elimination." Undeniably, they were taking steps to detect the disease and offer early treatment, but they were clearly working with no defined target in mind. Of course, I realize that reaching the WHO-defined target of elimination (fewer than one newly discovered case per 10,000) is not the entire solution. But a specific target does provide an essential motivating force. Brazil had agreed to be part of the whole effort organized by WHO that involved this benchmark, so it had a responsibility to make every effort to reach it.

That evening, I met with President Lula. Also present were Minister of Health José Gomes Temporão, Health Surveillance Secretary Dr. Gerson Oliveira Penna, Special Secretary for Human Rights Paulo de Tarso Vannucchi, national coordinator of MORHAN Artur Custódio, and seven people affected by leprosy. Originally scheduled to last fifteen minutes, our meeting lengthened to half an hour. I appealed to President Lula to improve the current situation of the people affected by leprosy in his country, and my sentiments were echoed by Artur Custódio and everyone else there with him.

The president had always been extremely interested in the quest to get rid of leprosy. Immediately after taking office, he had paid several public visits to leprosy facilities, and he had decided to pay financial compensation to people affected by leprosy who had suffered under Brazil's segregation policy through the 1960s. In 2006, he publicly proclaimed his support for improving the rights of people affected by leprosy in Brazil as a signatory to that year's Global Appeal. The president asked for an explanation from the health minister on the current state of affairs regarding leprosy, and he then stated he would do everything in his power to work for an improvement. It was a huge step forward to have people affected by leprosy making a direct appeal to the president and successfully extract a promise of help from him in this way.

This meeting with President Lula produced two significant results. First, it was decided that in January 2009, when the central govern-

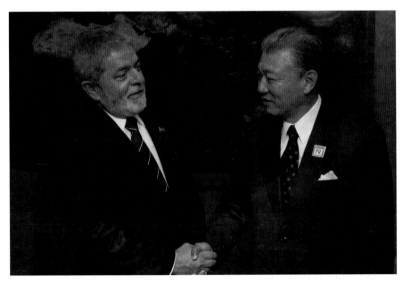

66. A handshake with President Lula (Brazil, November 2008)

ment announced the new year's primary objectives to the country's municipal leaders, the highest priority would be accorded to leprosy as a public health issue, alongside measures to combat dengue fever. Second, the Ministry of Health would ask the nation's governors, mayors, and other municipal leaders to submit written statements listing the efforts being undertaken in their municipalities to tackle the leprosy issue.

The next day, I flew on to São Paulo, where I went to the Padre Bento Hospital and the nearby São Francisco de Assis Home. The Padro Bento Hospital was built in 1931 and for thirty years was used as a segregation facility. After the policy of segregation was abandoned in the 1960s, it transformed into a general hospital. The city of São Paulo then offered a strip of land free of charge to be used for the housing of the people who had been living in the hospital, who had disabilities and had no place to go, and this was where the São Francisco de Assis Home was built. Afterwards, it became a home where elderly people could live, if they paid rent. At the time of my visit, eighty elderly residents were living there, and forty-two of them were people affected by leprosy. It was being run by a Catholic monastic order, and I remember well how gently and affectionately they treated the residents.

In the newly formed federal democratic republic—Nepal, December 2008

> Route: Narita→ Singapore (flight time: 7h 40m; one-night stopover) → Kathmandu, Nepal (flight time: 5h 25m)—one night—Kathmandu → Bharatpur (flight time: 45m)—one night—Biratnagar → Kathmandu (flight time: 50m) —one night—Kathmandu → Shimla (charter flight, flight time: 20m)—return same day—Shimla → Kathmandu (flight time: 20m) → Singapore (flight time: 4h 40m; 2h stopover) → Narita (flight time: 6h 40m)

In December, I made my second trip that year to Nepal. In May that year, the monarchy, which had ruled continuously for 240 years, was abolished and the country reborn as a republic. On my previous visit in February, I met with King Gyanendra and won his backing for our elimination activities, but now the political system had completely changed, as had Nepal's top health personnel, so I wanted to pay a visit as soon as I could, securing their strong commitment to leprosy elimination policy and encouraging them to meet the target as soon as they were able to.

On arrival, I was met by an old friend, Dr. Alexander Andjaparidze, the new WHO representative in Nepal. Dr. Andjaparidze, originally from Georgia in the Caucasus, had served as WHO's representative in residence in Timor-Leste from 2000 to February 2008, a period of great social upheaval. I have already written about how he had chosen to remain in the country when all other UN personnel had left, and how immediately above the desk in his office was a hole left by a bomb. He had moved to Nepal to become the WHO representative here in March. I was delighted.

Dr. Andjaparidze, ever passionate about his work, gave me a briefing in the airport lobby. He informed me that leprosy prevalence rates remained above two per 10,000 in eleven districts out of seventy-five, with the highest statistics recorded in the Terai belt in the country's south, on the border with India. Special teams had been formed to undertake intensive activities in the especially high districts, on a trial basis. If that approach proved successful, he intended to expand it to cover other districts as well. Dr. Andjaparidze said that he expected the elimination target to be achieved in Nepal at the national level by the end of 2009, but he had one major concern: political security. He could not be sure whether his staff would be able to safely undertake their activities in outlying regions. He was also worried about the possible rise of malaria. Previously, mosquitos had never been found in areas higher than 1,200 meters above sea level (Kathmandu was 1,300 meters above sea level), but now cases of both malaria and Japanese encephalitis had been diagnosed in areas at 1,400 meters, possibly as a result of climate change.

I then went to meet with Minister of Health and Population Dr. Pokharel. He was one of only a few members of the Council of Ministers under the monarch who had retained their position after the new government formed in August 2007, and I had met him a number of times at international conferences in Nepal and Geneva. He told me that "in the new republic there should be no place for leprosy," and made clear his resolve to achieve elimination in his country by 2009. Dr. Pokharel was supported in his position by two newly appointed deputies, a vivid indication of the changes wrought to Nepal's governing system. In a further development, to strengthen the country's elimination activities in earnest, just two weeks prior to my arrival Dr. Pokharel had appointed Dr. Garib Das Thakur, a highly skilled and experienced specialist, to serve as chief of the Leprosy Control Division of his ministry's Department of Health Services. It seemed that an ideal team of leaders had been put together, and this made me hopeful that major results would come of our activities in the near future. One of the suggestions made by Dr. Andjaparidze at this meeting for breaking down stigma was that patients who had been cured of leprosy should receive a "Treatment Completed" certificate bearing the minister's signature. This would also serve to let people know that leaders in government were committed to anti-leprosy measures. I thought this an excellent idea, and I was interested to see what would come of it. The minister accepted the idea on the spot. He also promised that he would accompany me on my next visit to places where leprosy remained endemic.

That same evening, I also called on Mr. Pushpa Kamal Dahal, the new prime minister under the interim government formed to draft a constitution, at his official residence. In Nepal, he was apparently better known by his sobriquet, "Prachanda." Between 1996 and 2006, he had gone underground as leader of the Maoist rebels seeking to topple the monarchy, a group that evolved into the People's Liberation Army in 2002, taking up arms against the military forces supporting the monarchy. At the time of our meeting, Mr. Dahal, still fresh from his role as the top guerrilla fighter, was now leader of the political party with the largest representation in the interim government, a position that put him in the prime minister's seat at the head of a new six-party alliance. (He was highly educated, a university graduate who had for a time been a professor. A true intellectual revolutionary.) The Maoists had been designated a terrorist organization by the United States. Face to face, however, this prime minister was a soft-spoken, gentle-looking man, perfectly at ease in a business suit. I found it altogether difficult to fathom that this person before me had been the leader of an armed insurgency that resulted in more than 13,000 deaths. Quite unexpectedly, he committed there and then to eliminating leprosy in his country by the end of 2009—the very next year.

This is off-topic, but Prime Minister Dahal, a Communist, would of course have been an atheist, and even though he had spearheaded the demand for a clear separation of government and religion in the upcoming government, he told me, no doubt trying to flatter me, that "I feel a bond with Japan, since Buddhism is strong in your country as it is in ours." As prime minister, Mr. Dahal had a responsibility to maintain agreement among the various parties in his government and, in keeping with his pledge to the global community (including acceptance of a United Nations mission to monitor the current ceasefire), to enact a new constitution. The issue of how to treat the 19,000 members of the People's Liberation Army who had waged a fierce war with the government forces during the years of the monarchy was apparently a source of conflict between the second and third most important parties in the six-party alliance. It had the potential to be the greatest factor destabilizing Mr. Dahal's interim government.

On this trip, I was able to visit two places in the southern and eastern regions where leprosy was endemic that had not been possible previously due to the political uncertainty: Birgunj and Biratnagar. I traveled to Birgunj on 3 December, accompanied by Dr. Andjaparidze and Minister of Health Dr. Pokharel. There we attended the opening ceremony for a workshop on women's empowerment organized by IDEA Nepal. This organization was formed in 1998 and works tirelessly in a whole variety of ways for the social and economic advancement of people affected by leprosy, including holding education and awareness campaigns and empowerment workshops. As of 2007, it had 120 lifetime members and 200 general members and now covered the whole of the country.

In the afternoon, I called at a leprosy clinic located within a primary health center in Gauriganj rural municipality, in Jhapa district. Here I found myself festooned with wreaths of marigolds, which in Nepal are flowers of happiness. I joined in the dancing of the local inhabitants, who are an ethnic minority, the Maithili tribe, dancing to the rhythm of drums. As part of my leprosy elimination activities, I always like to don the local attire and share in activities bonding with the people who live in these places. At the center, I chatted with each and every one of thirty or so people, offering words of encouragement, and I asked the health workers to tell everyone they could about our "three messages."

The following day, I went to visit the Indian border. Most national borders are areas of high tension (the Israel–Jordan border was particularly tense), but here even though pro forma there were checkpoints, everybody seemed to be just crossing and re-crossing as they liked. In addition to an immigration office, the boundary was marked by little pillars of stones every few hundred meters, with no barricades. Everything seemed quite calm and relaxed. People with leprosy used this border to cross from Bihar state to the hospitals in Nepal where they received treatment free of charge. No data was taken, which made it impossible to construct accurate statistical reports. The numerous ethnic communities, each with a different language, made for challenges in getting across accurate information about the disease. All sorts of factors combined to make eliminating leprosy a difficult task.

After that, we went to pay a visit to Mangalbari Primary Health Centre, in Morang district, traveling along barely passable muddy roads. The cars jolted around so much we felt that if we so much as opened our mouths we might end up biting off our tongues, so the journey progressed in total silence. So many places I go to in the course of my work have the most terrible infrastructure. My strategy is to think of the jolts of the car as an all-over body massage. I try to relax and give myself over completely to them as we move along.

The Mangalbari Primary Health Center operates 24/7, serving about 300 outpatients a day. Here I met fifty female volunteer health workers who distributed medicine and paid home visits to make sure that patients were continuing with their treatment. One of the women, who had been doing this for nineteen years, told me: "Your visit here to a country so distant from your own will fill our activities with light." As a show of thanks, she and others sang me Nepal's national anthem. I remembered a similar thing happened on a visit to India. I had promised some children that I would provide the support to build them a small school to save them from discrimination because their parents were affected by leprosy, and they had responded by singing me their national anthem. I had recently read a newspaper article about a Japanese high school student from Kyushu on a study-

347

abroad trip in Malaysia who had been the only one in a class of children who had been unable to sing his own national anthem—because he didn't know it. In most countries in the world, even if they are poor, the national anthem is something people take pride in.

In the Dhalkebar region, I visited the general hospital and learned that a ward specializing in leprosy had been added with funding from a Dutch charity. Some children had come here from across the border, more than an hour's walk. A woman from Bihar had brought her ten-year-old daughter for treatment. "I found some lesions on her," she told me, "and a family member advised me to bring her here." As someone who has repeated our set phrase "Early detection means a speedier cure" thousands of times, it felt good to hear these words. These children would have no aftereffects, and they would go on to lead lives that were free of any associated discrimination.

The following day, we headed to Lalgadh, in the district of Dhanusha. The first event on my itinerary was to watch a performance of street theater, supported by the Nepal Leprosy Trust. As we drove along, we passed a good number of hill tribespeople. Poppy flowers bloomed in the vegetable patches, and each house had harvested rice straw piled in bundles as high as the eaves. We reached Lalgadh just as the street theater began, with a circle of 300 or so villagers seated all around. When I joined them, a little child came and sat in my lap with a smile. The play was a family drama, the kind of story that always went down well in Nepal. It was a tale of diagnosis, rejection, understanding, and acceptance. A husband takes his wife, who he thinks has leprosy, to the hospital; a con man attempts to mislead a person affected by leprosy who has a disability, and so on. The script included facts that everyone should know about leprosy, and the dialogue was designed to expose mistaken notions and superstitions. The troupe apparently performs about 400 times a year in various places all over the country, and the actors put on a superb performance. Even the adult onlookers were enthralled, sometimes even shouting out their own questions about the disease into the mix. Literacy in Nepal remains at 47.5 percent, and activities such as these are a highly effective way of reaching people with information.

From there, I went to the Lalgadh Leprosy Services Center, built and run by the Nepal Leprosy Trust. The center is situated in neat, campus-like buildings, all connected by a covered walkway. It has fifty-two beds, and supported by the Sasakawa Health Foundation, it serves as a referral hospital for the surrounding five districts, handling leprosy reactions and other difficult cases. I formed a favorable impression of a well-run facility staffed by a dedicated and caring team.

On the flight back to Kathmandu, the secretary general of the Communist Party of Nepal was on board, so I explained to him all about the talks I had had with the prime minister and our leprosy elimination activities in Nepal. Such serendipitous encounters with world leaders are a truly enjoyable aspect of my work.

Countries visited in 2009	
January	Switzerland: (Discussions related to open-ended consultation on elimination of discrimination against persons affected by leprosy and their family members organized by the UN High Commissioner for Human Rights)
	● United Kingdom
February	● India
	Myanmar (Launch ceremony of "traditional medicine kits" project)
March	China (Visit to Yunnan prison; received honorary professorship at Yunnan University)
April	Jordan (WANA Forum)
	India (WHO conference; S-ILF board meeting)
	● Nepal
May	United Kingdom (International Maritime Organization)
	Hungary (Hungarian Academy of Sciences twentieth anniversary ceremony of SYLFF program)
	● Switzerland
June	China (Japan–China Field Officer Exchange Program)
	● Indonesia
	● Zambia

July	● Singapore
	Malaysia (Maritime navigational assistance fund)
August	Thailand (Asian traditional medicine projects)
	Denmark (Scandinavia–Japan Sasakawa Foundation board meeting)
September	Taiwan (Talks with Ma Ying-jeou of Kuomintang)
October	● United States
	Czech Republic (Forum 2000 International Conference)
	Myanmar (Launch ceremony of "traditional medicine kits" project)
	Philippines (Graduation ceremony of UN University of Peace)
November	France (Fondation Franco-Japonaise Sasakawa board meeting)
December	China (Yunnan University SYLFF projects)

● Indicates a trip that features in this section.

WANA: West Asia–North Africa, a non-profit think tank based in Amman, Jordan, comprising intellectual leaders in economic, environmental, energy, educational, and social spheres.

Forum 2000: An annual international conference launched in 1997 when Václav Havel, Elie Wiesel, and the author invited world leaders to Prague for open debate on the major issues and challenges of the new millennium.

SYLFF: Sasakawa Young Leaders Fellowship Fund program.

Global Appeal 2009 endorsed by religious leaders—United Kingdom of Great Britain and Northern Ireland, January 2009

Route: Narita → London, United Kingdom (flight time: 12h 35m)— three nights

For our fourth Global Appeal to End Stigma and Discrimination against People Affected by Leprosy, held every year since 2006, we asked seventeen religious leaders to lend us their endorsement. In many sacred texts of the world's religions, leprosy is used as a metaphor for impurity and sin, which has only served to increase the stigma pertaining to the disease, and for this reason we thought that the endorsement of faith leaders would be highly effective. The signatories included Vice President Ammar al-Hakim of the Islamic Supreme Council of Iraq; Archbishop Istrinsky Areseniy, vicar of Patriarchy Alexy II of Moscow and All Russia; the Dalai Lama; Cardinal Javier Lozano Barragán, president of the Pontifical Council for Health Pastoral Care, the Vatican; Chief Rabbi of Israel Yona Metzger; and Archbishop Emeritus Desmond Tutu of Cape Town, South Africa.

For the venue, we returned to London, site of the third Global Appeal: this time, a conference room in Church House, near Westminster Abbey, in central London. The walls were decorated with dozens of vibrantly colored paintings from the Bindu Art School, an initiative based in a leprosy colony in Bharathipuram in southern India, which promotes art for life by people affected by leprosy. Our audience was over 100 strong, with religious representatives, members of the media, and representatives of international NGOs. The launch opened with choral music. The dean of Westminster, the Very Reverend John Robert Hall, gave a welcoming speech, and I then gave a keynote address explaining the Global Appeal, after which the leaders of the various religious faiths in Britain and other visitors rose to voice their organizations' support.

In his address, Sanjay Jagaita, secretary-general of the National Council of Hindu Temples in the United Kingdom, related how in January 2002 he visited a leprosy colony at Tahirpur on the outskirts of Delhi. In one house, he had partaken of a cup of tea. The woman of the house had been so grateful, he said, thanking him as a "normal person" for coming to the home of one who was "not normal." Her words, he said, made him shed tears.

His Eminence Archbishop Gregorios of Thyateira and Great Britain recounted that he had relatives back in Cyprus, where he was born, who had been quarantined in a hospital for leprosy in the Nicosia region, and who were looked upon with prejudice even after they had been cured.

Finally, Kofi Nyarko, a teacher in Ghana, and Farida, a devout student of Islam from Indonesia, read out the text of the Global Appeal on behalf of people affected by leprosy all over the world.

S-ILF microfinancing begins—Republic of India, February 2009

Route: Narita → New Delhi (flight time: 10h 20m)—one night—New Delhi → Lucknow, Uttar Pradesh (flight time: 55m) → New Delhi (flight time: 50m; 9h stopover) → Narita (flight time: 7h 35m)

In February, I made a visit to Lucknow, the capital of Uttar Pradesh. This is a city with numerous historical reminders of the Islamic rulers who held sway in northern India from the eighteenth to nineteenth centuries. My objective was to participate in the National Forum's first Northern Regional Conference, along with about 330 representatives of northern India's leprosy colonies spread across ten states, which include not only Uttar Pradesh but also Delhi, Madhya Pradesh, and Bihar. In contrast to previous forums, which were attended almost exclusively by middle-aged and elderly men, I was pleased to

67. The author standing with leaders of the world's religions at the Global Appeal 2009 (United Kingdom, January 2009)

see that at this conference a good 30 percent of the delegates were women and younger people.

At this conference, ten award certificates from S-ILF were conferred for microfinance loans to colony residents and NGOs for projects that included dairy farming, candle-making and retailing—in amounts ranging from 23,500 to 309,000 rupees (around US$300 to 4,000), considerable sums in a country where millions live on the equivalent of US$1 a day. The loans were non-interest, and repayments would be made to the leprosy colonies, in a unique system set up with the idea of creating a wealth reserve that could be used for improvements in living conditions.

The next day, I went to visit the residents of the Adarsh Kusht Ashram, a self-settled colony about forty minutes' drive from the city. This colony comprised fifty-two households, about 250 people, of whom some ninety were people affected by leprosy. The residents lived in concrete tenements arranged around a wide-open space. The colony had its own water supply sourced from underground by means of a motorized pump. At first glance, it looked clean and tidy, but life

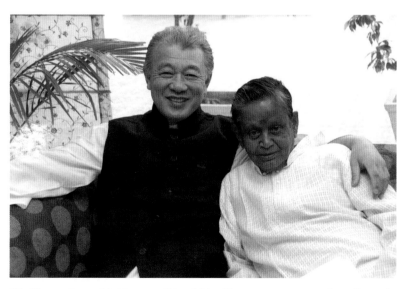

68. The author with his great friend Mr. Dutta, a representative of people affected by leprosy (Uttar Pradesh, India, March 2009)

for the people living here was quite evidently awful. Most of the houses were small, making it impossible for all the family to sleep under one roof, and 90 percent of the residents made a living from begging—which they did outside temples, restaurants, and shops in the city, earning an average of 50 rupees a day. These beggars carried a certificate to show that they were residents of the colony. In India, beggars with all kinds of diseases and afflictions live on the street, but these beggars were clearly making an excuse of their leprosy, and sadly I had to acknowledge that we had much more to do before my dream of getting rid of the need for begging altogether became a reality. I took comfort in the fact that even in such adverse living conditions, there were many residents who were keen to get proper employment and young people who had received an education at university or specialist training school that would enable them to look for jobs in the outside world.

Getting the media on board—Nepal, April 2009

> Route: Narita, Japan → Kansai Airport (flight time: 1h 15m; 2h stop-over) → Dubai, United Arab Emirates (flight time: 11h 15m; 2h stop-over) → Amman, Jordan (flight time: 3h 15m)—three nights—Amman → New Delhi, India (flight time: 5h 30m)—two nights—New Delhi → Kathmandu, Nepal (flight time: 1h 45m)—one night—Kathmandu → Dhanusha district (charter flight, flight time: 50m)—one night—Kathmandu → Bangkok, Thailand (flight time: 3h; 4h stopover) → Narita (flight time: 6h)

April 2009 saw me make a visit to Nepal, to follow up on my visit in December 2008.

In my role as Goodwill Ambassador, reaching out to the media is essential. Drawing the attention of the press to the issues surrounding leprosy and having leprosy covered in an appropriate way leads to a better-informed populace and a debunking of myths about the dis-ease, both of which ultimately mean that more people affected by leprosy seek treatment.

I was thus delighted that my visit to Nepal was spent in the com-pany of five local print, radio, and television journalists, who reported on my activities during my four-day stay. I took part in two events with journalists, one in the capital Kathmandu and the other in

Janakpur, Dhanusha district. These were designed to brief the media about the disease and to enlist their involvement in Nepal's leprosy elimination efforts.

Nepal's health authorities believed that they would be able to reach the elimination milestone of less than one case per 10,000 population by the end of 2009. As of mid-March, 3,165 people affected by leprosy were registered for treatment, and the prevalence rate stood at 1.16. The burden of the disease was mostly in the Terai belt and hilly districts in Nepal's midwestern and far western regions.

On arrival in Kathmandu, I paid a courtesy call on Minister of Health Dr. Pokharel, apologizing for visiting him on a holiday. "This is not a holiday for me," was his reply. "We don't take holidays when important work has to be done." In the afternoon, I attended a workshop at a local NGO, Rehabilitation Empowerment and Development Nepal (READ-Nepal). This NGO's mission is to improve the socioeconomic status of people affected by leprosy and disabilities. It was now working to ensure that their voices were reflected in Nepal's new constitution. READ-Nepal had recently completed an eight-bed ward for ulcer care, and I was asked to perform a ribbon-cutting ceremony. Joining me on the dais was Dr. Garib Das Thakur, director of the health ministry's Leprosy Control Division. He was one of the main speakers that evening at the first interaction with journalists, briefing them on the progress Nepal was making tackling leprosy.

The following day, Dr. Thakur also accompanied my team to Dhanusha and Mahottari districts in the Terai. Here we had a second get-together with local journalists. "This is a truly impoverished area," Dr. Thakur said to the assembled media. "But with your help we can achieve the elimination goal. Tell people leprosy is not a curse. Let them know that treatment is free."

Both the Kathmandu and Janakpur events were arranged in cooperation with the president of the Federation of Nepali Journalists, Dharmendra Jha. Addressing his Janakpur colleagues, he said that the Goodwill Ambassador had come all the way from Japan to fight leprosy, and it would not do for the media to remain silent on such an important issue. "As journalists, we have to discharge our social responsibility."

Dhanusha and Mahottari are among two of the four districts served by Lalgadh Leprosy Services Center, the NGO run by Nepal Leprosy

Trust, which I also visited. In addition to serving as a leprosy treatment and referral center, it performs many important functions, including capacity building of health workers and building community awareness through educational dramas.

Shortly after I left Nepal, the extraordinary news came that the prime minister had resigned, and the country was plunged into political chaos. Nevertheless, I was informed that the work that people were undertaking in the government's leprosy control program was continuing. I felt grateful to the journalists who accompanied me for their coverage of my visit, and I hoped that they would continue to keep leprosy in their sights.

Passion and persistence—Swiss Confederation, May 2009

> Route: Narita → Frankfurt, Germany (flight time: 11h 40m; 2h 20m stopover) → Budapest, Hungary (flight time: 1h 30m)—one night—Budapest → Geneva, Switzerland (flight time: 2h)—two nights—Geneva → Paris, France (flight time: 1h; 3h stopover) → Narita (flight time: 11h 30m)

In May, I traveled to Budapest, Hungary, to attend the twentieth anniversary of the SYLFF program at the Hungarian Academy of Sciences, and thence to Geneva, where I attended the World Health Assembly, as is my annual custom. I spent most of my time meeting with health ministers of governments, and international organizations, to discuss leprosy issues.

In a meeting with Francisco T. Duque, secretary of the Department of Health of the Philippines, I expressed my thanks to the Philippine government for its co-sponsorship of last June's Human Rights Council resolution calling for an end to stigma and discrimination against people affected by leprosy and their families. I also had praise for Dr. Arturo Cunanan, head of the technical division of the Culion Leprosy and Rehabilitation Program, for his work in the Philippines but also recently in Nepal, where he conducted technical training.

In a meeting with Dr. Suriya Wongkongkathep, senior health supervisor at the Office of Health Inspector General of Thailand's Ministry of Public Health, I thanked the Thai government for its support of the resolution. In turn, Dr. Suriya Wongkongkathep told me about some new developments in leprosy services in Thailand.

In a brief meeting with Zambia's health minister, Kapembwa Simbao, we discussed my forthcoming visit to Zambia, where I hoped to learn more about the leprosy control program.

During a working lunch attended by WHO Director-General Margaret Chan, WHO Regional Director for Southeast Asia Dr. Samlee Plianbangchang, and WHO Regional Director for the Americas Dr. Mirta Roses, Dr. Chan paid me the highest honor by praising my work as Goodwill Ambassador, and Dr. Roses joined in, saying that she appreciated my "persistence and patience." With reference to Brazil, which still has to deal with many new cases of leprosy each year, she admitted the difficult situation there, saying the country was using "a different language" in its approach to tackling the disease. However, she stressed that this did not signal a lack of commitment to reducing the leprosy burden and added that stepped-up surveys and investigations were being planned.

I then held a meeting with Dr. Kyaw Myint of Myanmar's Ministry of Health, who told me that the country was doing much better with

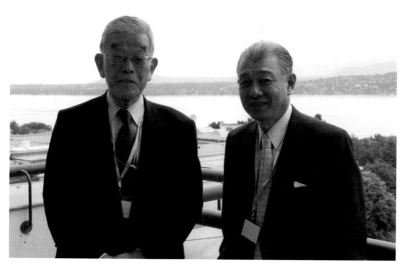

69. The author with his trusted advisor the late Kenzo Kiikuni, former chair, president of the Sasakawa Health Foundation, at the Palais des Nations, with Lake Geneva as a backdrop (Geneva, May 2009)

early detection, and the resulting early treatment meant that the number of people left with disability was falling. Professor P. I. Garrido, Mozambique's minister of health, told me that Mozambique had achieved elimination at the national level at the end of 2007, but that the president was waiting until the following year to make a formal announcement. By then, Mozambique had achieved elimination at the provincial level too. The country was now focusing on specific districts where the prevalence rate remained high, he said.

The next day, I met with the UN High Commissioner for Human Rights, Dr. Navanethem Pillay. Dr. Pillay, who had only recently (September 2008) been appointed, expressed her surprise that it had taken so long for leprosy to be viewed as a human rights issue. She commended my continuous efforts to draw attention to this and acknowledged the initiative taken by the Japanese government in overseeing the passage of the resolution. She said that she looked forward to the report that the Human Rights Council's Advisory Committee was preparing on leprosy and human rights and promised that her office would remain fully focused on the issue.

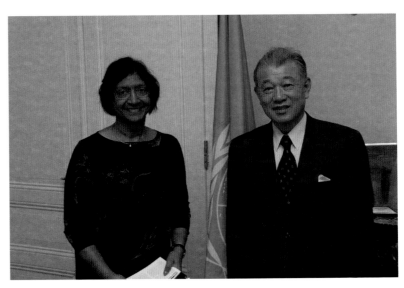

70. The author with UN Commissioner of Human Rights Dr. Naveneethan Pillay (Geneva, May 2009)

THE DRIVE TO SELF-EMPOWERMENT

Restoring the dignity of people affected by leprosy with PerMaTa—
Republic of Indonesia, June 2009

Route: Narita → Singapore (flight time: 7h; 7h stopover) → Surabaya, Indonesia (flight time: 2h 20m)—one night—Surabaya → Jakarta (flight time: 1h 20m)—one night—Jakarta → Narita (flight time: 7h 30m)

In June, I traveled to Indonesia. The main purpose of my visit was to attend the official launch of a new project on leprosy and human dignity—part of a totally new joint initiative of the Association of Southeast Asian Nations Secretariat (ASEC) and the Nippon Foundation—which we called ASEC-TNF—based on an agreement signed in June 2008, involving region-by-region projects over a period of five years aimed at restoring the dignity and realizing the social reintegration of people affected by leprosy. They would begin in Indonesia, where ASEC had its headquarters. It was an appropriate starting point, as Indonesia had the highest leprosy burden in all the ASEAN countries—17,000 new cases in 2008—and stigma remained a deep-rooted problem.

I arrived in the country a couple of days early, flying into Surabaya, the provincial capital of East Java. East Java had more new cases of leprosy than any other of Indonesia's thirty-three provinces, diagnosing about 5,000 new cases annually. Of these, roughly 600 were children, a ratio of 12 percent. Because of the strong stigma in Indonesia, the disease can affect their education and create problems for them later in life in terms of work and marriage. The proportion of grade 2 disability was similarly extremely high among new cases, at around 11 percent, placing a burden on families and communities. I was told that intensive surveys continue to uncover still more cases, with still more children, indicating that the disease was endemic and that there was an urgent need for information, education, and communication at the grassroots level.

Following a meeting with health officials, I visited a local convention center where I was asked to listen to stories in a writing contest to promote leprosy awareness, being run by PerMaTa (Perhimpunan Mandiri Kusta), an Indonesian advocacy organization of and for people affected by leprosy, and viewed paintings in an art competition. I also watched part of a drama about stigma and discrimination performed by high school students, in what turned out to be an unexpectedly lively few hours. In the afternoon, I traveled by car to Lamongan, about two hours from Surabaya, to an elementary school, where I sat in on a lesson about leprosy given by Ahmad Zainudin, president of PerMaTa. This was the school where he taught. Mr. Zainudin himself had been affected by leprosy just a few years previously. When his fellow teachers visited him in hospital and learned he had leprosy, the news quickly spread, and he was sacked from four of the five schools where he had worked as an instructor. At the one school that kept him on, he now taught every subject. As I listened to him explaining about leprosy and how it was spread, I wondered whether it might be a little too complex for his young listeners, but the pupils all listened attentively. At the very least, the most important messages, that people who have leprosy are no different from anyone else and that it is wrong to discriminate against them, came across loud and clear. I first met Mr. Zainudin in Manila, when he attended the launch of Global Appeal 2007. It was in the following month that he and Adi Yosep had established PerMaTa. Several members of PerMaTa accompanied me during my stay in East Java. Among them was Farida, who was one of two people affected by leprosy to read out the text of Global Appeal 2009 in London at the start of the year. I was delighted to hear that Farida's visit to London had inspired her to study English and to become active in PerMaTa as well.

On my last day in East Java, I traveled to Sumber Glagah hospital, about an hour's drive from Surabaya, in the company of representatives from five media outlets. Established as a leprosy hospital in 1995 by Dutch doctors, the 100-bed hospital now set aside fifty of its beds for people affected by leprosy and fifty for general patients. Anyone who recovered could immediately leave the hospital, while people with disabilities could get reconstructive surgery, and there was also a department that made shoes and prosthetic limbs. All in all, I found the hospital to be extremely well run, and I was impressed by what I saw.

A few minutes' walk from the hospital lay the village of Sumber Glagah. Its population included about 180 people affected by leprosy. Some ran their own small businesses or worked in the fields,

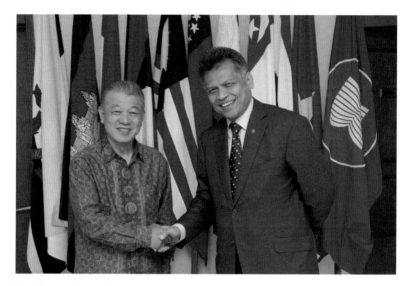

71. The author with ASEAN Secretary General Dr. Surin Pitsuwan (former foreign minister of Thailand) (Indonesia, June 2009)

but I am sad to say that most of the residents made a living from begging, traveling by motorcycle to nearby towns for that purpose. Just before I left, as I was addressing a group of villagers, one of them loudly announced that he was tired of visits such as mine that never amounted to anything. He demanded work. His anger was understandable. It is my role to make sure that the cries of people like this are duly conveyed to the country's leaders, and, through the media, to the general population.

After an inspection of the village, we headed for Jakarta. I was hopeful that the ASEC-TNF Project, which I explained above, would go some way toward providing a solution for people like the man I had just seen, who shouted for work, proof of how many people affected by leprosy were stymied, finding it impossible to become employed even after they were completely cured. It was the task of this initiative, together with the media, corporations, NGOs, and the government, to help improve the economic and social independence of people affected by leprosy. At the launch of this project, held in the ASEAN Secretariat in Jakarta, ASEAN Secretary General Dr. Surin Pitsuwan (former foreign minister of Thailand) was present, along with about 160 diplomats, dignitaries, journalists, and people affected by leprosy. Project-managing this event was PerMaTa's Adi Yosep. He had been diagnosed with leprosy when he was eighteen. He had developed lesions on his skin with swellings on his fingers, the same symptoms as his mother had several years before—and she recognized them. Unlike Adi, his mother hadn't received a correct diagnosis immediately and had been made to buy some expensive medication. Adi himself had fortunately received a correct diagnosis and received treatment and was now completely cured. "I was able to recover with the right information from people around me and the right kind of support," he said. "And now I want to devote all my energy into helping others affected by leprosy." That's when he decided to set up PerMaTa. When people affected by leprosy got up on stage, standing shoulder to shoulder with the ASEAN secretary general and officials from various governments participating in the project, it seemed a truly fitting symbol for the main objective of this new project, which was to have people affected by leprosy, and people who had leprosy in the past and are now completely cured, participating fully in society.

In the afternoon, we heard from a selection of people in an education and awareness workshop who reported on their experience and findings in different initiatives across a variety of sectors. Virendra S. Gupte of Tata International Ltd., India, who is providing support for the employment of people affected by leprosy in India, and who works as a counsellor on business ethics, gave a presentation on partnering with business. Ujjwal K. Chowdhury, a professor in media studies, gave a presentation on the involvement of the media in India. Ryotaro Harada, who works as a coordinator for university student volunteers to participate in what are called "work camps" improving the living conditions of villages affected by leprosy in China, gave a presentation on social changes related to leprosy in China. Aco Manafe, an Indonesian journalist, gave a talk on breaking the cycle of stigmatization through the media in Indonesia.

A change of heart from the president—Republic of Zambia, June 2009

Route: Narita, Japan → Frankfurt, Germany (flight time: 12h; 6h stopover) → Johannesburg, South Africa (flight time: 10h; 2h stop-

over) → Lusaka, Zambia (flight time: 2h)—three nights—Lusaka →
Johannesburg (flight time: 2h; 3h stopover) → Dubai (flight time: 8h;
5h stopover) → Singapore (flight time: 7h 30m)—one night (Visit to
Singapore Leprosy Relief Association (SILRA) home facility)—
Singapore → Kuala Lumpur, Malaysia (flight time: 55m)—two nights
(maritime projects)—Kuala Lumpur → Narita (flight time: 7h)

In June, after my visit to Indonesia, I flew to Zambia. Situated in the
center of the African continent, the Republic of Zambia comprises an
area roughly twice the size of Japan and is considered one of the most
peaceful nations in Africa. The Zambezi River that runs along its
southern border with Zimbabwe is famous for the Victoria Falls, one
of the three greatest waterfalls of the world.

With the DRC's and Mozambique's successful elimination of leprosy in 2007, every nation on the African continent had now reached
the WHO-defined benchmark for elimination at the national level.
Zambia had achieved elimination in 2000. On this visit, I wanted to
get an update on Zambia's situation. Accompanying me was
Dr. Landry from the WHO Regional Office for Africa. When I finally
arrived (after a succession of connecting flights) at a small airport in
Lusaka, the WHO's country representative Dr. Olusegun Babaniyi
and officials from the Ministry of Health as well as several representatives from the Zambian media were there to meet me.

Although on the surface all seemed to be well in Zambia, the truth
was that a corruption scandal had recently rocked the country: officials in the health ministry had been discovered to have embezzled the
equivalent of US$4 million of foreign aid donated for the govern-
ment's health projects, and twenty people or so, including a former
cabinet minister, had been thrown in prison. In June, a month-long
strike by nurses had left the hospitals barely able to cope. Perhaps
because of these factors, the officials we had to work with all seemed
jittery. The health minister met my request for sustained attention to
leprosy with a cagey answer: "I will definitely do all I can for this
cause—for as long as I have my job." From what I could judge, there
were gaps in the records on leprosy: data were missing for prevalence
rates and patient data for the last ten years—we could trust none of
the figures we were given. I advised the officials to construct policies
that would focus on areas where the numbers were high, to gather
accurate data, and to get qualified people to analyze them.

I then paid a courtesy call on President Rupiah Banda at his official residence. In the large grounds of his official residence were all sorts of wild animals, species I wouldn't be able to name, grazing on the grass, and I could see groups of monkeys jumping around in the trees unaware of anything going on in the human world below. But the peaceful scene belied the reality: our smart phones and cameras were confiscated as soon as we entered. I was shown into a sparsely furnished room, where the president sat alone on a sofa, his leg in a cast. I greeted him, and with some difficulty, he got up onto his feet to return the greeting. He told me he was recuperating from a knee operation, but he listened attentively while I told him there was still much to be done about leprosy, even though the elimination target had been reached; and about the need to wipe out the associated stigma and discrimination. He replied: "There is a lot of superstition about leprosy. Many people hesitate to shake hands with anyone who has had it. And I am no exception. Whenever my car passes a leprosy hospital, I always close all the windows and have my driver step on the gas. But if you're willing to shake hands with people affected by leprosy, Mr. Sasakawa, I will change my ways." And then, he joked:

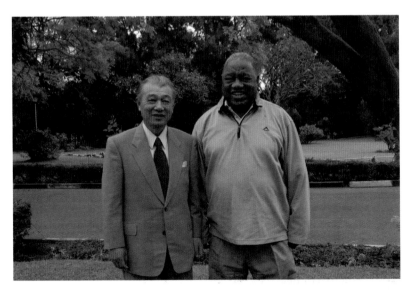

72. The author with President Rupiah Banda of Zambia (Zambia, July 2009)

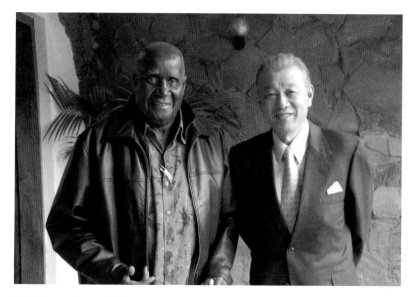

73. The author with former President Kenneth Kaunda, father of the nation (Zambia July 2009)

"Just a few days ago, during a press briefing outside, a monkey sitting above me in a tree urinated on my jacket!" I asked if I could have a photograph of myself with the president, and somebody brought in my confiscated camera. Indulging me, the president limped outside into the sunshine. I found him to be a very cordial, sympathetic human being.

That same day, I went to call on my old friend Kenneth Kaunda, independent Zambia's first president, and someone who is still thought of as the father of the nation today. Mr. Kaunda received an education in mission schools in colonial Zambia, and for a while he worked as a schoolteacher. After this, he became politically active, joining the independence movement and becoming a leader, for a time being imprisoned by the colonial powers, before becoming president, a position he kept for twenty-six years. Mr. Kaunda had since suffered some personal disappointments, having lost his eldest son to AIDS, but he now seemed to be living quietly out of public view. One particular memory of Kenneth Kaunda will always stay with me. In around 1986, Ethiopia was stricken by a famine, and

President Carter, Dr. Norman Borlaug, my father, and I used the presidential airplane to visit four countries in Africa, Sudan, Tanzania, Zambia, and Ghana, trying to work out a way of helping the poorer countries in Africa to increase their agricultural production. When we visited Zambia, a welcome banquet was held in our honor, with all the officials in attendance, and at one point President Kaunda rose to his feet calmly and, using his handkerchief to keep time, had everyone sing a song. It was a very solemn song, sung in low notes, with a strong rhythm designed to inspire fighters to victory in the battle held in the jungle against colonial oppressors. I well remember how moved I was to hear it.

On the third day of my stay, we visited Liteta Hospital, located less than an hour's drive out of the capital Lusaka. Built in 1959 as a national TB Center, in 1963 it was designated a leprosy center. Its proximity to the border with Mozambique meant that many people from that country came to it. At that point in time, there were seven people affected by leprosy undergoing treatment, all on an outpatient basis. In an attached compound for people affected by leprosy, thirteen people affected by leprosy were living quietly, along with their families—sixty people in all. They received food provisions from the government, and they had one well between them; but the houses weren't connected to the electricity grid. I saw people cooking meals, while others just sat staring through the windows. I could only assume that behind the welcoming smiles must lie some terrible experiences. I got a strong sense that this community was quite cut off from the rest of society and was being fast left behind by time.

On my final day in Zambia, I took time off from my role as Leprosy Goodwill Ambassador and went with Japanese Ambassador to Zambia Hideto Mitamura to take a look at some rural community development projects begun in 2002 in a joint aid initiative by the Japanese government with the Zambian Ministry of Agriculture, involving the construction of wells and community halls, and solar-powered milling plants. Development in Africa is not something that can be achieved through the efforts of a single private organization alone. It is only when NGOs are passionately concerned with achieving change on this vast continent, when leaders aspire to take their countries down their own unique path, and when committed efforts are made down on the ground that real breakthroughs occur. In Africa, political stability is such a precious and rare commodity. To our north and east, in the DRC and Angola, civil war raged, while to the south of us, in Zimbabwe, the people were governed by a dictator, and inflation was soaring. Since gaining its independence in 1964, under the government led by Kenneth Kaunda, Zambia was one of the few countries that had managed to achieve relative stability.

On my return, I went to Singapore via Johannesburg. Here I visited a facility for people affected by leprosy called the Singapore Leprosy Relief Association (SILRA) Home, originally built in 1951. There were fifty-one residents, the oldest ninety years of age, and the youngest fifty. In the 1940s, Singapore had a segregation policy, and anyone affected by leprosy had to live entirely cut off from their community.

After that, I made a brief stop in Malaysia, for a meeting for maritime safety in the Malacca Straits, in a project the Nippon Foundation has long supported. And then I was on my way back to Japan.

The vestiges of leprosy discrimination in a developed nation—United States, October 2009

> Route: Narita → Chicago, United States (flight time: 10h 40m; 2h stopover) → Atlanta (flight time: 1h 40m)—three nights (Visit to Carter Center)—Atlanta → Baton Rouge (flight time: 1h 10m)—two nights—New Orleans → Dallas (flight time: 1h 10m; 2h 30m stopover) → College Station (flight time: 3m)—three nights (Dr. Borlaug memorial service)—College Station → Dallas (flight time: 55m; 4h stopover) → Narita (flight time: 13h 30m)

In October, I visited the state of Louisiana, in the United States. There have been two leprosaria in the United States: one in Carville, Louisiana, the other in Kalaupapa, Hawaii. Carville National Leprosarium was established in 1884, and until Hawaii became a state in 1959, it stood as the sole facility in the United States where people affected by leprosy could be held. At 333 acres, it was a large institution and housed and cured many people with leprosy until it was closed in 1999. Leprosy was eliminated in the United States before 1990, but discrimination toward people with lived experience of leprosy persists. And still more than 100 cases of leprosy are diagnosed annually, mainly in the South.

On my arrival a little after midday at Baton Rouge Airport in Louisiana, I was met by Dr. James Krahenbuhl, director of Baton Rouge's National Hansen's Disease Programs. A leprosy researcher, Dr. Krahenbuhl treated many people affected by leprosy in Carville.

On the roughly 20-mile drive to Carville, we saw numerous dead armadillos. According to Dr. Krahenbuhl, Louisiana has huge numbers of these animals, and a good 25 percent of them carry the leprosy bacillus. Armadillos have a series of armor-like bands on their backs, the number varying with each species. There are two species in the American South, ones with six bands and ones with nine bands. Only the nine-banded armadillos (*Dasypus novemcinctus*) carry the leprosy bacillus.

Thirty minutes into the drive, the Mississippi River came into view. Dr. Krahenbuhl stopped the car. "Just here is where in 1884 the first people affected by leprosy came off the boats," he told me, pointing to the riverbank. We got out and walked to the spot. Autumn was definitely in the air, but mosquitos descended on us in clouds. In the old days, this area had been a swamp.

Five more minutes' drive brought us to Carville. Near the entrance was a building where the first patients were quarantined—standing just as it had been in the early days, along with several other buildings, including patient and staff residences, and other amenities that were added later, and a cemetery where 900 or so people who had died lay buried.

It was in the 1940s that they had the most patients—450 people affected by leprosy had lived here. Now, the buildings were used by the national guard, overseen by the state of Louisiana's Military Department. But a part of the facility still housed thirteen people affected by leprosy; their average age was seventy-nine years.

In the afternoon, I toured the National Hansen's Disease Museum, where I met Simeon Peterson, known as Pete, who worked as a guide there several times a week. Pete was now eighty-one and had lived in Carville for fifty-eight years. He and all the other people affected by leprosy who worked at the museum were paid for their work, Dr. Krahenbuhl told me. Founded in 1996, with the idea of preserving the site's history, the museum plays an important role in promoting people's understanding of the disease. At one point, barbed wire had surrounded Carville, residents were not permitted to leave, and they were forced to change their names on entry. The swimming pool on the premises was off limits until 1990. Laws prohibiting people affected by leprosy from having children (abolished in 1960) and withholding the right to vote (abolished in 1945) attest to the strength of the discrimination.

Pete told me he wanted to introduce me to somebody—Perry Enriquez, a person affected by leprosy who was 101 years old. We waited at the agreed meeting place, but Perry wasn't to be seen. People went to look for him, and then suddenly there he was—an elderly gentleman in a wheelchair. He didn't look much older than eighty. Out of curiosity, I inquired how old he was, and he replied, with absolute assurance: "How old am I? I'm going to be 101 this year!" The oldest person affected by leprosy I had ever met. He told me he hailed from the Philippines, and at age eighteen he had migrated to the United States and worked in the apple orchards in California—he had contracted leprosy during this time. He had been quarantined

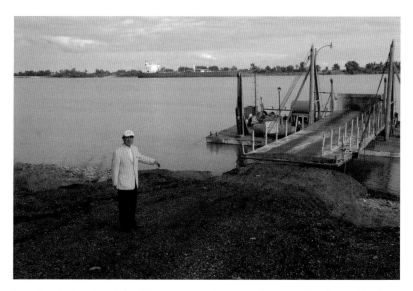

74. On the banks of the Mississippi, where the first people affected by leprosy to be put into Carville leprosarium came off the boats (Louisiana, United States, October 2009)

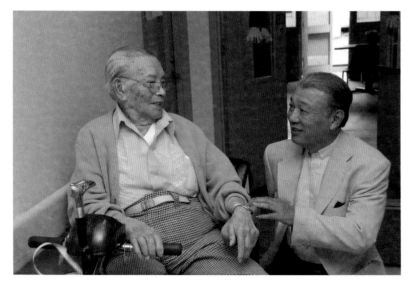

75. With Carville's oldest resident, Perry Enriquez, 101 years old (Louisiana, United States, October 2009)

in Carville in 1936, aged twenty-eight. When I asked him the secret of his longevity, he replied: "I guess, playing the guitar, and singing Frank Sinatra songs. Plus, I don't smoke, and I don't drink." He had grown habituated to the place and seemed very happy to be here.

With a sad expression on his face, Dr. Krahenbuhl told me: "There's still a huge amount of prejudice in the US. Part of it is fueled by the internet. High school students post images of people with disfigured faces and limbs with scare stories about leprosy that give the public the impression that leprosy is a terrible disease. One doctor who diagnosed someone with leprosy overreacted and posted a completely over-the-top, sensationalist account. As doctors, and as Americans, we should be doing our utmost to get the correct information out there about leprosy. There is a real need for it."

On the other hand, he told me a story about a high school student from a newspaper article published in November 2008. Diagnosed with leprosy, she was terrified at the thought of being left with disabilities. She had been shunned by her classmates. But with appropriate treatment she was cured, and then she started telling everyone proudly about her experience. "Catch it early and take the medication, and you really do get cured. It's no different from any other disease. Discrimination is utterly wrong." Once she started standing up for herself, the discrimination melted away. As Dr. Krahenbuhl said, people who are discriminated against can really make a difference to the way they are treated—if they want to.

I should also mention another resident, a Japanese woman, eighty years old, known as "Tokiko" (a pseudonym). Tokiko hailed from Kagoshima, and for a time she had worked in Okinawa—it was here that she caught leprosy, and she experienced discrimination. In 1969, she came to the United States for treatment, and she had been living in Carville ever since. Dr. Krahenbuhl had told her that I would be visiting, but she was unwilling to meet me because she didn't want anything about her to be reported to family and relatives in Japan. Tokiko was apparently a very cheerful person—she enjoyed cooking, baking cookies especially. But for forty years, there she had been, fearful to go home. I stood in front of the building where she lived and called out "How are you? I hope you're well!" any number of times, but there was no answer.

Most of the people (presently around 100) affected by leprosy in the United States originally went there from elsewhere for treatment. The armadillos that live in the Southern states, the only species (apart from some monkey species and of course humans) that carry the leprosy bacillus, are the reason that the research institute was located in Louisiana. Researchers at Louisiana University have conducted research into production of a vaccine based on bacilli derived from these armadillos. Thirty years previously, research was conducted by the Sasakawa Health Foundation into the practical application of an armadillo-based vaccine produced by renowned Venezuelan leprosy expert Dr. Jacinto Convit. Ultimately, however, it proved impossible to propagate enough bacillus from armadillos living in the wild, and they do not thrive in captivity—so we failed to get any results. The work led by the late Professor Tonetaro Ito of the Research Institute for Microbial Diseases, Osaka University, and carried out at the Sasakawa Research Building in Thailand to propagate the bacillus from genetically modified ("nude") laboratory mice also proved fruitless. It is perfectly possible to grow the influenza vaccine from chicken eggs, in vast quantities, but it seems that a vaccine for leprosy that would cure millions of people using armadillos and nude mice is not. The transmission pathways of the leprosy bacillus are still not fully understood. To truly eradicate the disease from the world, it will be essential to identify the transmission pathways and define ways to practically implement such a leprosy vaccine.

4

THE SOCIAL ASPECTS OF THE DISEASE

2010–12

Discrimination in legislation and in people's hearts

In December 2010, the United Nations General Assembly approved a resolution on the elimination of discrimination against people affected by leprosy and their family members. This development lent significant strength to our activities, particularly in our fight to eliminate the prejudice and discrimination that surround the disease—the social aspects of leprosy.

Despite the progress each country was making in achieving elimination (less than one case per 10,000 population, according to the World Health Organization (WHO) benchmark), discriminatory elements can still be found relating to leprosy in legislation and institutions in many countries throughout the world—even in the twenty-first century. In 2008, the Beijing Organizing Committee for the Olympic and Paralympic Games declared that people affected by leprosy would be prohibited from entering the country during the games. I immediately sent letters to President Hu Jintao, the mayor of the host city Beijing, and the president of the International Olympic Committee asking them to change this policy, and the problem was resolved—for the time being, at least. In the same year, India's

Supreme Court ruled in favor of an Odisha law that prohibits people affected by leprosy from standing for municipal elections or serving as councilors or local government heads. The Supreme Court's decision was an affirmation of the Odisha High Court's decision under a section of the Odisha Municipal Corporation Act that states that people affected by leprosy are not eligible to hold such positions. The affirmation stripped Dhirendra Pandua of his position as councilor and chairperson of the municipal council on the grounds that he was affected by leprosy. I sent a letter of protest to the chief justice of the Supreme Court of India and requested a new ruling. I could cite any number of comparable examples. The Western press inadvertently uses words such as "leper," and there are no end of films and other media that portray leprosy in a horrifying light.

Slowly and surely, once the UN resolution was approved, we began to see improvements in this state of affairs. From 2011, changes were made to legislation. Of particular significance were the repeals and revisions of discriminatory laws in India enacted during the period of British rule. The following list shows the main laws that were changed. The first date shows the year of enactment, the second the year of revision or repeal:

China: Marriage Law, 1980—Repealed 2011

India: Juvenile Justice, Care and Protection Act, 2000—Revised 2011

India: The Lepers Act, 1898—Repealed 2016

India: The Odisha Zilla Parishad Act, 1991—Revised 2016

India: The Odisha Gram Panchayats Act, 1964—Revised 2016

India: The Odisha Act, 1959—Revised 2016

India: The Rajasthan Panchayati Act, 1994—Revised 2018

India: The Bombay Prevention of Begging Act, 1959—Revised 2018

India: The Dissolution of Muslim Marriage Act, 1939—Revised 2019

India: The Special Marriage Act, 1954—Revised 2019

India: The Hindu Marriage Act, 1955—Revised 2019

India: The Hindu Adoptions and Maintenance Act, 1956—Revised 2019

India: The Divorce Act, 1869—Revised 2019

THE SOCIAL ASPECTS OF THE DISEASE

The Principles and Guidelines adopted by the UN, however, proved difficult for people who had recovered from leprosy to put to use. Many of the people affected by or recovered from the disease did not really understand what it means to have human rights. This was how deeply the prejudice and discrimination had taken root in these individuals' hearts and minds.

Countries visited in 2010	
January	● Nepal
	● India
February	China (People's Daily TV appearance)
March	● Ghana
	● Mozambique
May	● Sri Lanka
	India (Talks with Bihar state minister of health)
	Jordan (WANA Forum)
	● Timor-Leste
	● Switzerland (Attendance at WHO)
	● Sri Lanka (Talks with President Mahinda Rajapaksa)
	Philippines (Tenth anniversary of API (Asian Public Intellectuals) fellowship program)
	Malaysia (University of Malaya; twentieth anniversary of SYLFF program)
June	United Kingdom (Great Britain-Sasakawa Foundation board meeting)
	China (Japan–China field officer exchange program)
	United States (Washington, DC; Commemorative symposium for the fiftieth anniversary of the conclusion of revised Japan–US Security Treaty Symposium)
	● Ethiopia

	● Chad
August	● Indonesia
September	Sweden (Twenty-fifth anniversary of Scandinavia–Japan Sasakawa Foundation)
	● Norway
	China (Dalian: Japanese Language Education Program meeting)
October	France (Nippon Music Foundation concert)
	Czech Republic (Forum 2000)
	Philippines (UN University for Peace graduation ceremony; the Philippine School of Prosthetics and Orthotics)
	Myanmar (Nationwide ceasefire agreement: talks with government personnel)
	● Vietnam
November	● Palau
	China (Shanghai; United States–Japan Foundation board meeting)
	● Malaysia
	Cambodia (Opening ceremony for School of Traditional Medicines)
	Thailand (Myanmar nationwide ceasefire agreement: negotiations with Myanmar armed ethnic organizations)
December	● India
	● Egypt
	Lebanon (WHO Mediterranean Region Program Managers Meeting on Elimination of Leprosy)
	● Thailand

● Indicates a trip that features in this section.

WANA: West Asia–North Africa, a non-profit think tank based in Amman, Jordan, comprising intellectual leaders in economic, environmental, energy, educational, and social spheres.

API: The Nippon Foundation Fellowships for Asian Public Intellectuals, a fellowships program operated by five partner institutions across Asia.

SYLFF: Sasakawa Young Leaders Fellowship Fund program.

Forum 2000: An annual international conference launched in 1997 when Václav Havel, Elie Wiesel, and the author invited world leaders to Prague for open debate on the major issues and challenges of the new millennium.

Nepal after the elimination of leprosy—the Federal Democratic Republic of Nepal, 20 January 2010

> Route: Narita → Bangkok, Thailand (flight time: 7h; overnight transit) → Kathmandu, Nepal (flight time: 3h 45m)—two nights

Nepal had achieved its long-held goal of eliminating leprosy as a public health problem in 2009. On 18 January 2010, I visited Nepal to convey my congratulations at a ceremony scheduled for the following day, when the official announcement would be made. It was my first overseas leprosy activity of the year.

In this country in the Himalayan foothills, despite continuing political instability, concerned parties had worked together to make medicines available in all regions and promote disease control programs to enable the early detection of leprosy. The tireless efforts over the previous few years of the nation's Ministry of Health and Population and the WHO Nepal Office, in particular, had been awe-inspiring. The achievement would not have been possible without the work of Dr. Thakur, director of the Ministry of Health and Population's Leprosy Control Program, and Dr. Alexander Andjaparidze, WHO representative in Nepal. During the previous two years, I had visited Nepal every six months or so, but the unstable political situation seemed to bring a new minister of health every time I visited. I sometimes had to implore the minister not to transfer Dr. Thakur because the program would stagnate if he were removed from duty. I was glad I had done so, because officials were now conducting thoroughgoing monitoring of local health workers and volunteers to ascertain how accurately they understood leprosy, and the health services had seen a definite improvement.

I would like to make a special mention here of the help we received from the media, especially Dharmendra Jha, president of the

Federation of Nepali Journalists (FNJ). In April 2009, Mr. Jha took time out of his busy schedule to accompany me on a visit to the Terai belt in the country's south. There he gathered local journalists, and in his address he spoke strongly of the responsibility the media should assume in the fight to eliminate leprosy. A number of NGOs that had long been active in the region had of course also contributed greatly, among them the Netherlands Leprosy Relief (NLR) and the Nepal Leprosy Relief Association. Indeed, the elimination of leprosy in Nepal, despite all the political turmoil, was earned through concerted efforts taken by a full complement of organizations and groups.

When I went to convey my congratulations to President Ram Baran Yadav and Prime Minister Madhav Kumar Nepal in person and seek their ongoing commitment to further reducing the disease burden in their country, they acknowledged my request, both nodding in agreement. Prime Minister Nepal then gave the example of the ministerial meeting on the issue of climate change just recently held at Kala Patthar, over 5,000 meters above sea level, where he had to change planes several times to get to such a high elevation. "When you want to reach a high goal, you have to take things in steps. Eliminating leprosy as a public health problem is just the first step. What we want is to bring the number of patients progressively down to zero."

At a ceremony to celebrate Nepal's attainment of the elimination target held on 19 January and organized by the Ministry of Health and Population, several speakers took the podium, including Minister of Health and Population Umakant Chaudhary, senior officials Praveen Mishra and Sudha Sharma, FNJ President Jha, and Krishna Prasad Dhakal, the NLR country representative. At the end of the event, Minister Chaudhary declared that leprosy had been eliminated as a public health problem, and simultaneously the words "Congratulations Nepal, you have eliminated leprosy!" appeared above the stage. The audience erupted in applause.

The next day, I visited Panauti, a municipality in Kavrepalanchok (Kavre) district, about an hour-and-a-half's drive from Kathmandu. My visit coincided with Makar Mela, a Hindu festival that takes place every twelve years. A group of dancers, wearing wooden masks representing evil spirits, paraded before me, beating an array of percussion instruments. I later learned that among the dancers were individuals who had been treated for leprosy. The idea was that their participation in the ceremony would help change their self-perceptions and rebuild their confidence. Female volunteers working at the local sub-health post also performed a song that they use to raise people's awareness of leprosy. The lyrics of one of the songs went as follows:

> Without treatment, leprosy causes suffering
> Patches on skin that don't hurt when touched or pricked
> Are the most important symptom
> If you have leprosy
> Take the medicine the doctors gave you
> Don't think of leprosy as divine punishment

In rural areas of Nepal where people live far beyond the reach of television and newspapers, songs and plays like this are a very effective means of communicating information.

On the morning of my departure from Nepal, I appeared on a radio program with Raj Kumar Shah, leader of Rehabilitation

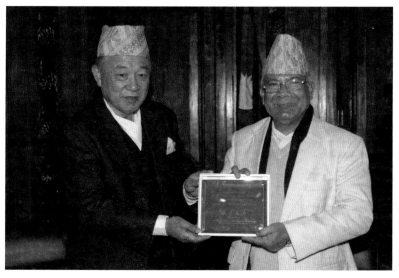

76. With a delighted Prime Minister Madhav Kumar Nepal, holding the commemorative plaque for the nation's leprosy elimination (Nepal, January 2010)

Empowerment and Development Nepal, an NGO established by and for people affected by leprosy. Still in his thirties, Mr. Shah had already linked up with organizations for people with disabilities, and the deep insight and passion fueling his work were clear to see. I always say that the words of those who have experienced discrimination are the most persuasive in eliminating it. One story from someone with experience of discrimination has far more power to reach people's hearts than 100 stories told by me.

Notwithstanding the achievement of the elimination target, the situation surrounding leprosy in Nepal was not resolved. The paths leading up to the famed Swayambhunath Temple in Kathmandu were still thronged with people affected by leprosy begging for alms, just as others had done for decades. It was part of my mission to find a way to change common perceptions about people with lived experience of leprosy so that they are not prevented from finding employment and living dignified lives as members of Nepalese society.

Finally, I would like to again give credit to Dr. Andjaparidze, a key figure in the fight against leprosy in Nepal, who would retire from the WHO in March. I have already mentioned Dr. Andjaparidze quite a few times, mostly in the context of my activities in Timor-Leste— how, while working there, this kind-hearted and generous man was completely unfazed by an explosive that rent a hole in the ceiling directly above his desk during the political unrest, and how he and his devoted wife worked tirelessly to direct WHO staff in dealing with the injured. I was aware too that he had refused to comply with a UN order to evacuate the staff and their families even though he had discreetly sent a parasite specialist from the Sasakawa Health Foundation back to Japan to safety. During this visit to Nepal, Dr. Andjaparidze invited me and my team to his home for dinner to celebrate the official elimination of leprosy. That night, he related an escapade that had happened in his youth, as we all listened, sipping on the wine we'd brought. "At the age of seventeen," he told us, "I was in Kyiv, Ukraine, and I got knocked down by a streetcar. Then the taxi I'd hailed got turned upside-down in a crash involving a bus and a truck. I was trying to make my way back to Georgia, but at the airfield, I got stabbed in the abdomen by thieves trying to steal the scarf I was wearing. The airplane I boarded got engine trouble halfway through the flight, and we had to fly on a single engine, only just making it to our destination. The unlicensed taxi I got at the airport was stopped at a checkpoint, and the driver fled. The taxi had been stolen, and I was taken to jail. And then, after my release, I had to undergo surgery at the hospital." In one day, he had been subject to six misfortunes. "I have survived by luck alone," he reflected. Of all the UN officials I have worked with, many of them in tough circumstances, Dr. Andjaparidze remains among those that left the most vivid impression. We have shared many good memories.

Issues and hopes for leprosy colonies—Tamil Nadu and Maharashtra states, Republic of India, January 2010

> Route: Kathmandu, Nepal → Delhi, India (flight time: 1h 15m; 2h 30m stopover) → Chennai, Tamil Nadu (flight time: 2h 30m)—three nights—Chennai → Mumbai, Maharashtra (flight time: 1h 50m)—two nights—Mumbai → Narita International Airport (flight time: 8h)

On 21 January 2010, I left Nepal and flew on to Chennai, Tamil Nadu, via Delhi. In Chennai, I attended the National Forum's Southern Regional Conference. Established in 2006, the National Forum had so far held two national conferences and three regional conferences, but this was the first conference in southern India. Some 350 representatives of the leprosy colonies spread across the southern states, including Tamil Nadu, Kerala, and Andhra Pradesh, attended the conference. Ms. Geetha Jeevan, Tamil Nadu's minister for social welfare, gave a somewhat hopeful (though perhaps less than inspiring) speech in which she stated: "The state government will continue to provide support, however modest."

After the conference, I paid one of my usual visits to a leprosy colony. This was my third visit to the colony in the Villivakkam area on the city's outskirts. With each visit, I noticed new buildings under construction, indicating that the residents' lives were improving. Home to some 100 households and around 300 people in all, this relatively large colony has gradually developed through support from NGOs and government agencies since its formation around 1980. Recently, many people who are not affected by leprosy also started to live there, making it an integrated community where people affected by leprosy and people who have no experience of leprosy live without division. The colony's leader, Mr. Prakasam, who himself was affected by leprosy, had united all the colonies in Tamil Nadu, having served for two decades at the helm of the Tamil Nadu Leprosy Patients' Rehabilitation Guild. The residents had received microfinance from the Sasakawa-India Leprosy Foundation (S-ILF) and had started up businesses to produce and sell items, including clothing, plastic goods, and automobile parts. With great pride, they showed me their wares—clothes, toys, cooking pots, shoes—all of good quality. A pair of sandals was selling for 100 rupees (around US$1.20), and a plastic cooking pot for roughly 400 rupees. The couple running the shop told me happily that their net profit of 300 rupees per month, after rent and expenses, was enough to send their two children to school. A woman who was selling saris and scarves and the like on the street told me how she researched the latest trends and put great effort into creating products that would please her customers. When I asked her how her customers paid, she answered, full of confidence, "The usual shops only accept cash, paid in full, but I allow customers to pay me in three installments, which they appreciate, and my business is doing well."

I next paid a visit to the Balpart colony, about thirty minutes away by car. This colony had thirty-five households, with some 110 residents in all. It had developed with support from a Christian charity. I was told that the houses had been constructed by younger residents who had learned how to build with support from the charity. However, the colony's financial situation was dire, and every day ten people departed and went to beg at temples, earning around 50 rupees (about US$1.10) per person. Some residents had applied to start businesses with microfinance from the S-ILF initiatives. But I could sense that they were still unaware of what it means to be self-reliant, so I told them, "I want you to draw up a solid business plan after proper consultations with the foundation's experts. We'll send someone to you. Don't give up." They showed their understanding by tilting their heads and wobbling them, an expression of affirmation in India.

While I was in Tamil Nadu, I went to two events that gave me particular joy. The first was a party celebrating the publication in English in December 2009 of the autobiography of Ms. Muthu

Meenal, a woman living in Tamil Nadu who had once had leprosy but had been treated and was now clear of the disease. In English, the book was titled *Thorn*. Initially published in her native Tamil as *Mul* in January 2009, the book became a bestseller, printed twice in six months. The author, Ms. Meenal, contracted leprosy when she was young and developed her writing talent despite suffering discrimination and social stigma. To make her autobiography known as widely as possible, the Sasakawa Health Foundation had supported the publication of this English-language edition. To the delight of those present, the event was attended by Kamal Haasan, a world-renowned actor, film director, and playwright who involves himself in a wide range of humanitarian work, including illness-related relief funds.

The second was a cultural event organized by the National Forum that occurs each year on the last Sunday in January in tandem with World Leprosy Day, featuring children and grandchildren of people affected by leprosy. It took place in an open-air hall built in memory of Mahatma Gandhi. First to meet my eyes was a bustling scene of stalls selling sari fabrics made by people affected by leprosy, a pop-up stall organized by the Hindu Art School selling pictures, and

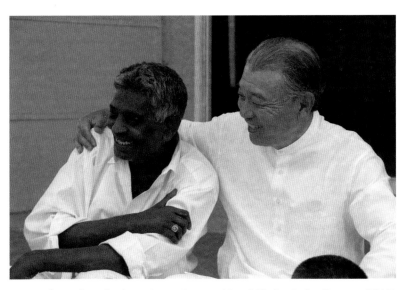

77. With a colony leader, Mr. Prakasam (Tamil Nadu, India, January 2010)

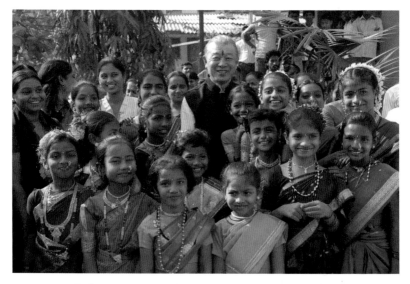

78. With the colony's children (Tamil Nadu, India, January 2010)

other stalls selling food and other items. On stage, the children of people affected by leprosy living in Chennai's colonies sang, danced, and performed magic tricks, and young people talked about all the languages and cultures of India to musical accompaniment. Some of the children were from the Villivakkam colony I had visited the day before. One girl whose grandfather had been affected by leprosy told me, "I want to become a doctor so I can be of help to people who suffer from sickness." She opened her eyes wide and shyly looked away.

During my stay in Chennai, I had all my meals at hotels due to safety concerns. I love Indian curries, and can eat way too much, so I make sure to watch my weight. The buffet-style meals are perfect for me because we can eat without delay. India has wonderful beer, but Indians themselves don't seem to care for it. As a result, it can be challenging to order beer before the meal starts, as one normally does in Japan. Usually, the first beer finally arrives around the time, tired of waiting, we have started to eat.

Incidentally, when working overseas, I make it a principle not to bring any Japanese food to eat, except for in emergencies. I also instruct anyone accompanying me to join me in experiencing the local food. Nothing beats eating the same food and singing and dancing together as a basis for communication. Sometimes we are served insects, but I enjoy such unexpected experiences.

On 24 January, I left Chennai for Mumbai in the state of Maharashtra. I was there to attend the launch ceremony of the Global Appeal 2010, the fifth such event, and to attend a workshop organized by the National Forum.

For the fifth Global Appeal, I asked business leaders from around the world to join us. People affected by leprosy should have the same rights as all other people and the same opportunities to contribute to society. I asked several of the world's leading companies to endorse the idea, with the implication that the business world should also adopt it. Representatives from fifteen of the world's largest companies, including India's Tata Motors, Mahindra Group, Japan's Toyota Motor Corporation, Mitsubishi Corporation, Canon Inc., Thailand's Siam Cement, France's Renault Motors, and Britain's Virgin Airlines, signed the declaration. The declaration ceremony was held at the famous Taj Mahal Hotel, directly in front of the Gateway of India. Co-sponsored by the Nippon Foundation and S-ILF—established to provide financial support to people affected by and recovering from leprosy—the event had around 120 attendees, including signatory company representatives and staff, people recovered from leprosy, NGOs, Japanese Ambassador to India Hideaki Dodo, Consul General of Japan in Mumbai Tamon Mochida, and media representatives. Following powerful speeches by one of the signatories, Mahindra Group Chairman Keshub Mahindra, and a guest from Thailand, Siam Cement Chairman Kan Trakulhoon, six young people living in colonies read out the declaration.

At the workshop sponsored by the Western Regional Division of the National Forum, several people affected by leprosy, as well as government and NGO representatives, participated in lively discussions on restoring dignity to people affected by leprosy. One of the guests, Member of Parliament (and former Minister of Petroleum and Natural Gas) Ram Naik, had been the lead signatory of a petition submitted to the Indian Parliament's Committee on Petitions in 2008, seeking to improve the lives of people affected by leprosy.

Mr. Naik is an influential figure in India who has always shown a deep understanding of my work.

I also visited a large colony with 720 residents located near Mumbai, Hanuman Nagar colony, which had received a loan from S-ILF and had residents raising water buffaloes. When I peeked into a barn, which I saw had been named Sasakawa Farm, I found eight healthy-looking buffaloes being kept there. The resident taking care of the buffaloes as if they were his own children was enthusiastic about expanding his business. "I want to eventually have around thirty water buffaloes," he told us. I got a clear sense of his bright hopes germinating. Next, I visited the Mahatma Gandhi colony, where another resident asked to submit a business plan to S-ILF. The S-ILF microfinance program seemed to have become widely known among colony dwellers.

Presidential babysitter—Republic of Ghana, March 2010

Route: Narita International Airport → London, UK (flight time: 12h)—one night—London → Accra, Ghana (flight time: 6h 30m)—three nights

In March 2010, I visited the West African nation of Ghana by way of London. Just a short walk in the capital city of Accra brings one out in streams of sweat due to the blazing sun, high humidity, and temperatures of around 30 degrees C. Even so, March is said to be the best time of the year to visit. The leprosy prevalence rate in Ghana had fallen to 0.29 per 10,000 population, but figures alone do not suffice. I visited two leprosy hospitals to ascertain the situation with my own eyes.

The first was Ankaful Hospital, about two and a half hours west of Accra by car. I had previously visited the hospital ten years prior, when it was called Ankaful Leprosy Hospital and was a focal point of the government's leprosy elimination program. The male and female wards were once packed with patients, but now I found only eight patients in the male ward, and the hospital had transformed into a general hospital that accepted patients with all sorts of different illnesses. I took some relief from this change. However, in a convalescent facility on the hospital grounds, the nearby Ankaful Camp for people affected by leprosy, I found around sixty people. These were people who could not return to society or the villages where their families lived due to prejudice and discrimination.

My second visit was to Ho Polyclinic, where here again there was a camp with around seventy people affected by leprosy, faced with the same sorts of issues. Ho Camp is about three hours northeast of Accra by car. When I arrived, I was greeted by a group of people affected by leprosy, with loud music blaring from speakers and an atmosphere resembling a festival. At first glance, the area looked like a typical rural farming village, but in reality most people were unable to find jobs and had no choice but to live on welfare. Their children receive only an elementary school education.

One person who has been working to improve these conditions is Kofi Nyarko, who accompanied me on this trip. As someone who has recovered from leprosy himself, he serves as the Ghanaian representative for the International Association for Integration, Dignity and Economic Advancement (IDEA), an international organization for people affected by leprosy. He also teaches children living in leprosy facilities, cares for the elderly, and helps those barred from going back to their homes and their villages. "Home is a special place," he told me, looking pleased. "So far, we have been able to return more than forty people from twelve colonies nationwide to their homes." My role is to support the work of people like Mr. Nyarko by visiting the front lines as often as possible, listening to the first-hand experiences of the people, and, if necessary, taking their voices to the heads of state to request that they do all they can to promote greater understanding of leprosy among the populace.

After this, I attended the Hideyo Noguchi Africa Prize Memorial Symposium, named after the late Japanese bacteriologist who died in Ghana in 1928 while researching a vaccine for yellow fever. The aim of the symposium is to work toward enhancing health research and systems in Africa. The symposium was attended by His Imperial Highness the Crown Prince of Japan (the current emperor). Medical researchers and health professionals working in the field discussed epidemic control. In a session titled "The Future of Africa: Poverty and Epidemic Control," I reported on my experiences in Africa with epidemic control, including leprosy, and our agricultural development project. The Sasakawa Global 2000 (SG2000) project, which teaches poor farmers in Ghana how to increase food production, is the most successful example of a program of its type in Africa. The then president Jerry Rawlings was also a strong advocate for our cause. Whenever we met, he would reminisce about the activities of SG2000 when he was in office. He had once told me that on his way back from a military exercise, he had happened to see a field of maize that looked quite different from all the others. He learned that it was an SG2000 field, which prompted him to reach out to us. SG2000 has enabled small-scale farmers to produce nutritious agricultural products, which has in turn led to a significant improvement in farmers' health and immunity, ultimately preventing epidemics.

However, just one month earlier, on 14 February, news had broken that President Rawlings's house had been destroyed in a fire. I had been looking forward to meeting him again, but in all the confusion, it had proved more difficult than I'd planned to get in touch with him. However, when I arrived in Ghana, I received a call from him. The president, whose whose residence doubled as his office, greeted me

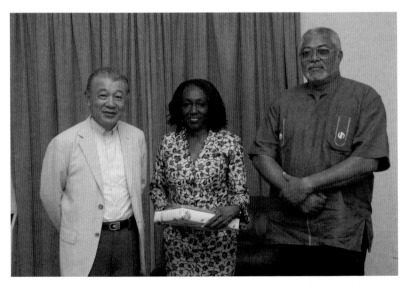

79. The author with former President Jerry Rawlings of Ghana and his wife Nana (Ghana, March 2010)

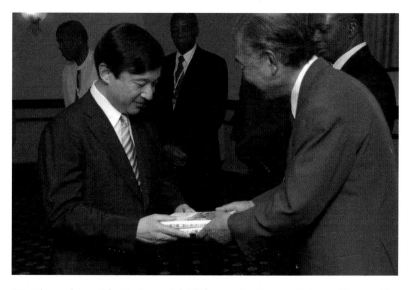

80. The author with His Imperial Highness the Crown Prince of Japan (the present Emperor of Japan) (Ghana, March 2010)

on my arrival with his wife Nana at his side. He showed me around his burned-out residence, which was now nothing but a frame. His exhaustion came through as he spoke. "Everything was burned. Photos, documents, and mementos too." But when he began talking about the political situation in Ghana, he was as passionate as ever, worrying that the people felt that things were hopeless and had nothing to keep their spirits up. Seeing the president like this made me remember how I had been when I started this work. Of all the presidents in office I had ever met, President Rawlings was the most keen and interested in my activities. Accordingly, the Republic of Ghana was one of the first countries on the African continent to eliminate leprosy as a public health problem. When I told him that I had just visited a leprosy facility, he told me: "Now that you mention it, I remember our baby-sitter was someone who'd once had leprosy—though that's more than twenty years ago now." I wondered if this had been why he had been so eager to cooperate in working toward elimination.

President Rawlings, the son of a Ghanaian and a Briton, became president in his twenties. He had the tragic experience of trying to visit his father in the UK after becoming president, only to be refused. During the SG2000 agricultural support program, President Rawlings launched into an anti-American diatribe in full military dress in front of President Carter. My father, Ryoichi Sasakawa, was present, and when he heard what was being said, he commented, loudly: "Stop being so rude. We did not come here to help you. We came to help the struggling farmers." At this, the president removed his sunglasses and stood stiffly to attention. Whenever we would meet, he would recount the episode to me: "It was terrifying. It was as if my own father was scolding me."

Toward eliminating leprosy in all provinces—Republic of Mozambique, March 2010

> Route: Accra, Ghana → Johannesburg, South Africa (via Lagos, Nigeria; flight time: 7h 45m; 4h stopover) → Maputo, Mozambique (flight time: 1h)—two nights—Maputo → Johannesburg (flight time: 1h; 6h stopover) → Dubai, United Arab Emirates (flight time: 8h; 3h stopover) → Kansai International Airport (flight time: 8h 50m; 1h 30m stopover) → Haneda International Airport (flight time: 1h)

On the afternoon of 11 March 2010, I landed at a small airport in Mozambique's capital, Maputo, after flying from Ghana via Johannesburg. It was my fifth visit to this East African nation since 2005, when I began making regular visits in support of its leprosy elimination activities. On my arrival, the humidity was fairly low, but the temperature was high, and the sun was scorching.

Mozambique reached the WHO's elimination target of less than one case per 10,000 population at the national level in 2007, but at the time, the Minister of Health Dr. Ivo Garrido, whom I knew well, was as cautious as ever, saying there would be no cause for celebration until this target was reached at the state level too. This was duly achieved at the end of 2008. In the capital Maputo, I joined Dr. El Hadi Benzerroug, the WHO's Mozambique representative, and Dr. Landry Bide, regional advisor of the WHO Regional Office for Africa, in commending Prime Minister Aires Ali, who had just assumed his post in January, and Vice President of the Assembly of the Republic Lucas Chomera and their officials on the country's success in eliminating leprosy, seeking their cooperation to further reduce the number of cases of the disease.

I later met with former President Joaquim Chissano, a wise man whom I have known for many years through his association with the SG2000 project, rekindling an old friendship after many years. That evening, I had dinner with Deputy Health Minister Jorge Fernando Tomo, Public Health Department Director Mourinho Said, and the WHO's Dr. Benzerroug and Dr. Bide at the official residence of Mr. Susumu Segawa, Japan's ambassador to Mozambique. Deputy Minister Tomo told us that the Ministry of Health was researching traditional medicines. When I asked for more information, he immediately put me in touch with a contact. The next morning, we visited the National Institute of Traditional Medicine within the Ministry of Health.

The institute was housed in a century-old building built during Portuguese rule and equipped with laboratories and instruments for analyzing substances. We were told that there are around 3,200 species of medicinal herbs in Mozambique, and about 75 percent of the population uses traditional medicines. Traditional medicines are low-cost and provide a valuable means for the rural poor to deal with the initial symptoms of fever, abdominal pain, and diarrhea. The Nippon Foundation has been working to enhance health care with traditional medicines in Mongolia, Cambodia, Myanmar, and other Asian countries, and now here in Africa, we were seeing new possibilities for this approach.

In the afternoon, there was a partners' meeting at the Ministry of Health attended by representatives from six NGOs involved in leprosy work and WHO officials. From the NGO side were Dr. Charles Phaff, NLR; Ms. Genama Salvetti, Amici di Raoul Follereau; Dr. Jean Marie Nyambe, Damien Foundation; Mr. Candido Raphael, British Leprosy Relief Association (LEPRA UK); Ms. Farida Gulamo, Mozambique Association of People with Disabilities (ADEMO); and Mr. Chamada Abibo, Mozambique Association of Persons with Leprosy (ALEMO)—the latter having traveled from the northern endemic region of Cabo Delgado.

Following the meeting, Health Minister Garrido gave a briefing on the current leprosy situation in the presence of TV and newspaper reporters. He announced that leprosy had been officially eliminated as a public health problem in every state, but the prevalence rate remained above one per 10,000 population in certain areas within a number of states. From now on, their efforts would focus on eliminating leprosy in each of these areas, reducing the number of cases by half. Regarding the situation in the north of the country, where the number of people affected by leprosy remained high, he said, "We cannot simply dismiss leprosy as a disease of the poor. There must be a reason why certain areas have a high number of patients. We intend to correctly analyze the situation and take the appropriate measures."

In the evening, the minister of health and about thirty others—including health ministry, WHO, and NGO staff and representatives—gathered for a banquet to celebrate eliminating leprosy as a public health problem. Minister Garrido gave a speech in which, with great sincerity, he paid tribute to my efforts. "Even I, as the chief administrator, always thought in the depths of my heart that it was impossible to eliminate leprosy in this country," he commented.

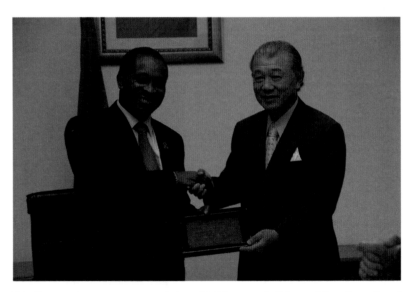

81. Presenting a commemorative shield to mark Mozambique's national elimination of leprosy to Prime Minister Aires Ali (Mozambique, March 2010)

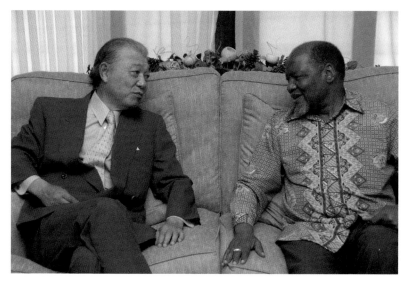

82. The author with former President Joaquin Chissano (Mozambique, March 2010)

"However, with the help of Mr. Sasakawa, who has come to visit us almost every year, traveling all the way from Japan on journeys that sometimes take as long as forty hours, to encourage us, and with the president too lending his support, somehow we did manage to achieve it. I have to say that without Mr. Sasakawa's efforts, we would not have been able to eliminate the disease."

Visiting states where leprosy officer positions remain vacant—Delhi and Bihar states, Republic of India, April 2010

Route: Narita International Airport → Delhi, India (flight time: 9h 20m)—two nights—Delhi → Patna, Bihar, India (flight time: 1h 30m)—three nights—Patna → Delhi (flight time: 1h 30m; 13h stopover, visited the WHO Regional Office for Southeast Asia and other WHO officials) → Singapore (flight time: 5h 40m; 2h stopover) → Narita (flight time: 7h)

During my April visit to India, I spent three days each in Delhi and the northeastern state of Bihar.

First, I attended a S-ILF board meeting in Delhi. Led by Executive Director Vineeta Shanker and trustee Tarun Das, we discussed the foundation's current status and future development. The expectations among residents in leprosy colonies were so high that it was not proving possible for S-ILF to meet all of their requests for loans. To do so, we realized there was an urgent necessity to solicit more donations from within India and to push forward with even more education and awareness activities.

The day after the board meeting was Sunday. I had some free time during the day, so I took a walk down the streets of Old Delhi for the first time in many years. This kind of free time is rare for me, as when I visit India, my schedule is almost invariably packed with minute-to-minute activities. Central Delhi is lined with neat, modern buildings, but the old city has an entirely different feel. Tangled electric wires hang down low over the narrow streets, while rickshaws carrying people and their belongings brush closely past vendors with vegetables laid out on plastic sheets. A cup of chai costs 6 rupees (about US$0.07). A bearded man thrust out a paper cup of chai at me with a sturdy arm, and I drank it right there in the middle of a crowded street. I typically avoid drinks and sweets that are too sugary, but the chai was surprisingly pleasant. Despite India's rapid economic growth, the scene before my eyes was no different from what it was ten years ago.

In the evening, I flew to Patna, the capital of Bihar state. Bihar has a population of about 100 million and is considered one of the poorest states in India. It is also one of the four states in India that had yet to achieve the WHO benchmark of eliminating leprosy as a public health problem. And yet, despite that, the state's leprosy program officer position was vacant at the time of my visit.

I wanted to visit three leprosy colonies in the East Champaran district, a two-hour drive from Patna, with guides from Bihar Kashta Kalyan Mahasangh (BKKM), an umbrella group of associations of people affected by leprosy in Bihar, established in December of the previous year.

The first stop, Motipur colony, was home to 158 people in fifty-five families, forty of whom had recovered from leprosy. Upon arrival, I heard the cheerful voices of children who were lined up in an outdoor hallway reading their textbooks aloud. In government schools, children are subject to discrimination simply for having family members affected by leprosy. Accordingly, the colony had opened its own school with the support of Little Flower, an NGO located on the border with Nepal. Nearly all the dwellings in the colony were simple, with roofs and walls made of straw, and some of the older women complained to me about their leaks and disrepair. Government support was not entirely absent. Families who were able to obtain certificates of eligibility for daily necessities for people on low incomes could buy 35 kg of rice for 70 rupees (about US$0.90) per month. Cooking oil and fuel were also available at lower prices than in the market. However, colony representatives complained passionately that many individuals affected by leprosy who have disabilities were seen as ineligible for disability pensions, and even elderly people eligible for old-age pensions of 200 rupees per month were not getting their benefit payments. Most of the population, I could see, supported themselves by begging.

My next stop, Chakia colony, was in a similar situation. This was a small community of thirty-five households and forty-five people, most of whom had to beg to make ends meet. The area is prone to frequent flooding, with many houses swept away in the great flood of 2009. The Sasakawa Health Foundation had assisted in reconstruction. The residents lived in simple huts constructed along the road but were now under pressure from the government to move because of a road-widening project. In response, they had been lobbying the government to provide them with alternative land to live on nearby, but the government had been slow to respond. An adjacent sugar company had even opposed an attempt to build sanitary facilities on the land, so the residents did not even have access to toilets.

My final stop was Pipra colony, home to thirteen households and twenty-two individuals. This colony had been the scene of a tragedy on 12 January 2010, when a neighboring landowner seeking to evict his tenants set fire to several houses. A five-year-old boy who failed to escape had lost his life in the flames. The aforementioned BKKM had just been established in December 2009, and it joined representatives from Bihar and the National Forum to negotiate with the police and the government. As a result, they obtained compensation of 100,000 rupees from the government and a promise to provide land and build housing in the neighborhood by April. So, the death of one

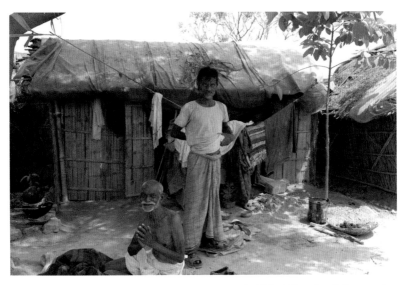

83. At the Pipra leprosy colony, where a child had lost his life in a fire (Bihar, India, April 2010)

small boy had, in the end, served to unite the Bihar representatives. It was the most heartbreaking story.

The following morning, I visited Vaishali district's Lalganj Primary Health Center, a small thirteen-bed hospital with minimal facilities and staff. It treats all sorts of patients, including those with leprosy or everyday ailments and those needing obstetrics and gynecology services. It receives an average of 200 outpatients a day. At the time, it was treating twenty-two leprosy patients with multidrug therapy (MDT). I was told that at private clinics where people got their first diagnosis, many doctors were still unaware that MDT is available as a free treatment. I was also informed that some people went all the way to Patna, the far-flung state capital, to receive treatment in order to avoid their neighbors becoming aware that they have leprosy. When we asked the hospital director about the activities of social workers whose job it was to detect patients, he explained confidently: "No such people exist. We don't need such social workers. Everyone knows about leprosy. We have done such a good job raising people's awareness that patients come here on their own accord." However, when I spoke to one man affected by leprosy, he said he received treatment without learning the name of the disease. His wife has the same disease, he said, but she did not want to come to the health center. This response from a single patient told us all we needed to know about the inadequacy of leprosy control measures in the region.

During my stay in Bihar, accompanied by BKKM representatives, I called on State Health Minister Nand Kishore Yadav. We asked him to appoint a suitably well-qualified person to fill the vacant position of state leprosy program officer, and to take steps to improve conditions for people living in the colonies. He replied by telling us that disability pensions only covered people with disabilities. Nevertheless, he said, he would look into establishing a special category of disability pension that would cover people affected by leprosy. He would also consider prioritizing people affected by leprosy in providing housing assistance to the poor. We took this as a positive response. I was the guest of honor at this meeting and sat in front of the minister. However, since Mr. Kamlesh Divyadarshi—the National Forum's representative for people affected by leprosy in Bihar—was sitting right next to me, I had him take a leadership role for the day. His face was flushed crimson with excitement at the prospect of being able to petition the health minister in person—the first time such a thing had ever happened, bearing in mind how the very existence of people affected by leprosy has consistently been ignored.

Next, I met with Sanjay Kumar, the executive director of the National Rural Health Mission and, to all intents and purposes, the head of the Ministry of Health. Mr. Kumar explained to us that there were twenty-seven colonies in Bihar. When I countered that, on the contrary, there were more than fifty, he promised that if we managed to provide him with a reliable list within the next two weeks he would deal with the issue of pensions for people recovering from leprosy.

I immediately conferred with officials of the National Forum, an organization of people affected by leprosy in India, and BKKM representatives, and we decided that we would draw up a list with the names of every person affected by leprosy in Bihar, conduct a survey of the living conditions of each colony, and present a report to the government. I provided $1,000 for the cost of the survey out of my own pocket. To ensure the cooperation of State Health Minister Yadav and Executive Director Kumar, I agreed to revisit the area and accompany them two weeks later when they handed over their fact-finding report.

Early in May, receiving word that the survey was completed, I traveled back to Bihar on my way back from a visit to Sri Lanka (see the following section). In the two weeks I had been away, the seven BKMM officials had raced around Bihar, an area larger than Hokkaido, literally spending every waking moment conducting the survey and finding out all they needed to know.

It was the hottest season of the year, particularly at the airfield where under direct sunlight it felt as if the temperature exceeded 50 degrees C. It was the kind of heat that made you sweat profusely and need to lie down after the shortest jaunt. Truly a scorching hell. In the hotel, on the other hand, the air conditioning was set to a very cool 18 degrees C. It is often quite hard for the body to keep up. I don't know why, but hotels in South and Southeast Asia seem to believe that the cooler the air conditioning, the better the guests' experience. Once during a meeting the air conditioning was so intense that the whole area from the back of my head down to my neck started to feel distinctly uncomfortable. I stepped away from the meeting to try and get some sunlight, only to be urged to return to the meeting. Anyway, the day before meeting the state health minister, I met with BKKM's leadership—Kamlesh Divyadarshi, Ram Barai Sah, and Braj Kishor Prasad—at the hotel and marveled at the detail of the survey report. In just fifteen days, they had gone door-to-door, visiting 997 households living in sixty-three colonies to find out about their land, houses, family structures, pension status, and more. Joking merrily about how much they had missed their wives, the three men glowed with satisfaction, despite the exhaustion written on their faces. Whereas the state government had recorded only twenty-seven leprosy colonies, this survey confirmed the existence of sixty-three.

The next day, the heavy survey report in hand, the BKKM leaders and I paid another call on Executive Director Kumar, State Health Minister Yadav, and Bihar Deputy Chief Minister Sushil Kumar Modi (whom we had not seen in April) to report on the current situation and petition for an increase in pensions. After Executive Director Kumar had heard us out, he said that he wanted to have discussions over four or five days between the BKKM representatives and the government. He gave us his word that the land and pension issues would be resolved within a month or so. I had met Deputy Chief Minister Modi at a ceremony marking Myanmar's leprosy elimination in 2003, and I remember he was able to recall in some detail the story I always tell of a beautiful young girl who lived in my father Ryoichi Sasakawa's hometown, which had inspired my father's involvement in leprosy. After asking just a couple of questions, like which regions had the most colonies and what he could do to help, Modi pledged his assistance to see that various issues were taken up.

On the last day of my trip to Bihar, I met with State Health Minister Yadav, and he scrutinized the report from beginning to end and said, "While existing measures may be able to deal with some of these issues, we will need to outline a completely new framework to extend assistance to people affected by and recovering from leprosy. I shall discuss this in detail with the appropriate officials." I also heard the good news that less than a month after my first visit, in April, the state had appointed a leprosy program officer. However, as I will explain later, it took another three years for the state to raise the pensions.

Suffering on "the resplendent island"—Democratic Socialist Republic of Sri Lanka, May 2010

Route: Narita International Airport → Bangkok, Thailand (flight time: 6h 30m; 4h stopover) → Colombo, Sri Lanka (flight time: 3h 20m)—two nights—Colombo → Jaffna, Sri Lanka (chartered flight time: 1h)—one night—Colombo (after returning by land) → Delhi, India (flight time: 3h 35m)—one night—Delhi → Patna, Bihar, India (flight time: 1h 30m)—two nights—Patna → Delhi (flight time: 1h 30m; 2h stopover) → Narita (flight time: 8h)

In May 2010, I visited Sri Lanka. The name "Sri Lanka" means "resplendent island" in the local Sinhala language. The country's inhabitants are mainly Sinhalese, 74 percent of whom speak Sinhala as their first language, and Tamils, 18 percent of whom speak Tamil. Sri Lanka gained its independence in 1948, after colonial rule by the Portuguese in the sixteenth century, the Dutch in the seventeenth century, and the British in the nineteenth century. A civil war

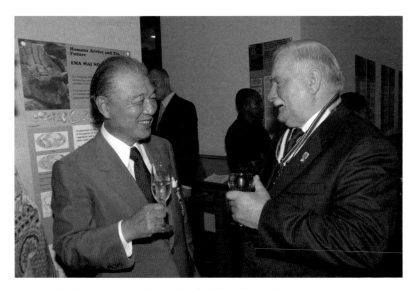

84. With former President of Poland Lech Walesa (Timor-Leste, May 2010)

between Sri Lankan government forces and the Liberation Tigers of Tamil Eelam, a militant Tamil organization, began in 1983, and by the time the war was declared over in May 2009, more than 70,000 people had been killed. Despite this conflict, the nation eliminated leprosy as a public health problem in 2005.

May 2010 marked my third visit to Sri Lanka and the first in three years. I visited just before the first anniversary of the declaration of the civil war's end. I aimed to observe the northern regions where the fighting was fiercest, assess the situation in the refugee camps, and survey leprosy conditions in the country. On my first day, I met with Health Minister Maithripala Sirisena, who had just been appointed to the post a week before (and who would later become president), to hear about the current leprosy conditions from the ministry's leprosy program director. Sri Lanka had eliminated multiple other diseases besides leprosy, including polio, filariasis, measles, and malaria. While dengue fever remained a threat, the nation's public health problems were now mainly non-communicable diseases, such as hypertension and diabetes, a rare situation for a developing country. Nevertheless, as many as 1,875 new leprosy cases were still being reported annually in Sri Lanka. It had yet to achieve district-level elimination in eight of its twenty-six districts, with a notable concentration of cases along its eastern and western coasts. I urged the health minister to maintain the country's progress in light of how well positioned it was to now bring the number of persons affected by leprosy down to zero.

That afternoon, I visited Hendala Leprosy Hospital, 9.6 kilometers north of the capital Colombo. Built by the Dutch in 1708 and said to be the world's oldest active hospital, Hendala continued to operate as a leprosy hospital after the British took over in the nineteenth century. In the days before the villages were built near the hospital, patients used to come by ferry across the Kelani River, which flows right in front of the hospital. The compound has many historic buildings and facilities, including a 115-year-old church and a manually operated washing machine made in 1935, still in use today. Surrounding communities do not discriminate against the hospital's residents, and believers come to the church from outside the village.

Within the large 8-acre premises, there were two wards, one for women and one for men. Colorful mosquito nets hung above the beds, and family photos and other personal belongings were on bedside tables. In the meeting hall, which also serves as a workshop, the hospital holds singing contests and Christmas parties, demonstrating the staff's care and dedication. The hospital houses forty-seven individuals who have recovered from leprosy, the youngest being just thirty-five. However, some residents came to the hospital at seven years old and had been living there for eighty years. Of all the people affected by leprosy I had met overseas, the oldest was a 101-year-old man at the National Leprosarium in Carville, Louisiana, United States. That day in Hendala, however, I met someone who was even older, a 103-year-old resident, Mr. Tisahami.

The following day, I flew to Jaffna, the northernmost city on the island, on a military plane provided by the government. I went to Kilinochchi and Vavuniya, which had been raging battlefields during the civil war. Fresh traces of fighting remained everywhere, and nothing was left but a few scattered scorched palm trees that still stood tall. Everyone said that the residents were terrified that the conflict could flare up again at any moment. In cooperation with its sister foundation, the Sasakawa Peace Foundation, the Nippon Foundation had been quietly conducting a project for peace talks among religious leaders for the past sixteen years. Such people exert significant influence on political leaders and citizens in Sri Lanka, which is a land of strong religious faith, and their cooperation is essential for building the foundations of society. Meetings had been held with Buddhist, Hindu, Christian, and Muslim leaders in both Sri Lanka and Thailand to continue efforts toward a ceasefire and a lasting peace. Despite the influence of these spiritual leaders, however, the conflict ultimately ended through the use of force, an unfortunate outcome.

Vavuniya in northern Sri Lanka has the Menik Farm Internally Displaced Persons Camp, one of the largest refugee camps in the country, where about 80,000 people still live. Ordinarily, outsiders were not permitted to enter the camp, but I knew from experience that accompanying a monk in a situation like this would work well. So I did so, and was able to enter the camp. Vinyl tents lined a vast expanse of land that had been carved out of the jungle, with whole families living inside each tent. Much of the land in the north remained riddled with landmines, and the residents had no option but to live here until it had been cleared and certified as safe. Temperatures reached more than 40 degrees C, and the heat inside the tents was unimaginable. However, international organizations and the government were clearly managing the area well, and so far, there had been no outbreaks of infectious diseases. There was a small school, a temple, a post office, and a bank, and all seemed to be running as it should be. International organizations were strongly urging that refugees return to their villages as soon as possible, but the government was prioritizing safety by ensuring that landmines were cleared in the areas where the refugees were returning. There was intransigency on both sides, but it seemed to me that the government probably had a better idea of what was going on and had the right intentions.

On the last day, I visited the Sri Lankan School of Prosthetics and Orthotics in Ragama, about 20 kilometers north of Colombo. The school was built in 2003 with the support of the Nippon Foundation to train orthotists, who create artificial limbs, for Tamil and Sinhalese soldiers injured in the conflict and people who have lost limbs in accidents, and aims to educate young Tamil and Sinhalese, who are on opposing sides in the conflict, in the same premises, conveying a message of peace and reconciliation between the two ethnic groups. The running of the school was shared between the Cambodia Trust, a British NGO, the Sri Lankan Ministry of Health, and the Nippon Foundation. In the beginning, it had nothing but a container to use as an office and instructor's room, and the heat inside it was searing—enough to make you faint. However, on my visit this time, there were proper school buildings and equipment, and twenty-three trainees. The Sinhalese and Tamils mostly live in separate regions of the country, and most of the students here would have never spoken to people in the other ethnic group until they entered this school. Principal Mike Scott commented: "The students come from areas where many people have lost limbs to landmines. It's like a microcosm of a war zone." In addition to this school in Sri Lanka, the Nippon Foundation has built prosthetist training schools in Cambodia and Thailand, with plans to build more schools in Indonesia, the Philippines, and Myanmar. I was told that in Cambodia, a Nepali woman who has recovered from leprosy was studying there and scheduled to graduate in the coming fall.

Very young patients in a small country yet to eliminate leprosy—Democratic Republic of Timor-Leste, May 2010

> Route: Narita International Airport → Dubai, United Arab Emirates (flight time: 12h; 3h stopover) → Amman, Jordan (flight time: 3h)—two nights (WANA Forum)—Amman → Doha, Qatar (flight time: 3h 30m; 6h 30m stopover) → Denpasar, Indonesia (flight time: 12h; overnight stopover) → Dili, Timor-Leste (flight time: 1h 50m)—two nights—Dili → Denpasar (flight time: 1h 50m; 9h stopover) → Narita (flight time: 7h)

In May 2010, I also made my third visit to Timor-Leste, landing in the capital Dili after trips first to Jordan and Indonesia. Timor-Leste was one of two countries in the world that had yet to eliminate the disease as a public health problem, the other being Brazil. Nepal, it will be remembered, had eliminated leprosy at the start of this year. In 2009, the prevalence rate of leprosy in Timor-Leste had fallen to 1.52 per 10,000 population, and thanks to efforts made by all concerned parties, it was expected that the elimination target would be reached before the end of 2010. The problem was the very high prevalence rate (6.39 per 10,000 population) in the Oecusse municipality, a coastal exclave of Timor-Leste within Indonesia with a population of around 60,000. On the last day of my trip, I flew by UN helicopter to this municipality, a fifty-minute trip just to get there, but since my visit was limited to about two hours, I managed to look round just one rehabilitation center. There, I met ten individuals affected by leprosy who were undergoing rehabilitation treatment. Most were elderly, but one was a twelve- or thirteen-year-old girl who had a severe disability in one leg due to the aftereffects of leprosy. In all my years of traveling the world, this was the first time I had seen such a severe disability in somebody so young. The villagers told me that in the Oecusse municipality, it sometimes happened that infants aged between three and five years old developed the disease, and they were at a loss as to how to handle these cases. They were hesitant to administer MDT, fearing it was too strong. MDT has regimens suitable for adults and for juveniles, with the latter suitable for children from around ten to fourteen years old. But what to do for children aged three to five?

When I learned about this, I felt it had been worth borrowing a UN helicopter to get to this site because it had allowed me to get a clear picture of the situation. If it really was the case that leprosy affected so many small children in this region, this was highly unusual, a most serious state of affairs; we had to immediately consider treatment methods and countermeasures. I contacted the WHO representative and requested that experts be dispatched to the Oecusse area as soon as possible to confirm the facts. The world is a huge place. This trip reminded me of the importance of in-person visits.

ALERT's achievements—Federal Democratic Republic of Ethiopia, July 2010

Route: Narita International Airport → Dubai, United Arab Emirates (flight time: 10h 50m; 5h stopover) → Addis Ababa (flight time: 4h)— six nights

In July 2010, I visited Ethiopia for the first time in four years, going via Dubai and landing in Addis Ababa. The day after arriving, I met with the WHO Regional Office representative Dr. Fatoumata Nafo-Traoré to hear the latest updates on the country. Born in the West

African nation of Mali, Dr. Nafo-Traoré had been on vacation in her home country. However, once she learned about my visit to Ethiopia, she interrupted her holiday to return to Addis Ababa. Concerningly, she told me that the annual number of new patients, about 4,000, had remained constant for more than ten years and that the severe disability rate among new patients was high, at 7 percent. Nearly 75 percent of the population lived in rural areas, which made detecting and treating patients challenging. Two health workers with one year of training had been assigned to each village to manage people's health, including people affected by leprosy. However, HIV/AIDS and tuberculosis were also significant social problems, and there was some concern that leprosy would not get much attention.

I immediately decided to pay a visit to Health Minister Tedros Adhano, accompanied by representatives from the Ethiopian National Association of Persons Affected by Leprosy (ENAPAL), and urged him to give sufficient attention to leprosy, which tends to be overlooked in favor of AIDS and tuberculosis.

Next, I visited the All Africa Leprosy, Tuberculosis and Rehabilitation Training Centre (ALERT) just outside Addis Ababa. ALERT was established in 1965 as an institution specializing in leprosy diagnosis, treatment, surgery, ophthalmology, and rehabilitation, built initially as a mission-sponsored leprosarium to shelter people affected by leprosy who had been subject to discrimination. It is jointly administered by the Ethiopian government, Addis Ababa University, and the International Federation of Anti-Leprosy Associations (ILEP). ALERT plays a leading role as a training institution for professionals in Ethiopia and English-speaking African nations. Today, its hospital and training department is overseen by the Ethiopian government, and it operates as a national hospital specializing in leprosy and general diseases (especially skin diseases). Half of the 300 outpatients who come to it daily and half of its 200 inpatients were people affected by leprosy with disabilities.

Near the training center was a colony that had sprung up spontaneously when people affected by leprosy who had come from all over the country seeking treatment ended up staying. Today, this community has grown to around 5,000 people, and it included people affected by leprosy and their families, as well as other residents who were not affected by leprosy at all. The community even has two elementary schools. In this colony—the largest in the world as far as I know—ENAPAL had started a number of income-generating projects aimed at helping people affected by leprosy become financially independent, with seemingly steady growth in projects that include weaving, embroidery, and oil-pressing. I spoke with a Ms. Mayagist, a woman who had once had leprosy but was now completely cured, who told me with a smile as she looked at the cow reposing in the next room: "I raised five children (two of them adopted) and now have grandchildren. I never quarrel with my husband, and I thank God daily." Her smile seemed even more precious when I imagined the difficulties she must have experienced in her life.

After this leg of my trip, I had some time to spare, so I headed to southern Ethiopia to meet the Mursi and Hamar peoples. I joined them in their jumping dance, with my shirt stripped off. I had in fact planned to visit one of the naked tribes who live deep in the interior, but I was told that that would be extremely hazardous because they drank homemade alcohol and randomly fired guns in the afternoon, so I had to abandon that idea.

Behind a colony relocation plan—Republic of Chad, July 2010

Route: Addis Ababa, Ethiopia → N'Djamena, Chad (flight time: 3h 45m)—three nights—Chad → Paris, France (flight time: 5h 45m; 7h stopover) → Narita International Airport (flight time: 11h 40m)

After Ethiopia, I made my first-ever visit to Chad, a Central African, landlocked nation. The country's northern half is an arid zone within the Sahara Desert. Conversely, the southern part is a fertile savanna region with relatively high rainfall. Chad gained independence from France in 1960, but its political situation is unstable, with conflicts between Muslim factions in the north and Christian factions in the south. Further disputes among the Muslim factions have also emerged since the 1980s. Chad is widely thought of as one of the most corrupt countries in the world, and foreign investment has been slow, also making it one of the world's poorest countries.

Chad eliminated leprosy as a public health problem in 1997, but in some parts of the country, especially in the eastern regions, prevalence remains high. The rate of severe disability among newly recorded patients is also high, and many new cases are children. There are various reasons for this, including inadequate organization and resources at the Ministry of Health, few medical facilities that can correctly diagnose leprosy, inaccurate patient data collection and communication, and frequent program director changes, which often results in inadequate patient monitoring and treatment interruptions. I had also received reports of human, financial, and material resource shortages, so I decided it was necessary to elicit a commitment from the government, which led to this visit to Chad.

On the afternoon of 18 July, I was met at the airport in the capital city of N'Djamena by Health Minister Dr. Toupta Boguena, WHO country representative Dr. Saidou P. Barry, and WHO Regional Office for Africa's regional advisor Dr. Bide. The weather was a bit drizzly, and when I apologized for bringing rain with me, they all smiled back at me, saying that those who come with the rain are thought to bring good luck.

The next day, paying a call on the health minister, I asked her to focus on fighting leprosy and spreading our three messages—that leprosy is a curable disease, that medicine is available free of charge worldwide, and that discrimination against leprosy is unacceptable. She told me she had a personal interest in leprosy: her own uncle had had the condition. Even so, with his family's help, she said, he'd led a prosperous life in the community without being isolated and ended up living to an old age. Whether this interest would actually impact policy, I couldn't tell. We would have to keep an eye on the situation.

I next went to a meeting with Assaid Gamar Sileck, the vice president of the National Assembly, who assured me he would take up the issue of leprosy in a National Assembly committee and that he would consider drafting and submitting a related bill if necessary. I also met with some members of the National Assembly and asked if they would promote correct information about leprosy among their local constituencies. In a country where the literacy rate is less than 50 percent, and television is almost nonexistent, dissemination of information necessarily depends on radio and word of mouth. I also met with Prime Minister Emmanuel Nadingar, who was busy preparing for a regional summit. He promised to take the necessary steps to ensure that Chad's future development would include both medical and social measures to combat leprosy. No doubt polite diplomatic language.

In a briefing at the health ministry, Dr. Moussa Djibrine Mihimit, the health ministry's coordinator for leprosy, explained that Chad had launched its leprosy elimination program in 1992 with the aim of eliminating the disease by 2000. At the time, there were 8,582 new patients annually, with a 14.4 per 10,000 population prevalence rate. But the country had managed to reach the target well ahead of schedule, reducing this figure to 0.96 per 10,000 population in 1997. Nevertheless, in the east and south of the country, there were still four regions where the prevalence rate remained high (1–2.75 per 10,000 population), and the rate of severe disability among new patients was unusually high at about 17 percent. There was a high proportion of children among the new cases, about 9 percent. The challenges cited included political instability in some areas, disease tracking among nomadic populations, and a lack of resources (human, material, and financial). Dr. Bide, the WHO's leprosy point man, who was present at the meeting, said that he thought entirely new initiatives were necessary to solve these problems in Chad, and work should begin immediately on specific measures.

On 20 July, my team and I boarded a UN plane early in the morning to visit more rural areas. Looking at the capital city of N'Djamena from above, I noticed that most buildings had just one story. In all the other African capitals I had visited, many buildings were at least ten stories high. This was just one feature that spoke of the reality of the conditions in this capital city, showing why Chad is ranked the fifth poorest country in the world according to the UN Development Programme.

Our plane arrived in Abéché, in the eastern Ouaddaï region, about 700 kilometers from N'Djamena. Chad's eastern border had seen an influx of more than 300,000 refugees from the Darfur conflict in neighboring Sudan, including large numbers of people affected by leprosy. Some of the patients pouring into Chad from Sudan were coming for treatment due to insufficient medical facilities back home. Ouaddaï is a region where prejudice and discrimination against leprosy remain entrenched, and the prevalence rate is very high at 2.73 per 10,000 population.

In Abéché, I paid a courtesy call on the governor before proceeding on to a local hospital. On the grounds of the hospital was a colony where people affected by leprosy and their families, 436 people in all, had taken up residence, their little huts with thatched conical roofs jostling for space. I was told there were plans to move this colony to a site 7 kilometers away. The colony's children had started to exhibit antisocial behavior with children from other areas whom they were bringing inside the colony, the governor told me in his explanation for the proposed relocation. Admittedly, the area chosen for the relocation had no water, he added, but the UN had plans for a well to be drilled, and the idea was to build a health center and elementary school at the new site. A local health official added that people affected by leprosy who had taken up residence on the hospital grounds were hindering proper patient care. I then heard a representative of the colony mention in his speech that the new location was far from the market, but the residents would agree to move so long as there was proper housing and water. I decided I had to visit the planned relocation site, which I discovered was in the middle of nowhere, far from the city, with vast grassy plains lying all around. A mere nine small brick houses, intended for the people who were to be relocated, were standing here and there. The original plan had been to build 116 houses, but construction had been abandoned due to rising costs. Claims that the area was completely arid—and that even if wells were dug, it would be no use—reached my ears. I could only conclude that the area chosen for the new site was totally unsuitable for its intended purpose and that it had been chosen for the purpose of segregating its residents. Clearly, there was some ulterior motive to this relocation idea. We frequently see forced relocations of colonies of people affected by leprosy—all over the world. There is no end to the number of cases of people affected by leprosy being forced to move without any respect being paid to their wishes and vested rights, whether the reasons are to do with land ownership, relations with local residents, or schemes for redevelopment.

The following morning, back in N'Djamena, I visited the parish of Habbena. About thirty years before, a health center specializing in leprosy had been set up here, and people affected by leprosy had settled in the area and formed a colony. Habbena means "abandoned land," but, I was told, as the community became increasingly mixed, the place name came to be pronounced differently, so that it meant "we love them." Currently, its population comprised 980 or so people—eighty-nine people affected by leprosy with disabilities together with their family members. The specialized leprosy health center is now a general health center, and they welcomed my arrival with a grand show of singing and dancing. The district had an elementary school with 2,000 pupils, with children of families affected by leprosy studying alongside children of families unaffected by the disease.

After Habbena, my next stop was Centre d'Appareillage et de Rééducation de Kabalaye (CARK), also in N'Djamena. This is a facility run by a Catholic NGO that manufactures assistive devices (artificial limbs, crutches, wheelchairs, shoes, and more) for people affected by leprosy and victims of war, traffic accidents, or industrial accidents, and also provides rehabilitation services. CARK works in partnership with the government's national leprosy program. The devices were extremely well made, not inferior in any way to ones I'd seen elsewhere, and the facility gave me a sense of hope.

In the afternoon, I headed to Koundoul, around 20 kilometers south of N'Djamena. Here, a local leprosy support NGO called the Association de Solidarité Avec les Lépreux du Tchad was running a project helping people who have recovered from leprosy become economically self-reliant, with financial support from the Fondation Raoul Follereau. People living in the Habbena district, where I had been that very morning, got the bus here every day to farm and raise sheep on about 20 hectares of land. The person showing me round explained that they consumed nearly everything they produced and sold the rest to generate cash income. I noticed many of the people working on the land had disabilities: the ideal would be to work where they lived. It seemed ridiculous in Africa to have to commute by bus to the fields, but I supposed there had to have been some appropriate reason for choosing this location.

The period of my visit coincided with a summit that Chad was hosting for the Community of Sahel–Saharan States, and Colonel Muammar Gaddafi of Libya was staying in a tent he had pitched on the grounds of the same hotel I was staying in. The hotel lobby was adorned with a huge photo of Gaddafi, and people were carrying

Gaddafi posters and paper Libyan flags—there was quite a bit of pageantry. The hotel manager explained to me that Gaddafi was considered a hero and a great leader in Chad. However, a year later, he was assassinated. I am no supporter of Gaddafi, but it is undeniable that since his death, the political situation in sub-Saharan Africa has become more unstable, with the emergence of all sorts of rebel militia and guerrillas.

Not to get off topic, but I sometimes see people in Africa with a gap between their front teeth. I once suggested to someone in the Sasakawa Africa Association who hailed from Burkina Faso that he should see a dentist to have his gap fixed, and he laughed at me. People with a gap in their front teeth are fortunate, he told me. When people bury their dead in his country, they first give the deceased a drink of water before putting them in the ground. Some people even have their teeth pulled, or the gap widened, in order to make it easier to get the water into their mouths.

The guilt of South Sumatra's governor—Republic of Indonesia, August–September 2010

Route: Narita International Airport → Jakarta, Indonesia (flight time: 7h 45m)—two nights—Jakarta → Palembang, Indonesia (flight time: 1h)—Palembang → Jakarta (flight time: 1h; 7h stopover) → Narita (flight time: 7h 30m)

Indonesia was still reporting a constant 17,000 to 18,000 newly recorded leprosy cases per year, with persistent prejudice and discrimination. There were sixty-nine leprosy colonies throughout the country. The first national organization for people affected by leprosy in Indonesia, Perhimpunan Mandiri Kusta (PerMaTa; meaning Leprosy Independence Association), was established in 2007. It had since made great strides in bringing the voices of people affected by leprosy to society and the government, mitigating the persistent prejudice and discrimination against people affected by leprosy, and working to restore dignity to those affected and their families. However, it was going to take much more time to build a substantial network in this nation, which, after all, consisted of thirty-four provinces (now thirty-seven) and more than 13,000 islands. Each island has dramatically different environments and living conditions, and many islands and regions are difficult to access. Efforts were going to have to be tailored to fit the requirements of each and every locality in detecting patients, delivering medicines, and providing effective support to people who had been treated. The difficulties in meeting all these local conditions had given rise to various self-help organizations and local associations of people who had been affected by leprosy in the past. I hoped that they would link up with PerMaTa and gain more strength.

On 30 August 2010, the annual meeting of the National Alliance for Leprosy Elimination and Yaws Eradication was held at the Hotel Cempaka in Jakarta. Before the meeting, Indonesia's minister of health, Dr. Endang Rahayu Sedyaningsih, expressed concern about the leprosy situation in Indonesia, especially the high number of new cases and the high rate of disability due to delayed detection and treatment. However, about any specific measures against leprosy, which was what I was waiting to hear, he said not a thing. For my part, I stressed that prejudice against people affected by and recovering from leprosy persists, and that in the future we must also put efforts into work restoring the human rights of everyone in any way affected by leprosy. The alliance meeting would also provide an opportunity to work out Indonesia's national action plan based on the WHO's Global Strategy for Leprosy, which was due to come into effect in January next year. We were planning to have efforts to eliminate discrimination against people affected by leprosy and their families included in the activities named by the project. The meeting's attendees included Health Minister Sedyaningsih, WHO Indonesia representative Dr. Khanchit Limpakarnjanarat, the West Java governor, medical officers from all of Indonesia's provinces, people affected by leprosy, members of the Human Rights Commission, and officials from the Ministry of Welfare. The discussion focused on the roles of central and local governments in formulating the national plan. Some of the officials said quite plainly that Indonesia, a multi-island nation, had undergone a decentralization process. As a result, even if the central government's Ministry of Health drafted a leprosy elimination plan and allocated a budget to each province, the power of local governors was such that budget money was often diverted from its original purpose. I realized I was going to have to pay regular visits to each and every province rather than simply visiting the central government, speaking directly to the governors and requesting their cooperation.

The next day, I took an early morning flight from Jakarta to Palembang, South Sumatra, which took an hour, and then traveled overland for two hours to visit the Sungai Kundur Leprosy Hospital. Health Minister Sedyaningsih joined me. The hospital was established in 1918 and currently had 450 beds, mainly for the diagnosis and treatment of leprosy, as well as for vocational training and social rehabilitation to improve the lives of patients. Only three hospitals in Indonesia provide such social rehabilitation services, including Sungai Kundur Leprosy Hospital. They accept people affected by and recovering from leprosy not only from Sumatra but also from the Kalimantan provinces. In the final stage of the process, people affected by leprosy are provided with a special facility designed to help them reintegrate into society, where they spend two weeks learning how to regain their lost self-esteem and interact with others.

After receiving a briefing on the hospital, I spoke with some of the people there. Many had completed their treatment and were engaged in rehabilitation and vocational training. They were enthusiastic about various exercises, including sewing with a sewing machine, training their fingers with various equipment, and playing musical instruments. While rubbing with my bare hand the foot of a middle-aged woman who had developed an ulcer in the ward, I spoke with reporters, imploring them to tell the public that leprosy is a disease that can be cured with medication and is not transmitted by touch.

Sungai Kundur Leprosy Hospital is hygienic and well equipped— one of the most well-equipped leprosy hospitals I had visited. However, it had only around sixty inpatients and ten to twenty outpatients, and most of its rooms and beds were unfilled. I admonished the hospital, declaring: "We now live in an era in which we have to actively seek out hidden and undiagnosed cases of leprosy. They're not going to come to us, you know, no matter how long we sit here and wait." I urged them to think of strategies for active case-finding.

The Sungai Kundur settlement adjacent to the hospital was established in 1914 and is currently home to about 2,000 people. One woman showed us around her house. It was spacious with four rooms and furnished with a bed, a TV, and a refrigerator. The other houses were about the same size as hers, judging from their exteriors. I got the impression that this settlement was not only materially blessed but also that the people were rich in spirit. During a discussion with the settlement residents, the people recovered from leprosy raised quite a few issues, including their worries about the lack of any assurance about their future—they were renting land from the government with no guaranteed rights—and Minister Sedyaningsih listened attentively. I explained that the UN Human Rights Council had passed a resolution on eliminating discrimination and was currently considering a draft resolution on a set of Principles and Guidelines, which, if passed, would definitely help improve the lives of people affected by and recovering from leprosy. I encouraged them not to lose heart and keep speaking up because this would help them find solutions to their problems.

In South Sumatra, I met with the province governor, Alex Noerdin. Governors had increased their authority dramatically in Indonesia with the spread of decentralization. That meant that the governor had the authority to prioritize health issues in the province. Since I knew that leprosy was not a high priority in South Sumatra, I asked Governor Noerdin to secure a budget to pay for education and awareness-raising to ensure that the province's population was correctly informed about leprosy. To which the governor replied that he was shocked to learn that leprosy was still such a significant problem in Sumatra. He could not help but feel personally responsible, he said, adding that he would take it upon himself to work to improve the situation by bringing the leprosy hospital in Palembang up to international standards and by focusing on the diagnosis, early detection, and early treatment. I suggested that one idea for early leprosy detection might be to have elementary school students check their mothers for the presence of leprotic patches as homework. The governor replied: "Schools can and should take a part in health management. Let my name be the first on the list when they check the fathers!" After my meeting with the governor, I spoke with a crowd of reporters waiting at the entrance of the state office building. I made it clear that the governor had promised to focus his efforts on leprosy.

THE SOCIAL ASPECTS OF THE DISEASE

The Leprosy Museum and Armauer Hansen—Kingdom of Norway, September 2010

Route: Narita International Airport → Paris, France (flight time: 12h 25m; 3h stopover) → Stockholm, Sweden (flight time: 2h 30m)—three nights (attended the Hiroshima Atomic Bomb Exhibition and the Scandinavia–Japan Sasakawa Foundation board meeting)—Stockholm → Oslo, Norway (flight time: 55m; 2h 30m stopover) → Bergen, Norway (flight time: 50m)—two nights—Bergen → Oslo (flight time: 50m)—one night—Oslo → Paris (flight time: 50m; 4h stopover) → Narita (flight time: 11h 25m)

Leprosy is thought to have first arrived in Norway around 1000 CE, having come from Ireland. From around the beginning of the sixteenth century, the number of people affected by leprosy in the various countries and regions in Europe declined dramatically. Strangely, however, in the early nineteenth century cases began to rise in Norway, particularly in areas along the west coast. The people affected were mostly farmers and fishermen living in dismal conditions in impoverished coastal communities. Bergen, Norway's second-largest city, was the first in the world to begin to keep a register of leprosy patients, which it did in 1856. This city was also where Dr. Gerhard Henrik Armauer Hansen discovered *Mycobacterium leprae*—the bacillus that causes the disease—in 1873. Thanks to this discovery, leprosy was shown to be neither a divine punishment nor a genetically passed-on condition but an infectious disease. It is this discovery that lies behind the other name by which leprosy is known, Hansen's disease.

In mid-September 2010, I visited Bergen's Leprosy Museum. Operated by the municipal government, the museum was established in 1970. It is housed in one of the buildings of what was formerly St. Jørgen's Hospital, the city's oldest leprosy hospital. Founded in around 1411, it had operated as a fully functioning hospital right up until 1946, when the last two patients living there died. At one time, in the 1600s, it had become a general hospital due to the decreased numbers of people affected by leprosy, but then in 1820, with the resurgence of numbers, it returned to being a specialized leprosy hospital, and at its busiest, in the 1840s, it had 179 patients. The hospital buildings were twice destroyed by fire, in 1640 and 1702.

Nine buildings were rebuilt in 1754, and the site is now registered for protection as a national cultural heritage building.

Two buildings are open to the public: the main building, where most of the patients lived after 1754, and the hospital church, the oldest building, built in 1707. The church, which has a beautiful painting above the altar of Jesus Christ blessing leprosy patients, has been open to the general public since it was built. For their part, up until 1891, patients were free to go into town to sell vegetables from the hospital's small farm and go shopping. Even after that, their livelihood continued to be guaranteed under government protection, and not one person had to beg.

At the museum, I was greeted at the main building's entrance by Grete Eilertsen, the only resident curator, and Sigurd Sandmo, the former director. It was Ms. Eilertsen's task to watch over the museum's materials, guide visitors, and teach at the school—which she did all by herself. The museum is a small facility, but in 2003, on the 400th anniversary of the public health system's establishment, the Norwegian government provided the museum with a fund for exhibitions and expansion. At the time, the museum was planning a new exhibition amid much talk about its significance in today's Norway. The basic idea was to make the museum a place where people could trace leprosy down through the ages rather than just focusing on the disease as a public health issue. "Rediscovering our forgotten history" is a byword of this museum, and it did seem as if many Norwegians were rediscovering Norway's history here. The interior of the museum was renovated to meet modern standards, with the atmosphere of ages past beautifully preserved, making it somehow more than just a museum and more of a building that paid homage to its patients and preserved the memory of their struggle. Today, information about the museum is included in textbooks and incorporated into school curricula. Around 3,000 schoolchildren visit the museum each year.

The museum is the oldest existing leprosy facility in Europe. Immaculately maintained, it looks just as it would have done in 1946 when the last patient died and the doors were closed. Until the mid-nineteenth century, it was the largest hospital in Western Norway. The inpatients all had to cook for themselves, and the kitchen still had over

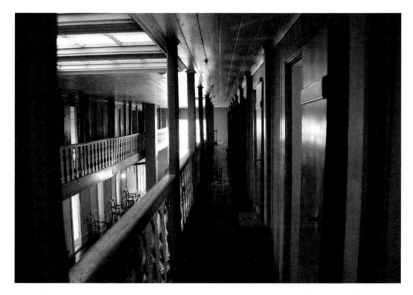

85. The interior of the leprosy hospital built in 1754 (Bergen, Norway, September 2010)

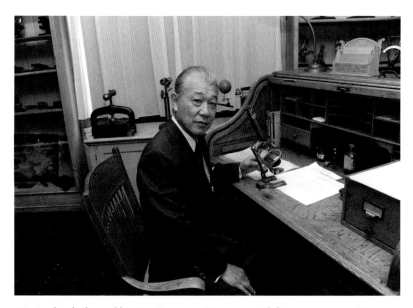

86. At the desk used by Dr. Armauer Hansen, with his microscope (Bergen, Norway, September 2010)

seventy or so pots and pans that they used: I could well imagine how busy mealtimes must have been. Numbered cupboards lined the walls, evidently with one to two patients to each one. I could still see the places worn down from use by patients' hands on those cupboard doors. "Were the patients referred to by their number?" I inquired. The answer came that no, they were all called by their individual names.

One room was decorated just as it was in the 1800s, with a report from 1816 written by a priest called Wellhoven on display. It contained information about hospitalized patients, including their names and photographs. It is considered the oldest preserved personal information on people affected by leprosy.

In another room, there was an exhibit about the work of two doctors, Daniel Cornelius Danielssen and Carl Wilhelm Boeck. These two men began their research in 1839 and published the first modern medical paper on leprosy in 1847, a breakthrough in leprosy research. Dr. Danielssen had argued that leprosy was a hereditary disease since many hospital patients were connected by birth. He used the terms "leprosy farm" and "leprosy family" to explain his ideas. It was Dr. Danielssen's son-in-law, Dr. Hansen, who then discovered the leprosy bacterium in 1873. Apparently, he had always said, right from the beginning, that he disagreed with his father-in-law's hypothesis.

One very important aspect of Norwegian leprosy history is the patient registration system—the Leprosy Registry, introduced in 1856. For this national register, doctors were required to register every case of leprosy, and regional hospitals had to forward all the information they recorded to an official in the central government, with everything managed centrally. In the Bergen museum, a panel displayed the names of 8,231 people affected by the disease. I couldn't help feeling that some present-day people might not appreciate their family names being included in such a display, but Ms. Eilertsen informed me that nobody minded in Norway. Americans see it as a tragedy, Africans are surprised that we have so many records preserved, while Asians are always astonished that we publicize the real names of patients, she told me.

The hospital's patient records fall outside personal data protection laws and are freely accessible to anyone who wants to see them. Quite a few descendants of patients, she told me, who previously didn't want to disclose the history of leprosy in their family, now request information. In responding to these requests for information from family members, the hospital saw its role as helping people identify lost relatives and accept them back into their family history.

Another place I visited was the Regional State Archives in Bergen, part of the Norwegian National Archives. It is here that the original documents from the National Leprosy Registry, introduced by royal decree in 1856, are housed. This was the first national disease-specific patient registry anywhere in the world. In 1856, it was found that 3.5 percent of 2,500 people living in a village in north Bergen were affected by leprosy (a prevalence rate of 350 per 10,000 population). These and similar kinds of data considerably advanced the epidemiological study of leprosy. The registry has been included in UNESCO's Memory of the World project. There were other interesting documents, including a record of a 1923 correspondence with a Japanese medical doctor. There is also a record of an international leprosy conference held in Bergen in 1909, with evidence showing Japanese experts participated, including Dr. Shibasaburo Kitasato, who discovered the plague bacillus and developed a cure for tetanus.

Hansen had his laboratory in Pleiestiftelsen No. 1 (the Nursing Institution for Leprosy Patients No. 1)—one of the leprosy hospitals established in the center of Bergen in the mid-nineteenth century. Today, it houses the University of Bergen's Department of Global Public Health and Primary Care. In Dr. Hansen's laboratory, I was able to look through the very same microscope Hansen used when he identified the leprosy bacillus for the first time. There, I met Dr. Lorentz M. Irgens—a professor at the University of Bergen and the director of the Medical Birth Registry of Norway—who is also a leprosy researcher and delivered a very interesting paper at an international conference on the epidemiology of leprosy held in Geilo, Norway, in 1981, which I attended with my father, the late Ryoichi Sasakawa. The professor cited malnutrition, poverty, and the effects of the use of peat moss unique to Norway's coastal areas as possible causes of Norway's leprosy epidemic and concluded that the sharp decline in the number of cases in the 1900s was due to improved material wealth and nutritional conditions.

I asked Dr. Irgens whether the fact that the disease has disappeared in the Global North while so many new cases are still seen in the warmer Global South was due to some difference in the leprosy bacillus itself. The professor replied: "There is still much to be done by way of analysis on the bacillus, including from the perspective of genetic research." He drew my attention to the possibility of emerging resistance to the MDT regimen. "It is something that is probably inevitable. So it's essential that we continue to advance our knowledge of the disease."

The last person affected by leprosy at Pleiestiftelsen No. 1 died in 1973. When the last of three elderly people in the same family who had been discovered in the 1950s to have leprosy died in 2002, there were precisely zero cases in the entire nation of Norway.

The Ba Sao shower room—Socialist Republic of Vietnam, October 2010

Route: Narita International Airport → Hanoi, Vietnam (flight time: 5h 40m)—three nights—Hanoi → Narita (flight time: 4h 50m)

During a visit to Vietnam at the end of October 2010, I took the opportunity to go to the Ba Sao Leprosy Treatment Center in Hà Nam province, 100 kilometers south of the capital Hanoi. A mere step out of the bustling, feverish streets of the city takes the traveler into a peaceful countryside landscape that must have changed little over the centuries. I took great delight in the two-hour drive along rural roads to the Ba Sao Leprosy Treatment Center, which though pleasant, involved numerous bumps of my head against the ceiling of the bouncy car.

The treatment center was home to about fifty people who were receiving treatment for leprosy, ranging in age from their fifties to their nineties. Just beyond it was a hamlet where about thirty of their family members lived. In a spacious room within the treatment ward, which had about six beds, sat a woman, Ms. Dao, who had artificial legs. She was sixty-one years old and had lived there for more than thirty years. Although her illness was completely cured, she was still here because of other chronic ailments. Now that her husband had died, she had no other family.

As I toured the center, I saw a white building with a newly constructed shower room. It had apparently been built the previous August with the help of Waseda University graduates from the leprosy support student NGO Qiao (meaning "bridge" in Chinese), at the university's Volunteer Center, along with a Vietnamese NGO called Hanoi Blue Dreams Volunteer Group, which aims to improve the lives of people with disabilities. The room had a mirror, a sink, and a railing—all extremely nice, and I couldn't believe that it hadn't been built by professional tradesmen. In one corridor, I met seventy-five-year-old Ms. Dai. Putting my hand on her shoulder, I asked how she was doing, to which she smiled and replied: "I have chronic problems and some ricketiness here and there, but I'm doing well." She said she could not use the shower room because of her prosthetic leg, but she had really enjoyed the exchange with the students this summer. "They were so kind, worked hard, and made us this great shower. I hope to see them again," she said fondly.

As I walked to the hamlet behind the treatment building, I was greeted by a woman, Ms. Be, smiling at us from a house with mud walls and a tin roof. She was nearly eighty years old but had no particular disability, she told me, and only a slight pain in her back. When I teased her that she must have been popular with men in her youth because of her beauty, she laughed and said with a touch of pride, "I was pretty, yes, and all the men used to chase after me." An older woman drying corn kernels outside the facility told me, "We had a good harvest this year because of the excellent weather. We are going to use these as feed for our pigs." Then she added, raising her eyes to the heavens, her back bent with age: "But my husband is at the hospital getting treatment, so I have to do all the work myself."

Then I caught sight of an impressive brick house under construction, and Ms. Qvet, a seventy-year-old woman, emerged from the back of the house. She told us the house under construction belonged to her daughter and her family. Her daughter's husband, who was working on the construction, then emerged, and next to him was a little girl of about three years old, her hair cut short and with a fringe. All around me, I could see the grandchildren of the people affected by leprosy playing, and I couldn't hide how pleased this made me—to see how people, whose lives must be filled with hardship, had pulled themselves out of it and finally managed to find happiness.

It seemed to me that people affected by leprosy in Vietnam lived in a much more pleasant environment than those in the Indian and

African regions. All the facilities I saw were clean, and while many of the people were elderly and were clearly having to deal with the aftereffects of leprosy and other chronic ailments, they received treatment from full-time doctors, nurses, and other staff. I got the distinct impression that despite being poor, these people were all cooperating and helping each other. Every month, they received 270,000 dong (about US$11) from the government, and they were also provided with two meals a day. However, this was still not enough to survive financially, so many of them made ends meet by raising chickens, pigs, and cows.

Here, I would like to share an anecdote about a certain mishap on this trip. Finding ourselves with some time on our hands, my team and I decided to take a trip to Ha Long Bay, a World Heritage Site. We rented a boat to go around Ha Long Bay, which involved a visit to a limestone cave along the way. When the boat's owner advised us to leave our luggage behind because the cave was slippery, telling us he would take care of it, we decided to do as he suggested. We assumed it would be all right since the boat was chartered, so we took the tour of the cave, leaving our wallets and passports behind on the boat. After returning from the tour of the cave, I checked my bag, just to be sure, and found that my wallet and passport were safe. We then had lunch on the boat, but when it came time to pay the bill, Natsuko Tominaga, the Nippon Foundation's photographer, looked in her wallet and saw that it contained only $70 when she was sure she had $300. Deciding she was probably mistaken, she collected cash from the other group members, and the bill was paid. Soon after we returned to Japan, we discovered that Tatsuki Nakajima, an accompanying staff member, had ¥40,000 missing from his wallet and that Kanae Hirano, an interpreter, also had ¥10,000 and $100 missing.

The boat owner and his team had pulled off quite a smart trick, taking small amounts out of everyone's wallets and leaving just enough money so that we could pay for the boat and meals. The point of leaving a bit of money was to allow us to pay the bill and so prevent us from immediately suspecting some kind of foul play. At any rate, this was my first experience of having money taken from me in a foreign country.

THE SOCIAL ASPECTS OF THE DISEASE

About the South Pacific Islands

Under Prime Minister Yasuhiro Nakasone, Foreign Minister Tadashi Kuranari announced what became known as the "Kuranari Doctrine," which laid out the key principles of Japan's cooperation policy with the Pacific Island nations. I took it upon myself to then organize the Pacific Island Nations Conference in Tokyo in August 1988, under the auspices of the Sasakawa Peace Foundation. The conference was attended by all sorts of top-ranking dignitaries and politicians, including the crown prince of the Kingdom of Tonga and the prime ministers and presidents of the Republic of Fiji, the Republic of Kiribati, the Federated States of Micronesia, Papua New Guinea, Solomon Islands, Tuvalu, the Republic of Vanuatu, Western Samoa (now the Independent State of Samoa), and the Cook Islands. Australia, New Zealand, Indonesia, and regional organizations in the South Pacific participated as observers. In 1989, in line with a resolution announced at the conference, the Sasakawa Peace Foundation established the Pacific Island Nations Fund with a total endowment of ¥3 billion to conduct specific regional projects. It has continued its activities to this day (the Republic of Palau, Niue, the Republic of the Marshall Islands, French Polynesia, and New Caledonia have since been added to the list of countries eligible for the fund).

Incidentally, at the time, Japan's Ministry of Foreign Affairs (MOFA) still used the colonial-era name, Pacific Islands Division, European and Oceanian Affairs Bureau, for its work in the Pacific. I had emphasized the Pacific Island countries' importance for Japan and urged the Japanese government to host a summit-level meeting, which finally happened as the Pacific Islands Leaders Meeting under Prime Minister Keizo Obuchi. The meeting was then held in Japan every three years. Before long, the MOFA changed the bureau's original name to the Asian and Oceanian Affairs Bureau.

After the Pacific Island Nations Conference in August 1988, which had been sponsored by the Sasakawa Peace Foundation, we took all the participants to China. Never before had so many foreign dignitaries visited China at the same time. Mercedes-Benzes from all over Beijing were assembled in a convoy that stretched more than 1-kilometer long. The meeting with Premier Li Peng at the Great Hall of the People combined a fascinating mix of leaders of countries with populations of a mere 20,000 to 30,000 and the premier of a country with a population of 1.3 billion. The countries all had one vote at the UN, however, which only served to underline how important the Pacific Island nations were. I have long been involved in various efforts to support this region.

The WHO definition of leprosy-free countries does not include countries with populations of less than 1 million. Nevertheless, there are still some small countries in the Pacific and Africa with prevalence rates of more than one person per 10,000 people, including the Union of the Comoros, Republic of Kiribati, Marshall Islands, Federated States of Micronesia, Republic of Nauru, and Tuvalu. These countries have not received much attention from the rest of the world, and they still face issues of prejudice and discrimination. The high proportion of young people affected by leprosy in many countries is also a concern.

The WHO Western Pacific Regional Office has jurisdiction over the many Pacific Island nations in Oceania, such as the Republic of Kiribati, which has islands scattered over 3,000 kilometers, and the Federated States of Micronesia, which consists of 607 islands (sixty-five of which are inhabited and have a total population of around 100,000). They are all difficult to access, so while the Sasakawa Health Foundation has supported leprosy control in the Federated States of Micronesia through more than twenty projects since 1988, those efforts have often proved extremely challenging. As a joint project of the government, WHO, and the Sasakawa Health Foundation, we provided preventive oral medication for the entire population from 1996 to 1998, during which health checkups were conducted semi-annually. Those diagnosed with leprosy were also started on MDT, while others were given prophylactic oral medication consisting of three different drugs. The first round of testing identified 322 new cases (a prevalence rate of forty-two per 10,000 population), of whom 36 percent were under fifteen years of age. At the second examination, the number of new cases decreased to eighty (prevalence rate of ten per 10,000 population), but 39 percent were under fifteen. In 2015, there were 141 new cases (prevalence rate of thirteen per 10,000), 38 percent of whom were under fifteen. This result indicates practically no change in the state of leprosy over the past twenty years in the Federated States of Micronesia.

During a previous visit to the country, the president and I campaigned by taking the MDT drugs in front of the TV cameras, but it had no significant effect. Another visit was scheduled but had to be postponed due to the president's sudden absence. I planned to revisit the Federated States of Micronesia as soon as it became feasible.

Traces of the past on Raibyo-Shima—Republic of Palau, November 2010

> Route: Narita International Airport → Guam, United States (flight time: 3h 30m; 4h stopover) → Koror, Palau (flight time: 2h)—two nights (attended a ministerial conference on maritime affairs)— Koror → Guam (flight time: 2h; 1h 40m stopover) → Narita (flight time: 3h 35m)

Palau is a republic with a population of around 20,000, consisting of islands surrounded by coral reefs and beautiful seas. It gained independence in 1994 after periods of Spanish and German colonial rule and Japanese and American administrations. During the period of Japanese rule, the South Seas Government administered a region known as the South Seas Mandate. During the Second World War, many Japanese soldiers lost their lives in fierce battles with American forces on Peleliu Island. The president of Palau, Mr. Thomas Remengesau Jr., told me that a recent visit of Their Majesties the Emperor and Empress (now the Emperor and Empress Emeritus) of Japan to Palau and their visit to the cenotaph on Peleliu Island had greatly moved the Palauan people.

The Nippon Foundation had donated two boats to travel between the main island of Palau and Peleliu Island, and when a typhoon damaged them, a further two. It also donated a maritime patrol boat to prevent poaching and maritime crime in Palau's vast waters and was trying to train personnel for this project.

The Palauan language has more than 1,000 words that originated in the Japanese language, a remnant of the Japanese colonial period. For example, the Palauan words for toilet and baseball are "benjo" and "yakyū," which are the same as in Japanese.

MAKING THE IMPOSSIBLE POSSIBLE

The main purpose of my visit this time was to attend an international joint public–private conference to improve Micronesia's maritime security, but quite unexpectedly I ended up making a rather precious discovery to do with the history of leprosy in the region. Somebody I was talking to during the conference happened to mention to me that there was a place called Raibyo Shima not too far from where we were. "Raibyo Shima?" At first, I thought it was a place name in the Palauan language, but then it hit me that these were actually Japanese words—and they meant "leprosy island." (*Rai* is the old Japanese term for "leprosy.") Immediately, a series of questions came into my head demanding to be answered, including how did it get this Japanese name, what is the island's history, and what is it like now?

I had less than twenty-four hours left in the country. Making use of a spare moment during the international conference, I had made a quick visit to the Belau National Hospital, the main medical treatment center on the island, to meet people affected by leprosy. Palau had six registered leprosy cases, with two people registered in 2009 and four in 2010.

When I arrived at the hospital, the six patients and their families were gathered in a coconut-palm-roofed outdoor rest area. As I greeted them one by one, I noticed a woman among them who seemed rather young. She told me she was just seventeen years old, and her name was Shosti. Her mother had brought her to the hospital, she said, because she'd found she had no sensation on the skin of her feet. Six leprosy patients in a tiny country with a mere 20,000 population. And why was the disease making an appearance in somebody in their teens? Once again, it struck me how so much about the transmission of leprosy remains unknown to us, yet to be proven scientifically.

Palau has a well-run healthcare system, and all six patients had taken their medicine from an early stage, had no physical disabilities, and would be completely cured in a few months. Connie, a nurse, said that she and a TB officer would be visiting the patients' homes daily to follow up on their condition. There were also plentiful supplies of MDT coming in from the WHO. It was during my visit to this hospital that I first heard about the leprosy island. A relative of one of the patients I met, Ella, had apparently been quarantined there. It appeared that the Japanese had instituted the policy of segregation in Palau when they had governed the island. And this had brought about discrimination and stigma for those affected by the disease.

Keen to pay a visit, I traveled to Raibyo Shima by small motorboat. It was less than a mile (1.5 kilometers) from Koror Island, which is the main island of Koror state. It was surrounded by shallow water, making it impossible for the boat to get anywhere near the shore, so I jumped into the water in my shoes and waded the roughly 10 meters to land. Keeping my eyes peeled for anything relating to leprosy remaining on the island, I eventually came across some rotting wooden steps and cautiously proceeded to climb up. Had these steps once been used by people affected by leprosy? Pretty soon, the steps petered out, covered with overgrown vegetation, and I was walking through what seemed like a thick jungle. I wandered around though there was nothing like a path, searching for remains of anything at all that might be related to leprosy—but found not a clue. With time running out, I regretfully returned to the boat and had the helmsman circle the island before heading back to the international conference hall. Here, I was pleasantly surprised when Minister of Foreign Affairs (and former Minister of Health) Victor Yano, who knew that I was the WHO Goodwill Ambassador for the Elimination of Leprosy, brought me a valuable document relating to the island I had just been to—a paper called "A Report on Ngerur Island," based on investigations carried out by Dr. Jolie Liston of the International Archaeological Research Institute in 1998.

Liston's report explained that the volcanic island's official name was, in fact, Ngerur Island. It is 4 acres in area, 350 meters north to south, and 250 meters east to west, rising at its highest point to 30 meters above sea level. The name "Raibyo Shima" derived from the Japanese government having used this island to segregate people affected by leprosy during its administration in the 1930s. Leprosy isolation facilities, consisting of three Japanese-style houses and a well, were established here in 1931. Initially, there were eighteen patients receiving treatment. It wasn't clear from the report how long the island was used as a leprosy treatment center, but it did note that former President Ngiratkel Etpison's family renovated the buildings in 1950. Photographs taken in 1998 showed houses where patients once lived as well as some graves. Apparently, they were to be found on the other side of the island to the slight rise with the steps I'd attempted to climb. I sorely regretted not having seen Liston's report before my foray to the island.

My stay had been exceptionally busy, as I'd arrived at 10 p.m. on 10 November, started working first thing on 11 November, and had to leave for the airport at midnight that night. I hope very much that I will get the chance to go to Raibyo Shima again.

After returning to Japan, I learned of the existence of a Palauan man in his eighties who had lived in the leprosy facility on the island and now lived on Koror Island. From what I was told, he had been confined to the island when he was ten years old, lived in the facility for several years, and then moved to another island as the war intensified. Once a month, a doctor brought medicine, the staff brought rice and canned food, and he and the other islanders grew their own taro, tapioca, and sweet potatoes. I had encountered the "leprosy → isolation → island" formula in nearly all the countries I had visited. Still, I thought Raibyo Shima was the tiniest leprosy island of them all, perhaps even the tiniest in the world.

Jerejak Island and Sungai Buloh—Malaysia, November 2010

Route: Narita International Airport → Bangkok, Thailand (flight time: 7h; 4h stopover) → Penang, Malaysia (flight time: 1h 45m)—two nights (API workshop)—Penang → Kuala Lumpur, Malaysia (flight time: 55m)—two nights—Kuala Lumpur → Bangkok (flight time: 2h; 2h stopover (interview with Kavi Chongkittavorn, API Fellow)) → Phnom Penh, Cambodia (flight time: 1h)—three nights—Phnom Penh → Bangkok (flight time: 1h; 4h 30m stopover) → Narita (flight time: 5h 40m)

In November, I visited the Malaysian island of Penang, which has long flourished as a commercial center, to attend a conference for the Nippon Foundation Fellowships for Asian Public Intellectuals (API Fellowship). I started from Japan, and the route involved going via Bangkok.

Penang Island is small, 24 kilometers long and 15 kilometers wide, and lies to the west of the Malaysian peninsula, and just off its coast lies Pulau Jerejak (or the "Island of Jerejak"). It is said that Captain

Francis Light, an Englishman who first arrived in Penang in 1796, stepped ashore at Jerejak Island in 1786. A very small island with an area of only 362 hectares, it was a place used to isolate leprosy patients. As many Chinese and Indian migrant laborers arrived on Penang Island and the number of leprosy cases increased, the government established a leprosy center here for forced isolation in 1871 and expanded it in 1880. And it remained a leprosy center right up until it was closed in 1969. Jerejak Island also served as a quarantine station for immigrant workers from 1875, with a hospital built to treat tuberculosis. However, with the start of the 1969 leprosy control program, the government transferred all remaining leprosy patients to Sungai Buloh and closed the island-based leprosy facilities. The tuberculosis hospital and quarantine station were also closed at this time. Between 1969 and 1993, the island served as a prison, and Jerejak Island was dubbed the Alcatraz of Malaysia after the infamous prison in San Francisco. Today, the island is home to a tropical resort and attracts many tourists, but its important place in the history of leprosy in Malaysia is not widely known. My guide to the island, twenty-nine-year-old Faisal Omar, who was born and raised on Penang, said he was taught nothing of this aspect of the island's history when he was at school. He had first learned about its leprosy connection when he had guided an Indian visitor to the island who told him he had once worked as a doctor at a sanatorium on Jerejak.

In 1933, Fumio Hayashi, a medical officer at Nagashima Aiseien Sanatorium, visited Jerejak and recorded his visit in his 1942 book, *Sekai Rai Ryokōki* (A journal of visiting the world's leprosy facilities). When he visited, there were apparently 765 people affected by leprosy; among them were 601 Chinese and 128 Indians. The book notes that there were 1,200 people affected by leprosy in Sungai Buloh at that time, 80 percent of them Chinese. There was a quarantine station with capacity for 4,000 people, which occupied half of the island. The other half was a leprosarium. This leprosarium was divided into different sections based on factors such as race and degree of disease severity. The only form of treatment was chaulmoogra oil, which was orally ingested, and there were large chaulmoogra trees growing on the premises.

Before the conference began, I hired a small boat and went to Jerejak Island. It is only about ten minutes away from Penang's harbor. The hospital is located on the back side of the island, out of sight of Penang. Along the grassy shoreline are only the ruins of the quay used for patient transport, a dilapidated leprosy hospital office building, and a guard's hut; no trace remained of any other old buildings. In the past, there was apparently a patients' wing, a shared kitchen used by people affected by leprosy, and residences for hospital staff. However, all traces of these buildings have been obliterated, and even the people of Penang do not know the details. In short, nothing remained of the island's leprosy past.

During my stay, I also visited the Sungai Buloh Leprosarium, about an hour's drive from the nation's capital Kuala Lumpur. Sungai means "river" ("kawa" in Japanese), and Buloh means "bamboo" or "bamboo grass" ("sasa" in Japanese), so in a sense, I visited Sasakawa Village. When I visited in 2002, it was tranquil, lined with plant and flower shops. However, in 2006, the government constructed a highway cutting through the Sungai Buloh Leprosarium. The landscape had changed completely, with a new hospital built at the same time.

The Sungai Buloh Leprosarium was once a self-supporting community, with its own school, hospital, movie theater, fire department, and training center for poultry farming and carpentry skills. Most of its current residents were over sixty years old and had disabilities, but those who could work planted trees and flowers for a living. At the time of my visit, there were 232 residents and 113 occupying some of the 409 chalets still standing, while the remaining 119 people were hospitalized with various ailments.

I met with five male residents, leaders of the community. The government had requested that they vacate their land to make room for the expansion of the university, with the assurance that alternative land and housing would be provided. They told me that the eastern side of Sungai Buloh had already been destroyed, and they were keen to make sure the remaining houses and facilities were not knocked down. They explained: "We have disabilities, few of us have families, and most live alone. We simply want to be allowed to live in peace." A Ministry of Health official gave the government's side of the story: the resident population, he explained, at one point 2,000, is now reduced to one-tenth of that number. The redevelopment would also bring other benefits besides the university campus expansion: a new health center that would promote the health of local citizens. The conflict between the importance of preserving the facility as a heritage site for its historical significance, respecting the residents' wishes, and allowing them to remain where they chose versus redeveloping the land in the interests of the population at large posed a difficult dilemma.

The history of discrimination against leprosy does not only concern events that happened in the past but also events happening now, in real time. It is a history of our own time. I feel we must do everything we can to make sure that the history of leprosy is not simply forgotten and continues to be told to all the generations to come—as one of the greatest errors committed by humankind. To do so, we need to preserve all historical evidence of the lives of those who suffered through leprosy, those who recovered from the disease, and their families, as well as the trajectory of their lives as they bravely fought against stigma and segregation. I am convinced that leprosy's history is as valuable as a UNESCO World Heritage Site in terms of what humanity should preserve.

After visiting all these leprosy sites, I had an audience with the current king of Malaysia and met with API and World Maritime University scholarship recipients. After that, I traveled to Phnom Penh, Cambodia, to attend the opening ceremony of a new building for a prosthetist training school and the opening ceremony of a traditional medical school.

Children's dreams of filial piety—Maharashtra, India, December 2010

Route: Narita International Airport → Mumbai, Maharashtra, India (flight time: 13h)—one night

In December, I visited Maharashtra, in Western India, where I went to Mumbai and Pune. I first visited some leprosy colonies in the Mumbai area. The Borivali leprosy colony in the northern part of Mumbai grew up spontaneously on the site of a former graveyard. During the 1940s and '50s, three or four families from minority tribes first settled here. Other marginalized people gradually moved in, bringing the total population to around 1,500 today. They eked out a living by cutting down trees or gathering nuts in the area and selling them. When I arrived, I found a great crowd of people waiting for me at the tin-roofed building that was the meeting place. I was greeted by some little girls who painted a bindi on my forehead and put a spoonful of sugar in my mouth. Each of them handed me a single red rose. Buying just one of those red roses would have involved spending a huge sum of money for anyone in this colony. The little girls may well have gone straight out to beg as soon as I left. I was grateful for the warm welcome, but it also, as always, pained my heart.

All over the world, people living in leprosy colonies are invariably kind and gentle. This kindness is the thing that strikes anyone who comes with me for the first time on these trips. Their kindness is so genuine that, at times, it makes them utterly defenseless. So occasionally, I feel as if my own conscience is being tested.

One of the problems the colony here faces is posed by the creek that runs next to it. During the monsoon, it overflows with untreated sewage, flooding houses and ruining sanitation. The colony's president, Bhimrao Madhale, was indignant that he had been ignored despite repeated requests to the proper authorities for improvements. According to him, land rights issues add to the colony's flood control and employment problems. The colony was originally located in the middle of a forest. However, after years of development, it is now surrounded by buildings and condominiums. Because there has been no legal procedure for land ownership, the residents do not legally own the land, so they have no legal protection. Despite their appeals, no specific solution was forthcoming from the authorities, and they were at their wits' end. Mr. Madhale told me passionately what he thought. "Even orphans have the means somehow to get help and protection from society. But we, on the other hand, are utterly alone, without any recourse."

The people at this colony spoke the Marathi language, and I had asked a local female graduate student to interpret from Marathi to English. Interpreting by my side the whole time, at one point suddenly her voice started to get choked with sobs, and then she confessed tearfully: "I have lived in Mumbai all my life, but I had no idea that people were living in such hardship and poverty. I am so ashamed."

Next, I visited the Panvel colony, about an hour's drive east of Mumbai. Established about thirty-eight years ago, the colony lies in two sections divided by a railway track. At the time of my visit, it was home to about twenty-eight families, totaling 150 people. A number of small-scale self-help groups operated there, supported by a Christian NGO. They produced household disinfectants and garments and provided financial assistance to elderly people affected by leprosy with disabilities. The women involved in these efforts proudly showed me around their clean though by no means spacious workshop. A woman named Shaila, who played a central role in the project, told me she lived with her husband's mother, who once had leprosy, though neither Shaila nor her husband has had the disease. Her mother-in-law had been forced to leave her hometown forty years ago due to leprosy and ended up in this colony. Another elderly woman told me that she went to beg at a nearby temple twice a week, where she made about 15 rupees (about US$0.20) a day. The practice of begging is alive and well even in colonies where efforts have been made to make people self-sufficient.

By contrast, the youngsters I met told me, eyes shining, that they wanted to become schoolteachers, cricketers, and the like. When one boy told me, "I want to grow up quickly so that I can ease the burden on my parents and pay them back for all they've done for me," they all raised their hands one after another, smiling and saying, "Me too!" "Me too!" Such filial piety, I thought. If only Japanese young people could take a leaf out of their books. At one point, it was decided that we should take a commemorative photo together. When I asked if anyone could not come to meet me because they were immobilized, they led me to a small barracks. Inside was an elderly man who had no limbs and had even lost his sight. He told me, "Everybody looks after me—that's why I've been able to survive." I realized that these youngsters who wanted to grow up fast so they could ease the burden on their parents were very likely empathetic toward everyone's plight, including severely disabled elderly people like this man.

The next day, I traveled to Pune, the second largest city in Maharashtra after Mumbai, to attend the "First International Workshop on an Inclusive Society: Leprosy and Human Rights," co-sponsored by the Sasakawa Health Foundation, the International Leprosy Union (ILU), and the National Forum, a national organization of people affected by leprosy in India. The ILU is an NGO founded in 1984 by my longtime friend Dr. S. D. Gokhale. It has a long history stretching over twenty years of diverse initiatives and social awareness campaigns to protect the lives of people affected by leprosy and their families, and in 2007 it was awarded WHO's Sasakawa Health Prize.

In this very month, a draft Resolution on the Elimination of Discrimination against Persons Affected by Leprosy and Their Families, accompanied by Principles and Guidelines, was proposed by the Japanese government and put before the UN General Assembly and approved on 21 December. WHO, which had been leading leprosy elimination efforts, had also announced a policy of actively involving people affected by leprosy in its activities to combat the disease. The purpose of this international workshop was to allow researchers and delegates to report on the current status of activities to eliminate social discrimination at the grassroots level, promote discussion, and formulate a concrete plan to ensure the elimination measures would take place and that people affected by leprosy could take center stage. It was attended by people affected by leprosy, NGOs, and government representatives from nine countries (Brazil, Colombia, Ethiopia, Bangladesh, India, Indonesia, Japan, South Korea, and the Philippines). Over the two days of the workshop, participants reported on discriminatory laws against people affected by and recovered from leprosy in their respective countries and on the history of efforts to restore the dignity of people affected by leprosy.

On the afternoon of the workshop's opening day, the participants visited another colony in the Dapodi district of Pune. Established in 1952, this colony was relatively large, home to about 400 people in 110 households. Like the Panvel colony I visited the day before, it had two areas divided by a railroad, and a public railway corporation owned the land. In recent months, with ILU's support, a flour-milling operation had been started there, and there were plans for a dairy farm nearby. Circumstances for these people living in extreme poverty, isolated from society, and in unsanitary conditions seemed to be gradually improving, and they could begin to feel some confidence and a glimmer of hope for the future.

THE SOCIAL ASPECTS OF THE DISEASE

Despair in the "Pearl of the Mediterranean"—Arab Republic of Egypt, December 2010

Route: Mumbai, Maharashtra, India → Dubai, United Arab Emirates (flight time: 3h; 4h 30m stopover) → Cairo, Egypt (flight time: 4h)—two nights—Cairo → Beirut, Lebanon (flight time: 3h)—one night—Beirut → Dubai (flight time: 3h; 1h 35m stopover) → Narita International Airport (flight time: 9h 30m)

I left Mumbai, India, shortly after 10 p.m. for Egypt and then Lebanon—via Dubai, where we had a wait of four hours for our onward connection. Just out of curiosity, I decided to wait sitting on the floor in a corridor in the airport. It might sound rude to people who have no choice but to beg, but putting aside the issue of the inherent indignity of having to do so, I wanted to see what it felt like (with my usual curiosity to experience everything I can) to have to sit on the ground as people passed by. All I can say is that I didn't find it too embarrassing—I suppose because I could only see the feet of passers-by and was spared having to look people in the eye.

Egypt eliminated leprosy as a public health problem nationwide in 1994. At the end of 2009, the prevalence rate was 0.13 per 10,000 population. However, it still had five governorates in the upper reaches of the Nile that had not yet eliminated leprosy at the provincial level.

On my first day in Egypt, I spent three hours in the morning visiting the Abu Zaabal Leprosarium in northern Cairo. Both sides of the road were lined with vast fields of cacti and mangoes. This leprosarium is a public hospital established in 1932 as a compulsory lifelong isolation facility. It currently houses about 700 people receiving leprosy treatments and people who had recovered but are suffering from its aftereffects and other ailments. It had a majestic appearance and could be mistaken for a palace from the outside. The facility is divided into three areas: one with a clinic, pharmacy, and offices, and separate wards for men and women. Inpatients seemed relaxed while sunbathing in the spacious garden. It looked more like a nursing home with medical facilities than a hospital, perhaps due to the large number of long-term inpatients.

From nearby, I could hear some sort of very shrill, drawn-out sound—like the cry of a large bird. I asked someone in my party who was familiar with Arab culture what it was and was told that it was "zagharīt," an ululation uttered, usually by women, in North African and Middle Eastern countries at ceremonies and as a sign of welcome. The sounds were coming from a group of women who quickly surrounded me, emitting this sound, produced by a high-pitched, loud voice, accompanied by a rapid movement back-and-forth with their tongue. The leprosarium was clean, the medical staff was well-liked by the inpatients, and the conditions were favorable overall. However, I would not want this medical facility to become a "permanent home," as the inmates say. What I really wanted to see was patients being allowed to spend time with their families once they recovered. The reason they were reluctant to return home was that society discriminated against and rejected them.

In the afternoon, I visited the WHO Regional Office for the Eastern Mediterranean, which is one of the six regional offices WHO has established worldwide, covering North Africa, the Middle East, and West Asia. It handles twenty-two countries, from Morocco in the west to Pakistan in the east, including conflict-ridden and politically unstable countries such as Afghanistan, Iraq, Somalia, Sudan, and Yemen.

The next day, I left at 6:30 a.m. for Egypt's second largest city Alexandria, about 200 kilometers from Cairo, a three-hour journey by car.

Alexandria is a beautiful city, much lauded as the "Pearl of the Mediterranean." On a small hill in the southwestern part of the city is the Amria Leprosarium. The building comprised a renovated British army barracks from the colonial era, and all in all, it gave the impression of a cold, inhuman concentration camp. The number of inpatients peaked about ten years ago, when there were more than 200, but now there were only twenty, with about four new admissions per year. A hospital was staffed by two doctors and six nurses, who lived in an attached wing of the hospital.

At the hospital, a doctor in a white coat showed me around. Just behind him was a man wearing sunglasses with his hands in the pockets of a leather jacket who did not greet me or ask me to shake his hand and kept following us at a distance. The doctor explained that he was the director, but the man did not crack a single smile the whole time. In the ward, there were people who looked terribly ill. They all appeared to be nomadic Berbers or Bedouins and were dressed in traditional costumes. Many had ulcers on both legs, which had been left without bandages. The air reeked of pus. Clearly, they were not getting sufficient medical treatment. The patients were nearly expressionless, and here and there outside the buildings, I saw the strange spectacle of four or five people just sitting on their haunches in silence. There was a sense of utter despair, as though their tears of pain, sadness, and even nostalgia had dried up. In all my travels around the world, I have never seen such a grim place. I had visited hundreds of other leprosaria, but the difference between Amria and those places was as stark as night and day. I was astonished by its lifeless and impersonal environment. Tears welled up when I thought of the future of the people confined there.

The Suzanne Mubarak Regional Center for Women's Health and Development, my afternoon visit, is a medical institution named after the former First Lady Suzanne Mubarak. It conducts training and research on childbirth, gynecological diseases, and related skill devel-

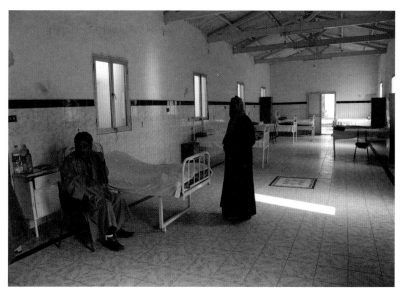

87. At the Amria Leprosarium (Alexandria, Egypt, December 2010)

437

opment, accepting trainees from Egypt and all over Africa. We spoke about improving medical standards in the Middle East and Africa.

On my last day in Egypt, I met with Deputy Health Minister Nasser El Sayyad to discuss leprosy and the state of insured medical care in Egypt. The private sector plays a significant role in the fight against leprosy. There are seventeen leprosy clinics in Egypt, and in many cases, nuns from abroad dedicate themselves to facility operations. Public health for children is another healthcare-related issue in the country. The government had partnered with universities on a planned program to mobilize 1 million students to establish habits including gargling and hand washing. It was also running a campaign to raise awareness about HIV/AIDS and hepatitis, having developed a strategy based on a maternal and child health survey. A medical insurance system covering 70 to 80 percent of the population was also about to be put into place.

That evening, I flew from Cairo to Lebanon, where I attended a WHO EMRO conference in Beirut on the following day. NGO representatives and leprosy officials from fourteen of the twenty-two countries under EMRO's jurisdiction were in attendance. We heard reports on leprosy elimination projects in each country.

The king and McKean—Kingdom of Thailand, December 2010

Route: Narita International Airport → Bangkok, Thailand (flight time: 7h; 1h 30m stopover) → Chiang Mai, Thailand (flight time: 1h)—one night—Chiang Mai → Bangkok (flight time: 1h 50m; 1h stopover) → Narita (flight time: 5h 40m)

The first leprosy facility built in Thailand was the McKean Rehabilitation Center. Leprosy facilities were then built across the country. The leprosy drug Promin was developed in 1943. In 1955, Thailand established a national leprosy elimination program, providing all leprosy patients with housing and dapsone (an oral drug synthesized from Promin). It also sent special treatment teams to forty leprosy-affected provinces in northern, northeastern, and central Thailand. As a result, the leprosy prevalence rate dropped from fifty per 10,000 people in 1953 to 12.4 in 1971. The Ministry of Health changed its policy to integrate leprosy facilities into general hospitals, ultimately eliminating leprosy as a public health problem in 1994.

THE SOCIAL ASPECTS OF THE DISEASE

In 1986, I organized a fundraising campaign to raise ¥870 million named after my eighty-seven-year-old father, Ryoichi Sasakawa, and endowed the Sasakawa Research Building to establish a medical research center for leprosy in Bangkok, Thailand. This facility was equipped with the latest advances to serve as a center for leprosy research primarily targeting Thailand and Southeast Asia. Professor Tonetaro Ito of Osaka University was appointed as its director. However, to my regret, the Thai government then decided to focus on HIV/AIDS research at the expense of leprosy due to the explosive HIV/AIDS epidemic that followed.

In December, I visited Chiang Mai in northern Thailand. The purpose of my visit was to attend the twentieth anniversary of the Sasakawa Young Leaders Fellowship Fund (SYLFF) established at Chiang Mai University. This is one of Thailand's finest national universities. It was twenty years since I had visited Chiang Mai and the first time since I initiated SYLFF. During that time, I visited the capital city of Bangkok many times and witnessed Thailand's remarkable economic development. However, I was amazed to see how much Chiang Mai had developed after an absence of twenty years.

In 1907, Dr. James McKean, an American Presbyterian missionary, appealed to the then king of Chiang Mai about the huge numbers of people affected by leprosy forced to live under bridges, whereupon the prince offered to give him the use of some land surrounded by a river and a canal. That was the origin of the McKean Rehabilitation Center. The land had at one time been where the king kept his elephants, and the local residents were terrified of using it, fearing the spirit of a white elephant that had died there. Dr. McKean built a few simple houses out of bamboo and wood and established the Chiangmai Leper Asylum in 1908. I was told patients flocked there from China, Laos, and Burma (now Myanmar). A clinic, an amusement center, a water tower, and other facilities were added later.

Before the Second World War, there was no effective treatment for leprosy, and the center used chaulmoogra oil. Even today, there are thirty chaulmoogra trees at the McKean Rehabilitation Center, allowing me to hold a real chaulmoogra fruit for the first time. In the past, those being treated for leprosy had to drink chaulmoogra oil or inject it into their muscles. However, there were no scientifically proven benefits from such treatments, and it is assumed that it was only effective in providing nourishment. After the war, when treatment with DDS (dapsone) was introduced, twice a week, an official would call patients to line up to receive their DDS medication, drinking water, and pocket money by tapping on a piece of bamboo. However, stigma was always a significant issue, with officials marking coins used by individuals affected by leprosy and issuing a special currency for use in the center (something similar was done in Japan).

During the Great Depression of the 1930s, McKean could no longer collect enough donations, and it became difficult to handle so many patients. It was at this point that relatively healthy and motivated patients moved to the surrounding land that McKean had purchased, cultivated fields, and began to build a new community. Today, there are twenty-two such communities in northern Thailand. The primary concern of those who moved to the new villages was their children's education. McKean built schools and provided educational support in all twenty-two villages. By the 1960s, more than 2,000 children had received an education in those schools.

In the 1970s, the WHO announced a policy of integrating leprosy treatment with general medical care. While many questioned whether such a thing was possible, McKean's staff took up the challenge of integrating rehabilitation and treatment in the most resolute way. McKean's medical team established outpatient clinics in five locations in Chiang Mai province, integrating leprosy and general wards. Doctors made regular visits to the clinics to treat leprosy patients who had returned to their families and the general population in the area. Above all, McKean's medical team worked to eliminate stigma and misconceptions about leprosy and conducted early detection awareness campaigns in schools and everywhere else to prevent disabilities from the disease. Alongside their surgical, regenerative, and psychological treatments, the team also conducted vocational training so that patients would not be a burden to their families when they returned home.

In 1978, King Bhumibol Adulyadej (King Rama IX) visited the site to recognize McKean's efforts. King Bhumibol's grandfather was King Chulalongkorn (Rama V, who died in 1910), one of Thailand's "three great kings," and his father, known as the father of modern medicine in Thailand, was the founder of Mahidol University, which boasts the country's best medical school. King

Bhumibol had a deep understanding of medicine thanks to his father's influence. The little houses of those who reside at the center hold the names of donors, and King Bhumibol Adulyadej added to one hut the name of his father.

In the 102 years since its opening, the McKean Rehabilitation Center has treated 13,000 people. Many have returned to their families and hometowns or moved to one of the twenty-two villages to start new lives. However, those who lost contact with their hometowns due to their long stays at McKean or who are too old or disabled to live independently after rehabilitation reside in the center's Northern Village. During my visit, forty-six people were living in these little houses built with donations. Five were in the hospital but were given three meals daily and a monthly subsidy of 2,000 baht (about US$60) from the government. However, each person needed at least 8,000 baht to live, and McKean made up the difference with donations and profits from arts and crafts sales.

It has been sixteen years since Thailand eliminated leprosy as a public health problem. However, as of early 2010, there were 762

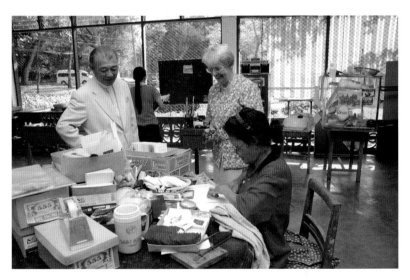

88. At the McKean Rehabilitation Center, people affected by leprosy engage in handicrafts. With Mrs. Heather Smith, of the Center (Thailand, December 2010)

registered people affected by leprosy, with 300 new diagnoses in 2009. The major challenge is to pass on the knowledge of early detection and the skills to provide prompt treatment.

Husband and wife Trevor and Heather Smith, who were my guides around the center, said that McKean would continue to play an essential role as a center for people affected by leprosy in northern Thailand. Heather mentioned that McKean had achieved three different kinds of community integration: integration with the community outside the center, integration with people with disabilities, and integration with elderly people. One of McKean's new initiatives was opening a nursing home for elderly adults.

I was impressed by McKean's progressive thinking and modest yet clean facilities. Center director Somchai Obboon told me that people who have had leprosy nowadays prefer to use the term "affected by" rather than "recovering from" leprosy. I could understand how the phrase "recovering from" might sound like they have recovered from a "bad" or "negative" situation. "Affected by," on the other hand, implies that leprosy is one of life's many possible experiences.

Thailand was my last stop of the year. It was here that I was informed that the UN General Assembly in New York had unanimously approved a draft resolution and the Principles and Guidelines for the Elimination of Discrimination against Persons Affected by Leprosy and Their Family Members. I savored a quiet joy to know that what started as a one-man effort had garnered the support of so many people to get approved by the UN General Assembly. Timor-Leste also eliminated leprosy as a public health problem in 2010 (officially announced in March 2011), leaving Brazil as the only country yet to achieve this goal.

Countries visited in 2011	
January	● China
February	● India
March	China, India, Timor-Leste trip scheduled, but cancelled due to Great East Japan Earthquake.
April	Philippines (Meeting with President Benigno Aquino)

May	Jordan (WANA Forum)
	● Switzerland (WHO General Assembly)
June	New Zealand (Massey University SYLFF twentieth anniversary)
	Australia (University of New South Wales Australia Business School SYLFF twentieth anniversary)
July	● Malawi
	Ethiopia (Sasakawa-Africa Association)
	● Central Africa
August	● India
September	United States (Washington, DC: Tokyo–Washington Dialogue)
	● India
October	Czech Republic (Forum 2000)
	Finland (Helsinki SYLFF twentieth anniversary)
November	● Mali
	● Burkina Faso
	● Brazil (São Paulo University SYLFF project)
December	Myanmar (Nationwide ceasefire agreement: talks with government personnel)
	Thailand (Myanmar nationwide ceasefire agreement: negotiations with armed ethnic organizations)

Indicates a trip that features in this section.

WANA: West Asia–North Africa, a non-profit think tank based in Amman, Jordan, comprising intellectual leaders in economic, environmental, energy, educational, and social spheres.

SYLFF: Sasakawa Young Leaders Fellowship Fund program.

SG2000: Sasakawa Global 2000 program. An agricultural project supporting farmers in need in Africa.

MAKING THE IMPOSSIBLE POSSIBLE

Forum 2000: An annual international conference launched in 1997 when Václav Havel, Elie Wiesel, and the author invited world leaders to Prague for open debate on the major issues and challenges of the new millennium.

The Universal Declaration and work camps—People's Republic of China, January 2011

Route: Narita International Airport → Beijing, China (flight time: 3h)—two nights—Beijing → Narita (flight time: 3h)

The People's Republic of China had manufactured the DDS (dapsone) leprosy drug domestically but relied on imports for other leprosy drugs. In 1980, a Lebanese-American who had participated in Mao Zedong's Long March, and was known in China as Dr. Ma Haide (his original name was Shafick George Hatem), made a request for cooperation from the then Sasakawa Health Foundation President Morizo Ishidate (first dean of the University of Tokyo's Faculty of Pharmacy and the first to synthesize the drug Promin in Japan), and a meeting took place in the province of Guangdong. Initially, the Chinese Ministry of Health denied that leprosy even existed in China and claimed that it was a type of skin disease, but thanks to Ma Haide's efforts, it came to recognize the existence of *mafeng* disease (leprosy). In those days, hotels were a rarity, and I still recall with nostalgia the scene of Chinese people sitting round eating at a standing buffet party at the hotel where the conference was held, not knowing how such a party was supposed to work.

In 1985, the Chinese Ministry of Health held the first International Leprosy Symposium in Guangzhou, Guangdong, China in cooperation with the international community, making a global commitment to work toward eliminating leprosy as a public health problem at the national level. In 1998, at the Fifteenth International Leprosy Congress in Beijing, China officially declared that it had eliminated leprosy and set its own high target of less than one case per 100,000 population to strengthen its efforts. Nevertheless, more than 20 percent of newly diagnosed patients in China develop disabilities. This figure, which is considerably higher than in other countries, indicates an average delay of about three years between the onset of the disease and the start of treatment. Furthermore, in fact forty-six areas in southwestern China, including Sichuan, Yunnan, Guizhou, Hunan, and the Tibet Autonomous Region, had yet to eliminate leprosy at the sub-national level.

On 25 January 2011, we held the Global Appeal 2011 launch ceremony in Beijing. It was freezing cold in Beijing at that time of the year, and a walk outside for fifteen minutes would make my ears sting. The theme of the sixth Global Appeal was education, with endorsements from the presidents of 110 universities in sixty-four countries, including Cambridge University, Yale University, Keio University, and Waseda University. The ceremony's co-sponsors were the China Society for Human Rights Studies, the Nippon Foundation, and Peking University, which served as the venue in light of its close relationship with the Nippon Foundation. Representatives from Peking University, Inner Mongolia University, Jilin University, Lanzhou University, Xinjiang University, and Yunnan University joined Paul Webley of England's School of Oriental and African Studies, University of London, and Chairman Hideoki Ogawa of Juntendo University in attendance. Other attendees included representatives of the Chinese Ministry of Health, WHO, the China Leprosy Association, local NGOs such as Handa Rehabilitation & Welfare Association (HANDA) and Joy in Action (JIA), and various media outlets.

The ceremony began with a speech by Dr. Min Weifang, then chair of Peking University Council, who said: "We may have succeeded in eliminating leprosy, but we cannot deny that few people know that this disease is curable. Let us continue to raise awareness and work together to build a better society." Following a message from Mr. Ye Xiaowen, the China Society for Human Rights Studies vice president, Dr. Hao Yang, deputy director general of the Bureau of Disease Control, announced that there were 611 settlement villages for people affected by leprosy throughout the country.

In his speech, Paul Webley, professor of economic psychology and director of the School of Oriental and African Studies, University of London, emphasized how prejudice is a terrible thing that can hurt people, ruin their lives, and even destroy their communities. He noted how "education and communication are essential to eradicating prejudice and bettering life chances." As an expert in both medicine and education, chairperson Hideoki Ogawa of Juntendo University stressed the need to propagate correct information through education and to disseminate a message to eradicate prejudice and discrimination as widely as possible.

At the press conference following the ceremony, we fielded a variety of questions from reporters. "Why are there so many people affected by leprosy in Sichuan, Yunnan, and other southwest regions?" "Why does it take two to three years from detection to treatment?" "How is the disease transmitted in the first place?" Many of the questions were right on target and demonstrated plenty of interest in leprosy.

Since 1984, the Nippon Foundation—through the Sasakawa Health Foundation—has provided leprosy medicines, vehicles, motorcycles, and training equipment for field activities to eight provinces along China's coast, contributing to and bolstering nationwide leprosy elimination efforts. It has also helped the work of local NGOs to support people affected by leprosy. Representatives of two of these, HANDA and JIA, were at the ceremony. Established in Guangzhou in 2004 and headed by Waseda University graduate Ryotaro Harada, JIA has been organizing workcamps in villages for people affected by leprosy in Guangdong, Hainan, Hunan, Hubei, and the Guangxi Zhuang Autonomous Region. This project involves Chinese and Japanese students who stay together in the villages and work to improve the living conditions of people affected by leprosy by repairing houses, installing running water and toilets, and paving roads. Initially, local residents were amazed to see the students linking arms and shopping with people affected by leprosy, but as the work camps took root, they began to treat this as normal. Carpenters who worked with the students on construction projects and drivers who took them to and from work were initially hesitant to approach the village, but today they willingly enter the rooms of residents affected by leprosy to drink tea, smoke cigarettes, and make small talk. Over the past ten years, more than 8,000 Chinese youth have participated in these work camps.

Around 20,000 people live in the 611 leprosy-affected villages throughout China. Many are over sixty years old and deprived of the opportunity to return to their hometowns due to deep-rooted prejudice and discrimination from families and local residents. With no relatives to watch them in their final moments, or to collect their ashes, most of them end up being given a shallow grave in a corner of the village. It is essential to provide the funding to find out about these leprosy-affected villages and see what we can do to improve the lives of the people who live there. Frankly speaking, the scenes I saw in the leprosy-affected villages in Guangdong were so appalling that I believe they are a disgrace to China. However, a major obstacle stands in the way of my work in that country: I cannot do even the slightest thing without permission from the authorities.

To not look away from failures—Delhi and Bihar, India, February–March 2011

> Route: Narita International Airport → Delhi, India (flight time: 10h)—one night—Delhi → Patna, Bihar, India (flight time: 1h 25m)—two nights—Patna → Delhi (flight time: 1h 30m)—one night—Delhi → Narita (flight time: 7h 20m)

On my March 2011 visit to India, my forty-first, I attended the first board meeting of the National Forum, an organization of people affected by leprosy. With its continued track record of successful initiatives, the National Forum registered as a trust on 21 February 2011, and this was the first board meeting held under its Articles of Incorporation. Dr. P. K. Gopal and the other eight trustees, all persons affected by leprosy, came from all over India to assemble in Delhi. This first board of trustees meeting was held at the offices of S-ILF. The agenda included approving the Articles of Incorporation, electing a chairperson (Dr. Gopal), opening a bank account, establishing offices, planning future activities, and establishing an advisory committee. Now that the National Forum had a foundation as a legal entity, I fully expected it to expand its activities, but it faced a mountain of challenges ahead. First, it had to strengthen its local organizations. Decentralization has been progressing in India, so action does not happen by direction from the central government but rather by state-level initiatives. Conditions had to be created to have the leaders of those affected by leprosy in each state unite their colonies and bring the voices of their people to the government and society at large. Another urgent task was to foster young leaders from among those affected by leprosy who could work at the state and national levels.

One of the National Forum's specific action goals was to establish a pension for people affected by leprosy. National and state frameworks for disability and old-age pensions existed, but only a very few states, including the capital Delhi and Uttarakhand, had pensions specifically for people affected by leprosy. In a report petitioning for the integration and empowerment of leprosy-affected persons to the Rajya Sabha Committee on Petitions, an independent committee of the Indian government, the National Forum had called for each state to establish a pension for people affected by leprosy of 2,000 rupees/month (about US$25). In 2010, I had joined people affected by leprosy to meet with Sanjay Kumar, the executive director of the National Rural Health Mission in Bihar. We petitioned the state government to establish a pension for people affected by leprosy (1,000 rupees per month, about US$12) and to improve their living conditions. However, the situation had seen no progress, and there had been no response regarding enhancements of help available for people affected by leprosy.

Thus it was that I decided hurriedly to head from Delhi to Patna, the capital of Bihar. On 28 February, I again visited Executive Director Kumar and Deputy Chairman Ganga Prasad of the Bihar Legislative Council. I appealed to them to urgently establish a pension system to resolve the current situation in which people affected by leprosy who are elderly or have disabilities must earn a living by begging.

I then met with Bihar's Deputy Chief Minister Sushil Kumar Modi, whom I had met in May 2010. His office had a bed set up for his use—I wasn't sure whether for daytime naps or nighttime sleep. The deputy chief minister offered us chairs, but there were not enough for everyone. Then, to my surprise, he had the three people affected by leprosy sit on the bed. I was amazed, knowing that some high-ranking officials would be reluctant to even let them sit at the same table. Deputy Chief Minister Modi then telephoned the director of the Social Welfare Department and instructed him to draft a detailed pension plan. He also assured me that he would personally persuade the chief minister on the matter. Obtaining the deputy prime minister's assurances was the most significant outcome of the visit.

THE SOCIAL ASPECTS OF THE DISEASE

On a suggestion from the deputy chief minister and with his help I also met with State Health Minister Ashwini Kumar Choubey that evening. I received an affirmative response from him on a number of matters—issuing the required pension certificates to people affected by leprosy, dispatching twice-weekly medical visits to the colonies, furnishing protective shoes, and providing medical benefits, as requested in the report to the Rajya Sabha Committee of Petitions—and finally, I could say that some progress was being made. I had hoped that the situation would immediately improve when we submitted our report, but in the interim elections were held, and ultimately it took three years for our requests to be implemented. Nevertheless, the Bihar state government eventually provided 1,000 rupees to each person affected by leprosy in Bihar, the poorest state in India at that time. This outcome positively impacted later efforts to increase pensions in other states.

The same day, I stopped by the Bihar branch of The Leprosy Mission (TLM) and received a detailed update on Bihar's leprosy situation. The prevalence rate was 1.08 per 10,000 population, with

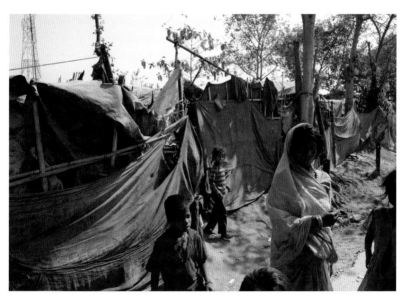

89. A visit to Jitwarpur colony in Samistipur. People affected by leprosy live in plastic sheets draped over a wooden frame. (Bihar, India, March 2011)

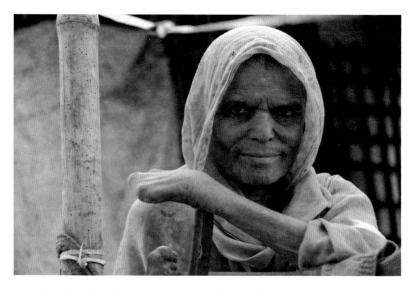

90. The deep, hard gaze of a person affected by leprosy. So much to tell (Bihar, India, March 2011)

more than 20,000 new cases per year (16 percent of them children). However, the small percentage (less than 2 percent) of new patients that developed disabilities indicated a favorable trend in detecting the disease early.

The next day, 1 March, I visited the public Tajpur Hospital, a two-and-a-half-hour drive northeast of Patna. The hospital serves a population of 150,000 and accepts four or five new leprosy patients every month; 150 volunteer health workers diligently check the villages to find most of these patients. Twenty or thirty patients come to the hospital twice a month to care for ulcers on their feet.

I then visited the Jitwarpur colony in Samastipur, a thirty-minute drive from Tajpur Hospital. This colony had moved to its present location about ten years before from alongside the tracks of a nearby railroad station. Eight families of people affected by leprosy and sixteen families of people with disabilities lived in a long, narrow plot of land alongside a road. While living conditions had gradually improved in the Indian colonies of people affected by leprosy in recent years, thanks to various support efforts, they still live in utter poverty and terribly unsanitary conditions compared to typical households. These people's dwellings were dust-filled tents and could not really be called "homes" at all—they were little more than plastic sheets draped over a wooden frame and weighed down with stones, offering little shelter from the wind and rain. Most people in the world have no idea that this kind of lifestyle exists; and even if they do, they are indifferent to the fact. The cruelty of such indifference can make me furious.

Just as I was about to visit another colony, word came that a meeting had been arranged with the minister of social welfare, so I hotfooted it back to Patna. Minister Parveen Amanullah was kind enough to give me time to meet with her even though the state legislature was in session. She had not yet been informed of my conversation with the deputy chief minister the day before, but she said she was open to the idea of setting up a pension for people affected by leprosy and promised to discuss it with the chief minister. This was not tantamount to success as yet, but I flew back to Delhi with a sense of relief that we had made the first step toward establishing a leprosy pension.

The next day, I had an early morning meeting with Dr. Nata Menabde, the WHO India representative, a Georgian who had arrived in India five months before, having chosen to move from her post as deputy director of the WHO Regional Office for Europe in Copenhagen. She seemed rather dissatisfied: "The Ministry of Health in this country seems to give all its attention to advanced medical technology and leaves basic public health unattended. If India wants to become a member of the UN Security Council, it has to first do something about basic sanitation. Even in Delhi, the national capital, there is garbage piling up everywhere in the streets." She was clearly feeling irritation at the way Western approaches do not always work in India and had not yet recovered from her culture shock. Before the meeting, Dr. Indranath Banerjee, a WHO leprosy officer, gave an update on the status of leprosy in the country. At the state level, two states (Bihar and Chhattisgarh) had yet to eliminate leprosy as a public health problem, while as many as 123 out of 633 districts (20 percent) in the country had not done so. Dr. Menabde and I shared our concerns about the declining priority given to leprosy by health authorities at the national and state levels in India and brainstormed how to work with NGOs to boost activities in the field.

That afternoon, I attended the S-ILF board of trustees meeting. At the meeting, the board reported on its activities in fiscal 2010. It noted that it had granted Rising to Dignity Awards to the most successful revenue-generating projects with microfinances: a dairy project (selling water buffalo milk), a battery project (rentals for electricity), and a silversmithing project (producing and selling silver goods). There were also detailed reports on the projects that had not worked out so well—something that gave me great hope, as I believe it is essential not to look away from failures but to analyze them, learn from them, and apply these lessons to the future.

To give an example of one project that had not gone as planned: S-ILF had decided to give support to a business in a colony that was raising goats. Soon after the business got going, a S-ILF representative visited to see how things were coming along and discovered that two goats were missing. When the person in charge was asked what had happened, he confessed that the goats had been eaten at a festival a few days before. "If you eat your livestock, you won't produce as much as you planned, and your profits will fall," the rep explained. The reply was: "There was a festival. When people came and said they wanted to feast on my goats, how could I refuse them? If you insist on making such a big deal of it all, I'll earn my living through begging. I'm good at that, and it's clearly much easier than raising goats." The rep didn't know what to say.

With every visit, New Delhi becomes more modernized and less like the India I once knew. Bihar, however, India's poorest state, which I visited on this trip, has bicycles, motorcycles, and automobiles running around on the verge of collision, people walking among the incessantly blaring horns, and cows reposing comfortably in the middle of it all. The uproar gives me a sense of a certain order amid the chaos, which is truly how I imagine India. Without it, I no longer feel like I am in the India I came to love.

Prejudice even among doctors—Swiss Confederation and French Republic, May 2011

Route: Narita International Airport → Frankfurt, Germany (flight time: 12h; 2h stopover) → Geneva, Switzerland (flight time: 1h)—

452

THE SOCIAL ASPECTS OF THE DISEASE

three nights—Geneva → Frankfurt (flight time: 1h; 1h 30m stopover) → Narita (flight time: 12h)

Geneva, Switzerland, is a city I visit frequently. Every year in May, at the World Health Assembly I get together with the heads of national health administrations to discuss efforts to eliminate leprosy. The Palais des Nations (the UN's European headquarters) in Geneva is a vast space, and the meetings usually take place as the officials involved move from place to place and are conducted extremely concisely, but I don't know of any other place that offers so effectively the opportunity to directly meet with health ministers from around the world and make my requests. I dare say that the sight of me rushing at breakneck speed through the corridors of the UN headquarters has become one of the fixtures of spring in Geneva. Along with attending the award ceremony of the Sasakawa Health Prize, which honors contributions to developments in primary health care, going to the World Health Assembly is for me an annual tradition.

In May 2011, I traveled from Switzerland to France. Between my visit to India in February and this visit to France, the Great East Japan Earthquake had struck on 11 March. In response, the Nippon Foundation was providing an array of relief efforts to the disaster's victims, with the emphasis on speed. Activities were still ongoing, but I decided to visit the World Medical Association (WMA) in Ferney-Voltaire, France, hoping to obtain support from national medical association representatives for the seventh Global Appeal, which was scheduled to be announced in January 2012.

Unfortunately, even doctors can be prejudiced against leprosy, and it is a sad fact that in many cases they refuse to treat patients. Furthermore, the vast majority of doctors in developed countries have no experience in treating the disease. But so many people affected by the condition still exist all over the world. It is so important that doctors learn that leprosy is no different from other diseases if we are to reduce the number of new cases. This is what I said to Dr. Katsuyuki Haranaka, president of the Japan Medical Association, and he immediately agreed to give his endorsement to the Global Appeal and contact the WMA. Through the good offices of the Japan Medical Association, I met the WMA's president, Dr. Wonchat Subhachaturas from Thailand; President-Elect Dr. Jose Luiz Gomes

453

do Amaral from Brazil; and Secretary General Dr. Otmar Kloiber from Germany. All three listened attentively to my argument and agreed with me that even if the world achieved a standard of eliminating leprosy as a public health problem, the issue would not be solved properly without eradicating prejudice and discrimination. They said they were more than happy to have the WMA lend its help to the Global Appeal 2012.

I then returned to Switzerland, to the Palais des Nations in Geneva. My first meeting was with Dr. Pe Thet Khin, Myanmar's health minister. He was the first minister of health of the democratic government that took office in November 2010 after the first general election in twenty years. At university, his mentor was Dr. Kyaw Myint, the former minister of health who served as rector of the University of Medicine 1, Yangon. Myanmar eliminated leprosy as a public health problem in 2003, but it still had around 3,000 new cases per year, requiring sustained elimination efforts. I urged Dr. Khin to focus even more efforts on promoting early leprosy detection to further reduce the figures.

I then met with Dr. Jarbas Barbosa da Silva, vice minister of health surveillance in Brazil, a country that is key in the fight to control leprosy. He has huge insight into leprosy and other public health issues, having served as the head of disease control at the Ministry of Health and then at the WHO Regional Office for the Americas. The prevalence rate in Brazil was 1.8 per 10,000 population, with some areas in the north as high as 8.5 to 9. The vice minister told me that the new president also had a strong interest in eliminating leprosy, and the Ministry of Health, mindful that leprosy is a cause of poverty, was preparing an action plan.

With grandparents who were affected by leprosy, Dr. Enrique T. Ona, secretary of health of the Philippines, talked about the problems that people affected by leprosy and their families face in society, where prejudice and discrimination prevent them and their children from having satisfactory educational opportunities. He stressed the need for support, such as scholarships, to enable them to get involved in society. The Philippines is the country of Dr. Arturo C. Cunanan Jr., a leprosy specialist with worldwide experience who hails from Culion Island and with whom I frequently work.

Nepal eliminated leprosy as a public health problem at the end of 2009, which would not have been possible without the steady efforts of the Ministry of Health and Population and the WHO country office, as well as the media's active awareness-raising campaigns. I said this to Nepal's Health and Population Minister S. B. Basnet, and I asked him to maintain his work on this issue as a top priority.

Indonesia's Director General of Disease Control and Environmental Health Dr. Tjandra Yoga Aditama stated: "Leprosy is a significant problem in our country, along with tuberculosis and HIV/AIDS." He also expressed concern that the number of new cases has leveled off in recent years.

My meeting with Sri Lanka's Secretary of Health Dr. Ravindra Ruberu was the first since May 2010. Sri Lanka was in the middle of reconstruction efforts after the end of its civil war in 2009, and the Nippon Foundation had been doing all it could to help, constructing a prosthetist training school and 100 elementary schools, mainly in the northern part of the country, the hardest hit during the civil war. Sri Lanka had eliminated leprosy as a public health problem in 2005. However, around 2,000 new cases are still confirmed annually, with several areas that have a high concentration of cases.

Malawi has also eliminated leprosy as a public health problem, but it confirms around 750 new cases annually. I told the country's Health Minister David K. Mphande about the importance of training personnel who can accurately diagnose leprosy and conducting surveys on actual case numbers and medicine distribution.

I asked Secretary of Health and Family Welfare Dr. K. Chandramouli of India, where 130,000 new cases occur annually, to hold a national meeting of health ministers and leprosy officials from states with high prevalence rates to discuss measures to reduce the number of cases. He immediately contacted the states and promised to convene the meeting in person.

Liberia, which eliminated leprosy as a public health problem at the end of 2004, is a small country with a population (at the time) of about 3.6 million, yet nearly 400 new cases are confirmed each year. This country also appears to have areas with high concentrations of cases, so I got the country's medical director of the Ministry of Health to agree to promote countermeasures, paying particular attention to such areas.

To each and every person I spoke to at these meetings, I made sure to repeat, again and again, the Principles and Guidelines for the Elimination of Discrimination against Persons Affected by Leprosy and Their Family Members, which had passed at the UN General Assembly in New York in December 2010, and ask them to take the measures necessary in the social sphere to restore the dignity and protect the human rights of people affected by leprosy in their own countries. When I first brought the issue of leprosy and human rights to the UN Commission on Human Rights (now the UN Human Rights Council), it was Dr. Bertrand Ramcharan, then the Acting UN High Commissioner for Human Rights, who listened to me earnestly and gave me advice. While in Geneva, I met him again for the first time in seven years.

In January 2011, Dr. Ramcharan became president of UPR Info, an NGO that works to raise public awareness of UPR (Universal Periodic Review), a mechanism of the UN Human Rights Council that periodically examines the human rights situation of all UN member states. I briefed him on the UN General Assembly resolution and

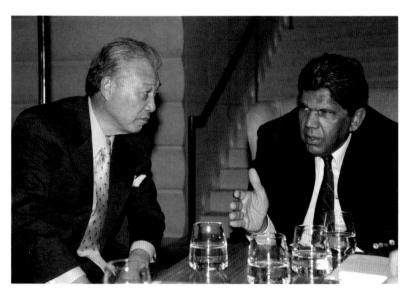

91. A reunion after seven years with Dr. Bertrand Ramcharan, a man whom I consider my mentor (Geneva, May 2011)

expressed my gratitude. Dr. Ramcharan vividly remembered the following words of one of the people affected by leprosy who visited his office with me: "For hundreds of years, society has excluded and neglected us. Now we are here in the Office of the UN High Commissioner for Human Rights."

The loneliness of refugees affected by leprosy—Republic of Malawi, July 2011

Route: Narita International Airport → Frankfurt, Germany (flight time: 12h; 6h stopover) → Addis Ababa, Ethiopia (flight time: 7h; 2h stopover) → Lilongwe, Malawi (flight time: 4h)—three nights

In July 2011, I visited Malawi in southeast Africa. It was my second visit since 2000. After a grueling thirty-two-hour journey from Japan, I finally arrived only to find that nine of my ten pieces of luggage were missing.

Malawi gained independence from the United Kingdom in 1964. It is a stable, peaceful country that has never experienced a civil war or coup d'état. It is known as "the warm heart of Africa" for its warm and friendly people. Seventy-five percent of the population is Christian, and Chewa is spoken as an official language alongside English. Its primary industry is agriculture, with 85 percent of the population producing tobacco, coffee, tea, cotton, and sugar.

Malawi eliminated leprosy as a national public health problem in 1994, but four of its twenty-six districts had not yet achieved this goal. The low priority given to leprosy in the public health administration had resulted in inaccurate patient data collection and communication, a lack of regular visits to each district for guidance and supervision, inadequate leprosy education for health workers, and insufficient medium- to long-term strategic planning. I had also heard reports of human, financial, and material resource shortages, so I decided it was necessary to elicit a commitment toward addressing leprosy from the government.

On the afternoon of 13 July, I arrived at the airport in the capital city of Lilongwe, to be met by Director Kabluzi of the Ministry of Health, WHO country representative Mr. Mushambosa, WHO regional advisor Dr. Landry Bide and tropical disease officer Dr. Shimizu of the WHO Regional Office for Africa. Malawi is in the southern hemisphere, so July is winter. Its capital is also over 1,000 meters above sea level, making for strong sunlight and fresh breezes. At the airport, a TV station interviewed me soon after landing. I told the interviewer that despite successfully eliminating leprosy as a public health problem, there was still work to be done to eradicate the disease and eliminate discrimination. I particularly wanted them to tell the people of Malawi about our three messages—that leprosy is a curable disease, that medicine is available free of charge worldwide, and that discrimination against leprosy is unacceptable.

That evening, Health Minister Mphande, whom I had spoken with in Geneva in May, hosted a welcome dinner for me, and we discussed the leprosy situation in the country, among other topics. To avoid hurting his pride, I spoke delicately about the need for prioritizing efforts to eradicate leprosy, despite Malawi's success in eliminating the disease as a public health problem and reducing the case numbers below those of HIV/AIDS, malaria, and tuberculosis. In every country, high-ranking government officials have a strong sense of dignity. It is counterproductive to be unnecessarily critical or loudly assert a legitimate theory. Negotiations that do not hurt their pride are a shortcut to achieving substantial results.

On the following day, 14 July, I visited the leprosy colony of Utale, located in the Balaka district, about 230 kilometers southeast of Lilongwe. As we sped along, sometimes at more than 100 kilometers per hour, I occasionally saw the odd power line, but most regions had no electric infrastructure, and the people lived without electricity or running water. The houses lining both sides of the road were small, some brick, but mostly made of dirt and dry grass.

Utale was established in 1946 as an isolated leprosarium by French Catholic nuns who arrived in the 1920s. Of the five facilities that existed at the time, only this one remains. When I visited, thirty-four people affected by leprosy lived in the rehabilitation center, while forty-three people had moved to a nearby village. A church led by Father Francis Kachere had built the residents' houses in the center and provided them with food and necessities. The houses were brick and more beautiful than any I had seen on the way to Utale. They had been personally built by Father Kachere and his team.

THE SOCIAL ASPECTS OF THE DISEASE

Most of the younger people affected by leprosy showed no signs of disability. Many elderly people had limb disabilities or audio/visual impairments, but most seemed cheerful and energetic, surrounded by their children and grandchildren. Among them, an older woman with a sad face caught my eye. She told me that she had fled alone as a refugee from the neighboring country of Mozambique, where there was a civil war. She had managed to reach this colony after her family abandoned her because of leprosy. Alone, and clearly lonely, she expressed her deep sadness yet some relief.

The next day, at a joint press conference with Health Minister Mphande, I urged the fifteen or so media outlets to disseminate correct information about leprosy to the Malawi people. I shared my impressions of my visit to Utale village and expressed my concern about the slight increase in cases but expressed my hope that the disease could be eradicated with future efforts. Minister Mphande admitted that the prevalence of leprosy was indeed on the rise. There were eight leprosaria in the country besides Utale, he said, and he would continue to do all he could to eradicate the disease. I could only hope these were not empty words.

On my last day in Malawi, I was supposed to meet with the president, but the meeting was canceled. It wasn't stated why, but it seemed that the thought of meeting with me was not something he relished. For the rest of the day, I decided to visit a market to get a feel for life in this country. I asked the local driver about something that had been bothering me for some time. "Is it true that the president has introduced a bill to fine people for farting?" The driver told me that it was indeed true. However, the National Assembly opposed the bill, and it was withdrawn. The bill had been introduced with the idea of protecting the environment, and apparently, the mere report of a fart could lead not only to fines but to arrests. I wondered how they would follow up on a report. I couldn't get over my curiosity, so I got my companion Natsuko Tominaga to try to extract more information from the young ladies at the hotel counter. She tried to explain what she meant using farting gestures, and the ladies at the counter were falling about with laughter.

At the airport, waiting for my flight out of the country, Dr. Bide of WHO told me something that took me aback. The Utale colony I had visited during my stay, he said, was in fact a general hospital. The people affected by leprosy whom I had met and talked to there had been brought in from other colonies for the day's visit purely to give the appearance of a beautiful, well-equipped leprosy colony. I had been completely duped. As I have noted already, in every country I go to, I have to be aware of people's sense of pride. With the exception of India, where I am generally permitted to arrange my own destinations, the people who show me round on my visits to various countries invariably try to show me the very best hospitals and facilities in a given region. I am always careful to make my own judgments about a country's actual situation from what I observe, but in Malawi, I was drawn in hook, line, and sinker.

Health centers lacking MDT—Central African Republic, July 2011

Route: Lilongwe, Malawi → Addis Ababa, Ethiopia (flight time: 4h)— one night—Addis Ababa → Bangui, Central African Republic (via Douala, Cameroon; flight time: 7h 20m)—four nights—Bangui → Paris, France (flight time: 6h 45m; 5h stopover) → Narita International Airport (flight time: 11h 50m)

After visiting the Republic of Malawi, I had a meeting in Ethiopia with members of the SG2000 agricultural project and then headed to the Central African Republic. The Central African Republic gained independence from France in 1960 but had long been embroiled in political instability due to repeated coups d'état and civil wars. In recent years, the government appeared to have finally stabilized and returned to normalcy. In 2005, the country eliminated leprosy as a public health problem at the national level, but four of the sixteen prefectures had yet to achieve the goal. Here, too, the number of cases was on a slight uptick due to the low priority given to leprosy in public health administration.

On the afternoon of 17 July, I arrived at the airport in Bangui, the capital. It was extremely hot and muggy, with the temperature over 30 degrees C and the humidity at 90 percent. I was welcomed by Health Minister Jean-Michel Mandaba; Social Affairs, National Solidarity, and Gender Promotion Minister Pétro Koni Zezé née Marguérite; Primary and Secondary Education and Literacy Minister

Gisèle Annie Nam; and Dr. Zakaria Maiga, the WHO country representative. Soldiers in camouflage with machine guns slung over their shoulders escorted the ministers. At the airport, I was interviewed by the media and explained that my visit to the Central African Republic was to encourage further efforts to eradicate leprosy and end discrimination, notwithstanding the fact that the country had eliminated the disease as a public health problem. I also appealed to the people of the country with our three messages.

As I stepped outside the airport, I was greeted by the sound of intense drumming and singing. People in colorful ethnic costumes sang and danced. I immediately joined in. Among the dancers were people affected by leprosy and people with disabilities. It was an unforgettable moment that relieved my fatigue from the long trip.

That evening, I received a briefing on leprosy in the country from Dr. Maiga, the WHO representative and the head of the national leprosy program. The Central African Republic is fighting against leprosy with the cooperation of Switzerland-based FAIRMED (formerly the Affiliation Leprosy Relief Emmaus-Switzerland), an ILEP member. At the time of my visit, the four prefectures of Ombella-M'Poko and Lobaye in the southwest, near the capital Bangui, and Vakaga and Haute-Kotto in the northeast had not yet eliminated leprosy as a public health problem. Dr. Maiga reported that the country's efforts would focus on these four prefectures.

On the following day, 18 July, I had an early morning meeting with Health Minister Mandaba. I expressed my appreciation for his efforts to combat leprosy, which affects fewer people than other infectious diseases, and asked that he continue to work with WHO to further reduce the number of people affected by leprosy.

After the meeting, I accompanied the health minister on a two-hour drive to the west to visit the village of Kaka, deep in the jungle of Lobaye prefecture, 160 kilometers from the capital Bangui. On the way to the village, the jungle suddenly opened into an area where we saw a massive, opulent building. It was Jean-Bédel Bokassa's palace. Bokassa, who styled himself the first emperor of the Central African Empire in 1977, built it on the model of the Palace of Versailles. The dictator Bokassa, who held an unprecedentedly grand coronation ceremony in the capital, was later ousted from power in a bloodless coup d'état and exiled to France.

Lobaye prefecture had a prevalence rate of 1.84 per 10,000 population. The surrounding area was also home to hunter-gatherers, commonly called pygmies, who lived by moving through the jungle. They slept in families of five or six on a bed of no more than 1 square meter, with dry grass on the floor and all around. Many pygmies do not come out of the jungle during the rainy season and rely on collecting caterpillars for food. In the village of Kaka, I shook hands and exchanged greetings with each of the fifty or so people affected by leprosy. Many were still suffering from the aftereffects of leprosy, but their wounds and injuries seemed to have been left untreated. In this village, there was a Belgian nun who had been doing what she could to examine and treat the villagers for about a year. She had been doing this kind of work in Central Africa since 1985 but had been shocked at how bad things were in this village, which was why she began work here. One of the people I greeted told us how sad people grew when they learned they had the disease, and how their suffering only deepened as the symptoms progressed to their hands and feet. Some people also asked us to help them get shoes. In this region, people live

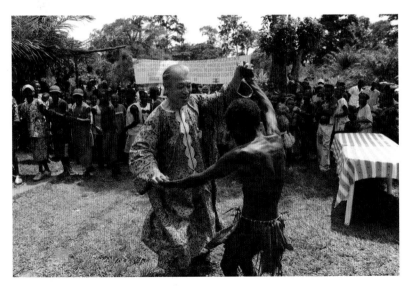

92. Dressed in the local garb and dancing with the pygmies (Central African Republic, July 2011)

barefoot with exposed wounds and injuries, exacerbating the disease's aftereffects. The health minister who accompanied me told me that when he saw me interacting with the people affected by leprosy, he said to himself, "We must do something too." At the end of the day, the local mayor, the health minister, and I joined the villagers in their dancing circle and worked up quite a sweat dancing together. Despite it being the rainy season, many pygmies also joined the dance. The pygmies came to the village the day before to build a makeshift grass hut in anticipation of the meal that would be served.

On 19 July, I met with Prime Minister Faustin-Archange Touadéra to discuss the leprosy issue. I also mentioned the Nippon Foundation's involvement in African agriculture and stressed the need for a large-scale agricultural development program to help people out of poverty. I informed him about an international conference to be held in Mali in November 2011 based on the experience of increased food production through the SG2000 project. I suggested he send a delegate to the conference. Later, I also spoke with National Assembly President Célestin Leroy Gaombalet and Social Affairs Minister Zezé, who met me at the airport.

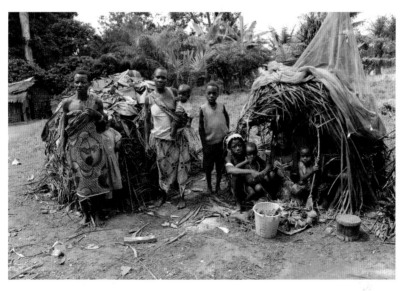

93. Pygmy dwellings, built as needed (Central African Republic, July 2011)

MAKING THE IMPOSSIBLE POSSIBLE

On 20 July, I met with three ministers from the Ministry of Education and Geographical Opening-Up: Higher Education and Scientific Research Minister Jean Willybiro Sako, Technical and Professional Education and Training Minister Djibrine Sall, and Primary and Secondary Education and Literacy Minister Nam. We discussed raising awareness of leprosy and human resource development. Next, I visited the UN Integrated Peacebuilding Office, where I heard about witchcraft and human rights issues in the Central African Republic from WHO representative Margaret Aderinsola Vogt, a human rights expert. She told me true stories of people affected by leprosy, people with disabilities, and sick women who were allegedly bewitched and sometimes killed. On the same day, I also visited a health center in the Damara sub-prefecture, 24 kilometers from the capital Bangui. This is one of five leprosaria in the Central African Republic, and it added general medical care in 2000. At the time, eight people affected by leprosy were outpatients at the center, but it had no MDT, medical records had been lost, and the staff had all fled due to the recent civil war, leaving the place in a state of disrepair, almost like an abandoned house.

Incidentally, the hotel where I stayed in Bangui was like a prison, surrounded by high iron walls, with all the windows protected by iron grates, and only one door large enough for just one person to barely pass through. Going outside at night was naturally prohibited. Here, too, I could feel for myself how dangerous things were.

At a dinner hosted by the government at the presidential palace, attended by Prime Minister Touadéra, almost all the country's ministers, and representatives of international organizations, I was awarded a medal by the government in recognition of my efforts to combat leprosy. I understood that this medal was awarded to all parties involved, including WHO, the Ministry of Health, NGOs, and above all, the people affected by leprosy themselves, for their efforts in the fight against the disease.

WHO begins to focus on discrimination—Delhi, India, August 2011

Route: Narita International Airport → Delhi, India (flight time: 8h 35m)—three nights—Delhi → Hong Kong, China (flight time: 5h 35m; 3h stopover) → Narita (flight time: 4h 20m)

464

During my trip to Delhi in August, I first attended the WHO's Global National Leprosy Programme Managers Meeting. This meeting was a crucial opportunity for leprosy program managers from nearly fifty countries in Asia, Africa, and Latin America to come together under one roof and decide on a global leprosy strategy. In the incoming five-year strategy, WHO had set a target of reducing the number of new cases with grade 2 (visible) disability by 35 percent between 2010 and 2015. Dr. Samlee Plianbangchang, regional director of the WHO Regional Office for Southeast Asia, reiterated this goal at the beginning of the meeting. He announced that although WHO's area of expertise is medicine and its mission is to eliminate leprosy, it would also focus its efforts on overcoming the problems of stigma and discrimination, referring to the results of my work at the UN Human Rights Council. For the first time, the meeting included a session on stigma and discrimination. This inclusion marked a shift in WHO taking the issue of discrimination against people affected by leprosy seriously. It also provided an excellent opportunity for senior officials from health ministries and international organizations to hear directly from people affected by leprosy.

In my keynote speech, I called for countries to apply and implement the Guidelines for Strengthening Participation of People Affected by Leprosy in Leprosy Services issued by WHO the previous year and introduce a three-pillar strategy to address social stigma and discrimination: approaching international organizations and government agencies, raising public awareness, and empowering the people affected. The first pillar is an initiative to appeal to governments to amend discriminatory laws and improve the lives of people affected by leprosy and their families, using as a catalyst the unanimous passage of the UN Resolution on the Elimination of Discrimination against People Affected by Leprosy and Their Family Members and its Principles and Guidelines. The second pillar uses our Global Appeal, endorsed by the WMA in 2012, as a steppingstone to eliminating prejudice against patients in the medical field. Finally, for the third pillar, I explained the movement for networking among interested individuals by the National Forum, a group of people affected by leprosy in India, and the microfinance program and scholarship initiative from the S-ILF.

After the morning meeting, we took a few moments to visit the Anand Gram colony in the Tahirpur area of Delhi, which encompasses twenty-eight colonies. Here, the residents are running a poultry farming project with the support of S-ILF, and 1,000 chicks were running around energetically. When they grow up, they are sold as chicken meat for 160 rupees (about US$2) per kilogram. I also met with representatives of fifteen colonies in the Tahirpur area. The representatives lamented that most residents live by begging, that their houses were old and leaky, and that they needed support to carry out their projects. It was a visit that made me realize how helpless I was.

I asked Minister of Law and Justice Shri Salman Khurshid for cooperation from the government of India regarding the UN resolution to eliminate discrimination against leprosy and the existence of discriminatory laws in India. The minister replied: "We respect the UN resolution. We will revise any laws that still have discriminatory provisions." While I managed to elicit this promise, I intended to monitor how India followed through.

Leaders increasing their presence—Chhattisgarh and Andhra Pradesh states, India, September 2011

Route: Narita International Airport → Delhi, India (flight time: 8h 35m)—one night—Delhi → Raipur, Chhattisgarh (flight time: 1h 30m)—three nights—Raipur → Hyderabad, Andhra Pradesh (flight time: 1h)—two nights—Hyderabad → Delhi (flight time: 2h)—two nights—Delhi → Hong Kong (flight time: 5h 35m; 3h stopover) → Narita (flight time: 4h 20m)

In September, I made yet another trip to India, following on from the one I had made in August. This time, I visited the states of Chhattisgarh in the east and Andhra Pradesh in the south. After arriving in Delhi, I woke up at 3 a.m. and hurried to the airport to fly to Raipur, Chhattisgarh, and then drove about four hours from the airport to visit the Bramba Vihar colony in Bilaspur to encourage the people there. The recent heavy rains had flooded the area around the colony, and sanitation conditions were bad. Established in 1979, the colony was home to forty-five people in twenty-three families when

I visited. TLM, which has been active for over 110 years, has assisted in forming four self-help groups in the state and also helped these groups open bank accounts. While living conditions seemed harsh, the colony seemed well organized around its leader, Mr. Chitra Singh. I introduced Mr. Singh to Mr. Ghasiram Bhoi, the president of the State Leprosy Rehabilitation Committee of Chhattisgarh. I explained to him the importance of unifying around the state leader and repeatedly petitioning the state government to improve the colony's poor conditions.

I then went to downtown Bilaspur to attend a meeting of about thirty leprosy officers from various districts, which Dr. D. Bhatpahare, the leprosy officer of Chhattisgarh, had organized in conjunction with my visit. Dr. Bhatpahare explained that the number of registered cases was steadily decreasing. At this point, Chhattisgarh and Bihar were the only two states where the prevalence rate exceeded one person per 10,000 population. Chhattisgarh, in particular, had the highest prevalence rate, and ten of the eighteen districts in the state were endemic, with a prevalence rate of more than one per 10,000 people. The doctor took me to the home of Mr. Harilal Kumhar, who had undergone reconstructive finger surgery and was now producing earthenware pots. He and his wife explained, giving each other glances, that they were doing good business in town, their storefront was filled with pots of all sizes, and there was considerable demand.

After that, we headed to State Health Minister Shri Amar Agrawal's official residence to meet him with Mr. Bhoi, the state leprosy organization president. A tremendous throng of people and cows blocked the road in front of the minister's residence—they had gathered to celebrate the minister's birthday, we were told. Everywhere we looked in the streets there were posters celebrating the occasion. For an official residence, the house was not luxurious. The room where we met was also small. Together with his daughter, a doctor, Minister Agrawal expressed his determination to make Chhattisgarh a model case for leprosy elimination and promised to cooperate with Mr. Bhoi.

The next day, we drove an hour to Ashadeep leprosy colony in the Durg district, where S-ILF supported small businesses. Women were weaving rugs on purchased looms. The recycled silk of five saris would make one rug. Sometimes they received orders from the government to make rugs for schools. Their earnings were about 4,500 rupees (about US$55) a month, allowing them to "put aside some savings, bit by bit," as they told me with a smile. They were working at other jobs too, such as broom-making and cleaning in town, and their children often helped them after school. Some of the colony's native sons and daughters had become doctors and engineers, they told me, and some of the men had earned the respect of women from outside the colony and married them. A good illustration of how it can be possible for people affected by leprosy to neutralize discrimination and gain respect through determination and hard work. Mr. Vishwanath Ingale, the colony's leader for several decades, is an activist who has been imprisoned nineteen times during the struggle to improve their lives. I was eager to hear his story, but his poor health made it impossible. He had apparently told a friend of mine who met him, "My work is finished." A few years later, I received news of his death.

In the afternoon, TLM and a state organization of people affected by leprosy co-sponsored a workshop that brought together NGOs working to combat leprosy. TLM operates two hospitals and three vocational training facilities here and has long provided dedicated services, including reconstructive finger surgery, counseling, and self-help group organization. A member of one NGO made a critical point during this workshop. He was skeptical about the fact that the previous year, the number of cases identified statewide was only ninety. When he had worked with members of the colony to find new patients, he related, they found 323 people in one day. Eliminating leprosy as a public health problem in Chhattisgarh still had a way to go.

On the next day, my last one in Chhattisgarh, we drove about an hour to Sant Vinova leprosy colony, a religious sanctuary located at the confluence of three rivers, including the Mahanadi, the largest river in the state. As a result of its location, many residents made their living begging from tourists, and the sanitary conditions were abysmal. I got the exact opposite impression from the colony I visited the day before: the residents looked downcast and had no apparent organization or leadership. Colony conditions are greatly influenced by the leadership skills of the colony leaders, so I keenly felt the need for a program to improve the qualities of leaders.

The day was busier than ever. I had a lecture at the Jivodaya Youth Dormitory, a school for about 400 children of people affected by leprosy, ranging from elementary to high school. I also had a press conference and meetings with related parties. Jivodaya Youth Dormitory's operator is a Catholic nun from Poland who uses a wheelchair. While I was in awe of her dedication, I had serious doubts about the idea of keeping children of people affected by leprosy all by themselves in one place. Surely, it was more important to allow them to attend public schools. Being segregated in this way would make them more likely to face discrimination when they became adults.

On 25 September, I flew to Hyderabad, Andhra Pradesh. Upon arrival, I immediately held a press conference at the Hyderabad Press Club, then drove three hours to Nizamabad to visit a colony. There was no traffic, which is rare in India, making for a smooth drive through beautiful rice paddies and forests. However, one region in the state, Telangana, had a separatist movement, and on this day there were public transportation strikes and violent demonstrations. I had considered abandoning the visit at one point due to safety concerns,

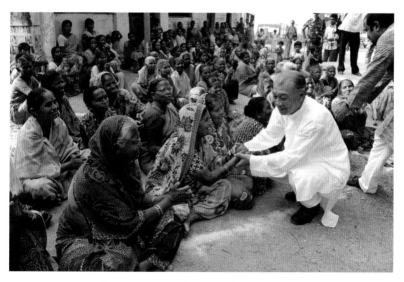

94. A visit to a colony in Nizamabad (Andhra Pradesh, India, September 2011)

but the locally elected member of parliament, Mr. Madhu Goud Yaskhi, who had requested the visit, guaranteed my safety. I was able to carry out my visit accompanied by a military escort. Devanagar colony in Nizamabad consists of 180 households, with 850 people making a living from farming or self-employment. However, around 10 percent of them survive through begging. S-ILF provided microfinances for beauty parlors, photo shops, laundries, retail stores, and water buffalo husbandry operations. In his speech at the colony, Yaskhi declared: "I will work for an increase in pensions, improved roads and infrastructure, and education for the children. I will set up an association of parliamentarians to fight for the elimination of leprosy-related discrimination."

In the afternoon, we participated in a leprosy-related human rights seminar. The agenda included discriminatory laws regarding suffrage, marriage, and the use of public facilities for people affected by leprosy. Mr. Yaskhi commented, "Love, not money, is what matters." I was impressed.

The day also included a meeting of representatives from thirteen colonies, where about fifty men and women gathered to report on their troubled living conditions. There are 101 colonies in Andhra Pradesh, the most in India. The meeting turned out to be a contentious affair, as the colonies faced various issues connected with land, housing, roads, sanitation, pensions, and children's education. However, the entire state is coming together under the leadership of Mr. V. Narsappa, president of the Society of Leprosy Affected Persons. Despite the confusion, this kind of exchange is vital to progress.

While traveling after the gathering, we encountered the aforementioned demonstration blocking traffic for the state secession movement, and our car could not budge. Following my motto, "You have to be there to understand," I squeezed through the crowd ahead of the demonstration. Among the demonstrators was a member of parliament with whom I had eaten breakfast at Mr. Yaskhi's residence that morning. When we noticed each other and shook hands, he motioned me to sit beside him. I had no choice but to decline. Had I been filmed sitting at the head of a demonstration, I may have been labeled a dangerous foreigner and banned from entering the country.

On my last day in Andhra Pradesh, I met separately with the CEO of the Society for the Elimination of Rural Poverty, Budithi Rajsekhar;

Andhra Pradesh's minister for social welfare, Pithani Satyanarayana; and the acting chairperson of Andhra Pradesh's Human Rights Commission, Kakumanu Peda Peri Reddy. Mr. V. Narsappa and other state leprosy group leaders joined me in attending all three meetings. Creating opportunities for them to speak directly with each other allows representatives to identify the conditions in colonies throughout the state, which in turn allows the representatives to set priorities and make precise petitions to the relevant departments, leading to a better government response overall. While I value the cooperation and support of Western philanthropic organizations in the leprosy issue, their efforts tend to only go so far, only rarely making petitions or requests to central or state governments. I believe it is the people with lived experience who should play the lead part in solving the issues that face people affected by leprosy, so I deliberately try to create opportunities that enable people affected by leprosy to have face to face meetings with government officials, be it national or local, as pioneers. I could explain what is happening a thousand times and not be nearly as persuasive as hearing the experience of just one person affected by leprosy. In India, where the caste system still retains its grip, it is essential that people affected by leprosy openly assert themselves and express their demands. All over the country, more and more successful outcomes are being achieved from such negotiations, and this only proves the validity of my belief, something that inwardly gives me great joy.

Andhra Pradesh is one of the places in India where the activities of people affected by leprosy are making progress. On that day, there was a meeting of young people living in the colonies, and seeing more than twenty young people discussing their desire to help their parents who they know have suffered so much, I was inspired to organize a youth section in the National Forum as a nationwide organization of resident colony youth.

Research efforts for the next generation—Republic of Mali, November 2011

Route: Narita International Airport → Paris, France (flight time: 12h 45m; overnight stopover) → Bamako, Mali (flight time: 5h 45m)—three nights.

In November, I visited the Republic of Mali in West Africa. It was my third visit and my first in five years. After gaining independence from France in 1960, Mali had gone through a long period of military dictatorship that has since been replaced by a democratic system based on a constitution enacted in 1992.

The primary purpose of my visit to Mali this time was to attend the commemorative symposium for the twenty-fifth anniversary of the Sasakawa Africa Association. My father, Ryoichi Sasakawa, started the SG2000 project to increase food production in Africa in response to the great famine that hit the region in the early 1980s. In 1986, he founded the Sasakawa Africa Association to promote this project. So far, it has been implemented in fourteen African countries, with

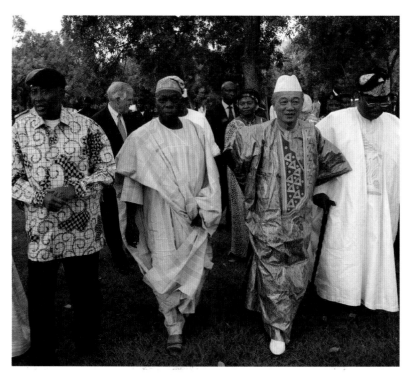

95. From right to left: former President Soglo of Benin, the author, former President Obasanjo of Nigeria, and President Touré of Mali (Mali, November 2011)

results. More than 100 people attended the symposium to discuss agriculture in Africa, including the president of Mali and other government officials, agriculture specialists, former presidents and agriculture ministers of African countries, representatives of international organizations and NGOs, and academics.

Another aim of my visit was to observe leprosy conditions in the country. Mali eliminated the disease as a public health problem nationally in 2001 and has maintained that status ever since. According to the Ministry of Health, this success was due to the ministry regularly educating doctors, nurses, and health workers about leprosy and having at least one health worker fully clued up on leprosy in each of the nation's health districts.

I arrived in the capital city of Bamako on the evening of 1 November. The next morning, I visited Kati Hospital in the city's suburbs with Health Minister Ousmane Touré. Five patients were waiting to be examined in the outpatient room. One or two of them had been left with disabilities, we were told, but they had completed their treatment. Nine others were currently undergoing treatment. In Mali, all hospitals can diagnose and treat leprosy, but more remains to be done about the physical and social rehabilitation of those affected by leprosy with disabilities.

Next, we visited the Center for Vaccine Development-Mali (CVD-Mali), formerly the Marchoux Institute. Founded by Dr. Émile Marchoux in 1931, the institute has served as a center for leprosy research, treatment, and human resource development in French Africa. Marchoux, a French-born tropical disease researcher, called for the humane treatment of leprosy patients at the Third International Leprosy Congress in Strasbourg, France, in 1923. He argued that isolating all patients was generally unnecessary, and that if necessary it should be done humanely. He later served as chair of the International Leprosy Congress and president of the International Leprosy Association (ILA).

I was given a tour of the center by its director, Dr. Samba Sow. There were about ten patients in the leprosy ward. Commenting on one young man's case, Dr. Sow said: "The inability of local doctors to recognize leprosy means that often by the time a diagnosis is made the disease is advanced. The numbers of cases might be decreasing, but we must keep the pressure on the education of medical personnel." He showed me around the research and experimental facilities, a ward for treating patients with Buruli ulcers—a type of bacterial infection that is on the rise in Africa—and other serious illnesses, a facility for making prosthetic limbs, and a laboratory for vaccine development. This is the only full-scale leprosy research facility in Africa and is of vital importance given the possibility that the disease will eventually develop resistance to the current MDT treatment.

We then took a tour of a livelihood improvement project where people affected by leprosy were raising and selling goats and cattle. Observing from the car, I was amazed to suddenly see a huge herd of goats—several thousand—on the sides of the road. Even more amazingly, I was informed that they all belonged to people affected by leprosy—140 people who sold an average of fifty to sixty goats per month. With support from the Fondation Raoul Follereau, an organization active in Mali for more than fifty years, this project had been started on their own initiative. It was rare anywhere in the world to have such large-scale projects succeed so well. An expert in agricultural engineering, director Timbo Oumou Ba of the Fondation Raoul Follereau Mali office, informed me that today's project was the result of several years of trial and error. The community has gained society's respect, and the efforts here could serve as a model for other countries. After my tour, I met with a group of people affected by leprosy. Their leader, Mr. Goulou Traoré, told me: "I think you have seen the smiles on our faces and how we live with dignity. There are 1,472 people in this community. We want to expand the project so that everyone benefits." His expression revealed a man full of self-confidence.

That afternoon, I met President Amadou Toumani Touré. I had not seen him in years. The president and I were old acquaintances, and he was a good friend of SG2000. I told him about the center I had visited that morning and also all about the goat raising project, which I considered extraordinary. "Ever since I was a child," the president told me, "people affected by leprosy have been everywhere. Hearing about that project makes me really pleased." He had a deep understanding of and interest in our efforts. President Touré was a leader whom former President Carter also held in high regard, but, regrettably, he was exiled to neighboring Senegal in a military coup the following year, in 2012. After the meeting, we attended a tree-planting ceremony held at the National Museum of Mali to commemorate the twenty-fifth anniversary of the Sasakawa Africa Association. Former President Olusegun Obasanjo of Nigeria and former President Nicéphore Soglo of Benin were also there, allowing us to renew old friendships.

Supporting agriculture helps people support themselves—Burkina Faso, November 2011

> Route: Bamako, Republic of Mali → Ouagadougou, Burkina Faso (flight time: 1h 20m)—three nights—Ouagadougou → Paris, France (flight time: 5h 30m; 5h stopover) → Haneda International Airport (flight time: 12h)

Late at night on 4 November, I arrived from Mali in Ouagadougou, the capital of Burkina Faso. Burkina Faso is a landlocked country where the majority are Muslim, 30 percent are Christian, and 10 percent adhere to traditional religions. In 1992, the nation eliminated leprosy as a public health problem, relatively early among African countries.

At the airport, despite my late-night arrival, I was greeted by Dr. Etienne Traoré, WHO's acting representative in Burkina Faso; Dr. Kafando Christophe, leprosy program director in the Ministry of Health; Dr. Landry Bide, regional advisor of the WHO Regional Office for Africa; and Mr. Tsutomu Sugiura, Japanese ambassador to Burkina Faso.

The next morning, on 5 November, I heard a briefing at the WHO Burkina Faso office. Many newly discovered cases were children, and the number of cases with severe disabilities was high, at 20 percent. There was clearly a need for the education of medical personnel about leprosy and a stepping-up of public awareness campaigns.

I expressed my gratitude to Health Minister Adama Traoré for the country's early success in leprosy elimination and reiterated the importance of educating the public about leprosy. He promised to continue being proactive and expressed his deepest condolences and sympathy for the victims of the March 2011 Great East Japan Earthquake.

After the meeting, I held a joint press conference with Minister Traoré. My visit to Burkina Faso took place during a significant

Islamic festival of sacrifice. Since it was also a weekend, neither political leaders nor the media could attend the meeting or the press conference. Nevertheless, about fifteen TV, radio, newspaper, and other media outlets gathered to cover the press conference with great enthusiasm. I mentioned that I had met President Blaise Compaoré many times in Tokyo, and he had told me about his deep interest in leprosy. It had stemmed from having frequent opportunities when he was young to meet with people affected by leprosy who lived next door to him at a military training camp. Unfortunately, he was exiled to Côte d'Ivoire due to the political uprising in 2014.

In the afternoon, I visited the Institute for Rural Development at the Polytechnic University of Bobo-Dioulasso, a school funded by the Sasakawa Africa Fund for Extension Education that operates in a number of African countries. When I arrived at the classroom building surrounded by millet and corn fields after an hour's drive, I was welcomed by the school's president, Hamidou Boly, as well as students, alums, village chiefs, and villagers.

On 6 November, I visited the western town of Koudougou, about two hours' drive away. Koudougou has the second largest number of people affected by leprosy after Dédougou, further west. With the support of the Fondation Raoul Follereau, about seventy people affected by leprosy are farming their own fields on a 1.3-hectare property. They lived far away from their fields, and some of them had been rejected by their families. Alongside the issue of discrimination, there is the problem of the distance to the fields and the technical challenge of having no agricultural leadership. They grew millet, corn, and rice, but there was little rain and a water shortage this year, so the fields had dried, and the rice plants withered. There was a pump well on the property, but it was either insufficient or not fully used. In any case, it was clearly not having much effect. The leader Simon Doran told me: "Our income is not sufficient, but we think having some kind of work is important." Working to help oneself is undoubtedly the first step toward living with dignity. However, earning a living through agriculture in a barren land with a poor climate is not an easy task. It will take time for the results of the agricultural extension education at the Polytechnic University of Bobo-Dioulasso and other institutions I visited the day before to spread to the entire nation. Still, I am committed to helping people affected by leprosy become self-sufficient.

In the afternoon, I returned to the capital city of Ouagadougou, where a small ceremony was held at the Japanese Embassy to commemorate the donation of 100 English-language books to the Polytechnic University of Bobo-Dioulasso as part of the Nippon Foundation's project for understanding contemporary Japan.

Parents and children reunite—Federative Republic of Brazil, November 2011

Route: Narita International Airport → New York, United States (flight time: 12h 50m; 11h stopover) → São Paulo, Brazil (flight time: 9h 30m; 2h 30m stopover) → Maceió, Brazil (flight time: 3h)—one night—Maceió → São Paulo (flight time: 3h 20m)—two nights—São Paulo → Rio de Janeiro, Brazil (flight time: 1h)—one night—Rio de Janeiro → Brasília, Brazil (flight time: 2h)—one night—Brasília → São Paulo (flight time: 1h 40m) → New York (flight time: 9h 30m; 6h stopover) → Narita (flight time: 14h)

In November, I visited Maceió and São Paulo, Brazil. This time, I had to fly first from Narita to New York, where I stayed overnight and took an onward flight.

Worldwide, people affected by leprosy are discriminated against in many aspects of their lives, including employment and marriage, even after they are cured of the disease. To change this situation, I have presented a Global Appeal every year since 2006. The presentation of the seventh Global Appeal 2012 was scheduled for 30 January 2012 in São Paulo, co-sponsored by the Brazilian Medical Association, with the endorsement of the WMA and other national medical associations.

After the Global Appeal ceremony, we planned to hold a human rights symposium on leprosy in Rio de Janeiro. It would be the first of a series of symposiums to be held in five global regions to inform the world about the significance of the UN Resolution on the Elimination of Discrimination against Persons Affected by Leprosy and Their Family Members and the accompanying Principles and Guidelines, which the UN General Assembly unanimously approved in December 2010.

It was very important that we would be having two major events take place in Brazil like this. At the start of 2011, the Brazilian Ministry of Health officially announced that it would eliminate leprosy as a public health problem by 2015. Achieving this goal in Brazil, the only remaining country not to have done so, was of huge significance in the history of humanity's fight against leprosy. In achieving this goal, it would be crucial to take all available opportunities to renew the world's awareness of the disease's existence and its social problems. In Brazil, the disease had recently received increased attention, with victims of past segregation policies raising their voices. The idea was to hold a symposium to call attention to leprosy as a human rights issue and create a significant wave of awareness originating in Brazil.

On 23 November, I arrived in Maceió, a city located along the northeastern coast of Brazil, via São Paulo. I went to Maceió to attend the ILA Regional Congress–Americas/twelfth Brazilian Leprosy Congress. The conference brought together doctors and scientists involved in leprosy research, as well as rehabilitation, nursing, and human rights specialists, historians, and NGOs, to approach the disease from a broad perspective. At the opening ceremony, an ILA representative and a leprosy official from the Ministry of Health expressed their commitment to eliminating the disease as a public health problem. They then pointed out the importance of the health workers who endeavor to find people affected by leprosy. In my speech, I described how I came to be involved in the fight against leprosy, the strategies needed to eliminate discrimination against the disease, and my thoughts on Brazil as it nears its elimination goal. Advisor Yo Yuasa of the Sasakawa Health Foundation, who had served as president of the ILA for two terms of nine years starting with the fourteenth General Assembly in 1993, also attended the conference, despite his advanced age of eighty-five. Dr. Yuasa, who had been involved in developing MDT with the WHO since the 1980s, was deeply moved by the progress in eliminating leprosy worldwide, with only one country left, Brazil. In a video message, Brazil's vice minister of health, Dr. Jarbas Barbosa da Silva Jr., expressed his determination: "Brazil is one step away from leprosy elimination, and we aim, working widely with various administrative authorities, medical personnel, NGOs, groups of persons affected by leprosy, and civil society organizations, to go beyond elimination at the national level to the state and municipal levels."

The next day, I visited the Oliveira Santana Rehabilitation Center, a thirty-minute drive from the hotel. The center, which has been in operation since the 1940s, had recently formed a team with the state government to identify and rehabilitate new cases of people affected by leprosy. It is dedicated to providing these people with accurate knowledge about the disease and the need for rehabilitation. In addition to providing computer and other vocational training, the facility also matches people with disabilities seeking employment with job openings at companies that register on its website, and it had begun to include people affected by leprosy in this framework. Motivating people affected by leprosy who can live on social security to enter the workforce is challenging. However, society must create an environment where they can work and achieve economic independence and are no longer held back from employment opportunities due to prejudice and discrimination.

After this, I returned to São Paulo to meet with the Brazilian Medical Association, the co-sponsor of Global Appeal 2012. I was greeted by Mr. José Luiz Gomes do Amaral, who served as president of the Brazilian Medical Association until the fall of 2011 and then became president of the WMA. I had not seen President Amaral since I visited the WMA headquarters in France six months before. At our first meeting, with my desire for doctors to be adequately informed about leprosy and provide treatment for the disease, I asked the WMA to support the Global Appeal. At its General Assembly in October, the WMA passed a formal resolution of full support. President Amaral and I were joined at the meeting by representatives of the São Paulo Medical Association and the Brazilian Ministry of Health's leprosy program director, who all pledged their cooperation in sending a message from Brazil to the world that discrimination against people affected by leprosy should be eliminated.

On 26 November, I left São Paulo for Rio de Janeiro. Waiting for me at the airport were members of the Movement for the Reintegration of Persons Affected by Hansen's Disease (MORHAN), an organization for people affected by leprosy, and a famous Brazilian actress, Ms. Elke

Maravilha. I traveled to Rio to attend an event organized by MORHAN to reunite people affected by leprosy who had been separated from their children by the former forced isolation policy.

In Brazil, a law enacted in the 1930s to isolate people affected by leprosy had been in place until it was repealed in 1962. While the isolation policy pertained, people with leprosy were taken by a state health police agency and forcibly placed in an institution and not permitted to bring their children with them. Any children born at these facilities would also be taken away as newborns. In many cases, the young children were taken to orphanages and grew up never knowing their parents. A harsh fate awaited the children. The following is the testimony of one of the survivors: "Before I was five years old, I had to care for the other younger children and infants. On the rare occasions when we were served any small things to eat, they were covered in mold. If I disobeyed an adult, I received corporal punishment and was thrown into a cell with no adequate toilet. I had to treat any wounds with coarse salt. I never expected to have time for studies and had to work all the time." The children were also sold to wealthy families as servants, no different from being trafficked.

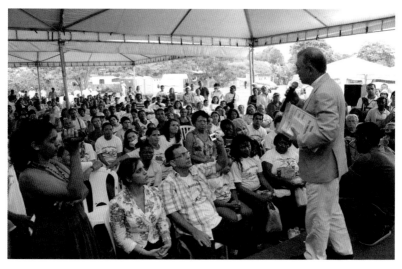

96. A reunion of children with their parents, from whom they were torn apart. The author giving a speech (Brazil, November 2011)

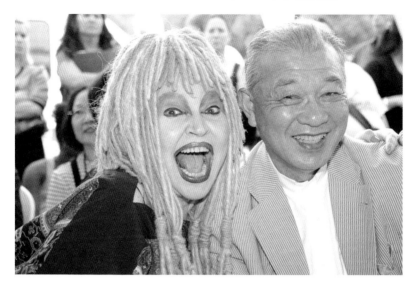

97. The author with the Brazilian actress and TV personality Elke Maravilha, a long-time passionate supporter of the fight against leprosy (Brazil, November 2011)

MORHAN is working throughout Brazil to reunite such parents and their children. I went to one such event that was held at a former leprosy colony called Tavares de Macedo, where many people affected by leprosy still live. A stage was set up in the event plaza, creating a lively carnival-like atmosphere. About 500 people affected by leprosy from four states, including Rio de Janeiro and São Paulo, were reunited with their children.

I then went to Brasília, where I discussed leprosy issues with key figures in government and international organizations. The WHO representative in Brazil, Mr. Diego Victoria Mejía, noted that President Dilma Rousseff, who took office in January of that year, had made leprosy policy a national priority, and told me that with the understanding of the federal government he would do his utmost to find patients at the local level. Health Minister Dr. Alexandre Padilha expressed his commitment to eliminating leprosy, saying that he had secured a budget for fiscal 2012 to eliminate the disease by 2015. He also promised to attend Global Appeal 2012 and the human rights symposium. Deputy Minister Ramaís de Castro Silveira of the Brazilian presidential cabinet's Special Secretariat for Human Rights noted that he understood the UN resolution on leprosy and mentioned that President Rousseff had positioned human rights issues as a key policy issue. He promised to attend the Global Appeal 2012 and the human rights symposium and cooperate in whatever way possible.

Such a long way from Japan, Brazil is a truly enormous country. On this visit, I saw São Paulo, Rio de Janeiro, Brasília, and Maceió. Of the total itinerary of about 200 hours, almost half (100 hours) was spent traveling. I slept on a plane for four nights.

Countries visited in 2012	
January	● Peru
February	United States (New York, United States–Japan Foundation)
	Mexico (El Colegio de México SYLFF twentieth anniversary)
April	● Bangladesh
	Thailand (Myanmar nationwide ceasefire agreement: negotiations with armed ethnic organizations)
May	Switzerland (WHO General Assembly)
	United Kingdom (International Bar Association)
	Czech Republic (Visit to Václav Havel's grave)
	Jordan (WANA Forum)
June	United States (New York UN Convention of the Law of the Sea thirtieth anniversary)
	Brazil (Rio de Janeiro: Rio+20 UN Conference on Sustainable Development)
	● Russia
July	● Ukraine
	Myanmar (Nationwide ceasefire agreement: talks with government personnel)

	Thailand (Myanmar nationwide ceasefire agreement: negotiations with armed ethnic organizations)
August	● India
September	Thailand (Chiang Mai: Myanmar nationwide ceasefire agreement work)
	Malaysia (University of Malaya honorary degree)
	Poland (Jagiellonian University SYLFF twentieth anniversary)
October	● India
	Thailand (Myanmar nationwide ceasefire agreement: negotiations with armed ethnic organizations)
	Myanmar (Nationwide ceasefire agreement: talks with government personnel)
	Czech Republic (Forum 2000)
November	Myanmar (Nationwide ceasefire agreement: negotiations with armed ethnic organizations)
December	Myanmar (Nationwide ceasefire agreement: talks with government personnel; ceremony marking rice delivery to internally displaced persons)
	Thailand (Myanmar nationwide ceasefire agreement: negotiations with Myanmar armed ethnic organizations)

● Indicates a trip that features in this section.

WANA: West Asia–North Africa, a non-profit think tank based in Amman, Jordan, comprising intellectual leaders in economic, environmental, energy, educational, and social spheres.

SG2000: Sasakawa Global 2000 program. An agricultural project supporting farmers in need in Africa.

SYLFF: Sasakawa Young Leaders Fellowship Fund program.

Forum 2000: An annual international conference launched in 1997 when Václav Havel, Elie Wiesel, and the author invited world leaders to Prague for open debate on the major issues and challenges of the new millennium.

MAKING THE IMPOSSIBLE POSSIBLE

Interaction of a kind with Che Guevara—Republic of Peru, January 2012

Route: Narita International Airport → Los Angeles, United States (flight time: 10h; 3h stopover) → Lima, Peru (flight time: 8h 30m)—four nights—Lima → Los Angeles (flight time: 8h 30m; 3h stopover) → Narita (flight time: 10h)

I began 2012 with a trip to Peru in January. It was my third visit to Peru and the first in four years. The last time I had visited was in 2008. While neighboring Brazil is the only country in the world that still faces leprosy as a public health problem, Peru has few people affected by the disease, with thirty-two registered cases as of early 2011 and no significant changes over the following ten years.

On 28 January, I traveled about an hour by plane from the capital Lima to visit the city of Pucallpa in the Ucayali region of the Amazon. Peru's northern Loreto region and the Ucayali region I visited have relatively high case numbers. At the Hospital Amazónico de Yarinacocha, a leprosy treatment center, the director and the regional nurse in charge of the leprosy program raised various issues. "The patients live far from the hospital, and some of them have to travel by boat for several hours. Most of our patients are poor. The regional government is hardly aware of leprosy, and we have no specialists." Although Peru's registered case numbers are low, it may have a significant number of unidentified patients in areas that are difficult to access, such as the Amazon basin.

I met around twenty patients in the hospital, people affected by leprosy, and their families from the neighborhood. Except for the older adults, their disabilities were not so noticeable, and they seemed to be taking the treatment well.

As I have mentioned before, *The Motorcycle Diaries* is a memoir of Che Guevara's motorcycle trip across South America with friends, and on the way he visits leprosy facilities in various regions. In the book's film adaptation, Guevara swims down a river to a leprosarium in the Peruvian Amazon region and meets with the patients. At a time when elsewhere patients were kept in segregation, and discrimination was rampant, Guevara's attitude to treating patients was impressive. The leprosarium is the San Pablo Leprosarium in Iquitos, Loreto, about a four-day boat ride along the Ucayali River from Pucallpa, where I visited this time. I had heard that it was now abandoned but hankered to see it nevertheless. But in addition to the San Pablo Leprosarium, Guevara had also spent two days at this hospital in Pucallpa. There was someone who had met Guevara during that period, I was told, but they lived somewhere rather far away, and, unfortunately, I was unable to meet them.

In his diary, Guevara wrote:

> One of the things which left a very strong impression on us … was the way the hospital patients paid us farewell. They had all chipped in 100½ soles, which they gave to us along with an effusive letter. Afterward, some of them came to say goodbye to us personally, and in more than one case, tears were shed as they thanked us for the little bit of life we'd given them. We shook their hands, accepted their gifts, and sat with them, listening to football on the radio. If there's anything that will make us seriously dedicate ourselves to leprosy, it will be the affection shown to us by all the sick we've met along the way.

I'm sure that Guevara's interactions with leprosy patients were a significant experience in shaping his outlook on life.

On my return from Pucallpa to Lima, I suddenly began to sweat profusely, and I collapsed at the airfield in Pucallpa. According to my team, I lost consciousness for a moment. After briefly resting at the airfield, I arrived at the airport in Lima, where an ambulance was waiting for me. I was scheduled to leave for Brazil the next day, but an executive of the Peruvian-Japanese Association bundled me into the ambulance and took me to the hospital for a thorough examination, where they found an irregular heartbeat. The doctor who examined me was adamant that I simply had to be fitted with a pacemaker. After consulting with my doctor in Japan over the phone, I decided to undergo surgery to have a pacemaker installed. Despite the critical events of Global Appeal 2012 and the human rights symposium coming up in Brazil, I had to cancel my trip there. I had the pacemaker installed and left for home the following afternoon. The Nippon Foundation had once supported the hospital where I underwent surgery. It was a curious coincidence. I ended up with a class 1 disability in Peru. However, thankfully, since it is mild, I'm still going strong and traveling worldwide.

MAKING THE IMPOSSIBLE POSSIBLE

Patients found in a tea plantation—People's Republic of Bangladesh, April 2012

Route: Haneda International Airport → Hong Kong, China (flight time: 4h 30m; 3h stopover) → Dhaka, Bangladesh (flight time: 4h 20m)—four nights—Dhaka → Bangkok, Thailand (flight time: 2h 30m; overnight stopover) → Narita International Airport (flight time: 6h)

In April, I visited Bangladesh. I arrived in the capital city of Dhaka via Hong Kong. Despite arriving in the middle of the night, I received a welcome from Dr. A. Mannan Bangali of the WHO Bangladesh Office and Mr. Saiful Ahmad, deputy director of the Ministry of Health.

On my first full day, I discussed the leprosy situation with Health Minister Prof. A. F. Ruhal Haque, who wore an impressive necktie. I asked him to have leprosy taught as part of medical education, as doctors are less likely to be exposed to the disease, and he agreed.

After lunch, I attended a partners' meeting with the Ministry of Health, WHO, and NGOs. NGOs are highly active in Bangladesh, including Grameen Bank, founded by Dr. Muhammad Yunus, a Nobel Peace Prize winner and endorser of Global Appeal 2010. Another one is the Bangladesh Rural Advancement Committee, one of the world's largest NGOs, with an annual budget of around $615 million. There are also around eight leprosy-related organizations working together. At the conference, there was a presentation of the five-year national strategy finalized at year-end 2011. The strategy called for continued efforts for early detection and treatment and a 35 percent reduction in the proportion of new cases with visible disabilities by 2005, compared to 2000. It also specified that people affected by leprosy should play a role in efforts to fight the disease. TLM Bangladesh reported on its human rights project and activities supported by the Sasakawa Health Foundation to help small groups of people affected by leprosy become self-reliant through microfinance. We also heard that parliamentarians and other interested parties worked together to repeal the Lepers Act, a discriminatory law that had existed for more than 100 years since 1898, at the end of 2011.

On the morning of my second day, I visited a clinic in Dhaka operated by the Salvation Army, an international Christian NGO headquartered in the UK. It was established in 1865 and is currently engaged in social welfare, medical care, poverty alleviation, and other activities in 119 countries. Its leprosy-related efforts in Bangladesh include operating a clinic in the Mirpur area of Dhaka, where it provides treatment for ulcers and disabilities, protective footwear, counseling, and small grants for technical training. It also operates traveling clinics, called "skin camps," four times a year in remote areas, where most new patients are found. In 2011, the thirty-two patients discovered had zero disabilities. At the clinic, I met Mr. Mohamed Arif, an eighteen-year-old whose illness was discovered at a skin camp. He had no noticeable disability other than a slight nerve palsy in his hand and was working as a cell phone repairman. A sari factory operated by a person affected by leprosy was a business born out of microcredits supported by TMI Bangladesh. The factory employs forty people, including the founder and operator Aben Taher, to sew saris. A sales outlet near the factory sells an average of 1,000 garments per month, making it one of the most successful examples of self-support activities for people affected by leprosy. In the afternoon, I visited the home of someone affected by leprosy who was taking a hand in organizing the finances of a small group of colleagues. Mr. Bilkes proudly told me that the sixteen group members, who lived in poverty in a slum, chipped in to put around $1,200 in a bank account, which they used to purchase fish and vegetables for sale, and save $1.20 each from their income. I sensed that his quality of life must have improved: the house had a TV, and the children were attending school. I could not drink the beer I always looked forward to at the end of a workday because it was a Muslim country, so I went to bed early.

The Bangladeshi New Year was on 14 April, and a festival began in a downtown park early in the morning. The roads—usually clogged with cars, three-wheeled cabs, and rickshaws—were designated for pedestrians only, and families and couples dressed in red ethnic clothing headed to the park to watch the festivities, looking festive and cheerful.

In the afternoon, we drove to Srimangal in the northeastern Sylhet district, about 200 kilometers from Dhaka. Srimangal is a tea production area famous for Assam tea and is one of the few hilly areas in Bangladesh. Due to traffic, it took us two hours to get out of Dhaka, and I finally arrived at my accommodation just before sunset, after more than six hours of our planned four-hour drive. Our driver, who told us he was an ex-police officer, coolly sped down roads in the lane of oncoming traffic in order to get round buses and trucks, and any number of times I was scared half to death.

The next day, I heard a report on the activities of Health, Education and Economic Development (HEED), a Bangladeshi NGO working in the area. HEED was established in 1974 after Bangladesh gained independence and began working on leprosy after finding and treating patients on a tea plantation in 1976. In addition to inpatient and out-patient treatment, physiotherapy, ulcer care and plastic surgery, provision of protective shoes, and vocational training, HEED has raised awareness through puppet shows, folk songs, and plays. However, due to financial difficulties, in recent years it has restricted its activities to providing therapeutic drugs. HEED's President Anwar Hossain, a pastor, said, "Please pray for Bangladesh and people affected by leprosy. Let us work together for their sake." I encouraged him to keep up the good work, saying that such grassroots activities in remote areas are essential.

I then shared inspiring words with the people at HEED's clinic, the hospital run by the tea plantation administrator, and the tuberculosis and leprosy clinic in the government hospital. About twenty people affected by leprosy had gathered at the tea plantation hospital, and I listened to their stories as they showed me the ways leprosy had affected them. There was a man with crutches making baskets, a woman who had received HEED vocational training sewing on a sew-ing machine, a man working on the tea plantation, and a girl whose mother had also been diagnosed with leprosy.

After the tea plantation, I visited the border with India, about 3 kilometers away. Both Bangladeshi and Indian sides had bamboo barri-ers, with a buffer zone of about 50 meters between the two sides. On both sides of the road, there was a high fence of 7 or 8 meters, quite different from the easily scalable fences I had seen before on the border between Nepal and Bihar, India, stretching away into the distance.

I then returned to Dhaka, which took a five-hour drive, and met with Secretary Khurshed Alam of the Ministry of Foreign Affairs. The next morning, I met with Dr. Gowher Rizvi, international affairs advisor to the prime minister, at the Prime Minister's Office to complete my itinerary in Bangladesh.

In a country where leprosy data disappear—Russian Federation, June 2012

> Route: Narita International Airport → Moscow, Russia (flight time: 10h; 5h 40m stopover (transfer to a domestic flight: 3h 30m)) → Astrakhan, Russia (flight time: 2h) → Georgiyevsk, Russia (travel by car: 11h) → Leprosarium Terski → Krasnodar, Russia (travel by car: 7h 30m)

Each year, WHO publishes the latest global leprosy data for each region under its jurisdiction. The six regions are Southeast Asia, Africa, the Western Pacific, the Americas, the Middle East (Eastern Mediterranean), and Europe. Nevertheless, huge amounts of the data from the European region—which covers the largest area, fifty-three countries stretching from Western Europe to Central Asia—are missing. Perhaps one of the reasons is the current lack of leprosy-related medical problems in Europe.

I visited Russia and Ukraine in June and July. In Russia, I saw three leprosaria (Astrakhan, Terski, and Abinski) in the southern part of the country.

Arriving in Moscow at 4 p.m., after a ten-hour flight from Tokyo, I drove directly to the domestic terminal. The distance was about 80 kilometers, but it took three and a half hours due to traffic. The flight departed at 10 p.m. and took me to Astrakhan. Since getting my luggage out of the newly opened airport in Astrakhan proved challenging, I did not arrive at the hotel until after midnight.

The Volga, Russia's great river, flows out of the northwestern part of Moscow and heads south into the Caspian Sea, 3,500 kilometers away. Astrakhan is located at the river's delta, and the white walls and pastel-colored spires of its Kremlin (fortress) define its skyline. Once you step out of the Volga Delta, you see a vast expanse of dry semi-desert. For some reason, both the airport and the city had a faint pungent smell of pesticide-like compost in the air.

Dr. Romana Drabik, a seventy-five-year-old German woman, accompanied and supported me throughout the trip. She had worked as a medical practitioner in Dinslaken, a western German town, until eight years prior and had been personally involved in helping people affected by leprosy for more than thirty years. She met people affected by leprosy for the first time on a sightseeing trip in Mombasa, Kenya. She was shocked to see them begging and went directly to the mayor, saying: "What is the government doing by neglecting these people?" After that, she vowed to live with people affected by leprosy and traveled around India and Africa with relief supplies. In the early 1990s, she broadened her scope to the countries of the former Soviet Union and continued to visit leprosaria throughout the region. She had many friends among leprosy specialists throughout Russia, and her personal connections were indispensable to my trip.

Our first stop was the National Institute of Leprosy Training and Research in Astrakhan. Built in 1948 as an annex to the leprosy hospital that opened in 1896, the institute became a center of leprosy research and technical guidance in the former Soviet Union. Under the current director, Dr. Victor Duyko, the institute serves as a base for fighting leprosy in Russia and other Commonwealth of Independent States (CIS) member countries.

The day after we arrived in Astrakhan, the institute hosted a meeting of Russian and CIS leprosy experts. Representing WHO was Dr. Sumana Barua, team leader of the Global Leprosy Program. He came from India to introduce WHO's leprosy program and stressed the need for meticulous information exchange with Russia and other CIS nations.

Astrakhan Institute staff reported that no new cases had been detected in Russia in the last three or four years, and as of early 2012, there were 382 registered cases. However, this figure is somewhat questionable. According to WHO standards, leprosy is considered cured after six to twelve months of medication, after which cured patients should be removed from registries. In Russia, however, once a patient is cured of leprosy, they remain on the registry, making it impossible to determine from what is noted there how many patients have completed treatment. WHO must conduct a thorough examination of the data.

The Astrakhan Institute also functions as a leprosarium. I spoke with people who had been living there for decades and those who had short rehabilitation or disease treatment stays. Sisters Maria, sixty-two, and Nina, fifty-eight, lived in one of the two-story rooms with bright blue exterior walls. It was a tasteful room with an easy chair, a simple bed, and a large carpet on the wall. They told me that Dr. Dukyo had improved residents' lives since his arrival. Indeed, the atmosphere was homey, with beautiful lawns, flowerbeds full of color, and a small pond surrounded by cranes and lotus ornamentation. There were also remnants of the Soviet era, including a 3-meter-tall white statue of Lenin and the ruins of a prison exclusively for people affected by leprosy.

About an hour's drive from Astrakhan lies the remote village of Vostochnoe, where people affected had completed their leprosy treatment. Later, people other than those affected by leprosy also began to move there. Today, only fifteen households of a community of 1,000 or so are families of people affected by leprosy.

When we got to the middle of the village, all we saw was a single wide gravel road stretching on for about 50 meters, completely devoid of people, and I was a little puzzled as to where the village was. Upon closer inspection, we saw that on either side there were

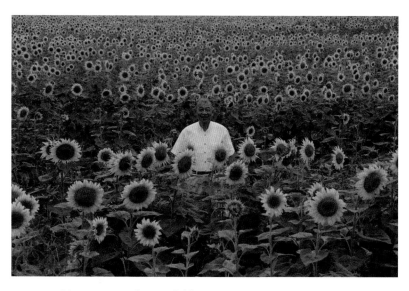

98. A vast sunflower field in Russia (Russia, June 2012)

old fences constructed with bits of wood and tin, and roofs peeking out from the bushes. Dr. Dukyo led us to one such fence, where an elderly couple appeared from their vegetable garden. Through a quick conversation, we learned that they were living there on a pension, and their teenage son practiced judo. In another house, a seventy-six-year-old widow lived alone on a monthly pension of about 6,000 rubles (around US$82). She had no gas or running water and had to live in quite difficult circumstances because she could not afford the 5,000 rubles (about US$70) to install pipes. She shared her plight: "During my short stay at the Astrakhan Leprosarium, I was robbed, and they took everything, even my iron and other necessities. Since the collapse of the Soviet Union, the village population has declined, with young people moving to the big cities and only the elderly remaining." Traveling the world, I fully comprehend how depopulation is both a Japanese and a global problem.

After two days in Astrakhan, we headed about 700 kilometers west in a nine-passenger minibus toward Georgiyevsk to visit the Terski Leprosarium, our next destination. This involved four hours of driv-

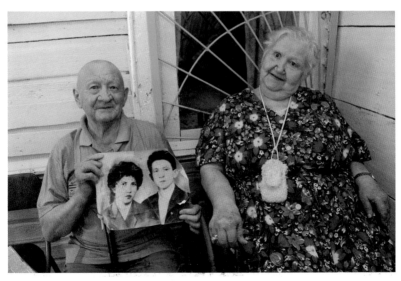

99. A husband and wife at the Terksi Leprosarium, with a wedding photograph taken years before (Russia, June 2012)

ing in the middle of the arid steppe, with a clear horizon as far as the eye could see. For lunch, we stopped in Elista, the capital of Kalmykia, an autonomous republic within the Russian Federation. Kalmyk is the only Buddhist region in Europe, with a population of less than 300,000. The name derives from a Turkish word meaning "those who stayed," referring to their choice not to convert to Islam. The Kalmyks were originally nomadic people who believed in Tibetan Buddhism. In the late eighteenth century, Russians, Ukrainians, and other settlers forced some of the Kalmyks to convert to Eastern Orthodox Christianity, so many emigrated to other countries. It is said that those who, for whatever reason, could not migrate stayed and formed Kalmykia. The director of the health department in Elista looked Japanese. At the Tibetan Buddhist temple with a statue of Shakyamuni Buddha, people with Asian faces prayed fervently.

We said goodbye to the Republic of Kalmykia and continued driving along a monotonous flat road with few oncoming cars when suddenly we came upon a vast sunflower field. For more than an hour, the road was lined with sunflowers on both sides, and strangely enough, not a single soul was to be seen in the fields. We had no idea why this should be. On the way, we passed a group of forty or fifty middle-aged cyclists from Beijing who were on their way to London by bicycle. A large truck was accompanying the group, probably to treat anyone who fell sick and to repair broken bicycles, but I wondered how many days it would take them to complete the journey. When I was young, there were so-called "magic buses" from London to Delhi. I remember the trip took about forty days, and I longed to take such a bus at least once. After an eleven-hour drive from Astrakhan, we finally arrived in Georgiyevsk a little after 7 p.m. After a simple dinner, I went to bed.

The next morning, 2 July, we went to the Terski Leprosarium. This is the oldest leprosarium in Russia, established 115 years ago. It is a beautiful facility surrounded by lush forests. At the time of my visit, it had fifty-one residents, forty-three staff, and the director, Dr. Mikhail Gridasov Ivanovic. Like the other leprosaria I visited on this trip, Terski is the final home for those who have been cured of leprosy but have chosen to stay here for family reasons or to escape social discrimination. One older woman said in hushed tones: "My children know I have leprosy, but my grandchildren and neighbors do not." Most people responded "niet" (no) to being photographed, seemingly fearing discrimination if their photos were made public.

As I walked through the dimly lit hospital entrance, I saw stunning landscapes and portraits decorating the walls. One of the paintings, depicting a lively scene on a boat, was a masterpiece so full of energy that the people seemed ready to jump out of the picture at any moment. The artist was a former leprosarium resident. I was amazed to learn that such a wonderful work was produced by someone in this community. However, no one had any idea of the name of the artist. Inadvertently, I realized, I had come up against one of the effects of an old, creaking bureaucracy.

On my last day in Russia, we headed toward the Black Sea and drove seven and a half hours, around 600 kilometers, to the Abinsky Leprosarium in the Krasnodar Krai of the western North Caucasus region. A military doctor built the leprosarium in 1905 to accommodate the rapidly increasing number of people affected by leprosy. A portrait of the doctor hung on the wall. Dr. Marina Georgievna had worked there for twenty-nine years, having succeeded her father as director of Abinsky after his thirty-year stint in the role. She said there were 500 residents when her father was director, but now there were forty, yet the number of employees was more than triple that, at 131. The most recent resident was admitted in 2009. I asked an older woman affected by leprosy her name and hometown. But before she could answer, a staff member beside her said: "Her name is Katya, and she has lived here for forty years. She's from Astrakhan." Even though I told the staff that I'd like to hear directly from the residents, they never had a chance to speak. The staff immediately interrupted them as soon as they started to say something. Regrettably, I never had a proper conversation with the residents there.

When I asked the staff why they did not treat patients with diseases other than leprosy, even though there were extra beds available, they replied in a firm tone: "We are not allowed to examine patients with other diseases because it is against the law." Russia had not yet implemented the WHO's integration policy by converting leprosy facilities into general hospitals. The nation's leprosy facilities lagged behind in the global leprosy treatment movement. The fact that 131 staff members were working with forty people affected by leprosy was not so much a reflection of the extensive care provided as of the fact that the employees had secure livelihoods due to the people affected by leprosy. The staff did not allow the residents to speak directly with me, reinforcing my impression of the facility. Was this really the right approach? Did the lives they had lived, so filled with hardships, mean nothing? Was it right that we just go on our way and forget about them? In addition to keeping proper records of events, we must pass on the evidence of each person's life in a tangible form before the memory fades. To this end, I wanted to hear how the people affected by leprosy I met there truly felt, even if just a little, about what kind of life they really wanted to lead. Did the unknown painters who surely existed at the Terski Leprosarium not want to express their feelings through their art?

What the white coat symbolizes—Ukraine, July 2012

Route: Moscow, Russia (flight time: 2h; overnight stopover) → Odesa, Ukraine (flight time: 2h)—one night—Odesa → Moscow (flight time: 2h; 1h 45m stopover) → Narita International Airport (flight time: 9h 25m)

After leaving Russia, I went to Odesa, a city in southern Ukraine. This is a port city on the Black Sea with a population of around 1 million. It is the third largest city in Ukraine after the capital Kyiv and the industrial center Kharkiv. Known worldwide for its art and culture, Odesa attracts many tourists every year to enjoy the beautiful cityscape, concerts, opera, and summer beaches. The long staircase from the film *Battleship Potemkin* is a symbol of the city. An hour-and-a-half drive from Odesa, at the edge of a fertile plain, is the Kutschurgan Leprosarium, Ukraine's only national facility for leprosy. Kutschurgan is the name of the region, originally established in 1808 by German immigrants fleeing war, and it currently has six villages with a population of 3,000.

During my visit, the temperature was 33 degrees C, slightly higher than in Japan, but the humidity was low, making it a pleasant stay. There were only seventeen registered patients in all of Ukraine. All of them were people affected by leprosy who had been fully cured.

Per the WHO's definition, once people complete their treatment, they are no longer called "patients." However, in Ukraine and Russia, those who have recovered continue to be registered as such.

Surprisingly, it was not the Ministry of Health that first brought the leprosy treatment regimen MDT to this country, but Dr. Romana Drabik, my companion whom I mentioned in the section on my trip to Russia. She brought MDT to Ukraine in 1997. "When I first brought MDT, I smuggled it through Odesa customs as if it were contraband. But when we gave it to patients in Kutschurgan, the treatment cured them perfectly. After that, I was able to bring MDT through customs with impunity," Dr. Drabik said, smiling mischievously like a little girl. At the time, the WHO was unaware there was a leprosarium there.

We arrived at the Kutschurgan Leprosarium after a 60-kilometer drive of about two hours from Odesa. The building brought to mind a school. According to Deputy Director Dr. Yuriy Rybak, the leprosarium was established in 1945 by a famous ophthalmologist from Odesa to treat leprosy patients, who were on the increase at the time. As a young man, this ophthalmologist treated leprosy patients in a hospital in Samarkand, Uzbekistan, leading to his decision to build a hospital in his own country. The leprosarium was built in an abandoned house and has treated 300 patients. Many of them came across the border from other countries. At one time, there were 150 patients, but now twelve people were living there, seven men and five women. The last time officials found a patient was in 2004.

The staff greeted me warmly in Japanese, saying, "Hello, welcome," using phrases that they must have practiced very hard. They showed us to a room in an old ward, where doctors and nurses in white coats surprised me by pointing to the room's wardrobe, saying, "Feel free to wear one of the white coats hanging there." I have visited leprosaria worldwide, but this was the first time I was asked to wear a white coat. Putting on that white coat creates a hierarchical relationship between the examiner and the person being examined (the patient), so I just could not bring myself to do it.

Dr. Vladimir Fedorovich Naumov, the director who had worked there for forty-three years, explained, "I wanted to help patients. Somehow it became my destiny. It used to be a very challenging disease. Many could hardly walk." When I asked him about his most memorable patient, he replied: "About ten years ago, a Korean patient with a very advanced disability suddenly received a visit from his son, aged sixteen or seventeen, all the way from Kazakhstan. The next day, the son was found murdered, and the investigation decided that his father, the patient, was the culprit. I insisted that the father could not have committed the murder because of his physical disability, but the court did not accept my argument. The father spent six years in prison. We continued to help him in prison, but he contracted tuberculosis after his health weakened, eventually dying here shortly after his release. He is now laid to rest in the leprosarium's cemetery. It is still unclear what really happened, as it was such a bizarre incident." His expression told me he was still disconsolate about the outcome.

The roads inside the leprosarium were well paved and lined with trees and flowers on both sides. I visited the home of eighty-year-old Anastasia, who had planted gooseberries and grapes in her front garden. She had decorated her house beautifully with family photos,

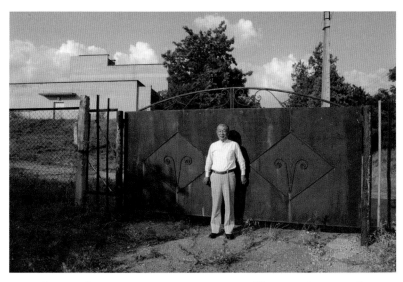

100. The Kutschurgan Leprosarium, once cut off by staunch gates (Ukraine, July 2012)

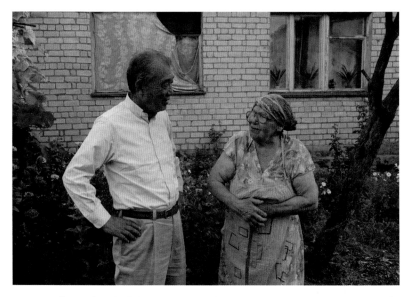

101. With an elderly lady at the Kutschurgan Leprosarium (Ukraine, July 2012)

carpets, and several portraits hanging on the walls. A widow, she said, "I live alone, but my son is in Odesa. Now I have four cats to talk to." I also met eighty-year-old Maria, who expressed her heartache over the news from distant Japan, saying, "I pray to God for the people of Japan who are suffering from the Great East Japan Earthquake."

The cemetery graves were magnificent, engraved with the names and portraits of those who had died at the leprosarium. The gravestone of the Korean man the director mentioned also had a picture on it. Many of the deceased were from Kazakhstan, Uzbekistan, and other foreign countries, having died alone and far from home.

His Holiness the Dalai Lama and leprosy—Delhi, Himachal Pradesh, and Madhya Pradesh, India, August 2012

Route: Narita International Airport → Bangkok, Thailand (flight time: 6h 30m; 1h 20m stopover) → Delhi, India (flight time: 4h 30m)—one night—Delhi → Dharamshala, Himachal Pradesh (flight time: 1h 30m)—one night—Dharamshala → Delhi (flight time: 1h 25m)—four

nights—Delhi → Bhopal, Madhya Pradesh (flight time: 1h 40m)—two
nights—Bhopal → Mumbai, Maharashtra (flight time: 1h; 5h stopover)
→ Narita (flight time: 9h)

In August, I visited India's capital Delhi, the northern state of
Himachal Pradesh, and the central state of Madhya Pradesh. The
morning after I arrived in Delhi, I traveled by air to Dharamsala,
Himachal Pradesh. Dharamsala is the heart of Tibetans in exile and
the current home of His Holiness, the fourteenth Dalai Lama, the
supreme leader of the Tibetan religion. The city is in a hilly area,
about 1,500 meters above sea level. Despite having been to almost all
twenty-eight states in India, it was the first time I had visited this
state, which has never had many people affected by leprosy.

At the time of my visit, the rainy season was just around the corner, so it rained heavily from time to time. The weather was rainy or
cloudy throughout my stay. The leprosy colony in Palampur, the only
one in the area, was established in 1917 by a Christian organization.
It once had thirty households, down to seventeen when I visited.
Some people moved there on foot via Delhi, crossing Nepal from
Tibet in honor of His Holiness the Dalai Lama. With support from
Christian organizations and the Tibetan government-in-exile, Ramish,
one of the colony's residents, told me: "It's a beautiful life here.
There's no discrimination. His Holiness, the Dalai Lama, regularly
sends me daily necessities, and I am living a happy life."

I had met His Holiness the Dalai Lama several times in Tokyo and
Prague, but this was the first time I met him in his hometown. He has
endorsed our Global Appeal twice and shown understanding and
cooperation in various ways with our fight against leprosy. This time,
I met with him to make a video to further spread the message that
discrimination against people affected by leprosy is unjust. His
Holiness the Dalai Lama said: "About twenty years ago, when I visited
the Indian state of Odisha with my late brother, there were 500,000
people affected by leprosy. I wanted to do something for them, but
the number was so large that I could do nothing. It is wonderful that
so many patients have been cured. I would like to pay tribute to those
who have been working on this issue. Each person's heart must
change if we are to change the world." For the video, he communicated this message: "We are the same human beings, brothers and

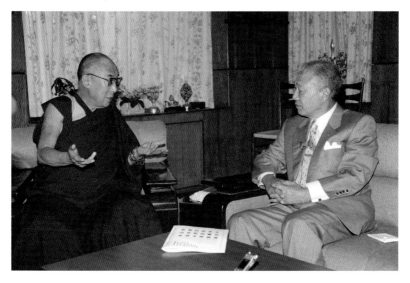

102. His Holiness the Dalai Lama, passionately discoursing on leprosy (Himachal Pradesh, India, August 2012)

sisters. Let us treat each other with compassion and love so that all can live happily as members of a community."

After meeting with His Holiness the Dalai Lama, I returned from Dharamsala to Delhi to attend a meeting of National Forum leaders. This meeting was held following the resignation of Dr. P. K. Gopal, who had played a central role in the organization since its founding, and the appointment of Dr. Vagavathali Narsappa from Andhra Pradesh as the new president. In Delhi, I met with the national health secretary, Dr. P. K. Pradan, and WHO's regional director for Southeast Asia, Dr. Samlee Plianbangchang. I also attended the S-ILF board meeting and gave media interviews before flying to Bhopal, the capital of Madhya Pradesh, early the next day.

In Bhopal, I asked the state government officials to work to reduce case numbers by ensuring early detection and treatment, to improve the lives of people affected by leprosy, and to eliminate discrimination. The state's pension for people affected by leprosy is as low as 150 rupees (about US$1.80) per month. In other states, the average is 500 rupees; in Delhi, a pension specifically for people affected by leprosy is 1,800 rupees per month. I immediately joined the National

Forum's President Narsappa and trustee and state leader Sarang Gaydhane to meet with Chief Minister Shivraj Singh Chouhan. Mr. Gaydhane presented a survey of the thirty-four leprosy colonies in the state and a proposal to the state government, which he had compiled in preparation for the day's meeting. I also brought up the example of Bihar, which had begun to increase its leprosy pension from 200 rupees to 1,000 rupees per month and asked the state government to continue negotiations with the National Forum to increase the pension payouts. Chief Minister Chouhan promised on the spot to increase the pension to 1,000 rupees as requested and also said that he would take good care of the other requests. After the meeting, I congratulated Mr. Gaydhane, saying, "That went well." He replied bluntly: "I won't be able to believe it until I get a response in writing." I understood his feelings, as so many petitions have been ignored in the past. "In Bihar, I made it happen through multiple visits. I'll come here as many times as I need to. Let's work together for the good of everyone." Once I said that, he finally looked relaxed.

After that, I met with Justice A. K. Saxena, the acting head of the state human rights commission, and held a press conference in front of about thirty members of the media. There, he explained the chief minister's promise to increase the leprosy pension, which was widely reported in the newspapers the following day.

On the following day, 31 August, we drove three hours from Bhopal, the state capital, to a city somewhat further afield, Indore. On the way, Mr. Gaydhane took us to see the Magaspur colony. He was on crutches that day. The day before, he had to endure the pain of wearing a prosthetic leg that did not fit because of the prominent role he had to play. The colony had a dairy business established with a microcredit from S-ILF that wholesaled 20 liters of milk a day to the state government and others. Each team of four people was earning about 18,000 rupees a month. In Ram Avtar colony, which we visited next, a team of thirty people was growing vegetables on government-leased land with a microcredit from S-ILF. There had been little rainfall and no harvest the previous year, but the rain had been heavy this year, promising a good harvest. When we spoke to Ms. Kalavati Wasuniya, who was studying to be a nurse on a scholarship from S-ILF, and told her that she was the pride of her village, she struck a determined pose and said: "I will study hard."

501

The last place we visited was the colony of Mr. Gaydhane, the state representative. I attended a meeting of nearly 100 residents and saw children who had been cured of leprosy, young people receiving scholarships to attend university, and the lively residents. I realized how indispensable the leadership and unity of each colony is to improving once abysmal conditions and inspiring children to have dreams and hopes for the future, despite their difficult lives. With his ability, Mr. Gaydhane should have been able to run a business with a microcredit from S-ILF. However, he secretly went begging once a week, saying he would be the very last one who would need to beg, and used the money he earned to unite the thirty-four colonies and serve as a unifying force for the organization.

The Second International Symposium on Leprosy and Human Rights—Delhi, India, October 2012

On 4 October 2012, the Nippon Foundation sponsored the Second International Symposium on Leprosy and Human Rights, held in New Delhi, India. The symposium was meant to promote a broader understanding of the Principles and Guidelines, encouraging governments worldwide to comply with and implement the UN resolution adopted in 2010 to "Eliminate Discrimination against Persons Affected by Leprosy and Their Families." The plan was to hold this international symposium once in each of the world's five regions (the Americas, Asia, the Middle East, Africa, and Europe). The first one was held in February 2012 in Rio de Janeiro, Brazil.

This second symposium for the Asian region was attended by key government officials from the host country, India, and representatives of international organizations and NGOs. Representatives from organizations for people affected by leprosy also came from India, Indonesia, the Philippines, and Ethiopia and participated in lively discussions.

Following video messages from UN Secretary-General Ban Ki-moon and His Holiness the Dalai Lama, I delivered a keynote speech in which I made a powerful appeal for abolishing discriminatory laws, institutions, and social practices that remain in India and other countries. India's Social Justice Minister Mukul Balkrishna Wasnik mentioned that the government recognizes the significant challenge in reintegrating people affected by leprosy into society. He also promised that the government would protect the human rights of people affected by leprosy and their family members and support them through various welfare policies. Adi Josep, a leader of an Indonesian organization for people affected by leprosy, pointed out the importance of community activities in motivating local governments in disseminating the Principles and Guidelines. Chuo University Professor Yozo Yokota, who promoted UN resolutions as a Special Rapporteur of the UN Sub-Commission on the Promotion and Protection of Human Rights, explained the resolution process and highlighted some of the articles in the Principles and Guidelines that he considered important. Stanley Prasejo, a vice chair of the Indonesian National Commission on Human Rights, introduced relief and welfare programs for people affected by leprosy and their families that public institutions offer in Thailand, Indonesia, India, the Philippines, and other countries.

The last session of the symposium was a statement by the Indian parliamentary group on their commitment to future efforts. Moderated by parliament representative Dinesh Trivedi, the session heard opinions from national Human Resource Development Minister Nandamuri Purandareswari and Mr. Madhu Goud Yaskhi, a key parliamentary group member, among others. Topics of discussion included the importance of resolving the non-medical issues associated with leprosy, improving the quality of life of people affected by leprosy and their families and reintegrating them into society, and communicating knowledge to and educating the general public.

Finally, the attendees decided to issue a resolution for the symposium. With Professor Yokota leading the discussion, the symposium resolved to form a working group of experts and concerned parties to examine and propose what was needed to put the Principles and Guidelines into practice. While we only had one day for the symposium, it was a very fruitful event.

5

OVERCOMING THE STAGNATION

2013–15

Accelerating the motorcycle of elimination toward a leprosy-free world

At the end of 2010, Brazil became the only country that had yet to achieve the leprosy elimination benchmark as defined by the World Health Organization (WHO) (less than one patient per 10,000 population). The UN General Assembly also adopted a resolution to eliminate discrimination against the disease. The "motorcycle" seemed to be making great progress, with treatment as the front wheel and human rights issues as the rear wheel. However, elimination in this final country was proving far from straightforward, and the success achieved in so many other countries had bred a sense of relief and complacency in the fight, with the result that leprosy elimination efforts showed signs of slackening worldwide. Many governments had become less mindful of the need for treatment activities and reduced the allocations in their budgets, which led to annual detection figures continuing to hover between 200,000 and 250,000. Delays in the detection of new patients meant that many new cases of leprosy resulted in disabilities, and case numbers among children saw no reduction. In countries where leprosy was still endemic, or high burden, there were still numerous inaccessible "hot spots," with extremely high prevalence rates. To break through this situation, in July 2013 the Nippon Foundation joined WHO in inviting health ministers and vice ministers of health from seventeen leprosy-endemic countries to Bangkok, Thailand, for an International Leprosy Summit. This resulted in the issuing of the "Bangkok Declaration: Toward a Leprosy-Free World," which aimed to give a boost to further efforts to overcome the remaining challenges. The Nippon Foundation announced that it would provide a total of $200 million over the next five years, starting in 2014, to revitalize activities in endemic countries.

The discovery of new patients usually means a temporary rise in prevalence rates, which in some countries is a source of shame because it shows that despite official elimination a lot of previously unidentified cases of leprosy yet remain. I call this attitude "elimination trauma." And yet, in other countries, like India, we see people proactively develop initiatives to discover new patients.

Following the 2010 UN resolution, we decided to organize a series of international symposiums on leprosy and human rights in five regions worldwide to inform as many people as possible about the "Principles and Guidelines" for eliminating discrimination against people affected by leprosy. The first of these symposiums was held in Rio de Janeiro, Brazil, in January 2012, the second in India, in October 2012, the third in Ethiopia, in 2013, and the fourth in Morocco, in 2014, with the final conference taking place in Geneva, Switzerland, in 2015. We then presented a report with follow-up recommendations and action plans relating to the UN resolution, based on the discussions that took place in these symposiums.

Countries visited in 2013	
January	Myanmar
	● United Kingdom
	Vietnam (Lecture at Vietnam National University, Hanoi)
	China (Hong Kong Third International Conference on Sign Linguistics and Deaf Education)

February	Myanmar (Nationwide ceasefire agreement: talks with government personnel)
	Thailand (Myanmar nationwide ceasefire agreement: negotiations with representatives of armed ethnic organizations)
March	Myanmar (two visits) (Nationwide ceasefire agreement: talks with government personnel)
	Thailand (Myanmar nationwide ceasefire agreement: negotiations with representatives of armed ethnic organizations)
April	● India
May	Greece (National and Kapodistrian University of Athens SYLFF twentieth anniversary)
	● Switzerland
	Thailand (two visits) (Myanmar nationwide ceasefire agreement: negotiations with representatives of armed ethnic organizations)
	Myanmar (two visits) (Nationwide ceasefire agreement: talks with government personnel)
June	Jordan (WANA Forum)
	United Kingdom (Great Britain Sasakawa Foundation board meeting; UK–Japan Global Seminar at Chatham House)
	Palestinian Authority (Jericho Agro-Industrial Park; Zaatari Refugee Camp)
	Thailand (Myanmar nationwide ceasefire agreement: negotiations with armed ethnic organizations for Myanmar ceasefire)
	Myanmar (Nationwide ceasefire agreement: talks with government personnel)
July	● Uzbekistan
	● Turkey

	● Tajikistan
	● Thailand
August	Thailand (two visits) (Myanmar nationwide ceasefire agreement: negotiations with armed ethnic organizations)
	● India
September	● Belgium
	● Ethiopia
	● India
	Thailand (two visits) (Myanmar nationwide ceasefire agreement: negotiations with armed ethnic organizations)
October	Myanmar (Festival of artists with disabilities; Myanmar nationwide ceasefire agreement: talks with government personnel)
	● India (Jadavpur University SYLFF twentieth anniversary)
November	Myanmar (Nationwide ceasefire agreement: talks with government personnel)
December	● Brazil
	● Colombia

● Indicates a trip that features in this section.

SYLFF: Sasakawa Young Leaders Fellowship Fund program.

WANA: West Asia–North Africa, a non-profit think tank based in Amman, Jordan, comprising intellectual leaders in economic, environmental, energy, educational, and social spheres.

Global Appeal 2013—United Kingdom of Great Britain and Northern Ireland, January 2013

Route: Narita International Airport → London, United Kingdom (flight time: 12h 40m)—three nights—London → Narita (flight time: 12h; 2h stopover) → Hanoi, Vietnam—three nights—Hanoi → Hong

Kong, China (flight time: 1h 50m)—one night—Hong Kong →
Haneda International Airport (flight time: 3h 40m)

The year 2013 began with the Global Appeal in January, in London, pressing for the elimination of discrimination against people affected by leprosy and their families. The eighth of our Global Appeals, this one was held at The Law Society building in London with the full endorsement of the International Bar Association (IBA) and was signed by forty-six law societies from forty countries worldwide. Despite the lack of any medical reason why people affected by leprosy should be segregated, laws around the world continue to penalize them for having the disease, and we were hopeful that the IBA's endorsement would go some way toward encouraging the repeal of as many discriminatory laws as possible.

This was the third time we held our Global Appeal in London. Following on from our appeal in 2008 with the endorsement of international human rights NGOs and the appeal in 2009 that had been endorsed by world religious leaders, this year we had the endorsement of the world's lawyers. Examples of discriminatory legislation relating to people affected by leprosy and their families include regulations in India used as a justification for divorce under Indian marriage laws, and in the United States where the fact that leprosy remains on the communicable disease list from the federal Department of Health and Human Services results in the blocking of issuance of visas. In my opening address, I called for the annulment of all the many ossified laws that remain in place but no longer have any practical application and continue to engender prejudice and discrimination by their existence. Among the more than 200 participants at the event was Baroness Helena Kennedy QC, co-chair of the IBA's Human Rights Institute, who said in her speech that lawyers have a responsibility to be the voice of the voiceless and to promote appropriate amendments to laws. Also present were President Vagavathali Narsappa and Vice President Guntreddy Venugopal of National Forum India (NFI), representing persons affected by leprosy worldwide. President Narsappa said: "I do not have the words to express how privileged and proud I felt to represent my country at the Law Society's hall here in London as a grassroots activist and as a person affected by leprosy."

MAKING THE IMPOSSIBLE POSSIBLE

The IBA's main representative was Tim Hughes, its deputy executive director. He went on to become a proactive partner in our efforts, among other things attending the International Symposium on Leprosy and Human Rights that followed Global Appeal 2013. To my great honor, in October 2014, I received the IBA's "Rule of Law" award during an annual meeting held in Tokyo.

From London, I traveled via Japan to Hanoi, Vietnam. In Vietnam, I had a meeting on educational issues for people with impaired hearing and then stopped in Hong Kong to attend the opening ceremony of the third International Conference on Sign Linguistics and Deaf Education in Asia.

Happiness is to see the joy of others—Jharkhand, India, April 2013

Route: Narita International Airport → Delhi, India (flight time: 8h)—one night—Delhi → Ranchi, Jharkhand, India (flight time: 1h 45m)—three nights—Ranchi → Delhi (flight time: 1h 45m; 4h stopover) → Narita (flight time: 8h)

In April, I visited the state of Jharkhand in eastern India. On my visit ten years prior, the prevalence rate (the number of registered patients per 10,000 population) in Jharkhand was extremely high, at 13.0. However, despite the difficult conditions—numerous hill tribes and lack of transportation—that figure had been successfully reduced to 0.7. The two main aims of my visit were to further boost these developments and to lobby for increased pensions for colony residents.

I arrived in Ranchi, the state capital, by air via Delhi. A week before, ten Maoist leaders were killed in a clash with another insurgent group. The Maoists shot four police officers on 4 April; two days later, they blew up a local railroad and called for a strike. Ranchi was seething with tension, and travel to the suburbs was restricted.

Nevertheless, I drove about an hour from the airport to visit the Murhu Community Health Center in Khunti district and offer words of encouragement to the eight people affected by leprosy who lived there and the female health workers caring for them. A ten-year-old girl and several people with limb disabilities were under the dedicated care of the health workers. In hospitals throughout the world, the work of women serves as a great asset.

Returning to the city center, in the absence of the state chief minister and other ministers, I met with L. Khiangte, the principal secretary of the welfare department, and K. Vidyasagar, the administrative head and principal secretary of the health department. The principal secretary of welfare responded coolly: his department was not directly concerned with leprosy but would do what it could. The principal secretary of health, in contrast, was enthusiastic: a drastic decrease in case numbers had been seen; his department would maintain this issue at the highest priority and promote further elimination measures. At both meetings, Mr. Narsappa, president of NFI, and Mr. Jainuddin, NFI's state leader representing fifty-eight colonies in Jharkhand, were present, and took a leading role in the negotiations. As WHO Ambassador for Leprosy Elimination, my role was to be a liaison, introducing the NFI representatives to the government and bringing them together.

I then attended a meeting with members of NFI state organizations. About thirteen people, including Mr. Jainuddin, were present and reported on their activities.

At a meeting with Mr. Ram Sewak Sharma, Jharkhand's chief secretary and number-two state official, I joined Mr. Narsappa and Mr. Jainuddin in an appeal for an increase in the disability pension, which is as low as 400 rupees (about US$5) per month. Chief Secretary Sharma promised to cooperate to the fullest extent. In my experience, getting pensions increased with one or two requests is impossible. However, if people affected by leprosy are persistent in negotiating with the government, and I show my willingness to visit frequently, the path to higher pensions opens wide. This is something I have learned through experience, which is one reason why "giving up" is not part of my vocabulary.

After a courtesy call on Justice Narayan Roy, the head of the State Human Rights Commission, I visited the Indira Nagar leprosy colony. This is a relatively large colony of 550 residents. I was looking forward to seeing the growth of the trees I planted there commemorating my visit ten years earlier. However, as the colony had developed and amenities improved, the barrack huts had transformed into rows of mud-walled houses, with no trace to be seen of the trees I planted. Despite the improved living conditions, wooden wheelbarrows still sat here and there in the corners and under the eaves of the houses, waiting to carry severely disabled and elderly people to beg, indicating that residents were still forced to do so to make ends meet.

The next morning, I visited the university dormitory, where I met Sonali and Sikha Mahato, two female students studying at a four-year nursing college on Sasakawa-India Leprosy Foundation (S-ILF) scholarships. At the 350-student women's nursing college, they told me, eyes shining, "We never imagined we would go on to higher education. We are so thankful to God and everyone. In the future, we want to work for the elderly and the disabled in the colonies." Meeting these girls reminded me of Tolstoy's words on happiness coming from seeing joy in others.

After that, I had a press conference before visiting Ranchi's Nirmala colony, where 150 people lived along a ditch running alongside the main road. The residents told me that in the past their huts would be affected whenever the ditch or the road flooded, but a recently built concrete levee had somewhat improved the situation. However, there had been no change in the stench from the garbage clogging the waterway and the clouds of mosquitoes.

It is no easy task to chat with people who live in despair, eking out a living by begging. No matter how much I tried to convince them that they could improve their lives, their eyes, full of distrust, would reject my words. One woman, who hugged her knees and cast her eyes downward while listening, had an expression that said: "Talk is cheap. We need to see change now. Show us change, and we'll believe you."

Preparing for the leprosy summit in Bangkok—Swiss Confederation, May 2013

Route (first trip, 5–7 May): Narita International Airport → Munich, Germany (flight time: 12h; 2h stopover) → Geneva, Switzerland (flight time: 1h)—two nights—Geneva → Munich (flight time: 1h; 2h 30m stopover) → Bangkok, Thailand (flight time: 10h 40m; 4h 20m stopover) → Yangon, Myanmar (flight time: 1h 25m)—four nights— Yangon → Bangkok (flight time: 1h 25m)—one night—Bangkok → Haneda International Airport (flight time: 6h)

Route (second trip, 21–3 May): Narita International Airport → Paris, France (flight time: 12h 35m; 2h stopover) → Geneva, Switzerland (flight time: 1h)—three nights—Geneva → Zürich, Switzerland (flight time: 50m; stopover) → Bangkok, Thailand (flight time: 11h; 2h stopover) → Yangon, Myanmar (flight time: 1h)—two nights (peace rally)—Yangon → Bangkok (flight time: 1h; 2h 40m stopover) → Haneda International Airport (flight time: 6h)

In May 2013, I visited Geneva twice. First, I took advantage of the annual meeting of the International Coordinating Committee of National Institutions for the Promotion and Protection of Human Rights to ask each country's representative of the National Human Rights Commission to endorse our upcoming Global Appeal 2014. I also raised awareness about leprosy at a lunch session co-sponsored by the International Coordinating Committee and the Nippon Foundation. The session was chaired by Dr. Mousa Burayzat from Jordan, the outgoing committee chair. Representing people affected by leprosy were José Ramirez Jr., managing editor of *The Star* newspaper in the United States, and Vagavathali Narsappa and Guntreddy Venugopal, president and vice president of NFI. They shared personal experiences of discrimination and the problems associated with leprosy. Mr. Ramirez related his anecdote about being transported to an isolation facility in a hearse.

I asked the representatives of the human rights commissions who took part to declare that they stand by the people affected by leprosy in their countries, as it would not only be of great encouragement to them but also be a tremendous step toward safeguarding their human rights and helping them to regain their dignity. I also mentioned the Principles and Guidelines for the resolution to eliminate discrimination against leprosy passed by the United Nations and asked the delegates to rectify any potential violations of these guidelines back home. Furthermore, Honorable Commissioners Ms. Bernadeta Gambishi from Tanzania and Ms. Ann Munyiva Kyalo Ngugi from Kenya made an emergency motion at the general International Coordinating Committee session, allowing me to speak for five minutes and ask the representatives to adopt Global Appeal 2014. It was my great pleasure to speak and see that all the participants welcomed our Global Appeal.

After Geneva, I went to Myanmar to mediate in a settlement between the Myanmar National Army and ethnic minority insurgency groups as Japan's Special Envoy for National Reconciliation in Myanmar. On my way back to Japan, I stopped in Bangkok to speak with Dr. Lalith Chandrakumar Weeratunga, secretary to the Sri Lankan president, and Mr. Harsha Navaratne of the Sewalanka Foundation on the current situation and future of Sri Lanka, before returning home.

Less than two weeks later, I was back at the UN European headquarters in Geneva. This time, I was to discuss eliminating leprosy with the world's health ministers assembled for the WHO General Assembly, give a speech at the Sasakawa Health Prize award ceremony, and attend the UN Sasakawa Award for Disaster Risk Reduction award ceremony.

In 1985, 122 countries had yet to eliminate leprosy, but now only one country, Brazil, remained. However, many countries still have endemic areas with many patient discoveries, and some nations have seen increases in the numbers of new cases. Others have fewer people affected by leprosy than those with other diseases, such as HIV/AIDS, malaria, and tuberculosis, and do not prioritize leprosy elimination in their health policies. Those involved in policy decisions must once again share a sense of crisis to further bolster our efforts. To this end, in July 2013, the Nippon Foundation partnered with the WHO Regional Office for Southeast Asia, which represents the most people affected by leprosy in the WHO's regions, to invite health ministers from eighteen endemic countries, where more than 1,000 new cases are found every year, to Bangkok, Thailand, for the International Leprosy Summit, with the full support of the Thai Ministry of Health. During my visit to Geneva, I met with representatives of twelve of the countries invited to the summit and asked them to come to Bangkok.

I met first with Secretary Keshav Desiraju of the Ministry of Health and Family Welfare, India, home to most new patients worldwide. India eliminated leprosy as a public health problem at the national level in 2005 and has continued to fight the disease since then, with only three states yet to achieve the elimination goal. Nevertheless, the new case figure had risen to 130,000 per year, so I wanted the nation to bolster its efforts, especially in endemic areas.

Next, I spoke with Dr. Enrique T. Ona, the Philippines secretary of health. It must have been challenging to distribute multidrug therapy (MDT) in a country consisting of more than 7,000 islands, but the efforts of all concerned had been successful, with the MDT supply system in the Philippines now serving as a model for other countries. According to Health Secretary Ona, the low prevalence rate had driven down concern about leprosy, making it difficult to detect remaining patients. He also indicated a need to train physicians and an interest in working with the Department of Health to promote efforts to enable people affected by leprosy living in leprosaria to return to their hometowns to live with their families.

Sri Lanka's Health Minister (later President) Dr. Maithripala Sirisena reported that several regions in his country had high patient concentrations and that the government was ensuring that every corner of the country was monitored.

Brazil's Dr. Jarbas Barbosa, the vice minister of health surveillance and an old acquaintance, reported on the latest leprosy news, both medical and social. Currently, Brazil was fighting leprosy by closely monitoring the situation in all of its states and through a drive to detect leprosy in schools involving 16 million students, with a report scheduled to be published in early June. With regard to human rights, the government had also begun to implement a bill to compensate people affected by leprosy and consider support for children who have been separated from their parents.

I had my first meeting with Health Minister Dr. Nafsiah Mboi of Indonesia, a country that has the third highest number of cases after India and Brazil. An expert in public health who had been appointed minister of health the previous year, she showed determination, saying, "Indonesia has endemic areas in fourteen of its thirty-four provinces. I have instructed leaders to strengthen efforts in the provinces of Aceh and Papua, where the prevalence rates are exceptionally high. In Papua, where I visited last year, I was surprised to find that 108 people were affected by leprosy in a village of 332. I am also focusing on protecting human rights."

Later, I met with Myanmar's minister of health, Dr. Pe Thet Khin. In February 2013, the Japanese Ministry of Foreign Affairs appointed me Japan's Special Envoy for National Reconciliation in Myanmar.

Since then, I had worked to achieve a ceasefire and peace in the seventy-five-year struggle between the government and separatist militia. I had also been working with the nation's Ministry of Health on policy related to leprosy and traditional medicine. Myanmar had made early efforts to integrate leprosy into general medical services, which WHO asks of countries worldwide. The minister, who provided a detailed report on recent developments every time I saw him, said that he intended to further raise awareness of leprosy and educate young doctors about the threat posed by the disease, necessary in view of stalled progress after leprosy elimination had been reached. I also accepted an invitation to a policy meeting scheduled at a former leprosy hospital (now a general hospital) in Mandalay.

Disability and discrimination issues were discussed with Bangladeshi Health Minister Prof. A. F. Ruhal Haque. We agreed that the country must reduce the occurrence of disabilities through early detection and treatment, as Bangladesh has a slightly higher disability rate than other countries, and also encourage acceptance, so people with disabilities do not suffer discrimination.

Deputy Director-General Li Mingzhu of the Department of International Cooperation in China's National Health and Family Planning Commission had attended the Global Appeal 2011 presentation ceremony in Beijing. He told me that, despite the low prevalence rate, the figure of more than 1,000 new patient detections annually was seen as a definite problem: further work was necessary on early treatment and detection by providing accurate knowledge to medical professionals and the general public. I informed him of the 1,600 Japanese and Chinese students who had participated in work camps in China, visiting villages of people affected by leprosy and eating and sleeping with the villagers.

I was also able to meet with representatives from four African countries. I thanked Ethiopian Health Minister Dr. Kesetebirhan Admasu Birhane for his cooperation as a local partner in hosting an African regional conference, the International Symposium on Leprosy and Human Rights, organized by the Nippon Foundation and scheduled for September 2013 in Ethiopia's capital, Addis Ababa.

I asked Tanzanian Health Minister Hussein Ali Mwinyi for regular status reports on his country's progress in eliminating leprosy, where case numbers had been reduced by just under 50 percent in the past seven years, so that Tanzania's achievements could be shared with other countries.

I also met again with Dr. Sira Mamboya, who once was the head of the leprosy elimination project in Zanzibar and had recently served as deputy minister of health. Dr. Mamboya spoke passionately about the situation in Zanzibar, saying that despite patient numbers falling, highly endemic areas still require the strategic promotion of active patient detection.

I then met with representatives from Mozambique and Madagascar, together with Madagascar's representative in Geneva. According to Juvenal Arcanjo Dengo, the Mozambican representative in charge of labor and social affairs, the minister of health and other government officials were proud that they eliminated leprosy in 2007. Still, they would not relax their efforts until the disease was eradicated at the provincial level. Mozambique had developed a patient detection method that was now used in other countries, whereby schools handed out human body diagrams on cards for students to take home and use to mark any skin patches, one of the early symptoms of leprosy, that have showed up on members of their family and return them to the school. I hoped that they would continue thinking up such unique initiatives. I made it clear to Solofo Andrianjatovo Razafitrimo, Madagascar's minister-counselor, that I had a significant interest in the country's leprosy situation and urged him to attend the Bangkok summit.

While staying in Geneva, I also met with UN High Commissioner for Human Rights Navanethem Pillay. Dr. Pillay mentioned the importance of the Principles and Guidelines and promised to send a representative to attend the symposium in Ethiopia.

The Land of Black Hats and Japanese patients—Republic of Uzbekistan, July 2013

Route: Narita International Airport → Seoul, South Korea (flight time: 1h) → Tashkent, Uzbekistan (flight time: 7h 30m)—one night—Tashkent → Nukus, Uzbekistan (flight time: 1h 45m)—two nights

In July, I visited Uzbekistan and Tajikistan in Central Asia. Uzbekistan, which has the largest population in Central Asia, borders Kazakhstan to the north, Kyrgyzstan and Tajikistan to the east, Afghanistan to the south, and Turkmenistan to the west. With around 9.5 million of its 30 million people aged eighteen or younger, its demographic makeup indicates excellent potential for development. It is one of the few countries in the world that is doubly landlocked, with no access to the sea without crossing two borders. It was my second visit to this country since 1996 and my first in seventeen years.

I had resolved to visit Uzbekistan after an encounter at the International Conference on Leprosy held in Astrakhan, Russia, in June 2012. The conference brought together people involved in leprosy from four countries that are members of the Commonwealth of Independent States (CIS): Uzbekistan, Tajikistan, Kyrgyzstan, and Kazakhstan, thanks to the efforts of Dr. Victor Duyko, director of the Institute of Leprosy Training and Research in Astrakhan, and Dr. Romana Drabik, a German physician. Two of the countries that particularly caught my attention were Uzbekistan, in which lies the shrinking Aral Sea, and Tajikistan, which has had an influx of people affected by leprosy from Afghanistan.

The WHO's European region, which includes Central Asia, has for a long time been thought of as a "blank zone," with no new cases of leprosy reported in WHO statistics. This made me want to learn more about the history of leprosy and the current situation in these countries. Following my visit to Central Asia in 2007, Dr. Drabik accompanied me again on this trip to unravel the history of leprosy in Central Asia.

I arrived at the international airport in Tashkent, the capital of Uzbekistan, from Japan via Seoul, Korea. The next day, I received an hour-long briefing on the health situation in Uzbekistan from Dr. Asmus Hammerich, a German national who works at WHO's Uzbekistan office. After Uzbekistan gained independence with the collapse of the Soviet Union in 1991, the central government implemented health reforms that transferred authority to the local governments, emphasizing maternal and child health in the early years. As a result, the newborn mortality rate decreased by about one-third in twenty-two years. Later, Dr. Hammerich and I called on Health Minister Alimov Anvar Valiyevich.

In the northwestern part of Uzbekistan, there is an autonomous republic with the unfamiliar name of Karakalpakstan. "Kara" means "black," "kalpak" means "hat," and "stan" means "country." In other words, it is the Land of Black Hats. Many people affected by leprosy currently living in Uzbekistan are from Karakalpakstan.

After leaving Tashkent, we flew to Nukus, the capital of the autonomous Republic of Karakalpakstan. From the air, Nukus looked to lie in the middle of a desert. At the airport, we were met by Dr. Khamraev Atajan Karimovich, the vice chairman of Karakalpakstan's Council of Ministers, and Health Minister Doniyor Khojiyev. From Tashkent, we were accompanied by Dr. Eshboyev Egamberdi Khusanovich, the chief leprologist of Uzbekistan's Ministry of Health.

No sooner had we arrived than Vice Chairman Karimovich and his team threw us a welcome banquet, with tables lined with plates full of fruit, bread, cucumbers, tomatoes, cheese, and salami. We ate for a bit, and were beginning to feel replete when we were told it was now time for the official dinner—soup, followed by the entrée, a meat dish. An interesting difference in food culture. As we sat at the table, Vice Chairman Karimovich and Dr. Khusanovich told us some interesting information.

After the Second World War, 140,000 Japanese POWs were interned in Uzbekistan and Tajikistan, which were then part of the Soviet Union. Among them were four or five individuals affected by leprosy—whose records, from their medical data to their shoe sizes, were kept at the Ministry of Health. Fortunately, they apparently returned to Japan in good health. Sadly, my schedule prevented me from taking a look at these records.

In the 1970s, there were twenty leprosaria in the entire former Soviet Union, and the leprosarium in Sergiev Posad (formerly Zagorsk), located northeast of Moscow, was exclusively for foreigners. Those that remain are the Astrakhan leprosarium in Russia, which I visited in 2012, and one each in Tajikistan, Uzbekistan, and Kazakhstan. There used to be leprosaria in Turkmenistan, Georgia, and Armenia. In Uzbekistan, case numbers peaked in the 1950s and 1960s. Samarkand in southern Uzbekistan once had a leprosarium with more than 1,000 people affected by leprosy. Its numbers decreased over time, and it closed in 2006. A total of twenty-eight new cases have been reported since 1991 across the entire country, nine of them relapses.

Karakalpakstan once had a large lake called the Aral Sea. During the Soviet era, the Amu Darya and the Syr Darya, the two major rivers that fed the Aral Sea, were diverted to provide irrigation for agriculture and cotton cultivation. As a result, the Aral Sea has now shrunk to a quarter of its former size. The lakebed has become a desert, and dust containing large amounts of salts and other chemicals is causing an increase in liver and respiratory diseases among the locals. The area is known worldwide as a symbol of large-scale environmental destruction, and I once visited the site from the Kazakh side.

I visited the former port town of Muynak, a two-and-a-half-hour drive north of the capital, Nukus. The town once flourished as an Aral Sea fishing port but was now a shadow of its former self. The former fishing port had dried up, and the wreckage of boats lay in ruins, with the lake shore now dozens of kilometers away. A leprosarium was once here but was demolished thirty years ago, leaving only a tuberculosis hospital on the site. During my visit, forty-nine people affected by leprosy were receiving treatment for the aftereffects of the disease at a skin and venereal disease clinic attached to the Muynak District Hospital. Many live peacefully at home with their children, grandchildren, and families. Dr. Aimurat, the head of the clinic, showed me a shelf that held the medical records of 400 people from when there was a leprosarium.

The next day, we visited the Krantau leprosarium, 40 kilometers northwest of Nukus. The leprosarium had first been built in Muynak in 1933, but frequent flooding had forced it to be moved to Karatau, near the southern quarry, and then to its current location in Krantau in 1952. The site covers an area of around 1.7 million square meters and is surrounded by taiga (coniferous forest zone). At its peak, there were about 700 patients, but today there are thirty-five residents. More than twice that number of staff members are on hand for care. In other words, just as in Russia, which I visited the previous year, a good number of medical personnel depended for their living on people affected by leprosy. The residents here received free room and board as well as a pension, but their personal belongings were of the barest necessities, and the only heating device I saw was a stove used for cooking. In winter, the temperature dropped to minus 10, very cold for the elderly. A woman—who moved to the leprosarium at nine years old and had lived there for sixty-seven years—smiled calmly as she told me that her grandchildren and great-grandchildren lived in a nearby village. When I asked the director how comfortable life was there, he replied that there were no water or sewage facilities and that the costly expense of pumping water from a nearby river was a problem. Since frequent power outages occur, the government was considering relocating the leprosarium for better services.

One of the candidate sites was an outpatient clinic located about an hour's drive from the Krantau leprosarium on the road back to Nukus. Combined, these two facilities must have had ninety-seven staff members working in shifts, including four doctors and forty-two nurses. The government's opinion was that the new location would be better for the second and third generations, since it was closer to the capital, Nukus. Vice Chairman Karimovich kindly found time to take me round the clinic. The outpatients crowded around us, asking "What's going to happen to *our* medical care?" It

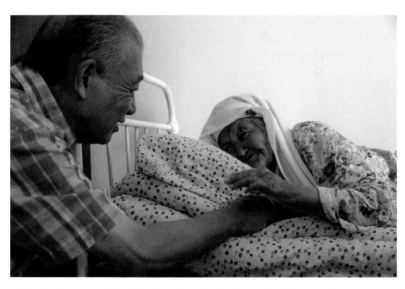

103. Visiting an elderly lady at her bedside in the Krantau Leprosarium (Uzbekistan, July 2013)

seemed there was a bit of a gap in communication between the government and the people who used the clinic on this question of relocation.

Helping people affected by leprosy from Afghanistan—Republic of Tajikistan, July 2013

Route: Nukus, Uzbekistan → Tashkent, Uzbekistan (flight time: 2h 15m; 2h 30m stopover) → Istanbul, Turkey (flight time: 5h 20m; 12h stopover) → Dushanbe, Tajikistan (flight time: 4h 30m)—three nights—Dushanbe → Istanbul (flight time: 5h 30m; 8h stopover) → Narita International Airport (flight time: 11h 15m)

Following my three-day visit to Uzbekistan, I next visited neighboring Tajikistan. Tajikistan borders Afghanistan to the south, China to the east, Kyrgyzstan to the north, and Uzbekistan to the west. About 9 million people live in Tajikistan, a country where 90 percent of the land is mountainous. After gaining independence from the Soviet Union in 1991, a civil war broke out between the communist government and rebel forces the following year, and by the time the civil war ended in 1997, more than 50,000 people had died.

In Tajikistan, I was accompanied by Dr. Drabik, a German physician. The distance from Tashkent, the capital of Uzbekistan, which we visited in the first half of the trip, to Dushanbe, the capital of Tajikistan, our next destination, is only about 300 kilometers as the crow flies, but security concerns made it dangerous to travel directly by car, so we had to make a detour via Istanbul, Turkey, 3,000 kilometers away. I arrived in Istanbul early in the morning after an overnight flight, and since I had a twelve-hour layover for the overnight flight to Tajikistan, I paid a second visit to the leprosarium I'd been to in Istanbul. There, I learned that Dr. Türkan Saylan, for whom I had great respect, had passed away. As I mentioned in Chapter 3, Dr. Saylan was a pioneer in her field, and the leprosarium's nurses looked just as busy as on my previous visit. I also went further into the city to visit the Topkapı Palace, where the Ottoman sultans resided from the mid-fifteenth to mid-nineteenth centuries.

I arrived at Dushanbe Airport in Tajikistan at 4 a.m. the following day and was met by Dr. Azizullo Kosimov, director of the Republican

Center of Venereal and Skin Diseases. It had been nearly a year since I met him in Astrakhan, Russia, last June.

On my first day there, Dr. Pavel Ursu, the WHO Tajikistan representative, briefed me on the state of health in the nation. He told me that the most headache-inducing problem is the influx of illegal drugs from Afghanistan. Tajikistan had become a relay point for drug smuggling, and the number of addicts was increasing among those who became drug couriers due to poverty.

I met Deputy Health Minister Dr. Rahmonov S. B. at the Tajikistan Ministry of Health. Deputy Health Minister Rahmonov is a Japanophile, having visited Japan in 1994 on a Japan International Cooperation Agency training program. I went to Tajikistan primarily to inspect the border area and learn about how people affected by leprosy flowed into Tajikistan from Afghanistan across a 1,000-kilometer border. Unfortunately, the government did not permit me to visit the area due to security concerns.

My original destination, Khorugh, was a forty-five-minute flight from Dushanbe. Situated 2,000 meters above sea level, this poor region borders Afghanistan on the Panj River, home to 28,000 people. Located in the Pamir Mountains, the region is said to be inhabited by the descendants of children born to local women and soldiers during Alexander the Great's eastern expedition. I heard many women there have blue eyes and dark hair, and it had long been one of my dreams to meet them.

Ministry of Health officials gave various excuses to prevent me from going to Khorugh. The flights to the city were irregular with uncertain departure times, they claimed. At the end of my tether, I told them that if that were the case, I would ask the minister of health to have the president arrange a helicopter for me when I met with him—only to be then told that my meeting with the minister of health was canceled. Khorugh is home to a leprosy hospital. I also very much wanted to visit because most of the information about Afghanistan comes from the capital, Kabul, with next to no communication from the regions where many Tajiks live.

The Ministries of Health of both nations regularly hold consultations, and more than 1,000 Afghans were receiving treatment at a Tajik border hospital. Dr. Rahmonov shared with me a Russian proverb, "Do not hold a wedding in your house if there is sorrow in your neighbor's." He added: "Afghanistan is a sibling nation, where many Tajiks live. It's one of my dreams to develop a facility in the border region so we can treat patients from Afghanistan." I fervently wanted to help him realize that dream. I hope the day comes when I can find out about the leprosy situation in Afghanistan with my own eyes.

An old friend of mine lost his life in Tajikistan. Yutaka Akino, a political scientist and a researcher in Slavic Eurasian studies whom Japan's Ministry of Foreign Affairs sent to the UN Mission of Observers in Tajikistan as a political advisor in 1998. He was killed in an attack by an armed group. I had heard that a memorial plaque could be found on the grounds of the United Nations Development Program Office in Dushanbe, so I took a detour to the site. A sturdy white fence surrounded the grounds, and on the wall of one building was the plaque inscribed with the names of the five people who had died together with the words "Died Serving the Cause of Peace." Not a day passes, I was told, without someone placing fresh flowers on the glimmering stone plaque as an offering. I placed my hands together and prayed for their happiness in the next world.

The next day, I visited Tajikistan's only leprosarium, the Honaka Leprosarium in Hisor district, about one-and-a-half hour's drive from the capital, Dushanbe. It was located within the city until 1928, when it moved to a leafier location on the outskirts. A short distance from the center of Hisor City, it stands on a vast plot of 50 hectares, with the Kofarnihon River flowing nearby and full of runoff streams from the Tian Shan Mountains. Fifteen people affected by leprosy lived here. Despite the presence of twenty-six nursing staff, the fifteen residents wore leather shoes over ulcerated, unbandaged feet. They were definitely not receiving the proper nursing care.

During the Soviet era, when a child was born to a person affected by leprosy, the government paid all boarding and childcare expenses and placed the child in a boarding home to prevent infection within the family. A couple from the Pamir district, named Sardor and Nizoramo, who had entered the institution at the age of fourteen, were now sixty-six years old. They had five adult children who were working outside the leprosarium. They kept up with what was going on in the world by reading Russian newspapers, they told me. "When we hear about the incessant conflicts, we are truly grateful for the peace that we enjoy here." They had been deeply moved by the Great East Japan Earthquake, which they had seen on TV. One of the elderly residents had once lived with three Japanese soldiers who had contracted leprosy. The soldiers were sent back to Japan around 1955.

In 1991, doctors from Astrakhan, Russia, carried out a survey to identify people affected by leprosy throughout Tajikistan. A Tajik doctor trained in Astrakhan conducted a second survey in 2001, finding only one new patient in the entire country.

There were forty-nine people affected by leprosy living in Tajikistan when I visited. However, only six dermatologists in the entire country could diagnose leprosy. "We need to conduct another survey to see if there are any new patients," Dr. Kosimov said, looking worried.

On the last day of my stay, I gave a lecture on the state of leprosy and discrimination worldwide at a meeting of 100 dermatologists and ophthalmologists at the Republican Center of Venereal and Skin Diseases in Dushanbe. The next day was Dr. Drabik's seventy-seventh birthday, and all the attendees surrounded her, dressed in ethnic costumes provided by Dr. Kosimov, and sang a chorus of "Happy Birthday," bringing my trip to an end with a smile.

According to an NGO survey, as many as thirty-eight new cases of leprosy were diagnosed in just five Afghan provinces in December 2012. The continuing chaos in Afghanistan means that people affected by leprosy are without access to medicine. Unfortunately, our relief efforts cannot reach them due to the deteriorating security situation caused by the conflict.

The Bangkok Declaration: breaking the stall in elimination—Kingdom of Thailand, July 2013

Route: Narita International Airport → Bangkok, Thailand (flight time: 6h 30m)—three nights—Bangkok → Narita (flight time: 6h 10m)

On 24 July, I visited Bangkok to attend the International Leprosy Summit, jointly organized by the Nippon Foundation and WHO. In 1999, the WHO General Assembly established a benchmark for leprosy elimination, defined as a prevalence rate of less than one new case in 10,000 population. This goal had motivated governments worldwide, driving the number of endemic countries from eighty-eight at the time to only one today. However, there was no room for complacency. During my travels around the world, I had discerned a definite diminishing of interest in leprosy among health ministries and officials. And this was reflected in the figures. The number of new cases had flatlined worldwide over the past few years, and in some countries the figures were even increasing. We could not overlook that people affected by leprosy are concentrated in certain areas, including urban slums, ethnic minority settlements, inaccessible mountainous regions, and remote islands. On the advice of Dr. S. K. Noordeen, an authority on eliminating leprosy who has long been a member of the WHO and shares my concern about these issues, I therefore organized a conference in cooperation with Dr. Samlee Plianbangchang, WHO's regional director for Southeast Asia, headquarters for the Global Leprosy Program. Thai Health Minister Pradit Sintavanarong offered to host the conference in Thailand. Health ministers, their deputies, and other experts from health ministries in seventeen countries with more than 1,000 new cases per year—India, Indonesia, Myanmar, Nepal, Sri Lanka, China, the Philippines, Bangladesh, Angola, the Democratic Republic of the Congo (DRC), Madagascar, Mozambique, Nigeria, Tanzania, Brazil, South Sudan, and Sudan—attended and discussed the future of leprosy elimination policies.

At the conference, we adopted the Bangkok Declaration, which commits its members to achieve the following: reducing the proportion of visible disability (grade 2 disability) among all new cases to less than one per 1 million people by 2020, detecting patients early in highly endemic areas, and encouraging people affected by leprosy to actively participate in elimination efforts.

Before the conference, WHO continuously worked with national health ministries at the secretariat level to formulate the draft. By the time the vote came to the table, representatives had developed positions, driving the discussion far beyond the original schedule. However, in the end the thorough debates were worthwhile, leading to a declaration that garnered everyone's agreement. To realize the goals in the Bangkok Declaration, we needed to lay out specific action plans as soon as possible. The Nippon Foundation started by announcing its willingness to provide a total of $20 million (about ¥2 billion) as a special fund for the Bangkok Declaration over the next five years.

The following is a summary of the main points of the Bangkok Declaration:

Bangkok Declaration toward a Leprosy-Free World (excerpts)

- We reaffirm the various global efforts that have been made to fight leprosy over the past twenty-five years and acknowledge with appreciation the enormous strides made by those involved, including in the widespread implementation of MDT among other prevention and care approaches and the significant reduction in case numbers.

- The long experience of leprosy-control initiatives in achieving the goal of eliminating leprosy as a public health problem globally will be used to improve the interventions against other neglected tropical diseases.

- However, there is a continuing occurrence of new leprosy cases being reported in a number of different countries, and also within certain countries a continuing existence of hyperendemic areas, that have led in recent years to the consequent stagnation in the leprosy situation.

- We note with concern that the decline in persons affected by leprosy has also led to a rise in government complacency and lower prioritizing, leading to fewer human and financial resources being made available to deal effectively with this public health problem.

- The seventeen countries assembled at this summit, in collaboration with WHO and other relevant partners, and in pursuit of our goal of achieving a leprosy-free world, declare that we will:

  * Work toward eliminating leprosy at the state and provincial levels, focusing on high endemic areas, by ensuring early diagnosis and treatment completion (so that no one stops treatment halfway through the course of the disease).

  * Aim to achieve the reduction by 2020 of the number of new cases with visible disabilities to less than one case per 1 million population.

  * Prevent the occurrence of disability through early detection and treatment. Curb any worsening of disabilities among those people who are already disabled.

  * Ensure that people affected by leprosy can participate from the planning stage in their care and socioeconomic independence programs, in accordance with WHO guidelines.

* Promote the empowerment of people affected by leprosy in accordance with the UN Resolution on the Elimination of Discrimination against People Affected by Leprosy and Their Families.

* Continue to monitor progress at the global level, with the support of WHO, to ensure that we stay on track toward achieving these goals.

• Finally, we reaffirm our will to further strengthen our political commitment, with the aim of achieving a leprosy-free world.

Following up on the Bangkok Declaration, and the Forum of Parliamentarians to Free India of Leprosy—Delhi, India, August 2013

Route: Narita International Airport → Bangkok, Thailand (flight time: 6h 40m; 2h stopover) → Chiang Mai, Thailand (flight time: 1h)—two nights (peace activism)—Chiang Mai → Bangkok (flight time: 50m; 4h stopover) → Delhi, India (flight time: 4h 30m)—two nights—Delhi → Narita (flight time: 8h 20m)

In August, after a meeting to discuss a ceasefire and peace agreement with Myanmar ethnic minority militia leaders in Chiang Mai, Thailand, I paid a visit to India.

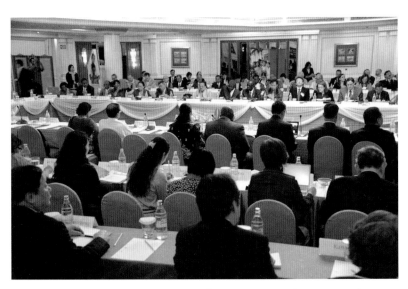

104. Country representatives at the International Leprosy Summit (Thailand, July 2013)

On the first day, I had an early morning meeting with Dr. Samlee Plianbangchang, someone responsible for worldwide leprosy elimination efforts. He reaffirmed his commitment to following up on the Bangkok Declaration, with particular emphasis on India, Brazil, and Indonesia, three countries with the highest number of people affected by leprosy.

I had been disappointed at the International Leprosy Summit in Bangkok by the absence of a government representative from India, which has the world's highest number of new leprosy cases. Thus, during this visit, I assembled government, WHO, and NGO representatives to report on the summit and I requested that India step up its leprosy elimination efforts from here on. The attending government officials included Secretary Keshav Desiraju of the Ministry of Health and Family Welfare, Joint Secretary Anshu Prakash, Additional Secretary-cum-Mission Director Anuradha Gupta of the National Rural Health Mission, Deputy Director-General (leprosy) Dr. C. M. Agrawal of the health ministry, Director General Dr. A. K. Puri, and officials from the Ministry of Health. The WHO representatives were Dr. Sumana Barua of the WHO's Global Leprosy Program, consultant Dr. Ranganatha Rao, Leprosy Program advisor Dr. Rui Paulo de Jesus of SEARO, and Dr. Nata Menabde, WHO representative to India. Vagavathali Narsappa, president of NFI, an organization for people affected by leprosy, was also present.

Since 2010, India had identified 209 districts with a prevalence rate of at least one per 10,000 population and had been focusing on these districts to detect new cases. Of the 130,000 cases reported in 2012–13, 20,000 were detected through home visits by health workers and volunteers, resulting in a 5 percent increase in patients from the previous year. I emphasized that while the increase in the number of patients might be cause for anxiety, it is an inevitable result of proactive patient detection efforts. The temporary increase is if anything welcome, as the number of patients will decrease once treatment is completed.

We had been presenting our Global Appeal every January to call for the elimination of discrimination against people affected by leprosy and their families. Next year, we would seek the endorsement of each country's national human rights commissions. As part of our preparations for this goal, I visited K. G. Balakrishnan, chair of the Indian National Human Rights Commission. The National Human Rights Commission had expressed sincere interest in the leprosy issue and sent a representative when the Asian meeting of the International Symposium on Leprosy and Human Rights was held in India in October 2012. In the same year, it also sponsored a leprosy workshop with representatives of state human rights commissions. Moreover, it was beginning to make progress in addressing prejudice and discrimination, albeit in a small way, by holding leprosy-themed sessions twice a year during the summer and winter internship programs for students majoring in law and human rights and having S-ILF conduct classes to raise awareness of the need to counter discrimination in junior high schools in the Delhi area.

In the afternoon, I again visited the WHO India Office to meet with Dr. Nata Menabde and discuss the current status of leprosy in India and measures to combat the disease. In the evening, there was a meeting of the Forum of Parliamentarians to Free India of Leprosy at the home of MP Dinesh Trivedi in central Delhi. Trivedi, who had served as minister of railways and minister of state for health and family welfare, had proposed the alliance, which brought together fifty-two MPs, including Madhu Goud Yaskhi, the forum's co-sponsor. Even though the parliament was in session, sixteen MPs attended, along with Mr. Narsappa, president of NFI. It was decided that the Forum of Parliamentarians would aim to actively raise the issue of leprosy as a priority in parliament going forward, to develop both medical and social awareness-raising programs for the general public, to formulate policies for low-income people, and to use community development funds held by each member of parliament to improve living conditions in leprosy colonies. A new initiative to improve the lives of people affected by leprosy and eliminate discrimination against them had been born. Unfortunately, however, little progress has been made since then in this effort, and work is underway to lend strength to this association of parliamentarians.

The next morning, I met with the NFI President Mr. Narsappa and trustee Guntreddy Venugopal and received a report on the NFI's activities. I then attended the S-ILF board of trustees meeting. With funding from S-ILF, about 150 small businesses had been established in sixteen states in India. In recent years, S-ILF had also focused on educational support for children of persons affected by leprosy. It had two educational assistance programs: a nurse training scholarship for women and a vocational training program for men and women. The program was funded by donations from the State Bank of India and the Sir Dorabji Tata Foundation. Since 2011, thirty-five women had taken a four-year, state-accredited nurse training course. Because nursing is traditionally a popular profession for Indian women, this scholarship is highly sought after. Unfortunately, in many cases, limitations in funds have meant that some of those who meet the application requirements have to be turned down. The vocational training program provides basic training for those who have completed education up to the tenth grade to facilitate their employment in the service sector where there is a labor shortage, including as retail assistants or fast-food delivery staff; and sixty-six young people had obtained jobs. The National Skill Development Corporation decided to donate the cost of training a further 350 people and planned to recruit applicants in each state.

Membership and ownership—Federal Democratic Republic of Ethiopia, September 2013

> Route: Narita International Airport → Frankfurt, Germany (flight time: 12h; 2h stopover) → Brussels, Belgium (flight time: 1h)—two nights—Brussels → Frankfurt (flight time: 1h; 3h 30m stopover) → Addis Ababa, Ethiopia (flight time: 6h 50m)—four nights

In September, I embarked on an extremely busy trip in which I visited Belgium, Ethiopia, and India in twelve days. Departing from Narita, I stopped first in Brussels, going via Frankfurt, and there I delivered a speech at the opening ceremony of the eighteenth International Leprosy Congress, which Princess Astrid of Belgium attended. This is a conference held every three years that brings together people from all over the world involved in leprosy-related activities. It allowed me to enjoy a reunion with people I had worked with worldwide.

Afterward, I headed to Ethiopia, going via Frankfurt. An African regional conference of the International Symposium on Leprosy and Human Rights was taking place in the capital Addis Ababa. The

Nippon Foundation had planned this symposium in five regions globally to encourage countries to implement the UN General Assembly's 2010 resolution to end discrimination against people affected by leprosy and their family members. The Ethiopian symposium was the third in the series, following Brazil in February 2012 for the Americas and India in October 2012 for Asia.

The symposium, held on 18 September, brought together about 200 people—people affected by leprosy, human rights experts, and representatives of NGOs and international organizations from thirteen countries, including the eight African countries of Ethiopia, Mali, Tanzania, Angola, the DRC, Niger, Ghana, and South Africa. Ethiopian Prime Minister Hailemariam Desalegn attended the opening ceremony and expressed his government's commitment to promoting the Principles and Guidelines associated with the UN resolution.

Prime Minister Hailemariam had taken up his post in August 2012, promoted from deputy prime minister and foreign minister after the death of Prime Minister Meles. I had met Prime Minister Meles many times and built a longstanding friendship, but I had just become acquainted with Prime Minister Hailemariam at the fifth Tokyo International Conference on African Development (TICAD V) meeting held in Yokohama in June 2013. He was also the residing chair of the African Union (AU) and said he would like to take up the resolutions of this symposium at the AU. Health Minister Kesetebirhan Admasu also expressed his commitment to advancing the fight for early detection and treatment of patients, social rehabilitation, and eliminating discrimination.

In my speech, I talked about the experience of Ms. Sinknesh, a twenty-eight-year-old woman affected by leprosy: "Ms. Sinknesh was diagnosed with leprosy at the age of twelve and went from her hometown in the west to a hospital in Addis Ababa for treatment, where she fully recovered after one year of treatment. However, her family disowned her, did not welcome her back home, and burned her belongings. She could not find work and had to make ends meet by begging. Fortunately, she was able to join a project of the Ethiopian National Association of Persons Affected by Leprosy [ENAPAL], allowing her to start an embroidery business and get an education. However, she still fears discrimination and has not been able to reunite with her family. To prevent more situations like hers, governments must work with NGOs, civil society, and the media to create concrete action plans based on the UN Principles and Guidelines to change social perceptions."

At the symposium, Deputy Executive Director Tim Hughes of the IBA called for eliminating or revising discriminatory laws and systems related to leprosy that remain in countries such as India, Nepal, and Singapore. Dr. Mousa Burayzat of Jordan—former chair of the International Coordinating Committee, of which each country's national human rights commission is a member—proposed that the commissions should address the human rights issues related to leprosy by monitoring government efforts and conducting educational and awareness-raising activities. ENAPAL's chairperson, Leulseged Berhane, made a powerful appeal to continue the fight against misunderstanding and discrimination. With the participation of the prime minister, the symposium was covered by nearly forty media outlets and became the top news story on Ethiopian television and in Ethiopian newspapers.

The day after the symposium, I traveled about an hour by plane from Addis Ababa to learn about the activities of ENAPAL's Bahir Dar branch in the Amhara region. Arriving at a colony where about twenty households of people affected by leprosy and their families lived, we were greeted by a throng of children. Despite their cheerful expressions, their living conditions were terrible. Some families had no income because the husbands had disabilities and the wives had just given birth and could not work, while others had no home and lived by begging. I derived no small relief to meet some people working hard to weave the straw mats for serving *injera* (a traditional Ethiopian flatbread), repair pots and umbrellas, or spin yarn.

Next, I visited a new settlement built with the support of UN-Habitat, which works to solve housing problems for the poor. The houses were solidly built, a far cry from the colony we had just visited, and some families were living in dwellings with TVs and sofas. The project began about four years earlier and brought some of the colony's most distressed people to this area, where thirty-nine families were now living. Residents saved money in bank accounts and used the funds to start small businesses, such as raising livestock or making and selling goods.

Such projects, which combined UN-Habitat's housing support and livelihood improvement assistance, had been developed in seven locations in Ethiopia, including Bahir Dar. According to my guides, ENAPAL's Managing Director Tesfaye Tadesse and the Bahir Dar branch representative, about eighty people affected by leprosy paid a monthly membership fee of 2 birr (about US$0.04) to participate in activities as members of this branch. Members were offered various training and business support opportunities, and there were 15,000 members nationwide who had paid their dues and were participating in activities. Half of the membership fee went to the sixty-three chapters nationwide and the other half to the head office. While not expensive, this system allowed each individual to take ownership and supported sustainable organizational management. I have seen organizations for people affected by leprosy in many countries worldwide, but this one seemed exceptionally well put together.

We stayed at Lalibela, also in the Amhara region. We were told in advance that there were many mites, and my companions were all very nervous, so I offered a prize to the person who got the most bites. Several young women were in the group, but for some reason, I, the oldest, came out on top with twenty bites. Nao Ozawa, one of my companions, did not get bitten at all, but after returning to Tokyo, he found that he had in fact been so severely bitten that he had to go to hospital. Some joked about how the Ethiopian mites must have wanted to hitch a ride to Japan.

Tears from an MP and a person affected by leprosy—West Bengal, India, September 2013

> Route: Addis Ababa, Ethiopia → Dubai, United Arab Emirates (flight time: 4h; 6h stopover (with a rest at the airport hotel)) → Kolkata, West Bengal, India (flight time: 4h 45m)—three nights—Kolkata → Bangkok, Thailand (flight time: 2h 40m; 1h stopover) → Narita International Airport (flight time: 6h)

From Ethiopia, we headed to India again. But it was pointed out to us at Addis Ababa airport that travel from Africa to India required a yellow card proving vaccination against yellow fever, without which no airline could issue a ticket. This was a bolt from the blue. My compan-

OVERCOMING THE STAGNATION

ion Natsuko Tominaga persistently negotiated for three hours, and as a result, we were able to get as far as the transit point of Dubai. After another two-hour negotiation, but with no breakthrough, Ms. Tominaga then suggested we enter the country once and exit again, which allowed us to obtain a boarding pass to India. When we later checked with the travel agency that had arranged our airline tickets, they told us they had no idea that the yellow card was required to travel from the African continent to India. Anyway, we arrived in Kolkata in the eastern Indian state of West Bengal. Despite our trepidation as we passed through immigration, the officers let us through without a word. Without Ms. Tominaga's persistence and sheer ingenuity, our work in Kolkata would have been impossible. West Bengal is contiguous with Bhutan to the north, Nepal to the west, and Bangladesh to the east. The official language is not Hindi, the familiar language of northern India, but rather Bengali. Because of its location connecting the northeastern states with the heart of the Indian subcontinent, West Bengal has long been a land of heavy human traffic.

Upon my arrival, Mr. Narsappa, president of NFI, an organization for people affected by leprosy, and NFI trustees Guntreddy Venugopal and Rambarai Sha came hotfoot from their respective states.

The next day, I visited two colonies in Asansol, Paschim Bardhaman district, 230 kilometers northwest of Kolkata. Joining me on this excursion were Dr. Pradip Kumar Mandal, the state leprosy officer for West Bengal's health ministry; Dr. A. K. Puri, from the Central Leprosy Division of the Ministry of Health and Family Welfare in Delhi; Dr. Saurabh Jain, the focal person for leprosy at the WHO's India office; and Dr. Vineeta Shanker, the executive director of S-ILF. It was the first time in ten years that an official from the national Ministry of Health had accompanied me on a regional visit. Dinesh Trivedi, an MP from West Bengal and a founder of the Forum of Parliamentarians to Free India of Leprosy, also joined us during our travels. An influential MP, he has served as the union minister for railways and the former union minister of state for health and family welfare. He is also the driving force of the Forum of Parliamentarians to Free India of Leprosy, established in October 2012.

From the hotel, we took a caravan of six vehicles for the four-hour drive to Asansol. Our first stop was the Rahmat Nagar Danda leprosy

535

colony. We were met by Malay Ghatak, a member of the West Bengal legislative assembly and state agriculture minister, and Tapas Banerjee, the mayor of Asansol.

We passed between rows of houses on the narrow plot of land, ducking below their eaves, which looked as if they might tumble down at any moment. In this colony of about 180 people living in sixty-five households, many people affected by leprosy were making a living by begging, as is typical. The second generation worked as day laborers and garbage collectors, earning a meager income to support their parents with severe disabilities. It was MP Trivedi's first visit to a leprosy colony. "I have to say," he told the accompanying media, and the residents, "that the government has been slow off the mark. People should not be allowed to discriminate against others in twenty-first-century society." At the time of the launch of the Forum of Parliamentarians in October 2012, he did not have much leprosy awareness, so I had to be thankful for his newfound zeal. He had clearly looked into leprosy and become more familiar with the suffering that the condition involved. In front of one house was an elderly

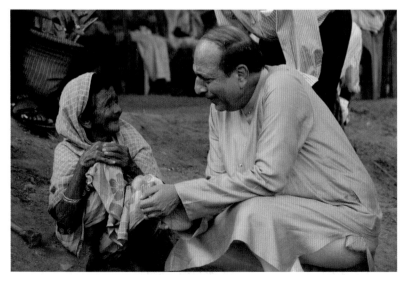

105. MP Dinesh Trivedi talking with a woman affected by leprosy, now cured (West Bengal, India, September 2013)

woman dressed in a traditional sari and holding the slender branch of a tree as a cane. She was blind and unable to walk on her own, and as Trivedi gently held her by the shoulders, she found it difficult to speak, and her eyes filled with tears.

Whenever I visit colonies around the world, I ask the media to accompany me. Broadcasting videos and images of me shaking hands with or putting my arms around people affected by leprosy allows us to get the message out to as many people as possible that leprosy is not contagious once it is treated; it is not the dreaded disease that superstition would have them believe. At this colony, we had an MP, a state assembly representative, and the mayor with us, and we were surrounded by journalists from nearly twenty media outlets.

Next, we visited Kankardanga leprosy colony, a twenty-minute drive away. We were greeted by children in clean white uniforms playing musical instruments. All the children attended a nearby public school. The colony had ninety families, with 254 people living there. Sixty of the houses were concrete units provided by the government's policy for low-income families. They had electricity and water, and the residents seemed more cheerful than in the previous colony.

The next day, my first appointment was a meeting with Justice Asok Kumar Ganguly of the West Bengal State Human Rights Commission at half past nine. As I listened to the petitions of NFI President Narsappa, Radhavallav Panda—the president of NFI's state forum in West Bengal—and four others who attended the meeting, I suddenly realized that my next scheduled appointment was approaching. I interrupted the discussion and stood up to leave, but Justice Ganguly said he wanted to hear more and told the others to stay. They later told me that they spent nearly an hour discussing how to guarantee livelihoods for those affected by leprosy and how to secure places for them to receive treatment for the disease's aftereffects.

Leaving Justice Ganguly and Mr. Panda at the hotel, President Narsappa and I headed for Jadavpur University, one of the most prestigious universities in India. Together with its sister foundation, the Tokyo Foundation for Policy Research, the Nippon Foundation has fostered international understanding and the next generation of leaders in solving social problems through a scholarship program it operates, the Sasakawa Young Leaders Fellowship Fund (SYLFF), for master's and doctoral students at sixty-nine universities in forty-four countries around the world, including Japan. Jadavpur University is one of those universities, and it hosted a ceremony to celebrate the tenth anniversary of the fund, which was established in 2003. The presentation I gave at the fund dedication ceremony ten years prior seemed to have left a strong impression, and they asked me to speak to the students about leprosy again this year. But I felt that a person affected by leprosy could speak more persuasively than I could, so I asked President Narsappa to talk about how he had previously been subject to discrimination but was now a leader of a movement, and how he has approached his work. Hundreds of students listened intently to a story that was unlike anything they had heard before.

After a sumptuous lunch provided by the university, we jumped in the car and drove to the West Bengal Ministry of Health and Family Welfare. We got through the terrible traffic in Kolkata and managed to get to our appointment a little before 2 p.m.

West Bengal has the country's fourth-highest number of people affected by leprosy. Most alarming is the high incidence of disability among new patients. The high incidence of visible disability is one indicator of slow progress of leprosy elimination measures. In Kolkata, the state capital, in particular, the incidence is 10 percent compared to a national average of about 3 percent across India. Despite that poor progress, more than half of the state's districts, including Kolkata, have vacancies in leprosy program officers. One factor is the low priority given by the state government to eliminating leprosy. At the state health ministry, I spoke with State Health Minister Chandrima Bhattacharya; Biswa Ranjan Satpathy, director of health services, West Bengal Ministry of Health and Family Welfare; and Sanghamitra Ghosh, director of the National Rural Health Mission. I opened by insisting that they resolve the vacancies in leprosy program director posts as soon as possible.

The meeting was followed by a stakeholders' summit attended by about thirty-five people, including senior officials of the state government's health ministry, a district leprosy officer, and a representative of a West Bengali NGO. The attendees declared their commitment to accelerate the efforts against leprosy discussed at July's International Leprosy Summit in Bangkok. After the summit, I had MP Trivedi join me for a press conference. About thirty reporters gathered, and the conference lasted much longer than scheduled.

My last meeting was with members of NFI's state forum and colony leaders, twenty-one of whom had traveled from across the state in conjunction with my visit. West Bengal's leaders, who play a more central role than in other states, were noticeably aging and were hardly what one might call active. However, I saw some young people at this meeting and hoped they would accelerate the movement to improve colony living conditions, increase pensions, and promote education.

A quick response—Uttar Pradesh, India, October 2013

Route: Narita International Airport → Yangon, Myanmar (flight time: 7h)—four nights (attended the opening ceremony for the Myanmar Arts Festival of Artists with Disabilities)—Yangon → Bangkok, Thailand (flight time: 1h 20m; 5h 30m stopover) → Delhi, India (flight time: 4h 30m)—one night—Delhi → Lucknow, Uttar Pradesh, India (flight time: 1h 45m)—two nights—Lucknow → Delhi (flight time: 1h)—one night—Delhi → Narita (flight time: 8h 20m)

After a busy September, I attended the Myanmar Arts Festival of Artists with Disabilities, co-sponsored by the Nippon Foundation, in October. After speaking with government officials on their analysis and strategies concerning the militant ethnic minority groups in the country, I once again headed for India, this time to the northern state of Uttar Pradesh. Uttar Pradesh is located east of Delhi and borders Nepal in the north. It is the most populous state in India, with around 200 million people. The state had the highest number of new leprosy cases in India, with more than 24,000 new cases per year.

Immediately after arriving at the airport in the state capital of Lucknow, I met with Shailendra Kumar Sonkar, the deputy commissioner for disabilities in the state's Department of Social Welfare. Deputy Commissioner Sonkar has a visual impairment. India's qualification for administrative officers, called the Indian Administrative Service (IAS), is said to be 100 times more difficult than the senior-level examination in Japan. Even after retiring, individuals with this qualification hold respected social positions, with "IAS" embossed on their business cards. Deputy Commissioner Sonkar was the first person with a visual impairment in Uttar Pradesh to pass the IAS exam. He listened to the petitions of the state leaders of people affected by leprosy who accompanied me and assured them that Uttar Pradesh's policies for people with disabilities, including pensions and loan programs for financial independence, would be extended to people affected by leprosy who have disabilities. He also promised to include people affected by leprosy in the disability councils in each of Uttar Pradesh's seventy-five districts.

In the afternoon, I attended a leprosy stakeholders' meeting aiming to accelerate measures against leprosy. Top officials from the Union Ministry of Health and Family Welfare attended, including Principal Secretary of Health Pravir Kumar and Special Secretary of Health Shashank Vikram. With its federal system of government, India requires the commitment of state governments to maintain a system that can diagnose new cases early and treat them promptly. Other participants included state leprosy officers, leprosy officers from thirty-seven districts of Uttar Pradesh with a prevalence rate of at least one per 10,000 population, NGO representatives, and people

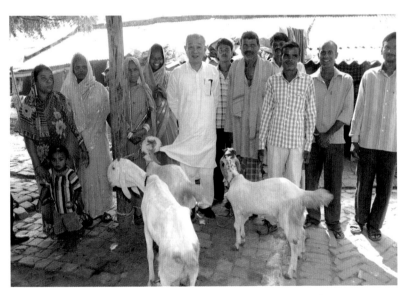

106. With a group rearing goats as part of a S-ILF micro-finance project (Uttar Pradesh, India, October 2013)

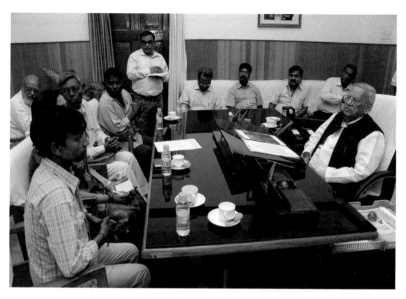

107. Leaders of the colonies directly putting their case to Health Minister Ahmet Hassan (Uttar Pradesh, India, October 2013)

affected by leprosy. Representatives from more than ten media outlets were also present.

The next day, I visited the Jay Durga leprosy colony in Raebareli district, about 80 kilometers south of Lucknow. Established in 1971, the colony is home to forty people who have recovered from leprosy and thirty-one children. Twenty-five of the houses are concrete buildings built by the state urban development organization, and the infrastructure is relatively well maintained, including wells with mechanical pumps and toilets. A total of thirteen members of the colony received support from S-ILF to engage in businesses, including bicycle rickshaw services and goat rearing. The cycle rickshaws earn an average of 200 rupees (around US$2.40) per day.

S-ILF is involved in about 150 projects in sixteen states across India. It is challenging to get people with limited literacy skills who have only ever begged involved in business, even on a small scale. The only way to encourage them is to send instructors to patiently teach them what to do. I will not be able to realize my dream of eliminating begging among people affected by leprosy unless they become self-reliant. I hope to see small businesses in all colonies as soon as possible.

Representatives from twelve colonies across the state attended the meeting and discussed the problems faced by their respective areas. Uttar Pradesh has a state organization for people affected by leprosy called the Leprosy Sufferers Welfare Association. In December 2012, they submitted a written request for better living conditions to the chief minister. It had five specific requests: establishing a leprosy pension of 2,000 rupees per month, expanding the state government's low-income housing scheme to leprosy colonies, improving infrastructure, providing higher education opportunities for the second generation, and supplying free medical equipment to the colonies. Since they had not received a response, they submitted the request again in September 2013 as an open letter through the media. They also provided copies to the relevant ministries and agencies of the state government. It was a well-thought-out action to see if their voices could get heard. In the evening, I returned to Lucknow with the state leaders and met with Anil Kumar Sagar, the director of social welfare for Uttar Pradesh. They handed him a copy of their written request and asked for his cooperation in establishing a special pension for leprosy. He commented that he would cooperate as much as possible.

The next morning, we met with Sunil Kumar, the principal secretary of the social welfare department. He said that despite having been in office for two months, it was the first time he had received a petition from a person affected by leprosy. Regarding higher education for second-generation children, one of the petition requests, Principal Secretary Kumar's advice was to apply for the state government's scholarship program for low-income families with annual incomes of less than 30,000 rupees. With regard to establishing a special leprosy pension, he said: "I will need each district to provide detailed data on who is eligible. The state government will use that data as a base for a verification survey. We will also need data on leprosy pensions in other states." He promised positive consideration. Later that day, I paid courtesy calls to Governor B. L. Joshi and Health Minister Ahmed Hassan and asked for their cooperation in solving the problems faced by people affected by leprosy.

To my surprise, we saw progress within a week of my return to Japan. Murari Sinha, secretary of the Leprosy Sufferers Welfare Association, sent me an email with a copy of the official letter sent out by Principal Secretary Kumar of the Department of Social Welfare. The letter addressed to the district welfare officers had a list of the names of children appended and stated: "With the completion of the verification survey, we would like the government to provide higher education grants to low-income families." I had traveled to various states to make similar requests but never before had I received such a prompt response. It was gratifying news.

Brazil's oldest leprosy isolation facility—Federative Republic of Brazil, December 2013

> Route: Haneda International Airport → Paris, France (flight time: 12h 50m; 4h stopover) → São Paulo, Brazil (flight time: 11h 50m; 3h stopover) → Brasília, Brazil (flight time: 1h 45m)—two nights— Brasília → Belém, Brazil (flight time: 2h 30m)—two nights

At the end of 2013, I visited Brazil and Colombia, first stopping in Paris. In Brazil, the momentum was building for the World Cup in 2014 and the Olympics in 2016.

The trip began in Brasília, the nation's capital, which took thirty-three hours from Japan. I visited the Ministry of Health and held discussions with a couple of old acquaintances, the health minister, Dr. Alexandre Padilha, and the vice health minister, Dr. Jarbas Barbosa. The Federal Ministry of Health is mindful of the importance of stepping up its fight against leprosy, and it outlined some specific examples of its work. In 2012, it ran a campaign to detect cases in schools, which, combined with parasite testing, resulted in the testing of 2.3 million children. If children learn about the disease, they will share what they know with their families, increasing public health awareness in the home. They also reported that the plan for the next year was to enhance leprosy training for doctors. Worldwide, far fewer people are affected by leprosy than malaria, HIV/AIDS, and tuberculosis, which impact millions to hundreds of millions of people each year. Doctors have very few opportunities to see patients with leprosy, and the disease tends to be left out of medical school curricula. Teaching doctors the signs of leprosy and how to diagnose the disease is thus crucial in preventing disability through early detection and treatment and eliminating discrimination. Health Minister Padilha requested that a WHO monitoring team be dispatched to Brazil. Finding leprosy patients living deep in the Amazon is immensely challenging due to the sheer vastness of the country, but the WHO and the Nippon Foundation have a wealth of experience and connections thanks to their many years of work toward eliminating leprosy globally. I expressed my willingness to take a positive approach and began coordinating with the relevant parties.

In addition to my medical discussions in Brasília, I made two significant advances regarding prejudice and discrimination. First, I spoke with Minister Maria do Rosário Nunes of Brazil's Human Rights Secretariat. This organ deals with various human rights issues and provides pensions under a law to compensate people affected by leprosy who were once forced to live in leprosy isolation facilities. The group that organized the meeting was the Brazilian NGO Movement for the Reintegration of Persons Affected by Hansen's Disease (MORHAN), the same organization that pushed for the compensation scheme and was also aiming to expand it to provide compensation for the second generation who were separated from their parents by the segregation policy. Thanks to these efforts, President Rousseff agreed to consider a compensation plan in August 2013. The meeting with Minister Nunes was attended by forty people who had traveled six hours by bus to Brasília. They included people affected by leprosy, their children, and their grandchildren, who all lived in a former colony known as Goiânia. They had all chipped in some money and chartered a bus to get to the meeting. I was impressed by the minister who welcomed them. When they entered the conference room, the minister said she first wanted to greet each and every one of the Goiânians, shaking hands and giving hugs to them all. She made it clear that the segregation policy was a mistake for which the government must take responsibility. She also gave high praise to MORHAN's efforts in bringing together the voices of many people affected by leprosy and their families and declared that the issue of compensating the second generation would be incorporated into the action plan. Moreover, she would join the endorsements of national human rights commissions and sign the Global Appeal 2014 to eliminate discrimination against people affected by leprosy and their families, which we would announce on World Leprosy Day in January 2014. She said she would add the Global Appeal to the Human Rights Secretariat's agenda. Even after continually meeting with leaders worldwide, I have rarely found anyone who makes such a clear commitment. I felt confident that we would get somewhere with the efforts with Brazil's leprosy and human rights situation.

The second advance stemmed from a meeting of legislators on the issue of leprosy. As far as I know, two other bipartisan groups of parliamentarians were working to improve the lives and restore the dignity of people affected by leprosy, in Japan and India, and the Brazilian group is the most recent, having been established in August 2013. As of December 2013, 180 Brazilian legislators had endorsed the group, meaning that one-third of the eighty-one Senate and 513 Chamber of Deputies seats were part of the endorsement. And more were expected to join. The leader of the alliance was Deputy Nilmário Miranda, the director of the Human Rights Secretariat during the administration of former President Luiz Inácio Lula da Silva. Deputy Miranda made this meeting happen because he felt that many people should have the opportunity to learn about leprosy and the alliance of legislators who were helping the fight against it. Even though it was the last day of the session, seventy legislators and many media representatives attended, indicating a high level of interest. In my opening remarks, I appealed to the legislators to share the issue's existence widely among their constituents.

I then flew from Brasília to Belém, the capital of the northern state of Pará. This state alone is about three times the size of Japan. Located at the mouth of the Amazon River, Belém is the largest city in northern Brazil, with a population of around 1.8 million. The first Japanese immigrants to the Amazon region arrived in 1929, and many Japanese-Brazilians still live there today. The city has roads lined with mango trees in a typical equatorial tropical rainforest climate. At 9 a.m. the following morning, I visited Pará's state government offices and met with Governor Simão Jatene. With its decentralized government, Brazil's state governors had significant decision-making authority. At a press conference following the audience, Governor Jatene opened with how the state's average income is half the national average. He then spoke on the urgency of improving public health in areas such as the Amazon backcountry, where eliminating leprosy was challenging amid the uncertainty about actual case numbers. He pointed out that many people affected by leprosy likely lived on the state's border, especially in the north, where populations move frequently. He promised to present concrete figures on the results of elimination measures and also appealed to the journalists packed in front of him that there should be no social discrimination.

I also traveled to several sites within Pará. The first stop was in Marituba, on the outskirts of Belém, at the Dr. Marcello Candia Reference Unit in Sanitary Dermatology. I heard that each month around 5,500 people affected by leprosy come for treatment at the facility, which is well equipped, including a workshop for making prosthetic limbs. At the leprosarium, a group of cheerful elderly people was enjoying a midsummer Christmas lunch. However, the facility was having difficulties getting MDT supplies. MDT, the drug used to treat leprosy, must be administered continuously for six

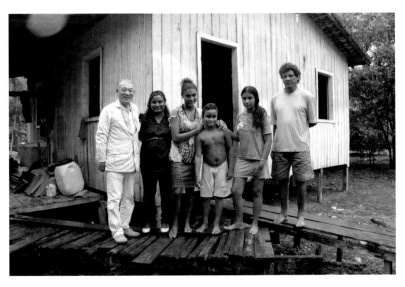

108. With Jose, Maria, and their three children who live in a solitary house overlooking the Amazon River (Brazil, December 2016)

months to a year until treatment is completed. I strongly felt the need for drastic measures to ensure that patients with the disease can continue receiving treatment. My conviction was reinforced when I visited a family of people affected by leprosy living in the middle of the state, along the Amazon River. I arrived there after taking two boats from a dock in Belém. The family comprised a couple, Jose and Maria, and their three children. José said he began treatment after developing limb disabilities and wished he had discovered the disease a little earlier. Maria had suspected that the spots on her body were cancer, but after receiving a leprosy diagnosis, she had treatment and was now cured. Their children were also undergoing, or scheduled to undergo, treatment. The state health ministry official who accompanied me expressed frustration at how some patients give up on treatment because of the distance to the hospital and the time and effort involved.

The small town of Santo Antônio do Prata is the site of Brazil's oldest leprosy isolation facility, which opened in 1924. The leprosarium, located in a town with a population of 3,000, is home to eleven people affected by leprosy, and about 200 people of the second, third, and fourth generations lived in the vicinity. The oldest resident was a healthy ninety-seven-year-old man. The residents all welcomed me cheerfully, singing and dancing, but when I thought of how they were languishing here in such an out of the way place, sent here due to a diagnosis of leprosy in the distant past, I was at a loss for what to say by way of comfort.

As I left the leprosarium, I was led to a small meeting place where the residents' thirty or forty children, grandchildren, and great-grandchildren were waiting for us. A woman, the daughter of a resident, complained mournfully about the emotional scars of having been separated from her parents and the discrimination she still suffers today because of her Prata background. I encouraged them, saying: "The words of people affected by leprosy are starting to reach Brasília. I hope those of you who have suffered will make your voices heard. Your efforts will give courage and hope to people in the same difficult circumstances worldwide. Brazil is the second country, after Japan, to compensate persons affected by leprosy, and if compensation for the generation that comes after becomes a reality, it will be the first time globally. Your struggle is leading the vanguard of a global fight. You must keep hope alive and make a solution happen with your own hands."

Preventing the same mistakes from happening again—Republic of Colombia, December 2013

> Route: Belém, Brazil → São Paulo, Brazil (flight time: 6h; 2h stopover) → Bogotá, Colombia (flight time: 6h 20m)—three nights—Bogotá → Paris, France (flight time: 10h 40m; 2h 30m stopover) → Narita International Airport (flight time: 11h 45m)

I followed my visit to Brazil with three days spent in the Republic of Colombia. This country had once required people affected by leprosy to isolate themselves from society, but in 1961 a law was passed abolishing this forced isolation. In 1963, one area that had a particular connection with this history became an independent municipality, seeking a way to develop without losing the memory of its past. That area is called Agua de Dios (literally, Water of God). In an age when leprosy was incurable, especially from the late nineteenth to the early twentieth century, all over the world hospitals and leprosaria were built to keep people affected by leprosy away from society. However, with the discovery of a cure, more and more of these places have been shuttered, which means we are losing valuable historical buildings. In Agua de Dios, there are efforts to prevent such history being lost. Yet the people originally sent there are now in their eighties or older. Their oral histories have to be recorded before it is too late. Humanity can learn much from the story of leprosy. In 2012, the Sasakawa Health Foundation organized an international workshop at the National Hansen's Disease Museum in Japan, bringing together people from the Philippines, Malaysia, Brazil, and Taiwan who share the same conviction.

Colombia's capital Bogotá lies at an altitude of 2,600 meters, with an oxygen level of about three quarters that of Tokyo. The morning after my arrival, a man came to meet me at my hotel. His name was Jaime Molina Garzón: he was sixty-seven-years old and a person affected by leprosy. I had first encountered him at an international conference on leprosy held in Pune, India, in 2010. He runs an NGO called Corsohansen in the town of Agua de Dios which works to restore the dignity of people affected by leprosy, raise awareness, and increase their income. We immediately set out by car and headed back to where he had come from—Agua de Dios. In Bogotá, police officers keep a watchful eye on people passing by, and the iron bars on the rows of stores in the streets brought home to me how unsafe it was. On and on we drove on a road that descended toward the town Agua de Dios, 400 meters above sea level. When the mist lifted, we were surrounded by pastureland. (Half of Colombia is covered by dense forests, one-third by pastureland, and the rest by farmland, with less than 1 percent made up of villages and urban areas.) About two and a half hours from Bogotá, I saw a sign for Agua de Dios. Fifteen minutes later, we arrived at the center of this "leprosarium town" where leprosy patients used to be sent to be kept in obligatory isolation.

Two leprosaria remained in Colombia. One is in Contratación, and the other is here in Agua de Dios. Agua de Dios was established in response to a decree passed in 1864 to set up a leprosarium in each department of Colombia. The first forty people were sent here in around 1870. At the time, the area was uninhabitable: the patients built their own huts, and began their lives there. The first hospital, Hospital San Rafael, was built around 1880, more than ten years after the settlement. Entering Agua de Dios required crossing a swift river flowing from the capital, Bogotá. In 1872, the Bridge of Sighs, now a Colombian national heritage site, was built on this river. The name comes from the fact that people affected by leprosy said their final goodbyes to their families before crossing the bridge. Until this bridge was built, a basket traveling along ropes suspended from both banks would ferry seven or eight people at once.

With time, the bridge deteriorated, and a new bridge was built a few dozen meters away in 2012. The water flowing under the bridge was black with wastewater from Bogotá. "It's the dirtiest river in Colombia," Jaime told me, with a wry smile. By the time the leprosy quarantine law was repealed in 1961, more than 6,000 people affected by leprosy had come to Agua de Dios. Some of them came from other countries, including Venezuela. Once they arrived at Agua de Dios, they were stripped of their IDs and issued with docu-

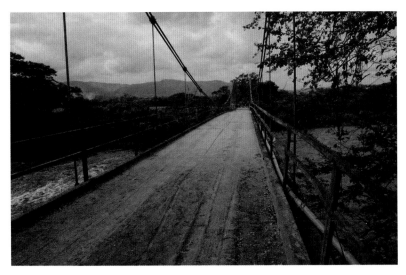

109. A bridge known as the "Bridge of Sighs": Once a person crossed it, they would never come back (Colombia, December 2013)

ments only accepted here. The leprosarium even had its own local currency. The purpose of the local currency was to prevent other people from touching the money touched by people affected by leprosy and to restrict the free movement of residents. When Agua de Dios was an isolation leprosarium, it was surrounded by a 4-meter-high barbed wire fence, and the government assigned guards to prevent escape.

The population of Agua de Dios was around 13,000 at the time of my visit. Of these, 85 percent were people affected by leprosy and their families. There are four leprosy-related museums in the town. The first is a museum attached to Jaime's Corsohansen office. Alongside photographs and other materials from the isolation period, there was an old, yellowed ID card of a girl named Emma, who had been ten years old at the time. She was still alive and in good health, and she greeted me with a smile that was the same smile of the girl in the photograph. Her daughter, Ana, worked for Corsohansen.

The second museum houses the belongings of the celebrated Colombian composer Luis Calvo. He contracted leprosy at the age of thirty-four and moved here to compose music.

The third is the Father Luigi Variara Museum, which is unique worldwide in that it is housed in a convent. It was the first time I had met nuns who had lived experience of leprosy (seven were present during my trip), and they were dressed in pure white habits, looking exceptionally mystical in their bearing. Father Variara came to Agua de Dios in 1894 at nineteen and devoted himself to educating children affected by leprosy. In the memorial hall, there were brass instruments that he had let the children use and a letter asking for a donation of "1 cent per Colombian citizen" for the construction of the facility.

The fourth museum, operated by the national leprosarium, aims to inform visitors about the history of leprosy in Colombia from an anthropological perspective and promote accurate knowledge of the disease. Its collection holds a large number of medical charts, with the oldest one dated 1903. The medical charts contained records of people who had escaped and were sentenced to labor, fines, and incarceration. The former prison was still standing, but some had suggested that it should be demolished. In response, the museum staff was working hard to preserve this invaluable historical facility. Many unorganized materials were deteriorating, and precious records were in danger of disappearing.

While all four museums showed how enthusiastic the people involved were in preserving and passing on the history of Agua de Dios, it was more than clear that there was a lack of funds.

The residents of the city's leprosaria were all elderly, so the facilities resembled nursing homes. At the San Vicente Women's Leprosarium, residents made handicrafts, watched TV, and enjoyed conversation with visiting family members, while at the Boyacá Men's Leprosarium residents played chess and other table games in the meeting room. They spent fulfilling days engrossed in their hobbies: one person read aloud a poem they had written, with feeling, while another presented a lovely handmade giraffe figurine, and a third showed off a bonsai-like plant they had tended. Many people affected by leprosy and their descendants worldwide have great talents, but rarely are they as famous as Luis Calvo (or, for that matter, the Japanese novelist Tamio Hojo). Many of their works are unknown or packed away out of sight and never see the light of day. I recalled the beautiful paintings by people affected by leprosy I had seen in a leprosy hospital in Russia.

Mayor Jorge Humberto Garcés Betancur, the son of parents who had been sent here, told me: "The history of leprosy is a stain on humanity, but the transformation of Agua de Dios from a city of despair to one of hope is a part of Colombia's proud history. I hope you will share it with the world. The related materials are our valuable heritage."

The reality was that the people here were still discriminated against simply because they hail from Agua de Dios, and its economic development lags behind other cities. Preserving their history and connecting it to the town's development and maintaining Agua de Dios as a place of hope into the future was a tremendous responsibility for the people of the town.

Countries visited in 2014	
January	● Indonesia
	Myanmar (Nationwide ceasefire agreement: talks with government personnel)
February	Myanmar (Nationwide ceasefire agreement: talks with government personnel)
	Thailand (Myanmar nationwide ceasefire agreement: negotiations with representatives of armed ethnic organizations)
March	● India
	● Nepal
April	● South Korea
May	Thailand (Myanmar nationwide ceasefire agreement: negotiations with representatives of armed ethnic organizations)
	Sri Lanka (Talks with President Rajapaksa)
	Latvia (SYLFF international conference at University of Latvia)
	● Switzerland
	● Romania
June	● Jordan

	Palestine (Talks with President Mahmoud Abbas)
	Israel (Talks with President Shimon Peres)
	● Myanmar (Nationwide ceasefire agreement: talks with government personnel)
July	Uganda (SG2000-related; Borlaug Legacy Symposium)
	Thailand (Myanmar nationwide ceasefire agreement: negotiations with representatives of armed ethnic organizations)
September	Thailand (Myanmar nationwide ceasefire agreement: negotiations with representatives of armed ethnic organizations)
October	Myanmar (two visits) (Nationwide ceasefire agreement: talks with government personnel)
	Thailand (Myanmar nationwide ceasefire agreement: negotiations with representatives of armed ethnic organizations)
	● Morocco
	● Spain
November	● Spain
	● India
	Myanmar (Nationwide ceasefire agreement: talks with government personnel)
	Thailand (two visits); Myanmar (Nationwide ceasefire agreement: negotiations with representatives of armed ethnic organizations)
December	Myanmar (two visits) (Nationwide ceasefire agreement: talks with government personnel)

● Indicates a trip that features in this section.

SYLFF: Sasakawa Young Leaders Fellowship Fund program.

SG2000: Sasakawa Global 2000 program. An agricultural project supporting farmers in need in Africa.

MAKING THE IMPOSSIBLE POSSIBLE

The loneliness of familial abandonment—Republic of Indonesia, January 2014

Route: Narita International Airport → Jakarta, Indonesia (flight time: 8h)—one night—Jakarta → Jayapura, Indonesia (flight time: 6h 45m)—two nights—Jayapura → Biak, Indonesia (flight time: 1h)—one night—Biak → Jakarta (flight time: 5h 50m)—two nights—Jakarta → Narita (flight time: 7h)

I began 2014 with a visit to Indonesia, my first in three and a half years and my fourteenth overall. The day after I arrived in Jakarta, I left my hotel at 3 a.m. and flew more than six hours to Jayapura, the capital of Papua province. The ethnic composition here is different from other regions, and many of the residents are not Muslim but Christian. Many people associate the word "Papua" with Papua New Guinea, which is a country on the eastern half of New Guinea island. Indonesia's Papua is on the western side of the same island.

After arriving in Jayapura, I visited the village of Hamadi, where many people affected by leprosy live. The residents performed a welcome dance, and one elderly man sang a song in Japanese. In return, my companion Kazunori Jotaki—the president of the Association of Professional Motorboat Racers (1,600 motorboat racers regularly donate to leprosy causes)—and I sang "Donguri Korokoro" with the message, "Let's all live together in harmony." Every family in the village has one person affected by leprosy. While early diagnoses seem to be progressing, children often develop the disease, and those with disabilities do not want to go outdoors due to embarrassment, so they did not show up at the welcome dance. This showed me that discrimination was still an issue here.

The next morning, I met with Papua's Vice Governor Klemen Tinal. I told him: "Many people do not go to hospitals because they feel ashamed of being affected by leprosy." When I added that I wanted him to promote accurate information about the disease, he confessed that he had been shocked to learn of more than 1,300 new cases confirmed annually in Papua province, which has less than 3 million people. He promised to implement immediate measures, report to the governor, and keep the twenty-nine regencies in the province well informed. I was shocked that the vice governor was unaware of the situation even though this was an endemic province, and based on my previous experience, I did not expect him to be proactive in this regard. It reinforced my belief that I would have to visit him again and again until I could finally motivate him to act.

In the afternoon, I visited the Hamadi health center in Jayapura. At the entrance, a young girl gave me a magnificent hat with feathers of the bird of paradise, which are common throughout the region, and a *koteka*, a penis sheath, which made me giggle. About fifteen to twenty people affected by leprosy visit the health center each week. Again, many are young people and children, including a four-year-old girl receiving treatment, the youngest person affected by leprosy I had encountered anywhere in the world. Vera Yok, the only nurse specializing in leprosy at the hospital, told me that many patients stopped coming to pick up their medicine during their treatment and that she had to visit them individually. She said that prejudice against leprosy is particularly widespread in mountainous areas, and they do not come to the hospital for fear of discrimination. She spoke frankly about how, if this situation continues, healthcare providers would have little hope of discovering patients hidden in remote areas, one of many examples of the lack of human resources and the challenges in their efforts. I was astonished at the severe conditions she had to handle alone on this island, which covers an area of 300,000 square kilometers and has a population of around 2.8 million.

After leaving the health center, I visited a boy who said he had contracted leprosy from his mother and had stopped attending school because he was ashamed. I sat beside him and tried encouraging him, but he remained dejected. My heart ached. My hope is to prevent even one more child from experiencing such sadness. After that, I repeatedly asked the Indonesian government to allow me to visit West Papua province. However, the violent independence movement and worsening security situation in the region meant that I was repeatedly refused.

The next day, I traveled an hour by plane to Biak Island. This small island was the scene of a fierce battle during the Pacific War, in which more than 10,000 Japanese soldiers died. The island's population is about 122,000, with around 150 new leprosy cases annually. I first visited a general hospital, where two patients were hospitalized, and

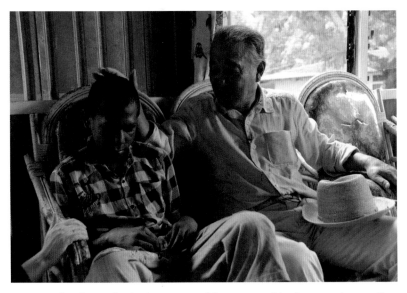

110. With a boy who had contracted leprosy and had stopped attending school out of shame (Indonesia, January 2014)

then a public health center with around seventy active patients on their records. After that, I visited Abia Lumbiak, a former fisherman who lived quietly by himself in an empty hut on the outskirts of a village. He developed the disease at fifteen, but despite being cured had lost feeling in the nerves in his legs. Five years ago, an injury left him with a disability. He now lived without visitors or anyone to converse with, except for his brother, who brought him meals. On days when he did not receive food from his brother, he slept on an empty stomach. After hearing his story, I visited Mr. Lumbiak again that night with a packed meal. We walked down the dark, mosquito-filled footpath and ate together. He broke his reticence to speak, saying, "It's been a long time since I had a meal with someone," before adding, mumbling to himself, "I want to be able to go outside on my own. I want to go out to sea again." However, his expression was vacant, as though he had given up on everything. Indonesia has many people affected by leprosy who live alone like this. A week before my visit, a local newspaper had reported the discovery in East Java of someone who had been living for five years in the forest, catching rats

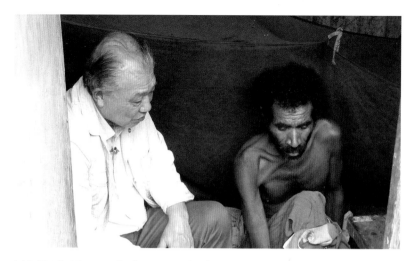

111. With Abia Lumbiak, a man who for years continued to live in isolation, despite being cured (Indonesia, January 2014)

and snakes to survive because his family had driven him away. Much later, I received some uplifting news. Mr. Lumbiak underwent leg surgery and, despite his disability, had resumed fishing and was now living with his family.

On 27 January, Jakarta played host to the ceremony for the 2014 Global Appeal to End Stigma and Discrimination against Persons Affected by Leprosy. This year's appeal, our ninth, was signed by national human rights institutions from thirty-nine countries and co-sponsored by the Indonesian Human Rights Commission. National human rights institutions (or national human rights commissions) are state institutions independent of the government that promote non-judicial relief from human rights violations and human rights guarantees. They play a crucial role in many countries worldwide, although they do not exist in Japan. The ceremony was attended by People's Welfare Coordinating Minister Agung Laksono, Health Minister Nafsiah Mboi, and Indonesian National Commission for Human Rights Deputy Commissioner Dianto Bachriadi, as well as representatives of other national human rights commissions from India, Jordan, Thailand, and the Philippines, and many members of Perhimpunan Mandiri Kusta (PerMaTa), an organization for people affected by leprosy. Speaking on behalf of President Susilo Bambang Yudhoyono, Minister Laksono said: "Many people still fear leprosy, and mistaken ideas and superstitions remain, including that the disease is incurable, genetic, or divine punishment. I would like to work with the National Commission for Human Rights and the Ministry of Health to correct these mistakes, eliminate discrimination, and ensure early detection and treatment." I requested that human rights commissions in each country protect the human rights of people affected by leprosy, investigate the various human rights violations they face, and advise their governments. I also asked them to work with domestic stakeholders and civil society to conduct ongoing awareness-raising initiatives and public campaigns.

Visit to a colony with His Holiness the Dalai Lama—Delhi, India, March 2014

> Route: Narita International Airport → Delhi, India (flight time: 10h 15m)—three nights

In March, I visited Delhi, on my fiftieth trip to India since my first in 1984. In some years, I have been there up to seven times, and it truly is like a second home to me. The day before my arrival was the Hindu festival of Holi, a time of great festivity to celebrate the coming of spring and pray for a bountiful harvest. Likely a remnant of the festival, red and yellow stains were conspicuous on people's clothes and the roads.

First, I attended a S-ILF board meeting. Under the leadership of Executive Director Vineeta Shanker, S-ILF had a small, elite staff of fourteen people working to support the self-reliance of people affected by leprosy and their families throughout the vast Indian region. It was operating 154 economic independence support projects in seventeen Indian states. We must remember that the success of these projects is due to the training provided before the project's launch, the extraordinary measures taken for cases where progress is slow, and the follow-up provided by S-ILF staff after projects get underway. Moreover, leaders are emerging from among those working on the projects, and I look forward to seeing further developments. What is even more commendable, however, is the attitude of publicly documenting failures and learning lessons for the next time. The accumulation of such expertise is one of S-ILF's strengths. In recent years, it has also been focusing on educational projects for children of people affected by leprosy and has expanded its scholarship programs to provide vocational training opportunities and train nurses.

After S-ILF's board meeting, I met with Mr. Javed Abidi, the chairperson of Disabled Peoples' International (DPI), an organization for people with disabilities. We discussed how to involve people affected by leprosy in the disability movement. In India, Mr. Abidi joins many other influential activists who have advocated for the rights of people with disabilities and negotiated with the government to achieve their participation in society. Their struggles and experiences can teach much to people affected by leprosy. Mr. Abidi also took time out of his busy schedule to attend the next day's meeting of state leaders of people affected by leprosy.

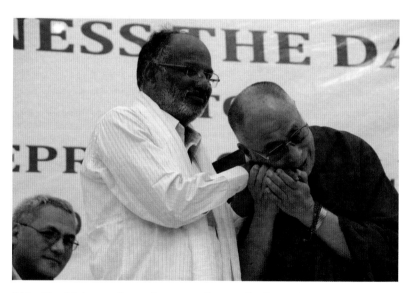

112. His Holiness the Dalai Lama laying the hand of Mr. Vagavathali Narsappa, president of the Association of People Affected by Leprosy (APAL; formerly National Forum India) against his cheek (Delhi, March 2014)

The next day, 20 March, I met with His Holiness the Dalai Lama, and together we visited a leprosy colony in Delhi. The impetus for this joint visit goes back to August 2012. I visited His Holiness at his office in Dharamsala in northern India, explained the fight against the discrimination experienced by people affected by leprosy in India, and asked him if he would like to visit a leprosy colony with me. He promised he would join me. It took some time to adjust his schedule, but he told me he could devote an hour and a half in Delhi, making this visit possible.

The Tahirpur neighborhood, about an hour's drive north of central Delhi, has a cluster of twenty-seven leprosy colonies, housing a total of about 10,000 people, including nearly 4,000 people affected by leprosy and their families. For this visit, the Kasturba Gram colony set up a special stage to welcome His Holiness. A large crowd filled the colony, which is usually sparsely occupied. Most were residents of the Tahirpur colonies, but some were state leaders of the Association of People Affected by Leprosy (APAL; formerly, National Forum India) from twenty states in India. Numerous domestic and foreign media representatives were also present. When His Holiness arrived at 9:30 a.m., he did not go to the stage, instead walking up to the assembled people affected by leprosy. After holding hands and hugging them for a while, he went on stage and received a welcome from children with songs and flower bouquets. He touched each of the children's faces as he greeted them, without hurrying. He held the hand of APAL's President Narsappa, who sat next to him, still with the aftereffects of the disease, and brought it to his cheek. His Holiness's empathetic gesture was more persuasive than the tens of thousands of times I had said in so many words that leprosy is not contagious; that once the disease is cured, it cannot be a source of infection; and that discrimination is unjust.

After listening to the plight of discrimination from people affected by leprosy, His Holiness said: "Seven billion human beings are all equal. Discrimination for any reason, whether caste, religion, or social, is a sin." He also encouraged the people affected by leprosy, donated 1 million rupees (about US$12,000) to the colony, and promised to continue to support it for the next five years. The media broadcast His Holiness holding the hands of people affected by leprosy and blessing them worldwide. More than 7 million people viewed his Internet streaming service. People who were not interested in leprosy issues became sympathetic to the cause. His Holiness is hugely influential, and his visit was truly appreciated.

In India's vastness, there are few opportunities for leprosy leaders from different states to meet each other, even if they belong to the same organization. After the ceremony, I had lunch with state leaders of people affected by leprosy who had gathered from all four corners of India and heard their thoughts and reports from the field. In the evening, I visited the Union Ministry of Health to call on Health Secretary Lov Verma. While he had just taken office this past February, he promised the Ministry of Health's cooperation in my efforts to eliminate leprosy.

Crossing a border for treatment—Federal Democratic Republic of Nepal, March 2014

Route: Delhi, India → Kathmandu, Nepal (flight time: 1h 50m)—four nights—Kathmandu → Delhi (flight time: 1h 20m; 3h stopover) → Narita International Airport (flight time: 7h 20m)

After leaving India, I headed to Nepal. It had been four years since I was invited to celebrate Nepal's elimination of leprosy. At the airport in Kathmandu, I was met by Dr. Lin Aung, WHO's representative in Nepal, and others. From the airport, I headed directly to the Nepal Ministry of Health and Population, where I met with Minister Khagaraj Adhikari, who was appointed to the new cabinet in February, along with Health Secretary Praveen Mishra. At a later meeting with Chair (and former Prime Minister) Pushpa Kamal Dahal of the Communist Party of Nepal (Maoist Centre), he spoke quietly and deliberately, saying, "On behalf of the people of Nepal, I would like to express my deepest gratitude for your support in eliminating leprosy as a public health problem. I will do my best to ensure that we make further progress both medically and socially."

The following day, I flew first thing in the morning to Nepalganj in the Banke district of Nepal's Mid-Western Development Zone. The leprosy community in the district's Saingaun village had a population of about 6,000 people, including many of the poorest people of the lowest caste in Banke district (the caste system also exists in parts of Nepal and Myanmar). More than fifty people affected by leprosy and their families lived there. Self-support groups had been organized, and businesses set up with microcredit from the government. Some of the self-support group members and community health volunteers had gathered together to meet me in a small concrete-built meeting-place. In Nepal, so-called Female Community Health Volunteers play a vital role in end-user government health services, including maternal and juvenile healthcare and infectious disease detection. Without their efforts, medical care in Nepal would not function.

I then traveled by car on rough roads for about two hours to the neighboring Bardiya district, where I visited another community of people affected by leprosy in the village of Taratal. In the Mid-Western Development Zone, the NGO International Nepal Fellowship (INF) has provided leprosy support for many years. Thirty-five years ago, INF took the lead in bringing together people affected by leprosy from all over Nepal who had been evicted out of their villages due to terrible discrimination. Eighty people affected by leprosy and their families still lived in Taratal when I visited. At first glance, they appeared to be leading a normal life, but I thought they were more than likely hiding a sense of homesickness deep in their hearts, and as always I couldn't help feeling sad for them.

In the evening, I happened to meet Dharmendra Jha, former president of the Federation of Nepali Journalists, at the hotel. Mr. Jha is a comrade in the fight against leprosy in Nepal, having accompanied me when I visited the Terai belt in 2009 and held an education session on leprosy for the local media there. I thought we could take some time to reminisce, but he was on his way out for a prior engagement and left the hotel with his customary briskness.

The next morning, I visited a clinic established in 1960 with the support of the German Leprosy and Relief Association. As a leprosy treatment facility in the Mid-Western Development Zone, the clinic sees patients from Banke and Bardiya districts. The staff of fourteen, including one doctor and six nurses, diagnoses and treats leprosy as well as its complications. There were eight inpatients. Because it had so few beds, patients could only stay for a maximum of two weeks.

Treating leprosy does not usually require hospitalization, and patients who cross the border from India or who require surgical treatment or long-term hospitalization are sent to the main treatment facility in the neighboring Surkhet district, about 120 kilometers away.

On my way to the airport to return to Kathmandu, I took a detour to the Indian border. The border was marked solely by a few stones on the grassy ground. I would have walked right past it without noticing if I had not been told it was there. On each side of the border, whether Nepal or India, I saw tranquil countryside. On the Indian side of the border is the state of Uttar Pradesh, with an exceptionally high number of patients in Bahraich district. Many people affected by leprosy come to Nepalese hospitals for leprosy treatment.

The next day, I visited a leprosarium in Khokana. Established by the king in 1857, this national leprosarium housed about 100 people affected by leprosy and their families. Initially, the government built separate leprosaria for men and women using both banks of the Bagmati River, a sacred Hindu river, but these were later consolidated on the right bank. Four residential buildings were constructed,

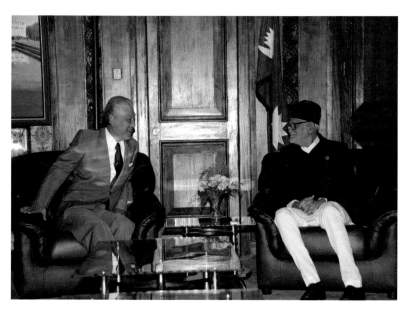

113. A meeting with Prime Minister Sushil Koirala (Nepal, March 2014)

but only one remains today. Since it was built eighty years ago, the leprosarium was dilapidated. With support from the Sasakawa Health Foundation, officials had constructed a new residential building nearby, and the residents had already moved in. While showing me around the dilapidated building, Chudamani Bhandari, director of the health ministry's Leprosy Control Division, told me of his dream of leaving the building as a museum to preserve this piece of leprosy's history.

On the way back to Kathmandu, we stopped by Bhandari's Leprosy Control Division in the Ministry of Health and Population. The building was initially constructed with the support of the Nippon Foundation in 1979 as a training center for people affected by leprosy. It had been renovated and was now used for the Leprosy Control Division.

In the evening, I attended a joint meeting with health ministry representatives, WHO officials, people affected by leprosy, and NGOs. It brought together members of organizations for people affected by leprosy from all over Nepal. To my delight, more than 30 percent of the leaders of these organizations were women. This is a progressive development compared to neighboring India, where most leaders of such organizations are elderly men and rarely women. One young female leader, Parwati Oli of the International Association for Integration, Dignity, and Economic Advancement (IDEA) Nepal, spoke fluent English and will play a significant role in the future. In promoting organizations of people affected by leprosy in various countries worldwide, young leaders are invaluable, so I have made it one of my missions to nurture young leaders wherever I go.

In Nepal, several local organizations of people affected by leprosy have emerged, including IDEA Nepal; Rehabilitation Empowerment and Development Nepal, which operates mainly in Kathmandu; the Nepal Leprosy Relief Association; and other grassroots self-support groups. Nevertheless, the incipient movement to establish a cross-sectional network of people affected by leprosy is, of course, a welcome development. A similar movement emerged in the Philippines, with the Coalition of Leprosy Associations of the Philippines launching in 2012.

On the morning of my last day in Nepal, I met with President Ram Baran Yadav at the presidential palace. The president—who had worked as a doctor at a hospital in the Terai belt of southern Nepal for more than twenty years before becoming involved in politics and serving two terms as health minister—had a keen interest in leprosy. He told Prime Minister Sushil Koirala, who had just assumed office in February, about the need for the government, legislators, and the media to continue working together to combat leprosy even after eliminating the disease as a public health problem.

While in Nepal, I read a local newspaper article about a low-income family with a person affected by leprosy confined to the village latrine for a week. In villages scattered in remote areas and deep mountains, many people remain ignorant about leprosy and so inevitably live under old customs.

The starting point of my fight against leprosy—Republic of Korea, April 2014

Route: Narita International Airport → Seoul, Korea (flight time: 3h)—one night—Seoul → Haneda International Airport (flight time: 2h)

South Korea's leprosy isolation island was created in 1916 under Japanese colonial rule. On the small island off the coast of South Jeolla province, in southern Korea, is a leprosarium, Sorokdo National Hospital. In 2002, I visited the hospital with Kazumi Sogano, Yasuji Hirasawa, Osamu Sagawa, and my late father Ryoichi Sasakawa's adopted Korean daughter, Kim Mi-ok (who was an opera singer in Korea). Kazumi Sogano was the head of the Japan Leprosy Association, while Yasuji Hirasawa and Osamu Sagawa were representatives of a class action lawsuit for damages against the Japanese government and instrumental in building the National Hansen's Disease Museum at the Tama Zenshoen Sanitarium. Officials had at one time had the residents expand the facility by their own forced labor, and at its peak in 1940 it held more than 6,000 people affected by leprosy. After the war, the Korean government took over the segregation policy but repealed the law in 1960.

In April 2014, I visited the Korean Institute for Leprosy Research in Anyang, a suburb of Seoul, South Korea. In 1974, my father, Ryoichi Sasakawa, decided to build the institute immediately after speaking with Masahide Kanayama, who served as Japan's ambassador to South Korea until 1972, who told him about the plight of people affected by leprosy in South Korea, and that Crown Princess Michiko was also concerned about the situation. The institute also had a hospital attached. In September 1976, I accompanied my father to the dedication ceremony and was startled to see him hugging a patient whose appearance had been changed by the disease, unconcernedly touching her wounds with his bare hands. So the institute had a special place in my heart as one of the sites that had led me to take up the fight against leprosy and the elimination of discrimination. Ms. Park Geun-hye (the former president), who was then twenty-four years old, also attended the dedication ceremony. At the time, she was deeply concerned that the eggs from the poultry farm run by people affected by leprosy would not sell due to social stigma, so she persuaded her father then President Park Chung-hee to purchase the eggs for the army. The people affected by leprosy thanked her for her efforts. When she came to Japan, I had lunch with her and found her to be a shy and gentle woman, a far cry from the woman she was when she became president.

When I visited the Korean Institute for Leprosy Research (my last visit had been twelve years previously), the cherry blossoms were in full bloom. The sapling my father had planted in commemoration of the facility's completion was no longer there, but the one I planted when I visited Sorokdo in 2002 had grown into a magnificent tree. Korea has seven leprosy hospitals besides this one, and the government reported 265 registered patients in 2012. The institute is adjacent to the village of St. Lazarus, a settlement for people affected by leprosy.

Such settlements were established in the 1960s to help people affected by leprosy reintegrate into society. They provided a way for groups of people affected by leprosy—who had had difficulty reintegrating into society due to prejudice and discrimination—to make a living by farming and raising livestock. At the time of my trip, there were ninety settlement villages, with populations ranging from twenty to 1,000. Around 12,000 people, 30 percent of all people affected by leprosy in South Korea, lived together with their 13,000 family members. Many made ends meet by raising pigs or poultry, and I heard that about 30 percent of all eggs produced in Korea come from the settlement villages.

Someone who has made great strides in fighting leprosy in Korea is Dr. Han Sang-tae, who took the trouble to return from the Philippines to accompany me during my visit to Korea. Dr. Han had served as the WHO Western Pacific regional director, contributing significantly to the fight against leprosy in the region. I remember when I visited the Federated States of Micronesia, I swallowed MDT, the cure for leprosy, together with the president and Dr. Han at a media event to educate the public about the drugs. However, until we had dinner together during this trip to South Korea, I had no idea that it was Dr. Han who had conceived of the idea of the settlement villages during his time at the Ministry of Health and Welfare. This project of villages, together with his projects of raising pigs and poultry, were hugely successful. If this model had been adopted worldwide, the lives of people affected by leprosy in many countries still suffering from poverty would have been considerably different.

At the institute, they were studying leprosy bacteria transplanted into zebrafish. Typically, researchers use armadillos or nude mice in their experiments, so this was an unusual trial.

At the hospital, I offered words of encouragement to more than a dozen patients, men and women, and noticed that there was one patient from Indonesia. The doctor in charge explained: "In recent years, foreign workers have developed the disease. We must keep an eye on the situation."

The visit also served to remind me of the flow of time. All signs of the once tranquil countryside were now nowhere to be seen, and the adjacent land bristled with any number of high-rise condominiums.

Talks with the world in Geneva—Swiss Confederation, May 2014

Route: Narita International Airport → Amsterdam, Netherlands (flight time: 11h 30m; 3h 45m stopover) → Riga, Latvia (flight time: 2h)— one night—Riga → Amsterdam (flight time: 2h 25m; 3h stopover) → Geneva, Switzerland (flight time: 1h 25m)—four nights

After attending the SYLFF tenth-anniversary celebration at the University of Latvia, I headed to Geneva. Every May in Geneva, I speak directly with the high-ranking health officials gathered from around the world for the WHO General Assembly. On the first day,

I spoke with Angola's Health Minister José Van Dúnem. He had accompanied me as a health secretary when I toured the country in 2003. After the nearly thirty-year civil war, the number of new leprosy cases exceeded 2,000. Since then, thanks to the efforts of the Ministry of Health and others, new cases had decreased to 400. The minister said: "We will never forget that you not only provided medicine but also visited the country during difficult times and traveled to remote areas. We want to repay you, Mr. Sasakawa, for your support." He waxed nostalgic about events from more than ten years prior and said he would work with other ministries to eliminate discrimination.

Next, I spoke with Dr. Enrique T. Ona, the Philippines secretary of health, for the fourth consecutive year. Typhoon Haiyan, which hit the Philippines in November 2013, caused extensive damage to the island of Culion, where many people affected by leprosy live. The Nippon Foundation had sent Japanese student volunteers to Culion Island to repair damaged houses. Secretary Ona told me that a staff member from the Department of Health had just visited Culion Island and expressed his gratitude for the Japanese assistance.

The following day, I met Brazil's Dr. Jarbas Barbosa, vice minister of health surveillance and an old acquaintance. Brazil is the only country that had yet to eliminate leprosy as a public health problem, but the vice minister reported that the latest statistics for 2013 showed improvement in all indicators.

According to Tanzania's Health Minister Seif Seleman Rashidi, the country's new cases had decreased from 5,000 to 2,000 in the ten years since 2004, and they were trialing further countermeasures.

I also had a series of meetings with the health ministers of Myanmar, Zanzibar, DRC, and Mozambique, as well as senior officials of the Ministries of Health of Morocco, China, and Sri Lanka. The WHO Secretariat set up a room and made appointments with the ministers of each country for me. The ministers came to my room in succession, so the meetings proceeded very efficiently indeed.

I also met with the regional directors-general responsible for the WHO's Americas, Western Pacific, Southeast Asia, Eastern Mediterranean, and Africa regions. These people are internationally elected and have a great deal of influence on public health policy in the countries of their respective regions. Their understanding and leadership are indispensable in promoting the fight against leprosy. We meet whenever I visit the WHO General Assembly in Geneva or the countries where the regional offices are located to discuss progress in eliminating leprosy. This visit was notable for allowing my first discussion with Dr. Poonam Khetrapal Singh since she assumed office as the newly appointed regional director for Southeast Asia, a region with many endemic countries, including India, which has more than half of the world's leprosy cases, and Indonesia, the third most endemic nation.

The Sasakawa Health Prize award ceremony at the WHO General Assembly is also an annual tradition. It has become WHO's oldest and most prestigious award, with cash prizes for NGOs contributing to regional healthcare. The uniqueness of this award is that the prize money must be used for healthcare-promoting activities. The 2014 prize was awarded to the Leprosy Control Foundation, Inc./Hubert Bogaert Institute of Dermatology and Skin Surgery in the Dominican Republic, which has been fighting leprosy for over fifty years. At a luncheon with the representative of the award-winning organization, WHO Director-General Dr. Margaret Chan was on hand to congratulate them. There was also a signing ceremony to renew my term as WHO Goodwill Ambassador for Leprosy Elimination for another two years. In lieu of a report on my activities, I handed Director-General Chan a list of the 320 people I have met since becoming ambassador in 2001, including presidents, prime ministers, health ministers, and provincial governors. She reacted with surprise, saying: "You are the most active ambassador of the World Health Organization."

Amorous advances at the Tichileşti leprosarium—Romania, May 2014

Route: Geneva, Switzerland → Munich, Germany (flight time: 1h 15m; 1h stopover) → Bucharest, Romania (flight time: 2h)—four nights—Bucharest → Paris, France (flight time: 3h 30m; 2h stopover) → Narita International Airport (flight time: 12h)

From Geneva, I went to Romania, going via Munich. While no new leprosy cases had emerged in Romania in recent years, there was still one leprosarium in Tichileşti in the eastern part of the country. From Romania's capital Bucharest, once called the "Paris of the East" because of its elegant architecture, a five-hour drive east took me to the Danube Delta, a beautiful wetland designated by UNESCO as a World Natural Heritage Site where the Danube River flows into the Black Sea. Thirty minutes more and we had reached a secluded area surrounded by acacia and lilac forests, the Tichileşti Hospital and Leprosarium. I had asked a Romanian resident in Japan to send an e-mail in Romanian to arrange my visit, but no reply came, as the person who saw the e-mail assumed it was a spam email—no one from Japan would be planning to visit a rural area in Romania. I had asked people on the streets of Bucharest about leprosy in Romania, but no one knew anything about it. So this was a place whose existence had been completely forgotten.

The Tichileşti Leprosarium was rebuilt once, in 1928. The number of patients at that time was about 180. It had forty-seven houses for patients and even a movie theater. However, at the time of my visit, there were a mere sixteen people affected by leprosy between the ages of forty-eight and eighty-six. In 2005, the disused residential buildings were rebuilt into a nursing home for the elderly, and the facility made available to all as a general residential home, in an effort to eliminate prejudice against leprosy.

The director, Dr. Rasvan Vasiliu, welcomed me at the leprosarium and showed me around the residential buildings, church, and other facilities. It was a beautiful day; the residents were sunbathing, chatting, and relaxing in front of their homes.

Wearing a beautiful dress with a red rose behind her ear, one resident named Maria had lived here since her leprosy diagnosis at fifteen in the 1970s. Her expression was cheerful, but she said, "I was widowed when my child was twelve, and it has been a hard life. My son got married and lives in the next village. I am bored here, so I want someone to take me away. I'm looking for a rich husband. That's why I always wear pretty clothes to attract others." She smiled mischievously. Jokingly, she added, "And today my dream came true. I won't wait any longer. Let's go somewhere together!" and we danced hand in hand.

Domnica's parents were diagnosed with leprosy, and her father and mother began living at the leprosarium when they were fourteen and twelve, respectively. They met here, married, and gave birth to Domnica. She was diagnosed with leprosy at the tender age of three and began treatment, but her hands remained slightly impaired. After attending school in the city, she worked for thirty years in the town of Tulcea in the Danube Delta, where she still lived with her son. Her parents had passed away, but she spent about half the year here. She told me: "My heart is connected to this place." Photos of her parents were displayed all over her room.

Finally, I visited the cemetery located within the leprosarium. Since its establishment in 1928, more than 100 people had been laid to rest here. Maria's husband, Domnica's parents, and their precious stories were buried there.

The WANA Forum—Hashemite Kingdom of Jordan, June 2014

In June, I traveled to Jordan to attend the sixth West Asia–North Africa (WANA) Forum. The WANA Forum is an opportunity for political leaders, international organization representatives, scholars, researchers, civil society delegates, and other cultural leaders in a wide range of fields to engage in cross-national dialogue on economic, environmental, energy, educational, and social issues in West Asia and North Africa. It is the Arab version of Forum 2000, the yearly conference for international intellectual dialogue that President Havel of the Czech Republic and I had conducted in Prague since 1997. In cooperation with Prince Hassan bin Talal of Jordan, whom I befriended through Forum 2000, six international conferences were held in Amman, the capital of Jordan, to which were invited cultural leaders from Arab countries, Turkey, Iran, Iraq, and other countries in South Asia. A renowned sage and Middle East representative, Prince Hassan has held such important positions as president of the Club of Rome and chair of the Independent Commission on International Humanitarian Issues.

The first meeting of the WANA Forum was held in 2009, and the sixth and final meeting was held on 11 June 2014. The themes of each meeting were as follows:

First Forum—Human Security

Second Forum—Pursuing Supranational Solutions to the Challenges of Carrying Capacity

Third Forum—Region in Transition
Fourth Forum—Identity
Fifth Forum—The Uprooted
Sixth Forum—Legal Empowerment

With around twenty countries participating in each conference, the meetings have been a great success, addressing various common issues. The creation of a transnational network of cultural leaders from Arab countries was significant and unlike anything seen before.

At these conferences, we focused on economic, environmental, energy, and civil issues facing the WANA region, and we also tried as much as possible to present examples from Japan and Southeast Asia. Speakers included leaders from Indonesia, Malaysia, the Philippines, and other countries we had invited to past conferences and Japanese governmental and academic representatives, including Ambassador Tatsuo Arima, Ambassador Mutsuyoshi Nishimura, Professor Seiichiro Yonekura of Hitotsubashi University, Vice President Keiichi Tsunekawa of the National Graduate Institute for Policy Studies, and Professor Tsutomu Kikuchi of Aoyama Gakuin University.

The following is the text of the speech that I delivered at the Sixth WANA forum.

It is a great pleasure to be back in Amman again this year to participate in the sixth West Asia North–Africa Forum. I would like to begin by expressing my deep gratitude to the host of this forum, His Royal Highness Prince Hassan, and members of the working group headed by Dr. Ahmad Mango and Dr. Erica Harper, for the contributions they have made and continue to make for the WANA region.

I have known His Royal Highness Prince Hassan for many years, and time and time again, I have been impressed by his wisdom and moved by his unwavering determination to realize peaceful, sustainable development for the WANA region.

There is no question that the WANA region is one of the focal points of the world's social, economic, political, and environmental activities.

However, longstanding conflicts and subsequent uprisings have mired the region with difficult challenges, including threats to human security and political instability. It is due to His Royal Highness' incredible foresight that this annual forum has served as a platform where stakeholders of the region can come together and address the very concerns that are impeding growth and making life difficult for so many.

"Legal empowerment" is the forum theme for this year. It is said that billions of people around the world live outside the protection of the law. The WANA region is no exception. Such exclusions from the rule of law can only have detrimental effects on factors such as economic growth and human development and deter the path to realizing an inclusive society.

I have witnessed this dark reality in my humanitarian work; people who have been excluded from society and the protection of the law; people who have been impoverished and unaware of their fundamental rights. I feel it has been most prevalent among people affected by leprosy.

I say this because leprosy is a disease that has been misunderstood and stigmatized throughout human history. Left untreated, it can cause external damage, such as deformities on the face, hands, and feet. The appearance of those affected by the disease struck fear in people's hearts and led many to believe that the disease was a curse or punishment from God. In various countries around the world, many people were forcibly taken away from their families and banished to solitary islands or to remote locations.

For many centuries, people affected by leprosy were forced to live outside the protection of the law. They were unable to access social services, unaware of their human rights and unable to free themselves from poverty.

Only recently has this situation started to improve. This has been promoted through the collaboration of various stakeholders, including international organizations, governments, NGOs, and those affected by leprosy themselves.

Among the various initiatives, it was legal empowerment that brought about one of the most positive outcomes. In many countries, discriminatory laws have been abolished. Moreover, organizations of and for people affected by leprosy have been established around the globe, and these people are working hard to be recognized as citizens with equal rights under the law. This has brought about tangible results, such as gaining access to public facilities and social resources, but most important of all, to bring the matter to the attention of the various layers of society.

However, I feel that in order to realize a truly inclusive society, efforts to transform the mindsets of the greater population must also take place. I have seen many societies where unjust practices are deeply woven into longstanding customs and traditions, so deep that the existence of such prejudice may be hidden from even the most conscious individuals. I would be pleased if such perspectives are explored in the upcoming discussions that will be held here at the WANA forum.

As leaders representing various countries and sectors of the region, you have gathered, not for your own benefit or the benefit of your country, but for a much greater purpose of attaining a prosperous future for the entire WANA region.

Let us hope that the success of this forum will bring us one step closer to realizing a brighter and more prosperous future for the people of WANA.

On 8 June, just before I had left Japan, it was reported that President Shimon Peres of Israel and President Mahmoud Abbas of the Palestinian National Authority had participated in a joint prayer for peace in the Middle East at the Vatican under the auspices of Pope Francis. Since US Secretary of State John Kerry's efforts to mediate had just failed, there was speculation that the pope's mediation could provide an opportunity to break the deadlock in the peace negotiations. Wanting to find out what was going on, I left Amman for the presidential palace in Jerusalem after my keynote address at the WANA opening ceremony.

The border between Jordan and Israel is the most heavily guarded in the world. The meeting that was about to take place would not have been possible without the excellent coordination between the Embassy of Japan in Jordan and the Embassy of Japan in Israel. Security at the presidential palace was also very tight, and as I had been fitted with a pacemaker, I had no choice but to expose my chest so they could check the implant location.

I had occasionally had the opportunity to speak with President Peres since our first meeting at Forum 2000 in Prague. He served as Israel's prime minister before becoming the country's ninth president, completing his seven-year term in July 2014. He was well respected by the people of his country, and there were strong calls for his reappointment, but he was adamant that it would not be a good idea to simply change the rules that had been decided by law.

Although the Israeli president is a symbolic figure elected by parliament, President Peres was exceptional. He would continue to have a say in reconciliation with Palestine. However, the fact that President Reuven Rivlin, who would assume the presidency in July, alongside Prime Minister Benjamin Netanyahu and Foreign Minister Avigdor Lieberman, were all right-wingers and tightening their grip on the Gaza Strip made the prospects for future peace negotiations bleak.

President Peres, who was ninety-one years old at the time, was in high spirits, having just returned from the Vatican. When I asked him about his impression of President Abbas, he said: "He is a fair and selfless man, and I trust him," and then added, "President Abbas and I have signed an agreement for a peaceful solution. There can be no solution to the Israel–Palestine problem except through peaceful means. At the Vatican, after the pope left the room, we stayed and talked. Israel and Palestine naturally have different cultural backdrops. We have to continue our dialogue in light of these differences. A peaceful society can be achieved only when we respect different opinions. I believe both countries' leaders will support the peace process and make the right decision."

He continued: "Currently, 60 percent of the Palestinian population is over twenty-five years old, promising rapid population growth in the future. If the population were to grow fivefold without commensurate economic growth, the number of people who are poor would grow fourfold. Assistance from the government and international organizations alone will not be sufficient to solve this problem. Support for entrepreneurship, especially in high-tech fields, will be crucial. In this regard, I look forward to the contribution of Japanese companies. Terrorists are like mosquitoes. They always swarm around us for blood, but we cannot shoot them all down with guns. It is more effective to create an environment where mosquitoes do not breed. From this perspective, we must support entrepreneurship targeting the younger generation." He was pointing out the importance of support from Japan, to which I agreed.

After meeting President Peres in Jerusalem, I returned to my hotel in Amman. The following day, I visited the presidential palace in Ramallah, the West Bank city of the Palestinian National Authority, to meet with President Abbas again. President Abbas was elected chairman of the Palestine Liberation Organization in 2004 upon the death of President Yasser Arafat, and the following year he won the presidential election and became the representative of Palestine in both name and reality. Amid his hectic schedule immediately after his return from the Vatican, I was able to meet with him thanks to Prince Hassan of Jordan, who personally negotiated the appointment by phone.

President Abbas spoke of his feelings toward Japan, including his experiences in the areas affected by the Great East Japan Earthquake and his visit to Hiroshima, and said: "President Peres is a good man and a peacemaker. We are close friends. I spoke with him about peace talks after the joint service at the Vatican the other day, and we found no differences between us," emphasizing his trust toward President Peres. He then clarified his outlook on reopening peace talks, saying, "We are ready and prepared to resume negotiations at any time without any preconditions."

The church in Mayanchaung—Republic of the Union of Myanmar, June 2014

Route: Haneda International Airport → Bangkok, Thailand (flight time: 6h 30m; 3h stopover) → Yangon, Myanmar (flight time: 1h 25m)—four nights—Yangon → Narita International Airport (flight time: 6h 30m)

Since its establishment in 1974, the Sasakawa Health Foundation has continuously supported the fight against leprosy in Myanmar (Burma). In 1963, Myanmar had an estimated 600,000 people affected by leprosy, with a prevalence rate (the number of patients per 10,000 population) of 250. The Myanmar government began actively combating leprosy in 1969, and the Sasakawa Health Foundation supported medical efforts for the first thirty years of the program, focusing on diagnosing patients and promoting MDT treatment. Since then, the foundation has invited Myanmar experts to conferences and workshops on leprosy elimination and treatments in Asia, supported the training of leprosy program officers and technicians for the Ministry of Health, and continued to provide medical equipment through the Ministry of Health. The foundation has also provided ambulances, motorcycles, bicycles (10,000), motorboats, and other equipment to enable health workers and nurses in the field to carry out their meticulous work in their assigned areas. Since 2003, when Myanmar eliminated leprosy as a public health problem, the foundation has also supported primary and secondary education for people affected by leprosy and their children living in settlement villages and helped bolster leprosy organizations.

In June 2014, I visited a village of people affected by leprosy called Mayanchaung on the outskirts of Yangon, Myanmar's largest city. In 1953, the government built a national leprosarium in this village to isolate patients. However, in 1989, the leprosarium was closed, and people affected by leprosy were resettled in the village since it was thought that isolation would be a barrier to their reintegration into society. A leader of this village once came to meet me at a hotel in Yangon during my visit ten years prior. Since then, I had wanted to visit the village someday, and my wish finally came true. On this visit, I was accompanied by journalists from ten media outlets, including local TV stations, newspapers, and news agencies.

Myanmar had eliminated leprosy as a public health problem, but it had roughly 300,000 people affected by leprosy, of whom 40,000–50,000 still had disabilities. Moreover, officials continue to discover 3,000 new patients every year. According to Dr. Min Min Htun, the leprosy specialist from the Department of Social Welfare and Health Planning who accompanied me to Mayanchaung, the immediate goal is to provide proper diagnosis and treatment for these new patients and to reduce the number of new patients to zero. As in other countries, many people affected by leprosy in Myanmar have formed communities to escape discrimination and live in seclusion. Mayanchaung is one of these settlements.

Mayanchaung has a population of around 1,600 people, about 120 of whom are affected by leprosy, and nearly half of them live at the Mitta Philanthropic Center at the entrance to the village. The Department of Social Welfare and Health Planning built this center in 1989 for those who could not live independently. When I arrived, many people affected by leprosy gathered in the village meeting hall. Most were elderly, and many used wheelchairs. Since some people may feel uncomfortable about my bringing the media along, I first informed them of the significance of the media presence, and they consented. For many of the reporters, this was their first visit to a leprosy facility, and they quickly began interviewing people. The next day's print and online news carried pictures of people affected by leprosy and their families living in Mayanchaung and messages such as "leprosy can be cured."

After the press event, I spoke to the people affected by leprosy living in the center. This was a simple one-story building with separate areas for men and women and beds in rows like a hospital. Its only other facilities were a dining room and kitchen. Most of the residents were elderly, but I noticed a few young men who were left with aftereffects of the disease in their limbs and faces. When I asked them why they had not received treatment earlier, they all spoke up and said they did not go to the hospital because they had to work to make a living. That was very likely true, but I suspected that the real reason was that they feared discrimination.

Next, I was led to a Christian church in the center of the village. The village's roads were terrible, and according to Dr. Min Min Htun, they used to be built as poorly as possible to prevent the resi-

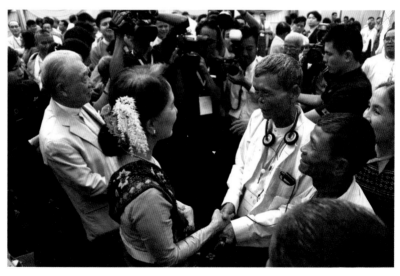

114. Aung San Suu Kyi clasping the hands of a person affected by leprosy (Myanmar, December 2018)

dents from coming and going. The Sunday church service was being held, and people affected by leprosy were present with their families and children. A woman with disabilities in both legs said: "I was affected by leprosy, and my family abandoned me. But thanks to God, I am alive with enough food and no other difficulties in my life." In response, the congregation all sang a hymn together. As I listened to them singing with all their heart and soul, I found tears running down my cheeks.

Postscript

On 12 December 2018, Myanmar held its first national conference for combating leprosy in the capital Nay Pyi Taw, with the support of the Sasakawa Health Foundation. In her opening speech, State Counsellor of Myanmar Aung San Suu Kyi encouraged the people affected by leprosy in the audience, saying, "It is essential that people with lived experience of leprosy like yourselves speak out."

A village without the word "leprosy"—Kingdom of Morocco, October 2014

> Route: Narita International Airport → Paris, France (flight time: 12h 45m; 2h 40m stopover) → Rabat, Morocco (flight time: 1h 50m)— five nights—traveled from Rabat to Tangier, with a stop at a village on the way

In October, my first visit was to Morocco, a constitutional monarchy in northwestern Africa, which I went to via Paris. For many people, Morocco may conjure images from the setting of the movie *Casablanca*. Morocco straddles the Mediterranean and Arab worlds as a member of the Union for the Mediterranean, the Arab League, and the Arab Maghreb Union. Its population is around 37 million. The first purpose of my visit was to host the International Symposium on Leprosy and Human Rights for the Middle East region, and the second was to investigate the leprosy situation. The Nippon Foundation had arranged for these symposiums to be held in five regions globally to encourage countries to implement the UN General Assembly's 2010 resolution to end discrimination against people affected by leprosy and their family members. The Morocco symposium was the fourth in the series. At the same time, working groups formulated concrete action plans, with the final action guidelines scheduled for an announcement at a symposium held at the European headquarters of the United Nations in Geneva in 2015.

A good number of Middle Eastern countries had shifted the focus of efforts from medical treatment to restoring human rights and preserving historical data and landmarks. Many of the countries that once had leprosaria now saw that their role had come to an end, and the main issues were how the elderly persons affected by leprosy could live out the rest of their lives and how the buildings and hospitals could be preserved. The symposium, held in the capital Rabat, featured lively discussions with speakers that included people affected by leprosy and experts from Morocco, Egypt, the United States, Ethiopia, and Brazil.

One of the speakers, Naima, a woman in her late thirties from Casablanca, held the microphone nervously as she began to share her own experience, looking as though it was her first time speaking in front of a large audience. Naima was diagnosed at nine and lost both her parents the following year. She was left completely alone after the marriage of her sister, who had taken care of her after she left hospital. She lived in a leprosarium with a residential facility and received training in sewing while earning a living as a housekeeper. In time, she married and had a son and a daughter. She now manages eighty people as the founder of an NGO that provides microcredits to people affected by leprosy so they can make small craftworks for sale. While she still had residual effects in her hands, she ended her speech by saying: "I am okay because I know Allah is with me. I am happy to have my first opportunity to talk about my experience at this symposium." Her initial expression of anxiety had faded, and the audience gave her a hearty round of applause.

The day after the symposium, I visited the National Leprosy Center in Casablanca, where Naima had been hospitalized. Established in 1952, at its peak the hospital had more than 200 patients, but it now had only eight to sixteen inpatients at any given time and about thirty outpatients per month. Three doctors, one of whom is a leprosy specialist, treat the few new patients discovered each year in the Western Sahara region and care for the aftereffects of the disease. With the decrease in the number of people affected by leprosy, the hospital had begun accepting general dermatology patients. The hospital had its beginnings when Dr. René Rollier, a French pioneer in treating leprosy in Morocco, turned a building that was once a military facility into a medical facility. Until French rule ended in the 1950s, patients were required to stay in the hospital for three months, a measure to ensure that treatment was completed. While in the hospital, they were provided with opportunities for cultural activities such as painting and education. Some patients had been hospitalized for more than twenty years, whether because their families had abandoned them or because they lacked the means to support themselves.

The leprosarium was a row of white-colored buildings in a quiet environment shaded by green trees. Dr. Eddaoula Asma, the female director who welcomed me, showed me to the building that had housed the medical records of every patient since the hospital's establishment. The yellowed medical records were carefully stored in drawers. I hope that officials will carefully maintain these medical records to preserve what happened here for future generations.

The men's ward had patients of all ages. One man born in 1940 had contracted the disease at sixteen and had his leg amputated at twenty-five, leaving an ulcer on the amputated surface of his knee. Despite the painful scar, the man was cheerful and reciprocated my handshake. A twenty-six-year-old woman I met in the women's ward told me she'd been the only one in her village who had contracted the disease: she'd had to conceal her illness when she developed a deformity in her hands. However, she was happily married with two children.

Dr. Asma, who was only around forty years old, used to work as a dermatologist before she started working at this hospital three years before. With large gestures, she confidently explained how rewarding it is to work with people affected by leprosy, how different their treatment is from mere dermatological therapies, and how financial support and, above all, psychological care are vital for patients, many of whom live in poverty. A Brazilian patient once lamented, "Doctors are only interested in leprosy, not in me as a person." I felt that the patients here were fortunate to be looked after by someone as caring as Dr. Asma.

The next day, we drove northwards, the Mediterranean Sea to our right, to visit a small village where people affected by leprosy lived, and a hospital. Morocco conjures an image of desert landscapes, but the northern part of the country facing the Mediterranean Sea is mild, and the 4,000-meter-high Atlas Mountains receive ample rain and snowfall. Our destination was a mountainous area 700 meters above sea level in Chefchaouen province. At the end of an ascent up a mountain road, we arrived at a small health center. I was welcomed by Mr. Ramadani, a nurse who specialized in leprosy. He had been fighting leprosy in northern Morocco, including Chefchaouen, for thirty-five years. In the days when four-wheel-drive vehicles were not available, he told me, he traveled by donkey to find patients and care for those affected by leprosy at his own expense. Today, his health center has jurisdiction over forty-eight villages and 31,000 people, some of whom come for medical care from 30 kilometers away at an altitude of 1,200 meters above sea level. It also provides maternal and child health care, vaccinations, and outpatient care. A 1980s general survey identified this area as a hot spot, with people affected by leprosy found at a rate of 4 to 5 percent of the population. However, the hard work of Nurse Ramadani and his colleagues had significantly reduced new patient numbers over the past ten years.

Led by Nurse Ramadani, I visited the home of Diab, an elderly man affected by leprosy belonging to an ethnic group in the village of Beni Bouhar. The village had a population of 232 people, all of whom were related to each other; they lived a self-sufficient lifestyle, raising crops such as olives, grapes, and figs, as well as livestock such as goats, chickens, and sheep. The house, which Diab had built himself, had stone walls with a roof of straw and soil, and it looked fairly stylish, painted white, in this rural setting. Nine members of a three-generation family welcomed us and served us traditional Moroccan sweet mint tea. Diab had been diagnosed with leprosy in 1999, but he recovered without any disability thanks to early detection by Mr. Ramadani. Diab seemed to revere Mr. Ramadani as a savior. He told me that he sometimes went all the way to the hospital where Mr. Ramadani worked, 80 kilometers away, just to see him. In this village, there was no word for "leprosy": it was simply regarded as a kind of skin disease. The low infectiousness of the disease was well known through experience, and people took it for granted that if symptoms appear, they should see a doctor, get cured, and return to the same life as before. The residents of this small Moroccan village proved firsthand that with the correct knowledge, leprosy is not a disease to be feared at all, and discrimination is unable to take root.

We then took another bumpy car ride and headed further north. Our destination was Tétouan, a town located 40 kilometers from the Strait of Gibraltar. The city's medina quarter, a unique neighborhood that reflects a mix of cultures from two continents and is registered as a World Heritage Site, is a labyrinth of low-rise white houses and home to various artisans. Because the northern tip of Morocco, including Tétouan, was Spanish territory (most of the southern part was French) until Morocco gained independence in 1956, most residents speak Arabic and Spanish.

The hospital I visited is the main leprosy facility in Morocco's northern region. It had no inpatient facilities, only outpatient services: diagnosis of people suspected of having leprosy and visits to their homes to confirm whether their families were infected. The hospital, with its white exterior and interior walls and stylishly shaped windows, served seven or eight patients on the day of my visit. Among them was a thirty-year-old woman who had just been diagnosed. She had driven an hour from the port city of Tangier. Her symptoms had appeared seven months earlier, and she had been to several doctors, but none had been able to diagnose the disease, leading her to this hospital. Her uncle's son also had leprosy, and the hospital's dermatologist would next investigate the whole family. Muslim women are reluctant to show their skin in public, so they can struggle to notice the early symptoms of the disease. Under such circumstances, Mr. Ramadani and his colleagues actively worked with local authorities to find patients, treat them, and prevent infection.

At a medical center in Tangier, I saw live leprosy bacteria under a microscope. The true form of the monster that has afflicted humankind for thousands of years looked like a tiny maggot.

Passing on leprosy's history to the next generation—Kingdom of Spain, November 2014

Route: (Traveled from Tangier to Spain via ferry) Málaga, Spain → Valencia, Spain (flight time: 1h 30m)—two nights

From the Moroccan port city of Tangier, I took the ferry across the Strait of Gibraltar to Spain. The ferry was largely empty of passengers, but the hold was full of cars and trucks. Thinking that I would probably never cross the strait again, I went out on deck to catch the sea breeze and was lucky enough to have a panoramic view of both Morocco and Spain, albeit for a short time. After a two-hour voyage, I arrived at the port of Algeciras, Spain. The Japanese Embassy in Morocco informed me that the day before I arrived, the militant group Islamic State of Iraq and Syria had called for a terrorist attack in the Strait of Gibraltar, and the alert level had been raised to the highest. I considered traveling by air, but doing so would have had a

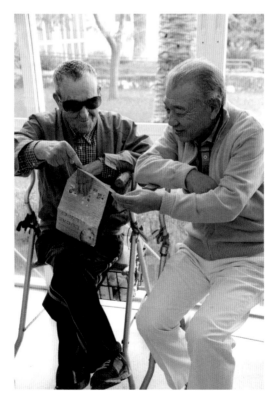

116. One resident at the Fontilles leprosarium, chatting with the author and showing him photographs (Spain, November 2014)

significant impact on my itinerary. My travel always involves some risk, and I had no choice but to travel by sea, as originally planned.

After a drive of one-and-a-half hours from the port of Algeciras to Málaga Airport and another ninety minutes in the air, I finally arrived in Valencia. After completing my journey by land, sea, and air, I went straight to my hotel and checked in.

The next morning, I headed to the Fontilles leprosarium, located less than two hours by car south of Valencia on Spain's Mediterranean coast. The leprosarium was built in a valley with vast grounds covering 700,000 square meters. Abounding in breezes, the place seemed the picture of cleanliness. Old buildings dotted the landscape around the leprosarium—which resembled an old castle with its bright orange roofs and white walls—giving an impression of how it once must have looked. This leprosarium was founded in 1909 by a Jesuit priest and a devout Catholic lawyer to help people affected by leprosy. In the 1920s, the surrounding villagers feared the disease's impact on their crops, so they built a 3-kilometer-long wall to enclose it. But it didn't take long for this mistaken notion to be dispelled, and the leprosarium became the villagers' primary source of employment. The highest number of inpatients was in the 1940s when 438 people lived there, with a church, theater, bakery, carpenter, beauty salon, gardener, and everything else necessary for daily life. Many buildings were no longer in use, and the number of residents had fallen to thirty-five. It still functioned as a leprosy research center, accepting many medical personnel for training. It also diagnosed and treated fifteen to fifty-five new patients found in Spain each year (many of them immigrants from South America and North Africa) and served as a general hospital and nursing home. Moreover, in 1989, the leprosarium began providing assistance overseas, with efforts currently expanding to India and Brazil.

After attending mass in the leprosarium's small cathedral with about forty people affected by leprosy, their families, and the staff, I spoke with some residents in a sunny corridor. Ginés García Mura—a physically fit man of sixty-eight who was a sailor in his youth and a native of Almeria, a port town in southern Spain—had lived at the leprosarium for the past eight years. He said he enjoyed watching soccer and ardently declared that he was a Barcelona supporter. A seventy-six-year-old woman had lived at Fontilles since being diagnosed at age sixteen, where she married and had many children and grandchildren. "When I got sick, I cried a lot because I was sad to leave my family, but now I am very happy, and I can go out and come back anytime I want," she said with a smile. In the courtyard, women in wheelchairs were enjoying a casual chat. Eighty-year-old Ms. Marmuela, in a pink wheelchair, said, "I came here when I was thirty years old after being diagnosed with leprosy. I was blessed with seven children but was devastated when I lost my daughter at thirty-nine. I now live for gossiping with my friends while thinking of my husband up in heaven," she told me, calmly.

The director then took me on a tour of the training facilities and the church. The library collects leprosy-related materials from all over the world and still attracts many researchers from home and abroad. I saw Dr. Kensuke Mitsuda of Japan in a sepia-toned group photo of participants at a leprosy conference once held in Germany. Eduardo de Miguel Selma, director of international cooperation, had explored potential collaborations by researching leprosy in Italy, Greece, Romania, and Portugal.

Fontilles has been engaged in a wide range of initiatives, including a final home for elderly people affected by leprosy, a center for preserving the history of leprosy and passing it on to the next generation, and support for endemic countries outside Spain, helped by its extensive experience and knowledge of the disease. The center was a pioneering and well-run institution that, from its early days, did not simply isolate patients from society but promoted activities that considered their humanity and created a place where they could live with dignity.

A kiss through the glass—Portuguese Republic, November 2014

Route: Valencia, Spain → Lisbon, Portugal (flight time: 1h 40m)—
two nights—Lisbon → Paris, France (flight time: 2h 30m; 1h 15m
stopover) → Haneda International Airport (flight time: 12h)

My visit to Spain over, I flew from Valencia to Lisbon, the capital of Portugal, about 220 kilometers away, and from there drove two hours north to reach the University of Coimbra, famous for its World Heritage Site. It had been thirty years since the Nippon Foundation began offering scholarships to outstanding students in the master's and doctoral programs at this university. I was surprised to hear that bats live in the university library. The bats prey on the insects that cling to the old books in the historic library building. It was daytime, though, so I did not see any. But come to think of it, I do wonder what they do about the bat droppings.

About an hour's drive west of Coimbra is the Rovisco Pais hospital-colony leprosarium, which I visited once in 2003. Established in 1947, the leprosarium was Portugal's first and only leprosy hospital and colony. It covers an area of 2 million square meters and is self-sufficient, with a hospital, residences, churches, and other facilities necessary for daily life. At its peak, from 1959 to 1960, it had nearly 1,000 residents. In Portugal, patients were mandatorily segregated until around 1980. The Rovisco Pais leprosarium was also known as a leprosy research center, where doctors advanced medical research and performed the first plastic surgery in the country. The last patient was completely cured in 1996, and the facility is now the largest rehabilitation center in Portugal.

With a snapshot of my visit ten years ago in hand, I went around the hospital rooms where elderly people affected by leprosy live. While there had been forty residents ten years ago, there were only twelve now, with seven men and five women. The youngest was seventy-five years old, and the oldest was ninety-three. During my last visit, I met a man who was the last new patient found in Europe. He was a slight man and lived to work in the fields. He was in the middle of his work, but he greeted me with a smile and a hoe in his hand. I had promised to visit him again and gave him a solar-powered wristwatch, which he held up to the sun with a curious look on his face. I hoped to see him again this time, but unfortunately, he had passed away several years before, at seventy.

It was teatime when I arrived, so three women and three men drank their tea in the dining room with some assistance. However, they had advanced dementia, making conversation a challenge. One of the people affected by leprosy recognized herself from ten years ago in the photo I was holding and nodded her head happily. A man sat in a wheelchair and stared outside from a hallway, and another made a strange face when he saw this unfamiliar visitor. The deep wrinkles on his scarred hands told me that this had indeed once been a leprosarium and also that it would soon come to the end of its original role.

This leprosarium had two unusual facilities. The first was an old V-shaped church. Usually, churches have an altar where the priest stands and pews for the congregation to sit in front of it. In contrast, this church's altar lay at the "V" base, with four or five pews in front of it so the altar could be seen from either side of the church. This arrangement was meant to allow women and men to attend mass without mixing, as one side was for men, and the other was for women, with the pews nearest the altar for leprosarium staff. As in Japan, it was customary to separate male and female patients to prevent anybody from getting pregnant. Even so, what happened to the children that were born? The answer lay in an old, dilapidated, one-story concrete building. It was about 81 square meters, dimly lit, with no electricity. The ceiling was high, and a glass frame divided the room into three sections. The glass had numerous holes about 3 centimeters in diameter. This place was where people affected by leprosy and their young children met. Church members raised the children nearby until they became independent, and they sometimes met their parents here through the glass. The children lived in beds stacked like silkworm racks, and when they became big enough, they were sent out to work as servants or maidservants.

"Children born to people affected by leprosy are not allowed to be raised by their parents." That notion went without saying everywhere in the world. In Brazil, Malaysia, and other countries that were once Portuguese colonies, children who were separated from their parents within a few days of birth went missing. The search for their immediate families is still underway in Brazil and other countries. The same tragedy occurred in Portugal. In June 2014, a local magazine published a feature article about them with testimonies: "Opposite glass partition walls, wooden benches line a wall with people sitting on them. A door opens, and children dressed in their Sunday best enter. They point to their parents behind the glass. The adult who brought the children picks them up and carries them close to the glass. The parent and child hold hands and kiss through the glass. The parent speaks through the hole in the glass, desperately asking, 'Are you eating? Are you being good? Are you doing well?' The child answers 'Yes' to every question. The children are taken back to their adult caretakers when visiting hours are over. Although they live only two miles away, they seem separated by a huge distance."

Establishing the H. H. Dalai Lama-Sasakawa Scholarship—Uttar Pradesh and Delhi, India, November 2014

> Route: Narita International Airport → Delhi, India (flight time: 10h 30m; 8h stopover) → Lucknow, Uttar Pradesh, India (flight time: 1h)—one night—Lucknow → Delhi (flight time: 1h 20m)—six nights—Delhi → Narita (flight time: 8h)

In November, following on from the previous autumn, I carried out work in the state of Uttar Pradesh in central India and the national capital of Delhi. On the morning of 18 November, I flew to Lucknow, the capital of Uttar Pradesh, going via Delhi. At the airport, I was met by APAL's President Narsappa and his advisor Uday Thakar, and the head of APAL's state committee Daylu Prasad and his deputy Murari Sihna. Principal Secretary Arvind Kumar, administrative head of the state's Department of Health and Family Welfare, told me: "Twenty thousand people affected by leprosy is not a significant number in a population of 200 million. Leprosy is not a paramount public health issue in this state. We do not have a leprosy officer in every district, and some officers even hold dual posts." This was frank, but to someone who had traveled all the way from Japan, his tone was uncooperative. I, for my part, pointed out that the state has the largest number of people affected by leprosy in India and strongly urged the department to hire more leprosy officers and assign them to all districts.

I also met with Akhilesh Yadav, the state's chief minister. When I spoke with Chief Minister Yadav—who had visited Japan ten years earlier as part of the India–Japan Strategic Dialogue Project organized by the Nippon Foundation's sister organization the Sasakawa Peace Foundation—Principal Secretary Kumar was also in attendance, so I repeated my request for the assignment of leprosy officers in each and every district. I also informed them that Bihar, a relatively poor state, had enacted a monthly pension for people affected by leprosy of 1,800 rupees (about US$22) and requested that the pension in Uttar Pradesh also be increased from its current level of 300 rupees. I introduced APAL President Narsappa and the young leader Vice President Sinha. They explained the current leprosy situation in the state and conveyed their requests directly to the ministers to increase the pension as soon as possible. The government later followed through on the petition, raising the pension to 1,800 rupees.

Next, I traveled on to Faizabad, a three-hour drive away. The following morning, on 19 November, I visited the Shri San Sewa Kush Ashram. This colony is home to sixty-six people, including fifty people affected by leprosy and their families. Their dwellings were all shacks with thatched and tin roofs that looked quite unable to keep out the rain. A few of the younger generation earned money by driving rickshaws and selling ornaments, but most residents begged by the nearby riverside. I walked with them to the river and watched them as they sat in place and began to beg from the people on the road, reminding me once again that my dream of eliminating begging from the lives of people affected by leprosy in India was still far away. Three years before, the colony applied for funding from S-ILF for a sustainable livelihood project, but a court case for land ownership was in its final stages, so the enterprise was abandoned. Now that the court case was over, the colony wanted to try again. They asked for financial support to enable them to sell firewood and weave, and I told them we would do our best to make it happen.

I returned to Lucknow with another three-hour drive and met with Governor Ram Naik. Governor Naik was interested in leprosy issues and had done his utmost to help when we submitted the Petition for Integration and Empowerment for Leprosy Affected Persons to the Rajya Sabha (Parliamentary) Committee on Petitions in 2008, and to follow through on the recommendations issued by the committee in response to that petition. A senior member of Prime Minister Modi's Bharatiya Janata Party (BJP), which became the ruling party in May 2014, Governor Naik promised his support, saying: "I have explained the issue of leprosy to the prime minister and obtained his pledge to hold a meeting with the relevant agencies to discuss the report of the Rajya Sabha Committee on Petitions. I hope to decide on something when setting the next budget."

In the evening, I flew to Delhi, and the next day, on 20 November, I held a press conference on establishing the H. H. Dalai Lama-

Sasakawa Scholarship to help young leprosy colony residents attend university. This was a new scholarship jointly established with the donation made by His Holiness the Dalai Lama during his visit to the Delhi colony in March 2014 and support from the Nippon Foundation. The scholarship provides tuition and living expenses to children of people affected by leprosy who have stopped attending university due to their economic circumstances with the aim of enabling them to pursue professional education in medicine, engineering, law, and other fields, become respected members of society, and even develop into leaders directly involved in leprosy issues.

The following day, 21 November, I met with His Holiness the Dalai Lama and reported the scholarship's successful launch. His Holiness provided encouragement, saying, "We must give them hope and pride." I remember when some years before I told His Holiness about my dream of eradicating begging in India, at first he had been gently doubtful. But in the end he had shown understanding, and promised to donate part of the royalties from his publications to support my efforts. It is rather unusual to receive charity from a monk— we usually give alms to them.

On 21 November, I attended a mid-term report meeting on the Indian Ministry of Health and Family Welfare's five-year plan to fight leprosy (2012–17), held jointly with the WHO. Despite the ministry's efforts over the past few years, case numbers in India had remained almost unchanged, with no progress in eliminating the disease in each district and 115 districts having a prevalence rate of more than one case per 10,000 people. I requested that leprosy officers go out into the field to break through this impasse. I also proposed that the top state public health policymakers come together in Tokyo for an Indian Leprosy Summit to make it a priority for the state governments. I later spoke one-on-one with Union Health Secretary Lov Verma and once again reiterated my request for a leprosy officer to be assigned in all districts of each relevant state.

On the last day of my stay, I met with Prime Minister Narendra Modi. We had spoken about leprosy issues in Tokyo when he visited Japan in September 2014, and he remembered my promise to introduce him to President Narsappa of APAL. It was a historic day when the two of them shook hands. Unfortunately, it was a private meeting,

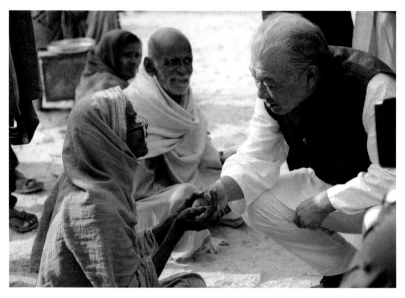

117. The author giving alms to an elderly woman who was begging (Uttar Pradesh, India, November 2014)

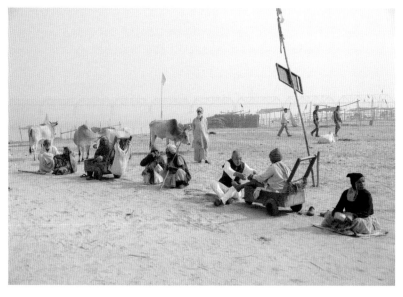

118. In a line of beggars (Uttar Pradesh, India, November 2014)

OVERCOMING THE STAGNATION

so we did not get a photo of the event. A picture of the prime minister and a person affected by leprosy shaking hands going public would have had a hugely significant impact, so this was somewhat disappointing.

Countries visited in 2015	
January	● Japan
	Thailand (Myanmar nationwide ceasefire agreement: negotiations with representatives of armed ethnic organizations)
February	Switzerland (Meeting with WHO Director-General Margaret Chan)
	Myanmar (Nationwide ceasefire agreement: meetings with government personnel)
March	● India
April	● Ethiopia
	● DRC
	● Republic of Congo
May	Sweden (Visit to WMU)
	● Switzerland
	Myanmar (Nationwide ceasefire agreement: meetings with government personnel)
June	● United States
	● Switzerland
July	Thailand (Myanmar nationwide ceasefire agreement: negotiations with representatives of armed ethnic organizations)
	Myanmar (Nationwide ceasefire agreement meetings: with government personnel)
	Sri Lanka (Talks with President Sirisena)
August	● Brazil

September	Thailand (Myanmar nationwide ceasefire agreement: negotiations with representatives of armed ethnic organizations)
	Myanmar (two visits) (Nationwide ceasefire agreement: meetings with government personnel)
	● India
	United Kingdom (UK–Japan Global Seminar)
October	● Kiribati
	● Fiji
	Myanmar (Nationwide ceasefire agreement: meetings with government personnel)
November	Myanmar (two visits) (Nationwide ceasefire agreement: meetings with government personnel)
	United Kingdom (International Maritime Organization International Maritime Prize Award Ceremony)

● Indicates a trip that features in this section.

WMU: World Maritime University.

Their Majesties the Emperor and Empress and people affected by leprosy—Japan, January 2015

On 13 January 2015, prior to Japan's first-ever Global Appeal conference to call for the elimination of discrimination against people affected by leprosy and their families, I had the privilege of briefing Their Majesties the Emperor and Empress (now the Emperor Emeritus and Empress Emerita) on the current state of leprosy in the world and the significance of the Global Appeal at their Imperial Palace. Their Majesties were deeply interested in the current state of leprosy around the world and asked a wide range of well-informed questions, including about leprosy medication and why Brazil has not yet succeeded in eliminating the disease. As a result, I talked with them for seventy minutes, far longer than the initially scheduled fifteen minutes.

594

On 28 January, the day after Global Appeal 2015, I then received an audience with Their Majesties the Emperor and Empress at the Imperial Palace, together with APAL President Narsappa and Vice President Venugopal; Kristie Lane Ibardaloza (a nurse from Culion Island, Philippines); José Ramirez, Jr. (from the United States) and his wife, Paulus Manek (from Indonesia); Legese Desta Sisulu (from Ethiopia); and President Kazuo Mori of the All Japan Council of Hansen's Disease Sanatorium Residents. Their Majesties talked with every one of their nervous-looking guests, giving them a handshake and enfolding their hands in their own. The meeting lasted for forty minutes, again, well exceeding the scheduled time. As the event ended, His Majesty said: "I hope that you remain active as leaders for those who are still suffering from discrimination as well as illness and that your lives improve."

I later wrote an article covering this audience with Their Imperial Majesties in January, which I published with accompanying photos in the autumn 2015 issue of *Our Imperial Family*. I will reproduce it here.

"The Day Their Majesties Took the Hands of People Affected by Leprosy from around the World"

The Nippon Foundation, of which I am the chairman, conducts a variety of humanitarian aid activities in the areas of social welfare, education, culture, etc. Since the mid-1960s, our leprosy-focused work has included grant support through the Tofu Kyokai, an organization that works for the betterment of the lives of people affected by leprosy in Japan, in building libraries and meeting halls at leprosaria and purchasing vehicles, etc. Overseas, my late father Ryoichi Sasakawa used his private funds to help build leprosy facilities in India, the Philippines, Taiwan, Korea, and elsewhere.

In 1974, the Sasakawa Health Foundation was established as an organization to work for leprosy elimination and support for people affected by leprosy overseas. Since then, in collaboration with the Sasakawa Health Foundation and with the World Health Organization as its main partner, the Nippon Foundation has cooperated with various nongovernmental organizations to expand its efforts, focusing on holding international conferences, training people engaged in eliminating leprosy, facilitating local technical cooperation, conducting leprosy research, developing and providing educational materials, pursuing publicity and awareness campaigns, and assisting with medicines and equipment.

MAKING THE IMPOSSIBLE POSSIBLE

During the five years from 1995 to 1999, the Nippon Foundation provided MDT, an oral medicine recognized as an effective treatment for leprosy, free of charge, to the world through the World Health Organization to help eliminate leprosy. Since 2000, the pharmaceutical firm Novartis succeeded the Nippon Foundation's mission and began distributing MDT free of charge to date, dramatically decreasing the number of people affected by leprosy worldwide. The WHO defines elimination of leprosy as a public health problem as bringing its prevalence rate to less than one case per 10,000 people. Brazil is the only country where leprosy has not been eliminated under this definition.

Every year, the Nippon Foundation presents a Global Appeal to end stigma and discrimination against people affected by leprosy and their family members to the world in conjunction with World Leprosy Day (the last Sunday in January). The first Global Appeal was launched in Delhi, India, in 2006. In 2015, the tenth Global Appeal was launched in Japan for the first time on 27 January. On 13 January, I had the opportunity to explain to Their Majesties the current situation of leprosy in the world and the significance of the Global Appeal at their Imperial Residence.

Their Majesties were deeply interested in the current state of leprosy around the world and asked a wide range of knowledgeable questions, including about leprosy medication and why Brazil has not yet succeeded in eliminating the disease as a public health problem. As a result, I talked with them for seventy minutes, far longer than the initially scheduled fifteen minutes.

On 28 January, the day after the Global Appeal, Their Majesties met with eight representatives of people affected by leprosy from Japan, India, the US, and other countries at the Imperial Palace. Their Majesties met them four at a time in two groups, then switched places, so that both of them could speak with everybody. Their Majesties took their nervous-looking guests' hands in their own, truly giving them all their attention as they spoke with each of them in turn. I am aware that Their Majesties kneel down beside the people affected by leprosy who are seated at leprosaria in Japan and take their hands as they speak to them, and they were treating all these people with just as much compassion and kindness. As I thought about all the challenges these people must have faced in their home countries, I could not help but be moved to tears by Their Majesties' noble nature. Some of these people had been abandoned by their parents and families and never had anyone hold their hands before.

The meeting lasted forty minutes, significantly longer than the scheduled fifteen minutes. As the event ended, His Majesty said, "I hope that you remain active as leaders for those who are still suffering from discrimination as well as illness and that your lives improve."

At the press conference that followed, a person affected by leprosy said, "I have never shaken hands with my parents or family, but Their Majesties the Emperor and Empress held my hand. In that instant, the suffering just evaporated." As they recalled their Imperial Palace experience, with tears in their eyes, they spoke about how it was like a dream and how Their Majesties listened with all their hearts. No dignitary in any country I have visited has ever shown as much love to people who have lived through the hardships of leprosy. Moreover, Their Majesties had invited these people affected by leprosy to the Imperial Palace. I could sense the genuine kindness of Their Majesties as they spoke intimately with their guests. I felt that they were the quintessence of selflessness, expressing their hopes for the well-being of the peoples of the world.

Truth to tell, my first encounter with leprosy happened through the guidance of Her Majesty the Empress [now Empress Emerita Michiko]. In 1965, Masahide Kanayama, who served as the Japanese ambassador to Korea at the time, visited my father and asked if he would help build a leprosy hospital in Korea.

My father immediately accepted the offer, and I attended the completion ceremony of the hospital with him. My father hugged patients who had despair on their faces, rubbing their ulcer-ridden feet and offering words of encouragement to each one. The sight of my father moved me, and that was the first step in my fight against leprosy, which continues to this day. When I mentioned my encounter with Ambassador Kanayama during a conversation with Their Majesties, the Empress said, "I am so glad to hear that."

The reason she said this was because when she was the Crown Princess she had received a letter from a nun working in Korea about the tragic situation of people affected by leprosy in that nation. She had then consulted Ambassador Kanayama about it, and so it was that he, considering her wishes, paid a visit to my father.

Actually, I was present at the time of this visit, and I have a clear memory of the Ambassador adding, "Her Imperial Highness is also concerned about the current situation in Korea." However, when I mentioned this in conversation with Their Imperial Majesties, I avoided saying this and merely brought up the name of Ambassador Kanayama. It was at this point that Empress Michiko told me about the nun who had written to her, and so on. As I listened to her story, it came to me that my long struggle with leprosy had actually originated in something Her Majesty had mentioned, which deeply moved me.

Since the time of Empress Komyo in the eighth century the Japanese Imperial Family has been devoted to the fight against leprosy. Seeing Their Majesties and witnessing up close their kind and gentle attitude toward people affected by leprosy, reaffirmed the significance of having a country like Japan, blessed with such an Imperial Family, appealing to the nations of the world to eliminate discrimination. At the same time, I felt a strong reaffirmation of the importance of promoting efforts to prevent the negative aspects of the history of harsh discrimination against persons affected by leprosy from fading away from memory.

Transforming the life of patients to change the country—Delhi, India, March 2015

> Route: Narita International Airport → Delhi, India (flight time: 10h)—three nights—Delhi → Narita (flight time: 7h 20m)

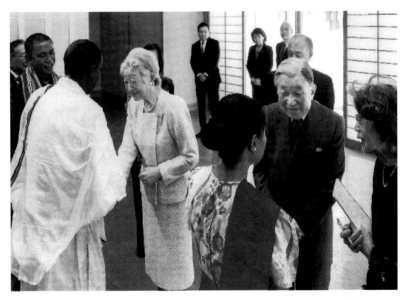

119. The Emperor and Empress (now Emperor Emeritus and Empress Emerita) of Japan, talking with persons affected by leprosy (Japan, 2015)

The Global Appeal 2015 we held in Tokyo in January went off very successfully. In February, I visited Geneva for a luncheon with UN Human Rights Council Advisory Committee members and a meeting with WHO Director-General Margaret Chan. In March, I went to India where I attended a conference hosted by the Union Ministry of Health and Family Welfare in the national capital, Delhi. The Union Ministry of Health and Family Welfare's National Leprosy Eradication Program (NLEP) had developed a Five-Year Plan to Eliminate Leprosy (2012–17), an action plan filled with specific achievement targets. In 2014, independent experts conducted a mid-term evaluation of the current plan. The measures being put into action by NLEP included carrying out special programs that concentrated on endemic provinces, going door-to-door to find children affected by leprosy, and disseminating leprosy knowledge to paid volunteers among the Accredited Social Health Activists (ASHA). The key to implementing programs lies in having a leprosy officer in each state health department, who is the person responsible for developing and implementing effective strategies by checking the central government's plan against actual conditions in their state.

When I entered the hotel conference room for the state leprosy officers (SLOs) meeting, about 100 people had already gathered. Dr. C. M. Agrawal, deputy director general for leprosy, Ministry of Health and Family Welfare, opened the meeting by strongly emphasizing the need to share awareness of the problem and to make further efforts to address it. WHO's representative to India, Dr. Nata Menabde, suggested that mapping was needed to identify areas with large numbers of cases and where the disability rate and rates of leprosy in children were high, so that attuned measures could be put into place. At the same time, she stressed, the issue of human rights is vital: until discrimination against people affected by leprosy ends, elimination in the true sense will not be achieved. I focused on the importance of treating children, especially before they develop disabilities, and the role that people affected by leprosy have in detecting new patients. Later, the SLOs made presentations, and APAL President Narsappa offered his cooperation in finding and counseling patients through a network extending across the country.

The following day, there was a national stakeholders' meeting for a leprosy-free India. This was the first attempt to bring together a wide range of stakeholders, including the Ministry of Health, SLOs, WHO, and people affected by leprosy who had attended the previous day's meeting, as well as NGOs representing people with disabilities and media experts, to discuss ways to end the disease and discrimination.

Health Secretary Bhanu Pratap Sharma said that he was determined to make leprosy programs sustainable, using all the tools and methods at his disposal, with measures concentrated on hot spots. I quoted Mahatma Gandhi's words: "If you can transform the life of a patient or change his values of life, you can change the village and the country," and reiterated the close connection between leprosy and human rights issues.

Microfinance for self-reliance—Federal Democratic Republic of Ethiopia, April 2015

> Route: Narita International Airport → Paris, France (flight time: 12h 35m; 5h 30m stopover) → Addis Ababa, Ethiopia (flight time: 7h)—two nights

In April, I embarked on a trip to Ethiopia and the two Congos, the DRC and the Republic of the Congo. I landed in Addis Ababa, the capital of Ethiopia, having flown from Narita via Paris. It was cool in high-altitude Addis Ababa. I went to the WHO office to hear from WHO Country Representative Pierre M'Pelé and the leprosy program coordinator on the situation in Ethiopia. The number of new patients had been hovering around 4,000 for the past ten years, and 13 percent of the patients were children, which indicated a stalling in elimination efforts.

The Ethiopian Ministry of Health had come to the 2013 International Leprosy Summit held in Bangkok, Thailand, and was due to implement programs to bolster leprosy elimination efforts through the Special Bangkok Fund for Eliminating Leprosy, an initiative the Nippon Foundation set up on that occasion. The focus of the plan for the next three years was to promote new case detection by training health workers to visit each household. At present, the health workers had insufficient knowledge: they did not even know how to adequately diagnose the disease. Health Minister Kesete Admasu stated that the leprosy distribution survey conducted by his ministry had identified problem areas, so he would intensify elimination efforts there, training 5,000 nurses on leprosy and involving them in these activities.

When I visited the office of ENAPAL, I found a commemorative photo of a meeting between me, former Prime Minister Meles, and then-Chair Birke Nigatu. Executive Director Tesfaye Tadesse proudly told me that, despite being ten years ago, that meeting was a historic moment for people affected by leprosy in Ethiopia, as it was the first time they had the opportunity to directly explain their situation to the prime minister.

The next day, we visited the villages of Tesfa Hiwot and Addis Hiwot to see how ENAPAL managed the microfinancing provided by the Sasakawa Health Foundation. We left Addis Ababa at 6 a.m. and arrived at the village of Tesfa Hiwot four hours later. Here, I visited the house and fields of the Mekonnens, who had been able to send their two children to university by cultivating vegetables on a plot bought with microcredit. The plot was large, and the onions were growing well: apparently they earned about US$2,500 from harvesting three times a year. Since the minimum wage for civil servants was around US$16 per month, this was a more than adequate income. However, I met another man, who had not used microcredit and spent most of his time in his home. "Truthfully," he told me, "I want to go out and work. But if I borrowed money, I worry whether I could repay it." I encouraged him to listen to stories from successful people and have hope in his work, but I keenly felt that working amid deep-rooted prejudice and discrimination from the villagers requires the presence and cooperation of excellent mentors and supporters.

The village of Addis Hiwot was located along a river. The villagers ran a chicken farm funded by the Sasakawa Health Foundation and managed to secure their daily meals from the income. The villagers had arranged a meeting to coincide with my visit and used the opportunity to make a number of requests, including for a replacement generator to operate the pump to draw water from the river, since the old one had broken down, and for free health care, which, unlike in the past, was now only available at cost. I said that it was crucial to work for solutions to their problems in collaboration with ENAPAL, and for each and every person to have a sense that they have a stake

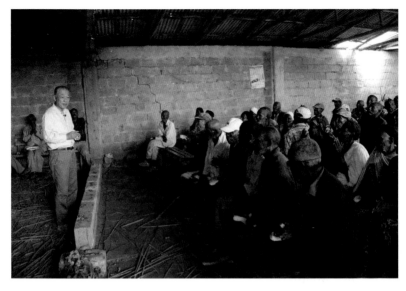

120. At a meeting in Addis Hiwot village, in a room unlit by electricity, giving a cheering speech (Ethiopia, April 2015)

in what happens in their community. Seeing these people doing their level best despite poverty, despite all the challenges—traveling 70 kilometers to find a health post, a lack of jobs for young people, and insufficient access to secondary education—my heart truly ached. I wanted to do everything I could to help. On the other hand, there were limits to my power.

During this visit, the Sasakawa Health Foundation agreed to help ENAPAL build a new headquarters with accommodation. It is my hope that this facility can play a part in uniting people affected by leprosy from all African countries.

Reuniting with the pygmy people—DRC, April 2015

Route: Addis Ababa, Ethiopia → Kinshasa, DRC (flight time: 4h 20m)—five nights—Kinshasa → Brazzaville, Republic of Congo (boat to Brazzaville: 30m) → Paris, France (flight time: 8h; 7h stopover) → Narita International Airport (flight time: 11h 50m)

After my visit to Ethiopia, I traveled to the DRC. While the DRC has eliminated leprosy as a public health problem, it has the second-highest number of new cases in Africa and the fifth highest world-wide. The vast country still has some hot spot endemic areas with high prevalence rates.

At the WHO country office, I was briefed on the leprosy situation in the DRC and received a more detailed report from Dr. Jean Norbert Mputu Luengu, the Ministry of Health's leprosy program manager. Dr. Mputu was responsible for the frontline leprosy elimination efforts in the DRC and had assisted me in every visit to the DRC since my first in 2005. According to him, 3,744 patients were registered in Congo in 2013, and there were eight provinces with an exceptionally high prevalence of patients (more than five per 10,000 people). Moreover, some states did not have up-to-date data. The Ministry of Health was planning to identify patients in these eight provinces as part of its intense elimination efforts, and I decided to visit one of these provinces, Équateur, where hunter-gatherers live.

The DRC Ministry of Health had attended the 2013 International Leprosy Summit held in Bangkok, Thailand, and had decided, like Ethiopia, to implement programs to step up leprosy elimination efforts through the Special Bangkok Fund for Eliminating Leprosy, provided by the Nippon Foundation. The ministry had set a new target: to increase its new patient detection by 50 percent per year. After eliminating the disease at the national level, many governments turn all their attention to elimination at the local level, doing everything they can to reduce patient numbers. I had supported the idea of the new target in patient detection, even though for officials, once elimination at the national level has been achieved, increases in numbers of newly discovered patients are actually the last thing that they want. Oftentimes officials tend not to put much effort into new detection, in a phenomenon I call "elimination trauma," and statistical data show that patient numbers flatline. However, early detection of the patients who will infect others is crucial to eliminating the disease. Indeed, a significant increase in patient numbers in a region or country is inevitable when health officials exert themselves in their job. Ultimately, however, it can only lead to an overall decrease in cases, which is to be welcomed. I told the DRC's Ministry of Health officials that I fully supported them in setting the target. Dr. Mputu had formulated a meaningful strategy after many years of dealing with leprosy.

With Health Minister Dr. Felix Kabange Numbi Mukwampa, I next paid a call on National Assembly Speaker Dr. Aubin Minaku. I asked Dr. Minaku to communicate our three messages—leprosy is a curable disease, medicine is available free of charge worldwide, and discrimination against leprosy is unacceptable—to all members of the National Assembly so that they could then pass them on to their constituents. Speaker Minaku immediately replied: "I will have the minister of health prepare a brief statement for each National Assembly member to communicate to their constituents. I will instruct them to issue this statement during the recess from June through September." I reported the speaker's promise to the media.

The next day, I left for Mbandaka, the capital of Équateur, with Health Minister Kabange, Dr. Mputu, and the WHO country representative. The purpose of the trip was to meet people affected by leprosy among the pygmy people. We flew to Mbandaka on a chartered United Nations plane. The only other way to reach Mbandaka was by boat up the Congo River, one of the world's major rivers, on a par with the Nile. This was not an unattractive option, but it would take two weeks one way. The thirty-one-seat twin-engine propeller-driven plane to Mbandaka was almost filled to capacity with passengers. We arrived at our equatorial destination in around ninety minutes. As we stepped off the ramp, we were greeted by the Équateur Province Health Minister Mpetsi and other provincial officials. The unpaved road from the airport to the hotel was lined with little shops, and gusts of dust rose with every passing car, unheeded by the women who ran the stores. Most buildings were single-story. The same day, after meeting with Health Minister Mpetsi and Provisional Governor Sébastien Impeto Mpengo, I spoke to the local media and voiced the same request that I have repeated hundreds and thousands of times before: to give the people accurate information about leprosy. Our accommodation was a lodging house—extremely rudimentary. It had about fifteen rooms. Our departure would be early the next morning, without breakfast, not unusual for us.

The next morning, there we were, bright and early at 6 a.m., without breakfast but waiting to leave—only to be told that our guide had gone off to have a bite to eat, we would have to wait a while. We took this in our stride—what passed for courtesy was different here.

Once we were all together, we headed out in four Land Cruisers to make an excursion to meet the people affected by leprosy living deep in the jungle. According to the health minister, the outbound journey would take about two-and-a-half hours. In contrast to the previous day's sunny weather, it was going to rain all day. I'd been told that rain in Africa is welcomed as a good omen. Pretty soon, we found ourselves going along a single red-earth dirt road. We were in the middle of the jungle going along the Congo River. The rain was coming down quite heavily, and the road was getting worse. Thunder began to rumble, but still the four-wheel-drive vehicles kept up their brisk speed. Then, I heard what sounded like the report of a gun. The car directly behind mine had been struck by lightning. Fortunately, not one of the passengers was hurt. The route passed over numerous small creeks that flowed into the Congo River, and many of the bridges that crossed them, constructed of simple lined-up wooden logs, looked in a parlous state due to the rising water, some with sections washed away. We proceeded onward, doing what we could to rebuild the bridges so they were passable by dint of collective

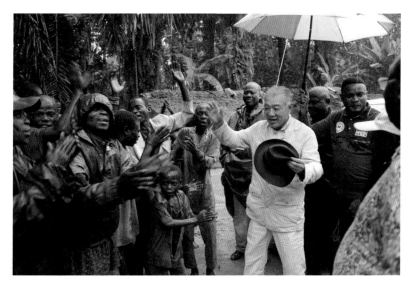

121. With residents of the village of Boimbo who provided a welcome despite the pouring rain (Democratic Republic of the Congo, April 2015)

effort. It was past noon when we arrived at our first destination, a health center in a village of Bokatola, Ingende, after more than five hours of travel instead of the scheduled two and a half.

Waiting for us were two people affected by leprosy of the Batwa tribe, commonly known as pygmies, a man around sixty-five years old and another around twenty years old. They had walked 45 and 21 kilometers, respectively, to meet me. They looked healthy, with no aftereffects in their limbs.

Our next stop was at the village of Boimbo, also a Batwa village, where the villagers welcomed me with singing and dancing in the rain. I danced with them, getting soaked through. I always make a point of mingling with the local people—I eat their food, listen to their stories, and join in with their dancing, and I always love doing so. One woman had the distinctive patches of leprosy on her abdomen, and she looked concerned that she had not yet heard anything about any possible treatment. I tried telling her that medicine was available to cure her, but the local interpreter knew nothing about leprosy, so whether the woman understood me I couldn't tell.

It was almost an hour before we reached our final destination, but by now, the time was already around 1 p.m. The rain was just getting heavier and heavier—it was torrential. The return trip would also take well over five hours, and if any one of the log bridges had been washed away, the fear was that we might end up being marooned. We should turn back now, or we would be driving in the dark, which would be dangerous. The thought of all the people I knew who were waiting for me to come and see them pulled at my heart strings, but I followed the advice of the health minister, who said the safety of our companions came first.

On the way back, we found that one log bridge that we had repaired had been completely swept away by the water. Here again, we did what we could with a collective effort. It was nighttime when we arrived back at the hotel. That day, we had driven more than ten hours and simply made a round trip through the jungle. I knew that we would have been able to find many more people affected by leprosy there at our destination, and was bitterly disappointed that the bad weather had prevented me from making an on-site investigation. It is of utmost importance to detect new patients, even in hidden endemic areas, to prevent disability through early treatment, even if, as Dr. Mputu said, this would lead to a temporary increase in new cases. I could only hope that early detection and early treatment would be made available to all those people affected by leprosy living deep in the jungle.

We had all skipped breakfast and lunch that day and were looking forward to finally having a chance to eat. However, nothing had been prepared for dinner at the lodging house, so we had to settle for some of the *sekihan* (red bean rice) we brought for such a rare emergency.

The next day, I returned to Kinshasa from Mbandaka, took my first warm shower in two days, and attended an afternoon press conference organized by WHO. In the evening, a great friend paid me an unexpected visit at my hotel in Kinshasa. It was Victor Makwenge Kaput, a former health minister who had done his utmost to eliminate leprosy and even accompanied me into dangerous jungle zones during my visits in 2007 and 2008. He was now vice chair of the National Assembly's Health Committee. Dr. Kaput promised to handle the message that I asked Mr. Minaku to convey to all National Assembly members. He suggested creating a leprosy information day for members of the National Assembly. In the DRC, he told me, superstitions abound, and leprosy is often thought to be a shameful disease or a witch's curse. Nevertheless, many people were gradually learning the facts—that medication is available for free, and it is possible to live at home while on a course of treatment. A good friend is a blessing indeed. His visit was a wonderful gift to me at the end of my trip.

The next day, I took a thirty-minute boat ride from Kinshasa to Brazzaville, the capital of the Republic of Congo, just a stone's throw away. I visited the WHO Regional Office for Africa and had time to discuss the leprosy situation in Africa with Regional Director Matshidiso Moeti. That evening, I made my way back to Japan via Paris.

Meeting with health ministers from around the world—Swiss Confederation, May 2015

Route: Narita International Airport → Copenhagen, Denmark (flight time: 11h 25m; drove from Copenhagen to Malmö, Sweden)—one night—drove from Malmö to Copenhagen → Geneva, Switzerland

607

MAKING THE IMPOSSIBLE POSSIBLE

(flight time: 2h)—three nights—Geneva → Copenhagen (flight time: 2h; 2h 45m stopover) → Narita (flight time: 11h 50m)

In May, after a visit to the World Maritime University in Malmö, Sweden, I went to Geneva, Switzerland, to speak at the annual Sasakawa Health Prize award ceremony during the WHO Assembly. I also spoke with health ministers and government officials of the countries gathered for the assembly to discuss leprosy issues.

The winner of the 2015 Sasakawa Health Prize was Poland's Childbirth with Dignity Foundation. This organization provides pregnant and nursing mothers with hospital information to enable them to make birth decisions, legal advice to protect their rights, and educational activities to foster respect for the human rights of pregnant and nursing mothers in hospitals and the workplace.

Next were the meetings with health ministers. This time, I had meetings with health ministers and senior government officials from the DRC, Madagascar, Indonesia, Myanmar, Brazil, Mozambique, Sudan, South Sudan, the People's Republic of China, India, and Tanzania. I also spoke with the International Federation of Anti-Leprosy Associations (ILEP) and regional directors from the WHO's Southeast Asia and Africa offices. A key goal of these meetings was to request support for a draft resolution on eliminating discrimination against leprosy, which the Japanese government planned to submit at the twenty-ninth session of the UN Human Rights Council in June 2015.

The DRC's Health Minister Dr. Felix Kabange Numbi Mukwampa had accompanied me and cooperated with my inspection during my visit to his country in April. He said: "Despite the significant decline in patient numbers over the past ten years, I have received many reports of people with grade 2 disabilities, and 10 percent of the patients are children. However, the reality is that our leprosy elimination budget is insufficient, so I would like further financial support to reduce our case numbers." I informed him that the DRC had applied to the Bangkok Declaration Special Fund, which the Nippon Foundation established under the WHO in 2013, to provide financial assistance to countries with many people affected by leprosy, and that the application was currently under review.

Madagascar eliminated leprosy as a public health problem in 2007, but its case numbers had flatlined since then. I conveyed my

608

concerns about this to Madagascar's Health Minister Mamy Lalatiana Andriamanarivo.

Indonesia is an indispensable nation in the fight against leprosy. I asked Health Minister Nila Djuwita Farid Moeloek to make sure that the money provided by the Nippon Foundation's Bangkok Declaration Special Fund was put to effective use. I also told her about my visit to Papua province, where I was surprised to see a case of leprosy in a four-year-old child, as the disease is believed to have an incubation period of several years, and asked for her cooperation in my efforts in Papua and other island regions. The minister expressed her gratitude for the approval of the application for the Bangkok Declaration Special Fund. Leprosy was still highly prevalent in fourteen provinces, she told me, including Papua and Java. She asked that she be informed when I next visited these areas.

Myanmar successfully eliminated leprosy as a public health problem in 2004, but its case numbers had remained stagnant since then. I asked the country's health minister, Dr. Than Aung, to use the Bangkok Declaration Special Fund to bring leprosy numbers down to zero. He promised to further step up efforts, and thanked me for the support the Nippon Foundation had provided for the Training School of Prosthetics and Orthotics.

I informed Brazil's vice minister of health surveillance, Dr. Jarbas Barbosa da Silva, that I would be visiting Brazil with WHO Director-General Margaret Chan in August and hoped to see concrete results by that time.

Mozambique's Deputy Health Minister Mouzinho Saíde remarked: "We are grateful for the support in eliminating leprosy. I know that patient numbers have remained unchanged after we hit the WHO prevalence target, with figures remaining high in some areas, but I want to ensure that drugs properly reach those who need them."

I told India's Health Minister Jagat Prakash Nadda that I was aware that various initiatives across several states were making headway, but that I wanted to see more measures for early detection to ensure early treatment. We also discussed the dates of the Tokyo Summit scheduled for July with the Indian state health ministers. He replied: "Prime Minister Modi has made it one of his pledges to eradicate leprosy. We aim to do everything we can to detect people affected by leprosy and provide them with the proper medication. In the next two months, we will be revamping our leprosy elimination measures aiming to ensure that we wipe leprosy out completely." The Tokyo Summit, he said, would be more convenient in September or later. I told him we would reschedule, but unfortunately, the event never materialized—for various reasons, including the minister not being able to find time for it.

An address at the Voices of People Affected by Leprosy event—United States, June 2015

> Route: Narita International Airport → New York, United States (flight time: 13h)—three nights—New York → Narita (flight time: 13h 45m)

On 15 June, we held a side event at the Conference of States Parties to the Convention on the Rights of People with Disabilities at the UN Headquarters in New York City. Mr. Javed Abidi, the global chair of DPI, planned the event to give people affected by leprosy an opportunity to stand up and have their say in the disability community, from which they had previously been absent. UN Assistant Secretary-General for Economic Development Lenni Montiel attended on behalf of the UN secretary-general, while Ambassador Yoshifumi Okamura, deputy permanent representative of Japan, delivered an address on behalf of the Japanese government. Dr. P. K. Gopal and Mr. José Ramirez Jr. shared their stories as people affected by leprosy. My address was as follows:

> Today, I am very grateful that we are able to hold the very first event that combines disability and leprosy. I hope we can all take the time to explore the possibilities of how people with disabilities and people affected by leprosy—people with lived experience of these conditions—may collaborate to strengthen the collective voices of both communities.

> I first met Mr. Javed Abidi, the global chair of DPI, three years ago. The Nippon Foundation organized a symposium in India on leprosy and human rights, and Mr. Abidi was a participant.

> As you saw in the video earlier, leprosy has been one of the most misunderstood and stigmatizing diseases known to humankind. Now, effective treatment is available, and leprosy has become a curable

disease. At the conference, Mr. Abidi said to me, "Regardless of the differences in how we became disabled, people who have disabilities are all allies, and together we ought to be able to achieve things." And he proposed that we explore how to strengthen the ties between people affected by leprosy and people with disabilities.

Mr. Abidi's offer was very encouraging, and it reconfirmed my thoughts that although the circumstances of the organization he heads and the issues faced by the community of people affected by leprosy are different, our goals and visions are very similar.

The disability community and the leprosy-affected community are both aiming to achieve an inclusive society. And over the years, we have met successful milestones toward that end. Around the world, the two groups have been advocating for a greater say in government policies, as well as reaching out to communities to help improve quality of life.

In terms of our global fight for human rights, people with disabilities succeeded in getting the UN Convention on the Rights of People with Disabilities in 2006, and the people affected by leprosy won the Resolution to End Discrimination against Persons Affected by Leprosy and Their Family Members in 2010.

However, if you look at the living conditions of these concerned groups around the world, I think you will all agree that there is still a long road ahead of us until we see a truly inclusive society.

Last year, the Nippon Foundation and DPI started a new project to explore ways to strengthen collaboration between people with disabilities and people affected by leprosy. Details of these developments will be shared later on, but to give you an example, in the case of India, Mr. Abidi and Dr. Gopal, who is the co-founder of the Association of People Affected by Leprosy or APAL, are looking into possibilities of collaboration.

In India, people with disabilities and people affected by leprosy have finally begun to work toward linking up their activities and efforts. In the case of Ethiopia, there is already a strong relationship established between the disability group and the group representing people affected by leprosy.

On the other hand, there are many countries where no such organizations currently exist. In these countries, possibilities should be explored on how to get these organizations up and running. As you can see, circumstances vary in countries and regions. That is why I believe it is best to tailor each case accordingly.

611

Through these efforts, if people with disabilities and people who became disabled from leprosy can come together, the cries for human rights can be amplified.

I truly hope that this event will offer new opportunities for people with disabilities and people affected by leprosy to form cooperative relationships and new possibilities where together, we may shorten the long road ahead to realizing an inclusive society.

The final International Symposium on Leprosy and Human Rights— Swiss Confederation, June 2015

Route: Narita International Airport → Paris, France (flight time: 12h) → Geneva, Switzerland (flight time: 1h)—two nights—Geneva → Paris (flight time: 1h; 2h stopover) → Haneda International Airport (flight time: 12h)

The International Symposium on Leprosy and Human Rights, which the Nippon Foundation had held five times since 2012, concluded in June 2015 at the Graduate Institute of International and Development

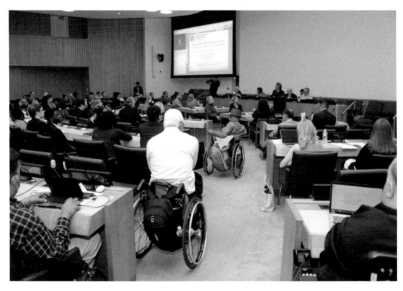

122. Delivering a speech at the Conference of States Parties to the Convention on the Rights of People with Disabilities (New York, United States, June 2015)

Studies in Geneva. This international conference brought together people from five continents to examine what governments, international organizations, NGOs, and others should do to put into practice the resolution to eliminate discrimination against persons affected by leprosy and their family members and its accompanying Principles and Guidelines, adopted by the UN General Assembly in 2010. The first and second symposiums were held in Brazil and India in 2012, the third in Ethiopia in 2013, and the fourth in Morocco in 2014. The ultimate objective of this series of meetings was to set forth an action plan and mechanism to put these Principles and Guidelines into practice. At this fifth and final meeting, representatives presented a follow-up plan. This symposium was attended by people affected by leprosy, human rights experts, lawyers, medical professionals, and UN officials worldwide, and featured video messages from the UN Secretary-General Ban Ki-moon and the WHO Director-General Margaret Chan.

Among the participants were leaders of organizations of people affected by leprosy from Indonesia, Morocco, Colombia, India, China, Brazil, Ghana, and the United States, as well as representatives from the IBA, the International Federation of Human Rights Organizations, the UN Human Rights Council Advisory Committee, ILEP, the International Nurses Association, and the World Medical Association. Professor Barbara Frey of the University of Minnesota Human Rights Center—representing an international working group of human rights experts organized after the first symposium in 2012—gave an address and reported on the working group's studies. The working group's main proposal was to create a mechanism to monitor how various stakeholders, including states, implement the Principles and Guidelines. It also presented a model for developing national action plans. Among other things, the working group proposed that a new resolution should be adopted by the UN Human Rights Council Advisory Committee to conduct a study on developing a follow-up mechanism. In 2017, the Japanese government then submitted this proposal to the Human Rights Council, which unanimously approved the resolution.

Alongside the symposium, the Nippon Foundation's Natsuko Tominaga exhibited her leprosy and human rights photographs at the UN in Geneva from 17 to 24 June.

Medical examination in a "silent area"—Federative Republic of Brazil, August 2015

> Route: Haneda International Airport → Paris, France (flight time: 12h 30m; 7h stopover) → Brasília, Brazil (flight time: 11h)—three nights—Brasília → Cuiabá, Mato Grosso, Brazil (flight time: 1h 30m)—four nights—Cuiabá → Brasília (flight time: 1h 30m; 2h stopover) → Recife, Pernambuco, Brazil (flight time: 2h 30m)—two nights—Recife → São Paulo, Brazil (flight time: 3h 30m; 2h stopover) → Paris (flight time: 11h 20m; 6h stopover) → Narita International Airport (flight time: 11h 50m)

In August 2015, I visited Brazil for the first time in a year and a half. Brazil was the only country in the world that had not yet met the WHO goal of eliminating leprosy to less than one case per 10,000 population. Brazil is one of my priority areas, but for some unknown reason, the Brazilian government seemed reluctant to allow me to visit. It seems that the efforts of MORHAN, an organization for people affected by leprosy that supports my work, were a source of embarrassment for government officials.

This time, I flew from Tokyo to Brasília, the capital of Brazil, via Paris, where I stayed two nights in transit. In Brasília, I was attending

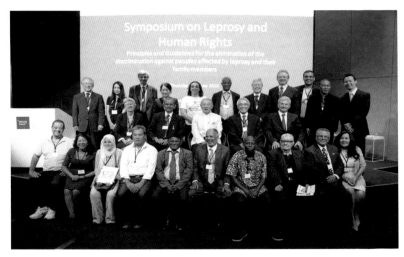

123. Country representatives at the International Symposium on Leprosy and Human Rights (Geneva, June 2015)

a leprosy convention organized by the Novartis Foundation. In between meetings, I tirelessly visited the Ministry of Health, the Human Rights Agency, legislators, and other prominent officials, repeatedly telling them that I would spare no effort to cooperate with and support them.

At a meeting with Health Minister Ademar Arthur Chioro dos Reis after a conference, I immediately noticed an acrimonious atmosphere, with MORHAN representatives and journalists being barred from the discussion for reasons unknown to me. The skinny minister's face stiffened as he abruptly stated that Brazil would officially announce eliminating leprosy as a public health problem by the end of this fiscal year. I asked him if this was really the case, and if I could convey this information to WHO Director-General Margaret Chan. "Absolutely!" he said, emphatically, as if I was wrong to doubt it. This should have been big news, but I felt compelled to make sure because the expression on his face was so utterly gloomy. I'd never received such a curt response from an official in all the days I'd spent in leprosy work. I later found out that an official of the Ministry of Health had alerted this minister to a comment I'd made in an earlier meeting about why Brazil, a World Cup and Olympic Games host, was the only country in the world that had not eliminated leprosy despite its abundance of human resources and funds. But if his declaration was true, it would seem that my dream of eliminating leprosy worldwide would soon be realized. However, I quickly learned that the minister's statement that leprosy would be eliminated by the end of the year was not in fact true. He resigned immediately after my return to Japan, although I do not know why.

After a meeting with officials and dignitaries in the capital, I visited the state of Mato Grosso the next day. The state governor of Mato Grosso paid a visit to me at my hotel with his wife, in contravention of the health minister's demands, and even though it was a Sunday. Mato Grosso is a vast state, the third largest in the country, in the western central region bordering Bolivia. Many tourists stop by the state capital, Cuiabá, to visit the Pantanal, a UNESCO World Heritage Site. However, compared to the nation's coastal areas, Cuiabá's economy has developed more slowly, with inadequate transportation and infrastructure, resulting in insufficient medical services. This state had the largest number of new leprosy cases in Brazil. In the endemic region of Mato Grosso, there was a "silent area" where no new cases had been detected for many years. I observed doctors and nurses working to quickly detect and treat patients in this silent area.

The Sucuri district, a twenty-minute drive from Cuiabá, had data showing zero new cases for two years, but people affected by leprosy live in the surrounding area, so some of them had to be unconfirmed cases. Cicero Frasa de Melo, a nurse that works as the state health department's leprosy program coordinator, questioned the data and got to work.

First, I observed Cicero examining about ten residents suspected of having leprosy at a clinic. The examination consisted of a medical interview to check for symptoms such as diminished sensation and limpness, to ask about any family members with leprosy, to check for nerve swelling, and to examine the sensory nerves by applying hot or cold water to the skin or lightly applying a needle to the foot or other parts of the body. While I was at the clinic, he examined four people, one diagnosed with a strong possibility of leprosy and another with a near-confirmed diagnosis. The twenty-one-year-old man diagnosed with leprosy was gently told that he would be cured after twelve months of medication, that he could continue with his everyday life, and that his family and neighbors would also need to come in for an examination. Cicero also explained that the medication has side effects, including difficulty breathing and purple lips, in one out of every 100 patients, but that the treatment must continue. Some patients will discontinue taking the drug if they are not informed of the side effects beforehand.

I accompanied Cicero to two homes with people affected by leprosy and witnessed him diagnose their families. The first stop was home to a seventy-three-year-old man who had been diagnosed with leprosy. He had lived in Rondônia state but could not get treatment, so he moved to where treatment was available in Mato Grosso to live with his younger brother. When we visited, Cicero examined the man's sister, brother, and niece. The sister and niece were diagnosed with leprosy, and both broke down in tears, but they seemed relieved after hearing the nurse's kind explanation. Our second stop was the home of a seventeen-year-old boy who had been diagnosed with leprosy fifteen days earlier. After examining his family, Cicero determined that his father and two brothers also had leprosy.

In the half-day I was there, we discovered six new cases. Getting serious about early detection would lead to many more patients being identified in this area. According to Cicero, frequent medical personnel changes and a shortage of doctors create these silent areas. He put it plainly: "These areas are not silent. They are screaming, crying." My driver, who was being treated for leprosy, told me that he was almost finished with his six-month course of MDT and was feeling well with no aftereffects. He drove me over rough roads with nimble hands at the wheel, telling me, "You should not hide your illness."

During my stay in Cuiabá, I met with Governor José Pedro Gonçalves Taques of Mato Grosso and state assemblyman Leonardo Ribeiro Albuquerque. The governor was particularly enthusiastic about the leprosy issue, so much so that he pledged to prioritize the issue during his election campaign and said he would do everything in his power to follow through on his promise during his remaining three years in office. I told him that I was ready to cooperate with the governor and the politicians if they were serious about tackling the problem, but unfortunately, I have not heard from him since then.

I also discussed specific measures with Dr. Werley Silva Peres, the former city health department director, who is as enthusiastic as Cicero about finding new patients. According to Dr. Peres, intensifying discovery efforts would double patient figures for the first three years. However, the numbers would surely decline after that. Having many people affected by leprosy is not something of which countries should be ashamed. It is shameful to neglect them. It is extremely difficult to explain this in an easy-to-understand manner to leaders who value prestige, and it is frustrating to have to use indirect expressions to persuade them.

While in Mato Grosso, I also attended a meeting of IDEA, an international organization for people affected by leprosy. IDEA was working to improve the lives of people affected by leprosy at a local Catholic church. Around fifteen people affected by leprosy joined thirty residents with no experience of leprosy to make handicrafts that would stabilize their income and to take part in exercises to improve their health. Many people affected by leprosy live in the neighborhood, but their disabilities make them reluctant to go outside because they fear being seen. Therefore, IDEA members visit their homes to encourage them to join the activities. The group's leader Alzira Rodriguez introduced the organization to me. She was diagnosed with leprosy at fourteen, and one day her parents asked her to go to São Paulo to work. They wanted to hide their daughter's illness. She married in the colony and had two children, but they were taken from her to be raised by her parents. Ms. Rodriguez, who still has severe disabilities in her limbs, told me emphatically that she would like to further bolster IDEA's efforts, despite the difficulties, so that people affected by leprosy in similar circumstances can regain their dignity and lead stable lives.

My final destination was Recife in northeastern Brazil. I briefly returned to Brasília from Cuiabá, Mata Grosso, before heading to Pernambuco. At the state health department, I learned about its SANAR program for identifying and treating patients affected by leprosy and other neglected tropical diseases. It is natural for the state health department to take the initiative in efforts like this, but it is also cooperating with various institutions, including working with educational institutions on detecting diseases early in children. For leprosy, children are shown pictures of early symptoms, such as skin patches, and asked to check for similar symptoms in themselves and their families. In 2013, the program targeted 240,000 children, with 20,107 children tested, of whom fifty-seven were infected. An additional 650 prisoners were tested for leprosy, and fifty-five were confirmed to be infected.

Next, I visited the Hospital Geral Mirueira on the outskirts of Recife. Established in 1941, it housed people affected by leprosy who had been shunned by their families and society. The residents began cultivating fields and raising poultry and pigs on the grounds. They built places of worship and theaters, and the approximately 10,000 hectares of land resembled a small town. Some residents even made a name for themselves through music or literature. One nurse carefully preserved records of these events. Concerned that the history of those days would be lost, the nurse interviewed people affected by leprosy and hoped to publish their stories. At its peak, there were around 500 residents in the hospital. However, the number of beds had been reduced to sixty-one by the time of my visit. About 200 outpatients came per month, a significant number for a single hospital compared to hospitals in other countries.

A nurse showed me around the medical records room, outpatient ward, rehabilitation room, inpatient ward, resident quarters, and theater. One man who had lived here alone for forty-three years remarked sadly: "I've lived here ever since I was admitted at twenty-seven. My whole life is here." The woman living alone next to him sang as best she could in a heartfelt voice for her guests who had come from the other side of the world.

Later, I attended another meeting for people affected by leprosy and their families held by the Brazilian leprosy organization MORHAN. In Brazil, those affected by leprosy were separated from society and their families and forced to live in institutions until forced segregation was legally prohibited in 1962. Those admitted as children were not allowed to attend school, marriage was limited to others in the institution, and children born to them were sent to outside institutions or adopted. MORHAN is doing its utmost to demand compensation for these inhumane policies and that the central government implements measures to improve their lives.

Cut off from the village for thirty years—Odisha, Uttarakhand, and Bihar, India, September 2015

In September, after taking part in peace talks with senior government officials and ethnic minority militia leaders in Myanmar, I visited Balangir, Odisha, in eastern India. I was met by Umesh Nayak, the state leader of APAL. As I left the hotel the next day, I saw people from the Kallaripalli colony begging in the street. One elderly woman told me she made 30 to 50 rupees (about US$0.40 to 0.60) per day. Since Odisha's special monthly pension for people affected by leprosy is 300 rupees (about US$4), she earned two to three times that in twenty days of begging. It was clear that the special pension needed to be raised. The special monthly pension in Bihar was 1,800 rupees, which was enough to keep an elderly woman from begging. I walked to the colony with Umesh. After walking for about fifteen minutes under the blazing sun, we found women drawing water from a well at the entrance. Men and women, young and old, gathered around and greeted us. They had primitive houses with brick walls and black coverings weighed down with stones instead of roofs. The windows were small, and temperatures inside must reach over 50 degrees C. Even though it was midday, the homes were pitch black inside.

I approached one woman who lived in a house whose roof had collapsed due to heavy rains two weeks before. She appeared to have been inside when it happened, and the memory of it had traumatized her. A young couple were nearby. The husband, who was not from the colony, told me the fact that his wife was affected by leprosy made it impossible for him to find work outside. This was clear discrimination, but they had torn down one wall of stigma by getting married. I then went to meet some beggars at a nearby Hindu temple. It was only nine in the morning but already hot. Other beggars had taken the side of the road suitable for begging, so the colony residents went to the other side. Did discrimination exist even in the world of begging? Krishna, the colony's leader, hung his head as he said, "No one enjoys begging. We have to do it to survive."

My final stop in Odisha was a house on the outskirts of a village, about a ninety-minute drive from Balangir, where a man affected by leprosy lived. I greeted the village head and went with Umesh to the man's house. The villagers seemed surprised at our sudden visit, but some of them followed us to the man's house. It was simple, with mud walls and a straw roof. A gray-haired man emerged from the dark house, propping up his severely emaciated body with a thin cane. He said he had lived in this house, which he had built himself, for thirty years. His wife still lived in the village, but he lived alone to avoid disturbing the other villagers. His wife sometimes brought him water and vegetables but never touched him. His two sons and grandchildren seldom came to see him. No one had held his hand in the thirty years since he left the village. The villagers believed the gods had punished him. I remember on Indonesia's Biak Island, too, I met a lonely old man who had lived in a hut for many years, with only his brother to bring him meals; he went to sleep hungry on the days his brother did not come. There must be many such people in the world—who knew how many? I felt my determination to fight on surge.

I returned to Delhi and traveled four hours to Haridwar, Uttarakhand. Uttarakhand was created in 2000 when it broke off from Uttar Pradesh. It is the source of the Ganges and attracts many Hindu pilgrims. The Ganga Mata Kusht Ashram is located on the bank of the Ganges River. Its houses were simple, with corrugated tin roofs and walls made of plastic sheeting. When I arrived, I was greeted by Keshav Choudhary, the Uttarakhand colony leader. He cut a charismatic figure, clad in an orange robe.

In Uttarakhand, the monthly state pension for people affected by leprosy is 1,000 rupees (about US$12). The colony residents had more stable livelihoods than those in Odisha. Santosh Gupta, forty-eight, was originally from Kolkata and said he knew Mother Teresa. He had four children and eight grandchildren, all of whom attended school. Ten-year-old Bhim told me he was learning to write his name, and while we were talking, his eighteen-year-old brother Vikash came home from school. A handsome young man, he had never experienced discrimination in the colony. He told me about his dream of going to a technical college. I heard that the colony attracts people from all over the country, too many for the land area.

For the final leg of my trip, I traveled to the state of Bihar, where I visited the Prem Nagar leprosy colony in Patna, the state capital. Located next to a bridge construction site, the colony's air was dusty from all the construction materials. This colony had existed for sixty years but was forcibly moved from its original location two years prior in order to make way for the bridge. According to Saudagar, the seventy-five-year-old colony elder, the new location was a swamp. They were using soil to fill in the land, and the space for their housing was minimal. Fifty-year-old Sheetal started his business with microcredit from S-ILF. His business was making *chaat*, fried dough stuffed with mashed potatoes, and he had a cart outside the colony's entrance. Watching from afar, I saw adults and children purchase food from his cart, one after another. His business was doing well, thanks to S-ILF, he told me. All the families in this colony had the ability to be independent. What they lacked was the opportunity to work and an environment where their children could receive an education. S-ILF's role here was massive. We had to continue our efforts to expand it further.

MAKING THE IMPOSSIBLE POSSIBLE

Boys and girls affected by leprosy on a small island—Republic of Kiribati, October 2015

> Route: Narita International Airport → Yangon, Myanmar (flight time: 7h)—four nights—Yangon → Singapore (flight time: 3h; 6h stopover) → Brisbane, Australia (flight time: 7h 50m; 4h 30m stopover) → Nadi, Fiji (flight time: 3h 30m; overnight stopover) → Tarawa, Kiribati (flight time: 3h)—three nights

In October, after holding separate discussions in Myanmar with the government, the national army, and armed ethnic minority groups regarding a ceasefire and peace, I headed to the Republic of Kiribati, an island nation located in the middle of the Pacific Ocean. With the world's largest coral reef, Kiribati consists of thirty-three islands scattered south of the Marshall Islands, east of Nauru and the Solomon Islands, and north of Tuvalu and the Cook Islands. While the total area of all the islands is about the size of Japan's Tsushima Island, going from one end to the other by sea takes a week. Rising sea levels due to global warming have become a serious problem, and while driving around the island, the driver stopped the car at the top of a small hill, saying, "This is the highest point on the island, 2.4 meters above sea level." Sea levels are expected to rise by nearly 30 centimeters by 2055. According to the World Bank, 50 to 80 percent of the islands around the capital Tarawa could be inundated. In response, the government has decided to purchase land in Fiji and is drawing up a plan to relocate the population in case of an emergency.

It took three full days to reach Kiribati from Myanmar via Singapore, Australia, and Fiji. Many people had gathered at Bonriki International Airport in Tarawa to watch the plane, which has only two weekly flights. The journey from the airport to my accommodation was taken by microbus, along a single road. Incredibly, it had the sea on both sides, and at its narrowest, the land was a mere 5 meters wide.

In a deep-roofed meeting hall unique to this country, called a "mwaneaba" in the native language, I was briefed by the WHO representative and Ms. Erei Bonebati Rimon, the leprosy program manager under the Ministry of Health. She told me that 100 to 200 new leprosy cases are discovered annually in Kiribati's population of about 100,000, and that, as of October, 121 people were undergoing treatment. The prevalence rate was more than ten cases per 10,000 people. However, since the total population is less than 1 million, Kiribati is not on the WHO list of countries that have not eliminated leprosy. People affected by leprosy are still mostly poor and concentrated in South Tarawa, but I was told that other areas had them too, but they were simply undetected. With only three leprosy program officers that have jurisdiction over far-flung islands, follow-up is a major challenge, especially in the heavily populated South Tarawa and the islands surrounding the main island chain, called the outer islands. We discussed the care that they might provide to people affected by leprosy to improve their future, including finding hidden patients and giving hope and courage to those they know about.

The following day, I had a meeting scheduled with the minister of foreign affairs, but he failed to show up. This didn't often happen to me. However, one saying here was apparently: If you come to Kiribati, do not get angry. This accorded with my own belief, which is to respect the customs and values of every country I visit. My next appointment was at a clinic in Nawerewere, a district of Bonriki, near the airport, and there I was kept standing outside for more than thirty minutes. It was sweltering, even at ten in the morning. The humidity was high, and the sweat dripped in beads down my face. When I finally got inside, where a New Zealand leprosy support group was working, three people affected by leprosy were there. An eleven-year-old girl brought by her mother showed few symptoms on her face or hands. A sixteen-year-old boy had side effects from the medication all over his face and nose, but he managed a broad smile when I encouraged him to stick with the drug and assured him that he would recover. Ms. Rimon of the Ministry of Health told me that the high number of youths affected by leprosy is typical of the Pacific region, where 20 to 40 percent of patients are children. They have a database of disease detection methods, ages, and locations; if one family member shows symptoms, the whole family is supposed to be examined.

My next stop was the village of Bonriki, right in front of the airport. The village had huts on stilts and a *mwaneaba*. It looked a peaceful place, with children napping and men lolling in hammocks. In one hut, a twenty-six-year-old man affected by leprosy was living with his father. He was divorced, he told me—his marriage had ended before he got leprosy. (I was glad to know that the disease was not the reason for his divorce.) He had relatives living in the village, he said, and his friends took him out occasionally, though he did have some aftereffects in his legs. He pulled out an MDT blister pack from his pocket, saying, "I take my medicine with me wherever I go."

After taking my leave of him, I went to meet a man who had started a business with the support of an NGO. With his tin-roofed store under a roadside tree, sixty-two-year-old Kimwaere Mikaere had a slight disability in his hand, but with the help of a New Zealand leprosy support group, he had bought an electric compressor pump, and he now inflated tires and washed cars, earning at least AU$20 (about US$14) a day, or on a good day AU$30 (about US$20), for twelve hours work. The national average is AU$12.50 (about US$9), and he spoke proudly as he stopped his busy work and looked out at the ocean, saying that his job enabled him to live confidently. According to Wayne Uan, the New Zealand-based Pacific Leprosy Foundation (PLF) field director, they were currently training thirty-nine people in growing fruit trees, catching and drying fish, and book-keeping.

In the afternoon, I visited the village of Teaoraereke, where PLF was conducting medical examinations to detect new patients. About 100 villagers gathered in a *mwaneaba* in the village center. At the back of the *mwaneaba* were four medical checkup rooms separated by blue tarps. Here, Dr. Arturo C. Cunanan Jr., a well-known leprosy doctor from the Philippine island of Culion—once called "the island of despair"—was treating patients. We were delighted to see each other again in such an unexpected place. On the day of my visit, he found one new person affected by leprosy. The girl had symptoms on her face and would stay at the center for a while for treatment. PLF refers to its efforts here as "skin camps." They don't like to call their work a "leprosy exam" and prefer "skin care" to avoid any potential stigma.

Before returning to the hotel, I visited the Betio area, the site of fierce fighting between the United States and Japan during the Second World War. A former Japanese gun emplacement and a 1-meter-thick reinforced concrete fortress remained where the Japanese Army headquarters was located. The sea view from the gun emplacement was so calm and beautiful that it was hard to believe that 4,500 Japanese soldiers died rather than surrender here.

On the third day, I set out for the island of Abaokoro in North Tarawa. The landing site is on a shallow lagoon, where boats can enter only at high tide, and there was an incredibly long wait for a boat. I do a lot of waiting in my work. Finally, a small six-passenger boat arrived, and I boarded it. The open-topped boat was swelteringly hot, but the emerald-hued sea glistened magnificently. Our guide threw a sacred object into the sea and said one word: "Mauri." Residents of North Tarawa strongly believe in spirits and pray to their ancestors in the sea for safe navigation.

After an hour, we reached the island's shallows, where I had to get out and wade ashore, knee-deep in the water. Piling into the trailer of a truck that went along what seemed like a dirt track, after about five minutes we finally arrived at the only clinic on the island. At the entrance was a poster about the harmful effects of tobacco and a weekly schedule packed with appointments and events. A single glance was all I needed to see that the staff there took their work seriously. The hospital's warehouse also stored the therapeutic drug MDT, and several patients had come for treatment.

A six-year-old boy living in a nearby shack had white patches on his arms, legs, and back, an early sign of the disease. He apparently was not bullied or called names at school. According to Ms. Rimon, discrimination in the old days used to be rife, but nowadays advanced cases were rare, and there was better understanding of the disease. Dr. Nobuyuki Nishikiori, a WHO Western Pacific Regional Office coordinator, accompanied me and examined a sixteen-year-old girl who had just arrived at the hospital with her mother, finding two areas where she had no feeling, raising suspicion of leprosy. Her great-grandmother had been interned on Makogai, an island used to keep people affected by leprosy in isolation in faraway Fiji, and her mother knew that leprosy could be cured if detected early, so she immediately brought her daughter to the hospital.

In the afternoon, I had a meeting with President Anote Tong. In recent years, the president has been vociferously raising the issue of climate change, fearing that Kiribati could disappear due to climate change-driven sea level rise. The president was a Japanophile who had visited Japan several times. He obtained a black belt in Kyokushin karate while studying in New Zealand, and his favorite book was Musashi Miyamoto's *The Book of Five Rings*. The three leprosy officers in Kiribati were doing their job well, I reported, despite the shortage of human and budgetary resources. Though the case numbers were low, not amounting to a public health problem, I asked that the government continue to keep their eye on this issue along with other public healthcare concerns. The president thanked me for our work. "Leprosy used to be feared when I was a boy. But recently it seems to be seen merely as just one of many curable diseases." That evening, the president hosted a welcome banquet in the garden of his official residence. We were treated to a whole roasted pig, the highest mark of hospitality.

In Kiribati, the efforts that were being made for early detection had resulted in fewer cases with disabilities, and it seemed to me that one effect of this was less prejudice and discrimination than in other endemic countries. Notwithstanding the chronic shortage in human resources, they were coping well. Dr. Nishikiori told me, however, that there were many sparsely populated remote islands where there were no doctors at all, and many cases where treatment was delayed. Kiribati needed a comprehensive approach to address infectious diseases, he said, including tuberculosis and neglected tropical diseases, to improve cost efficiency in the leprosy elimination effort. The situation on the farthest islands was very different from the main island and the capital, he said. There, health services were virtually nonexistent, and to get angry. This main island it was quicker to first head to Hawaii and then fly in via Fiji than to go directly by boat.

Memories of Makogai Island—Republic of Fiji, October 2015

Route: Tarawa, Kiribati → Nadi, Fiji (flight time: 3h)—two nights—Nadi → Suva, Fiji (driving time: 3h 30m) → Nadi (flight time: 30m; 3h 30m stopover) → Auckland, New Zealand (flight time: 3h; 8h stopover) → Narita International Airport (flight time: 11h)

After completing my work in Kiribati, I visited the Republic of Fiji, located in the western South Pacific. It was my third visit to Fiji.

An island nation consisting of more than 330 islands, Fiji borders Vanuatu to the west, Tonga to the east, and Tuvalu to the north, with a total area of about 18,000 square kilometers, slightly larger than Japan's Shikoku Island. Called the "Crossroads of the South Pacific," Fiji has long served as the intersection of the peoples and cultures of the South Pacific, playing a central role among these countries. Major industries include tourism, sugar, and apparel. Makogai Island, once known as an island where people affected by leprosy were kept in isolation, is also in Fiji.

I arrived in Nadi, the country's third-largest municipality, and then immediately drove three and a half hours to the capital, Suva. Suva is Fiji's legislative and administrative capital and the largest city in the South Pacific. However, the weather is not so good as on the island's eastern side, and it has few resort facilities, so tourists rarely see the city.

At the WHO's Suva office, the staff, including WHO representative Dr. Liu Yunguo, gave me an enthusiastic welcome. I told them: "Leprosy has been almost completely eradicated in Fiji, but there are still some South Pacific countries where leprosy still frequently occurs. As the heart of the South Pacific, I hope that Fiji will play a role in monitoring the situation in these countries." Representative Liu responded: "Leprosy is still a vital issue in the South Pacific, and we intend to step up our health programs in the region." During a meeting, Health Minister Jone Usamate said that "Fiji has few new cases but we are also strengthening our outreach and early detection programs to proactively find people affected by leprosy." At the post-meeting press conference, I asked him to use Fiji's knowledge to benefit its neighboring island countries, as they still have many undetected people affected by leprosy.

The following day, I visited P. J. Twomey Hospital in Tamavua, Suva. In this hospital, with its bright green roof and yellow walls, people affected by leprosy were receiving treatment for their disabled limbs. With the development of modern medicine, the P. J. Twomey Hospital began treating leprosy patients around 1969. Previously, Makogai Island served this role. I chatted with Harrietta Tonu, a gray-haired eighty-one-year-old woman with a bright hibiscus-patterned blue dress and a friendly smile. She told me her memories of when she was sent to Makogai Island and separated from her family. Nanise Moala, a seventy-five-year-old woman dressed in bright yellow, had been diagnosed at twenty-five. She told me how shocked she was to learn she had the disease, but her family understood and accepted her situation. Sixty-six-year-old Peni Vuniciva showed me a painting he had done based on his memories of Makogai Island. He had disability in his hands, but the painting was magnificent. Coming to the island must have been heartbreaking for everyone, and they must have gone through many hardships there, but no one I spoke to had anything bad to say about the place.

I decided I wanted to pay a visit to Makogai Island. Our team departed from Suva on a small, ten-passenger motorboat. Since we could not reach the island before sunset, we decided to stay overnight on Leleuvia Island, about an hour and a half from the Suva wharf, which was where we would be setting off. Leleuvia Island is tiny, and takes about twenty minutes to walk around. We enjoyed a relaxing dinner in a small rustic cabin while listening to the sound of the waves. The next morning, we took a small motorboat from there to our destination. Fortunately, the weather was good, the waves were calm, and we were bathed in tropical sunshine.

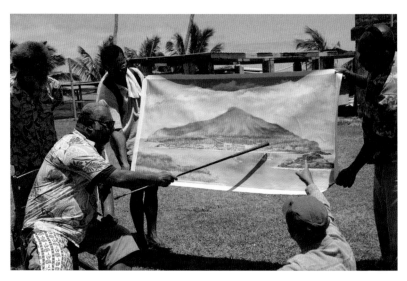

124. Mr. Peni Vuniciva, a person affected by leprosy, recounting memories of his life on Makogai Island, using one of his own paintings (Fiji, October 2015)

OVERCOMING THE STAGNATION

The first transfer of leprosy patients from Fiji's main island to Makogai Island took place in 1911, and the island operated for fifty-eight years. Several Catholic missionaries moved to the island and provided services to improve the lives and treatment of the people affected by leprosy. Later, as its reputation grew, people migrated from neighboring countries, increasing the number of residents to a peak of 742. During its fifty-eight years in operation, the island was home to a total of 4,500 people. Of these, 2,500 returned to their hometowns after treatment, 500 returned to their home countries (or neighboring islands), and about 1,500 ended their lives on the island. The island still had a cemetery where people affected by leprosy and the nuns who had served them were laid to rest side by side. In most isolation facilities, patients and medical personnel are buried separately. This island's gravestones did not segregate patients from staff, just as at the Koyama Fukusei Hospital in Gotemba, a private facility in Japan.

Peni Vuniciva showed us around. Walking with a cane because of disability in his legs, he spoke of his memories of the island, every now and then welling up with tears. He recounted: "I came here in 1968. The weather was gorgeous, just like today. There were rumors that patients were shot, and I thought I would never make it home alive. But in reality, it was all quite different. There were other children of about the same age as me, and the nuns, who worked as nurses at the time, cared for us lovingly, as if we were their own family. I had been told that I would never be able to go to school since I had leprosy, but here I was able to study properly. In particular, Sister Siena taught me how to paint, which led me to my current job." When he left Makogai Island, he said, he had felt as bereft as when leaving his parents. That was how much the nuns had loved him. He brought out the painting of the island I had seen the day before and showed it to me again. I could see all the landmarks, vividly rendered, including the red-roofed church, the Kiribati people's residential area, the mountainside cemetery, the movie theater, the hospital.

Another sixty-two-year-old man then showed us the rest of the island. This man had lived there since the age of two. The isolation wards (with men and women in separate buildings), movie theater, prison, and other facilities were just as they used to be. Security was

629

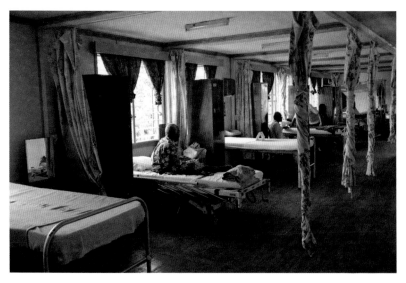

125. A cool-looking ward in the hospital, as one might need in the south Pacific (Fiji, October 2015)

good on the island, he told us. The rare crimes that occurred were minor ones, such as a drunk man chasing after a woman. Even though Makogai Island was a facility to keep people affected by leprosy isolated from the world, the loving care of the nuns and Irish doctors had given the residents plenty of happy memories.

At one time, I frequently played golf with President Kamisese Mara of Fiji, who was once considered a great president. He was over 1.8 meters tall and a gentleman in the English style. I fondly remember, when playing a round at Tokyo's Koganai Country Club, he asked me why the rules prohibited the use of drivers at certain holes. I explained that Communist Party members lived near where the ball would land and would immediately complain to the club if a ball landed on their property. The president laughed mischievously and replied: "Then let's play with a red ball!" Kamisese Mara's daughter is the wife of President Epeli Nailatikau, who was president of Fiji at the time of my visit, so this trip allowed me to renew an old friendship.

HOPE AND COURAGE LEADING THE WAY TO THE FUTURE

2016 AND BEYOND

From Japan to the world

The Japanese government played a vital role in the 2010 UN resolution on the elimination of discrimination against persons affected by leprosy and their family members. This was followed, in January 2015, by the news that people affected by leprosy had been given an audience with Their Majesties the Emperor and Empress of Japan (Emperor Akihito and Empress Michiko; now Emperor Emeritus and Empress Emerita), which brought great courage and hope to communities affected by leprosy worldwide.

In Japan, as in other countries, leprosy was historically referred to as a "karmic" disease, that is, a sickness resulting from sinful deeds in a past life, and this had fueled discrimination against people affected by leprosy for centuries. It was also often regarded as a blood (or genetic) disease, so the families and relatives of those affected were also subject to discrimination, commonly leading them to abandon those who had contracted the disease, who as a result had to lead lives of vagrancy. On the other hand, in the Nara period (710–94), Empress Komyo sponsored welfare facilities such as the Seyaku-in and

Hiden-in to provide relief for people suffering from diseases—including people affected by leprosy. Emperor Akihito and Empress Michiko have similarly shown a deep concern with the plight of people affected by leprosy, visiting all fifteen leprosaria in Japan and conversing and corresponding with residents and patients. In 1975, when the emperor visited the National Sanatorium Okinawa Airakuen, His Majesty presented the residents with a *ryuka* (Okinawan folk song) with lyrics he had composed. The residents began to sing this song to the tune of a well-known folk song, and eventually some said, "If only there were a unique tune for this song." Upon learning of this, the emperor encouraged the empress to compose music for the words. Thus was born "Utagoe no Hibiki" ("Resonance of the Singing Voice"), with words written by His Majesty and music composed by Her Majesty, published as a CD book in November 2015 as part of the celebrations of Their Majesties' longevity—they were now both in their eighties.

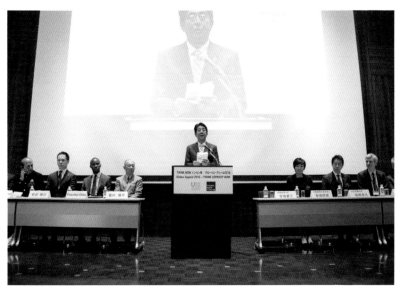

126. Prime Minister Shinzo Abe giving his speech at the Global Appeal 2016 (Japan, January 2016). Launched in partnership with Junior Chamber International, at the Sasakawa Peace Foundation Building in Tokyo (Japan, January 2016)

Countries visited in 2016	
January	● Japan
	Myanmar (Nationwide ceasefire agreement: talks with government personnel)
	Taiwan (Meetings with key persons)
February	United Kingdom (Attended former President Jimmy Carter's speech at the House of Lords)
	Palau (Maritime security support measures-related naming ceremony)
	Thailand (Myanmar nationwide ceasefire agreement: negotiations with representatives of armed ethnic organizations)
	China (China Disabled Persons' Federation)
March	● Indonesia
	Myanmar (Nationwide ceasefire agreement: talks with government personnel)
April	United States (Washington, DC: Mental Health Conference; Howard University SYLFF project)
May	Iran (International Conference on Women, Peace, and Sustainable Development)
	India (S-ILF and APA board meetings)
	Taiwan (President Tsai Ing-wen inauguration ceremony)
	Switzerland (WHO General Assembly and Sasakawa Health Prize award ceremony)
June	Thailand (Myanmar nationwide ceasefire agreement: negotiations with representatives of armed ethnic organizations)
	Myanmar (Nationwide ceasefire agreement: meetings with government personnel)
	Bulgaria (Conferred Doctor Honoris Causa degree by Sofia University)

	● Vatican
	Monaco (Forum for Future Ocean Floor Mapping)
July	● Cameroon
	Myanmar ((Nationwide ceasefire agreement: talks with government personnel)
August	United States (Florida: World Blind Union and International Council for Education of People with Visual Impairment Joint Assembly)
	Kenya (Tokyo International Conference on African Development VI)
	Myanmar (Nationwide ceasefire agreement: talks with government personnel)
October	Myanmar (Nationwide ceasefire agreement: talks with government personnel)
	● Ecuador
	Peru (Visit to former President Alberto Fujimori)
	Switzerland
November	India (S-ILF tenth anniversary)
	China (Beijing University SYLFF tenth anniversary)
December	● Indonesia

● Indicates a trip that features in this section.
SYLFF: Sasakawa Young Leaders Fellowship Fund program.
S-ILF: Sasakawa-India Leprosy Foundation.

In 2016, the Vatican and the Nippon Foundation co-sponsored an international symposium titled "Toward Holistic Care for People with Hansen's Disease, Respectful of Their Dignity." The symposium's conclusions and recommendations began with the statement: "Every new case of Hansen's disease is one case too many." The guidance that followed included ceasing the use of discriminatory words such as "leper," and avoiding the use of "leprosy" as a discriminatory metaphor. The statement also declared: "The leaders of all religions—and this is an essential and urgent matter—should, in their teachings, writings, and speeches, contribute to eliminating discrimination against persons affected by leprosy by spreading awareness that leprosy is curable and stressing that there is no reason to discriminate against anyone affected by leprosy or members of their families."

Those who are spiritual pillars to many people—including His Majesty the Emperor, His Holiness the Pope, and His Holiness the Dalai Lama—understand the situation of people affected by leprosy and the need to eliminate discrimination against them, and they shine a hugely significant light on our work to eradicate the disease.

Global Appeal 2016—Japan, January 2016

In January 2016, we announced the 2016 Global Appeal to End Stigma and Discrimination against People Affected by Leprosy and Their Families, the eleventh such appeal, in Tokyo. The 2016 Global Appeal received endorsement from Junior Chamber International—a non-profit NGO, whose members, aged eighteen to forty, are active in 130 countries worldwide. The event was attended by about 300 people affected by leprosy and their supporters from thirteen countries. Prime Minister Shinzo Abe, his wife Akie Abe, and Minister of Health, Labor, and Welfare Yasuhisa Shiozaki were among the guests of honor. It was followed by an international symposium titled "Discrimination and How to Prevent It: Lessons from Leprosy," featuring a panel discussion on leprosy and the broader issues of health and discrimination, with invited speakers including experts on HIV/AIDS, albinism (congenital leukoderma), intellectual disabilities, blindness, and deafness. A discussion between writer Fumihiko Takayama and religious scholar Tetsuo Yamaori cast new light on discrimination against people affected by leprosy from historical and spiritual perspectives.

The "Let's Find a Patch!" dance—Republic of Indonesia, March 2016

Route: Haneda International Airport → Jakarta, Indonesia (flight time: 7h 30m)—one night—Jakarta → Surabaya, Indonesia (flight time:

1h 30m)—two nights—Surabaya → Singapore (flight time: 2h; 2h 30m stopover) → Narita International Airport (flight time: 6h 30m)

In March, I carried out work in Indonesia. Leprosy was eliminated in Indonesia at the national level in 2000, based on the World Health Organization (WHO) benchmark of less than one case per 10,000 population. However, twelve of its thirty-four (now thirty-eight) provinces had not achieved this benchmark. East Java, my destination for this visit, had an exceptionally high number of cases, accounting for 40 percent nationwide. The WHO Indonesia leprosy officer explained that the number of new cases detected in East Java over the past ten years had flatlined, and early patient detection rates were also significantly lower than we would have liked. The Indonesian government had apparently just implemented a new "zero strategy," a plan to eliminate disease, infection, disability, prejudice, and discrimination. I could only hope that it would not end up as a pipe dream, but based on Indonesia's past leprosy initiatives I couldn't help being skeptical and had to wonder whether the words would be backed up by actions. Still, I wanted to hold out some hope.

Erwin Cooreman, the WHO Global Leprosy Program team leader, who had traveled from Delhi, India, observed how promoting patient detection is crucial even if it leads to a temporary increase in newly diagnosed patients: the goals should be to achieve early diagnoses, control the spread of infection, and reduce the rate of long-term disability. I spoke about the vital role that the media play in helping to raise awareness of the disease, the importance of eliminating ignorance about leprosy among physicians, and the value of screening family members who live with people affected by leprosy.

After the meeting at the WHO office, I traveled to Surabaya, the second-largest city in Indonesia and the capital of East Java province. I then went to the village of Sumber Glagah, where ninety-three people affected by leprosy and their families live. About 100 people, from the elderly to small children, gathered in the small hall built with the support of the Ministry of Social Affairs. My message was that leprosy is a curable disease. I said that anyone who sees any skin patches on children's bodies should contact a doctor immediately—for those are signs of leprosy. I also asked for the assistance of the journalists who were accompanying me in communicating this message.

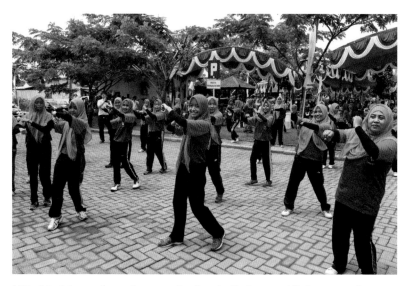

127. Health workers dancing the "Let's find a patch" dance (Indonesia, March 2016)

At the adjacent Sumber Glagah hospital, I was welcomed in the courtyard with singing and dancing from the staff. They had choreographed a dance to go with the song titled "Let's Find a Patch!"—a song that encourages people to look out for the patches of light or darkly colored skin that are one of the signs of leprosy, both on themselves and other family members, to be used in awareness campaigns. It was a pretty good effort, and I even joined in myself. A fifty-year-old man named Sugino admitted to this hospital two weeks before had ulcers on his right hand and right leg. He had neglected his illness for five years because he thought that treating it would cost too much. The delayed treatment had left him with aftereffects, and, he told me, his wife and children had abandoned him. A pair of brothers, aged thirty and thirty-six, were washing each other's feet in the courtyard, and the younger one had a prosthetic left leg. Had the brothers and Sugino come to the hospital immediately after their symptoms first appeared, their lives would have been so different. No matter how many times I hear of such tragedies, they always make feel acutely conscious of my powerlessness and lack of effort. The two brothers let me wash their feet with my bare hands.

637

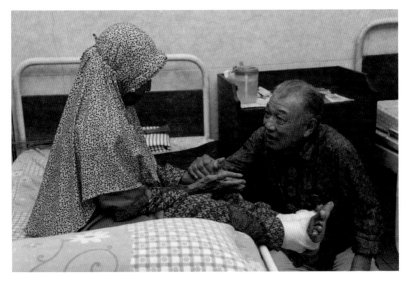

128. The author visiting a muslim woman affected by leprosy at the Sumber Glagah hospital (Indonesia, March 2016)

The next day, I left my accommodation early, at 5 a.m., and headed for Madura Island by microbus. After an hour or so, we passed the Suramadu Bridge, the longest in Indonesia, and the misty island of Madura came into view on the other side of the strait. After another hour's drive beyond the bridge, we arrived at the Sampang city hall with its large red roof, a traditional Indonesian structure. Dr. Firman Pria Abadi, head of the Sampang District Health Office, explained the problems faced by the island: "There is still a strong stigma attached to leprosy, but you have to keep in mind that 30 percent of the population lives in poverty and most children get an average of a mere four years of education. Some can't read or don't understand what's being said, making it hard to spread knowledge about leprosy."

We then transferred to an open space for an event to mark this year's World Leprosy Day in January, where a tent decorated with red and white cloth was set up outside. About 800 people, mainly elementary and junior high school students, had gathered there. In his greeting, Vice Health Minister Subuh spoke enthusiastically about the World Leprosy Day awareness campaign. Afterward, the Ministry of Health staff, the many children who had gathered, and guests, including myself, joined in the "Let's Find a Patch!" dance. It was a lot of fun, and we were drenched in sweat under the hot sun. The campaign was going to start in East Java, be implemented in South Sulawesi and Central Sulawesi, and eventually expand all over Indonesia. I could only pray that it would not end merely as part of a ceremony to welcome me.

In April, I visited Gallaudet University in Washington, DC. This is the world's largest university for people with impaired hearing, and since 2003, the Nippon Foundation has provided scholarship support to outstanding young international scholars with impaired hearing, with a total of 223 students receiving the scholarship. I then attended a World Bank-sponsored mental health conference at Georgetown University. I had dinner with Chairman Dennis Blair (a former admiral and commander in chief of US Pacific Command) of the Sasakawa Peace Foundation USA.

> Route: Narita International Airport → Washington, DC (flight time: 12h 40m)—three nights—Washington, DC → Narita (flight time: 14h)

In May, I attended an international women's conference in Iran and the S-ILF board meeting in India.

> Route: Narita International Airport → Dubai, United Arab Emirates (flight time: 11h 15m; 3h 30m stopover) → Tehran, Iran (flight time: 2h)—three nights (attended a conference for the advancement of women with Akio Abe, the prime minister's wife, and met with Iranian Vice President Masoumeh Ebtekar)—Tehran → Dubai (flight time: 2h; 2h stopover) → Delhi, India (flight time: 3h 25m)—three nights—Delhi → Narita (flight time: 7h 45m)

In the same month, I attended the Sasakawa Health Prize award ceremony held during the WHO General Assembly in Geneva and spoke with health ministers from countries worldwide.

> Route: Haneda International Airport → Frankfurt, Germany (flight time: 10h; 3h stopover) → Geneva, Switzerland (flight time: 1h)—two nights—Geneva → Frankfurt → Haneda (flight time: 11h)

An international leprosy symposium at the Vatican—Vatican City State, June 2016

> Route: Haneda International Airport → Bangkok, Thailand (flight time: 6h 30m; 3h stopover) → Chiang Mai, Thailand (flight time: 1h

20m)—one night (Myanmar ceasefire and peace talks)—Chiang Mai → Bangkok (flight time: 1h 10m; 2h 30m stopover) → Frankfurt, Germany (flight time: 12h; 4h stopover) → Sofia, Bulgaria (flight time: 2h)—two nights (received an honorary degree from Sofia University)—Sofia → Rome, Italy (flight time: 2h)—six nights (Vatican symposium)—Rome → Nice, France/Monaco (flight time: 1h)—three nights (attended an ocean forum)—Nice → Frankfurt (flight time: 1h 30m; 2h 20m stopover) → Haneda (flight time: 11h)

In 2013, Pope Francis had used a discriminatory metaphor: "Careerism [in the Vatican] is a form of leprosy. Leprosy!" He did the same thing again later the same year, likening pedophilia in the Church to leprosy. In response, I sent a letter of protest petitioning him not to use such phrases, as they might contribute to the public's misperceptions regarding the disease. Acknowledgment came, but I had the feeling that His Holiness had probably not perused my letters himself, so I rethought my strategy and proposed an international conference co-sponsored by the Nippon Foundation and the Vatican, which was readily agreed to. The symposium would serve as a social awareness event aimed at dispelling society's misconceptions about leprosy and eliminating discrimination against people affected by the disease and their families.

This international symposium took place in Vatican City, the seat of the Catholic Church, for two days on 9 and 10 June 2016. Titled "Toward Holistic Care for People with Hansen's Disease, Respectful of their Dignity," it was co-sponsored by the Pontifical Council for the Pastoral Care of Health Care Workers, the Good Samaritan Foundation, and the Nippon Foundation. The event marked the first time that people affected by leprosy and religious leaders from around the world had come together to discuss the relationship between religion and leprosy. I would like to note that the symposium's success was due in no small part to the truly prodigious efforts of the Nippon Foundation's Tatsuya Tanami, who worked tirelessly to make it happen.

When the pope came around to greet us after a mass in St. Peter's Square on the day before the conference, I handed His Holiness a sheet of paper with a message in Italian to him saying, "Please do not use the term 'leprosy' as a negative metaphor." The pope listened to the interpreter's brief explanation, smiled, and slipped the note into the folds of his gown.

About 250 people from forty-five countries attended the symposium, including people affected by leprosy, religious leaders, UN Human Rights Council Advisory Committee members, medical personnel, and NGO representatives. Representatives of the Roman Catholic Church, Judaism, Islam, Hinduism, and Buddhism each presented their religious interpretations of leprosy and examples of relief efforts. I was truly moved by the Islamic leader's speech, in which he stated: "It is the teaching of Islam to treat the sick with compassion, and it is written in the Quran that family ties must not be severed and the sick must be healed." Once again, I observed that religion can play a truly significant role.

People affected by leprosy from Japan, India, Brazil, Ghana, China, South Korea, the Philippines, and Colombia talked about their life histories and efforts to eliminate discrimination. Masao Ishida from Nagashima Aiseien Sanitorium, a national leprosarium in Okayama prefecture in Japan, gave an overview of the history of leprosy in

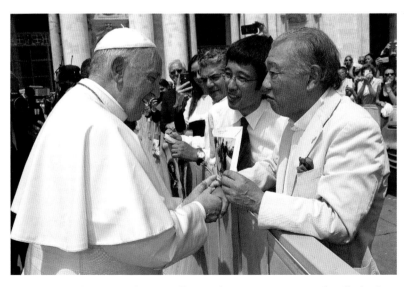

129. "Please do not use the term 'leprosy' as a negative metaphor!" Pleading with Pope Francis (Vatican City, Rome, Italy, June 2016)

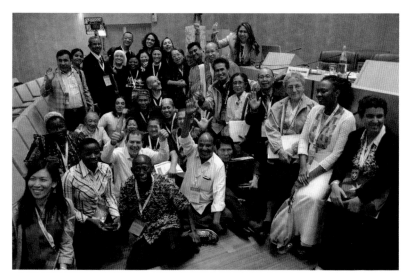

130. A gathering of participants celebrating the successful conclusion of the international symposium (Vatican City, Rome, Italy, June 2016)

Japan from the postwar period to the present. He told the participants: "We are currently working to register Japan's leprosy museum as part of UNESCO's Memory of the World. We believe our mission is to prevent the repetition of this cruel and tragic history."

In the closing event on the second day, the symposium presented its "Conclusions and Recommendations," a compilation of the discussions and remarks from the two-day event. They began with the statement: "Every new case of Hansen's disease is one case too many." The recommendations that followed included ceasing the use of discriminatory words such as "leper," and avoiding the use of "leprosy" as a metaphor for things to be avoided. It also declared, "The leaders of all religions—and this is an essential and urgent matter—should, in their teachings, writings, and speeches, contribute to eliminating discrimination against persons affected by leprosy by spreading awareness that leprosy is curable and stressing that there is no reason to discriminate against anyone affected by leprosy or members of their families."

On the following day, 11 June, we held a session for people affected by leprosy and the UN Human Rights Council Advisory Committee members. It was a meaningful session where human rights experts heard directly from people affected by leprosy, who were provided with an opportunity to share the discrimination they have experienced in their countries, allowing the UN Human Rights Council Advisory Committee members to confirm the extent to which the Principles and Guidelines have been implemented. In the latter half of the session, people affected by leprosy from around the world introduced their own issues and efforts, with a participant from Colombia stating: "The government is not making any progress. We ourselves must take the lead in taking action to eliminate discrimination." These words seemed to have inspired many of the people affected by leprosy who were present.

On Sunday, 12 June, I attended the extraordinary mass for the jubilee of the sick and disabled, which was held in St. Peter's Square as a papal event for the Extraordinary Jubilee of Mercy. About 70,000 people with disabilities, medical and welfare professionals, Christians, and general participants from all over the world gathered to listen to Pope Francis's homily with great interest.

At the mass, Pope Francis said: "An international conference took place in Rome this past week dedicated to the care of people affected by Hansen's disease. My gratitude goes to the organizers and participants of this conference, and I hope for a fruitful commitment in the fight against this disease," drawing loud applause from the audience. The audience was especially moved by the message from those affected by the disease in South America and the Philippines, home to many Catholics. The message from the Vatican—the seat of the Roman Catholic Church and its 1.3 billion believers worldwide— about eliminating discrimination against people affected by leprosy surely had a tremendous impact.

Afterward, Msgr. Jean-Marie Mupendawatu, secretary of the Pontifical Council for Health Care Workers of the Vatican, who chaired the symposium, said the following in an interview: "This symposium allowed us to learn for the first time about the full extent of the atrocious consequences of leprosy. The pope has over the past two days been praying for the symposium's success … We have been so ignorant about leprosy. We were amazed to hear the stories of those affected by the disease. I could not believe that when people affected by the disease died, their bodies were left to pile up on church grounds for years and then taken elsewhere … Surely more dignified arrangements could have been made. Truly, we have been benighted."

Discrimination in a community of twenty-three—Republic of Cameroon, July 2016

> Route: Haneda International Airport → Paris, France (flight time: 12h 30m; 9h stopover) → Yaoundé, Cameroon (flight time: 6h 30m)—seven nights—Yaoundé → Paris (flight time: 6h 30m; 7h stopover) → Narita International Airport (flight time: 11h 30m)

In July, I visited Cameroon in west-central Africa. Cameroon is one of Africa's most ethnically diverse countries, with around 250 different ethnic groups. At the end of 1998, the country supposedly eliminated leprosy as a public health problem at the national level, but 70 percent of its administrative units have no reported leprosy data available, so the actual number of cases is unknown. Cameroon has no facilities to deal with leprosy's aftereffects or to prevent cases from deteriorating, and medical services appear to be scant for hunter-gatherers, which include the Baka (commonly known as pygmies) and other ethnic groups, and for internal refugees.

On 3 July, I traveled to the capital, Yaoundé, via Paris. At my first stop, the Ministry of Health, I passed through a corridor barricaded with heavy wooden walls, and three heavy wooden doors in the space of 10 meters, to enter Health Minister André Mama Fouda's office. After greeting one another, we headed for the office of Dr. Ernest Nji Tabah, the leprosy officer. His office was in the corner of a building that was once an inpatient facility for leprosy patients. Another room had a great pile of mosquito nets that had not been distributed to the people—aid supplies for malaria control. Such things are not unusual in developing countries. The principle of aid to developing countries is that simply sending funds and supplies to a site is insufficient. It is incumbent on donors to visit these sites, on the ground, and confirm that aid is reaching its intended targets. As an aside, I once discovered that multidrug therapy (MDT), used to treat leprosy, had not arrived in Mozambique on schedule. I immediately reported the delay to the local WHO office and instructed them to expedite arrangements for the drug. My field-oriented approach is based on the idea that the field holds both problems and their solutions.

Early the next morning, I departed for Bertoua, the capital of the East Region. It was the last day of the Islamic month of Ramadan (fasting), and the town was filled with Muslims dressed in bright colors and celebrating. Houses with mud walls lined the roads, and children used large banana leaves as umbrellas in the sudden showers of rain. The view from the car window was delightful. However, the most worrisome part of visiting Africa is traveling to the countryside. Despite the paucity of vehicles, there are many traffic accidents. We encountered many trucks that had overturned due to overloading and excessive speed.

I arrived in Bertoua after a six-hour drive from Yaoundé. The East Region is the largest of Cameroon's ten regions but has the smallest population. And because it borders several perennially weak countries in Central Africa, a fifth of its population of 1 million are refugees, making food and health problems severe. The governor prepared a dinner party to welcome me. During the meal, I learned that the governor was an avid reader of Yukio Mishima's *Kinkaku-ji* (The Temple of the Golden Pavilion) and was interested in Kyoto. We got along so well on our first meeting that he gave me a ballpoint pen to commemorate the occasion.

The following day, I headed for a village that was home to the Baka, a hunter-gatherer tribe living in the forest. After about an hour and a half drive from Bertoua, I first went to the Abong-Mbang Health Department for a briefing on the region's leprosy situation and then drove almost two hours from the health department to Menzoh village. About 100 people from the Baka tribe and the Bantu tribe of farmers living nearby had gathered in the plaza, and they welcomed me with drums and dancing, while the women added to the excitement with strange ululations and hand clapping. As usual, I joined their circle and broke a sweat dancing. Ellen, the leader of the Baka tribe, introduced me to three people affected by leprosy. The first was a thin, gray-haired old man with a cane; the second was a toddler with spots on her back that appeared to be early signs of leprosy; and the third was a middle-aged woman with ulcers on her hands, thin legs, and a lingering scar around her nose. When I asked her if anything terrible had happened to her, she complained with tears streaming down her face, "Every day they bully me, and I am thinking of suicide. My hands are useless, I am told to go back to the forest, and my family shuns me." I took her arm and told the assembled villagers that leprosy was a curable disease and that they should not be mean to her as she was a human being and one of them. When I said, "Raise your hand if you pledge not to discriminate against people affected by leprosy," most of them raised their hands. I could only hope that they would keep this promise after I left. Discriminatory practices do not disappear immediately after a brief explanation by an outsider like me. However, we will never solve the problem if we stop trying.

Next, we drove for about thirty minutes through the roadless jungle mud to a facility in the village of Kwamb. Here, the villagers welcomed me with another dance. According to the village head, this leprosarium was established in 1936 to treat and hospitalize the nearby Baka people affected by leprosy. In the 1970s, it had over 600 patients. Abong-Mbang once had a hospital, but it was relocated deep in the jungle due to opposition from nearby residents who feared leprosy. The road here was built as part of a national policy to settle

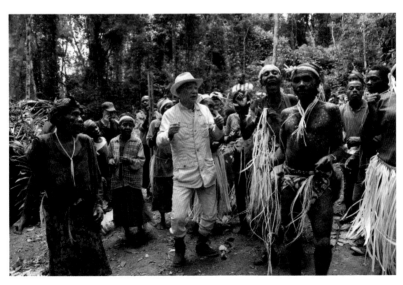

131. A welcoming ceremony deep in the jungle (Cameroon, July 2016)

the Baka people out of the jungle, and along the road there were settled and semi-settled Baka people living in miserable huts.

One of the village's four people affected by leprosy, a blind old man dressed in bright blue, welcomed me with a song. I am not sure whether he had prepared the song in advance or if it was improvised, but I heard "Sasakawa" frequently in the lyrics, and his thick, low voice echoed through the forest. I hugged the old man, saying, "You have an incredible voice. I salute you for enduring so much sorrow and suffering for so long." He responded with a powerful handshake, his sightless eyes wide open.

I then spoke with Justin, a middle-aged man who lived in a dilapidated building. He said he had contracted the disease as a child and had been chased from the jungle where he lived with his family, leaving him to live alone. Having been cured with therapeutic drugs, he wanted to return to the jungle, but he looked dejected, saying his community would probably not accept him.

On the last day, I sought out and visited a settlement deep in the jungle. Like an explorer, I put on boots and gloves and carried a long walking stick as I made my way along an unmarked path in the dense forest. I heard the sounds of unfamiliar birds from all around. The jungle was so deep that I lost sight of my guide while slowing my pace due to fallen trees and swampy areas. I heard strange voices and emerged into a narrow clearing. The place looked like something out of a Weissmuller Tarzan movie I had seen as a child. There were five small domed huts made of wood and leaves, with two families and twenty-three residents. According to the group's leader, they shared any animals they hunted and killed. Among them were three people affected by leprosy and two with albinism, who were not allowed to join the family circle and stood off to the side. Whispering, I asked the three people affected by leprosy if they had ever been bullied. The three fell silent after saying they had experienced it so much that they did not want to say anymore. When I asked the other family members how they thought the three had contracted the disease, one man answered loudly and clearly: "It was either God's punishment or the devil's possession." The fact that there was such severe discrimination so deep in the jungle, even among a small group of twenty-three people, shocked me and made me rethink the human condition. I said: "Leprosy is neither a divine punishment nor a curse; it is just a disease. If it is treated quickly, there will be no aftereffects, and I want everyone to live in harmony. Raise your hand if you promise to stop discriminating." Everyone raised their hands, but I was still doubtful. Five of the twenty-three lived as hunter-gatherers, moving through the deep jungle and suffering discrimination daily.

Whether on a small island or in a large forested area, prejudice and discrimination against leprosy occur wherever there are people, even in the twenty-first century. Even those who swear in front of me that they will not discriminate against people affected by leprosy cannot change immediately. Here were twenty-three people who moved through the jungle as hunters in search of prey. They were adults and children, yet the two people with albinism and the three affected by leprosy had to walk behind the rest of the group. I could well imagine that for food they had to subsist on what the others left. Whether in a modernized metropolis with its vast maze of information or in a jungle isolated from it, the common denominator is that people discriminate against each other.

The problem of albinism, like leprosy, is particularly acute in Africa. In the belief that white skin possesses magical powers, people cut off albinos' fingers and arms and use the bones as amulets for good luck, sometimes even taking their lives. It is an especially severe issue in Tanzania. Once I learned about this African problem, I started activities to support those with albinism.

In August, I visited Orlando, Florida, in the United States, to attend an international conference for the deaf. The conference's hotel venue, with its vast conference hall, was nearly overflowing with attendees from all over the world.

After the conference, I went to Nairobi, Kenya, via London. The Tokyo International Conference on African Development, sponsored by the Japanese government, had been held in Yokohama every three years, but 2016 was the first time it had been held in Africa. The Sasakawa Africa Association (SAA), a sister organization of the Nippon Foundation, was given an opportunity as an NGO to deliver a short speech at each plenary session, but it also hosted a significant side event, since the conference was being held in Africa and the SAA had conducted projects in fifteen African countries. The event was well received, with speeches from Prime Minister Shinzo Abe and Akinwumi Adesina, president of the African Development Bank.

I then traveled to Myanmar, where I held discussions relating to a ceasefire accord with the government and the national army.

> Route: Narita International Airport → Chicago, United States (flight time: 11h 30m; 3h 30m stopover) → Orlando, United States (flight time: 2h 30m)—three nights—Orlando → Miami, United States (flight time: 1h; 3h stopover) → London, UK (flight time: 8h 40m; 2h stopover) → Nairobi, Kenya (flight time: 8h 30m)—four nights—Nairobi → Dubai, United Arab Emirates (flight time: 5h; 4h stopover) → Bangkok, Thailand (flight time: 6h 30m; 2h 20m stopover) → Yangon, Myanmar (flight time: 1h)—two nights—Yangon → Narita International Airport (flight time: 6h 30m)

A quarantine facility just ten minutes from the heart of the capital—Republic of Ecuador, October 2016

> Route: Narita International Airport → Houston, United States (flight time: 13h 30m; 6h stopover) → Quito, Ecuador (flight time: 5h)—three nights—Quito → Lima, Peru (flight time: 2h 20m)—one night—Lima → Houston (flight time: 6h 40m; 4h stopover) → Narita (flight time: 13h 30m)

In October, just as Japan's autumn winds began to blow after the sweltering heat of summer, I visited Ecuador. Located in western South America, Ecuador has the Galapagos Islands, famous for their role in Darwin's theory of evolution, about 1,000 kilometers west of the mainland. The Nippon Foundation had previously donated a surveillance boat to monitor poaching in the nation's abundant fisheries, and I had visited the islands on that occasion. I still remember the cries of the giant tortoises echoing in the forest.

My visit was to attend the Third United Nations Conference on Human Settlements (Habitat III) to discuss solutions to issues related to human settlements. One of the Nippon Foundation's objectives is to create inclusive communities where people with and without disabilities can live together without discrimination.

In keeping with my usual practice, after attending the conference, I visited the Hospital Gonzalo González, a leprosy facility with nearly 100 years of history. Located in the capital city of Quito, on the map the facility was only a ten-minute drive from my hotel. Most leprosy facilities worldwide are built on the outskirts of cities in order to keep residents and patients separate from the general population, so I was somewhat surprised. At any rate, we set off in the car, and indeed it only took us ten minutes to reach the hospital—however, the city itself is small, and so crossing a few hills from the town center took us outside the city limits, where the Hospital Gonzalo González was located. The hospital entrance had a sturdy iron gate, and the place was surrounded by a wall. Another facility built with the idea of keeping people affected by leprosy shut well away. According to the hospital director, the number of leprosy patients has been decreasing in recent years, and the hospital now has resources for drug addicts and alcoholics as well. Its history as a leprosy hospital dates back to 1929. Until the 1920s, as in Japan, the policy was to have the police forcibly isolate patients, with many people confined at the hospital.

In 2009, the government built twenty-three housing units on the hospital grounds, and twenty people affected by leprosy lived in them at the time of my visit. Their average age was sixty-five, with the oldest at eighty-four. There were eighty beds in the inpatient facility for leprosy patients, but they were rarely used anymore. The baroque buildings on the hospital grounds retained the aura of times past, and I could even see the ruins of an old theater.

I was shown into the home of Yolanda Toro, the unofficial leader of the residents. She had lived there for twenty-five years and loved sewing and basket weaving. Her works were displayed throughout her tidy house. Ms. Toro is from southern Peru, where her father also had leprosy. She moved to the facility at thirty and quickly began treatment, so she had few aftereffects of the disease. However, she divorced before moving to the hospital and has had no contact with her family since.

The residents' biggest concern was apparently a disagreement with the hospital. The hospital authorities wanted it to be rebuilt as a general hospital due to the declining number of people affected by leprosy, but the residents were worried about losing their homes. It was perfectly natural for them to be concerned about being forcefully evicted after having experienced forced isolation.

As I was leaving, one of the residents handed me an old magazine, saying, "Don't forget about us." It was a magazine for people affected by leprosy throughout Ecuador, and the first issue was published in 1961. It contained articles about illness and love, poems, memorials to those who had passed away, and daily life. It was published by the Hospital Gonzalo González, and the contributors were residents and the women's association that supported them. In Japan, many magazines for and by people affected by leprosy have been published in leprosaria, and in Ecuador too, more than fifty years ago, such magazines were published to provide emotional support to the residents.

In October, I again visited Geneva for a meeting with WHO Director-General Margaret Chan.

> Route: Haneda International Airport → Paris, France (flight time: 12h 30m; 2h 20m stopover) → Geneva, Switzerland (flight time: 1h)—two nights—Geneva → Paris (flight time: 1h; 2h 20m stopover) → Haneda (flight time: 12h)

In November, I attended a board meeting of the S-ILF and a reception to mark its tenth anniversary in Delhi, India.

> Route: Narita International Airport → Delhi, India (flight time: 10h)—two nights—Delhi → Narita (flight time: 7h 30m)

Toward eliminating leprosy in all provinces—Republic of Indonesia, December 2016

> Route: Narita International Airport → Jakarta, Indonesia (flight time: 8h)—one night—Jakarta → Padang, Indonesia (flight time: 1h 50m)—one night—Padang → Jakarta (flight time: 2h)—three nights—Jakarta → Surakarta (Solo), Indonesia (flight time: 1h 20m)—same-day return—Surakarta (Solo) → Jakarta (flight time: 1h 15m) → Narita (flight time: 7h).

My last trip in 2016 was to Indonesia. In December, I visited Jakarta; Padang, the capital of West Sumatra province; Subang Regency on the island of Java; and the ancient capital city, Surakarta (also known as Solo). At the WHO office in Jakarta, the country representative, Dr. Jihane Tawilah, and other officials from the Ministry of Health joined me for a meeting. When I asked the leprosy officer about the government's budget for eliminating the disease for the current fiscal year, she replied vaguely that it was left to local administrators and that the exact budget for leprosy was unknown. No matter how many times I visited this country, I could see no progress in the Indonesian Ministry of Health's efforts to take the fight against leprosy further. I was greatly disappointed and discouraged, but I felt that if I gave up at this point, all my efforts would be for naught. I decided to visit the provincial governors with the authority to make decisions on leprosy budgets and appeal directly to them.

After leaving the WHO office, I flew two hours to Padang city in West Sumatra province, the western neighbor of Java. The island of Sumatra is larger in area than Japan, and although a significant earthquake had just struck on 7 December, Padang appeared free of any signs of substantial disruption. There are various ethnic groups living in Indonesia. The Minangkabau people live in Padang and its surroundings. They are known for their spicy local cuisine and have a matrilineal society that is rarely seen worldwide. When marrying, the man joins the woman's side of the family, takes the mother's family name, and the daughter inherits the property.

In general, mornings start early in Indonesia. The next day, there was a leprosy awareness meeting for West Sumatra province in Padang at 8 a.m. While the chairs of the meeting—the deputy governor of West Sumatra province and the director of the Health Department—were men, I noticed many attendees were women. I wondered whether that might be related to it being a matrilineal society.

Regardless of concerns about effectiveness, the provincial health office was conducting a campaign with motorcycle and cab drivers, mosques, and women's associations. They also briefed me about an organization for people affected by leprosy called Input, which provides early detection and advice on recovering from psychological damage.

After leaving the meeting, I visited the Enam Lingkung health center in Padang Pariaman Regency, which has the greatest number of new cases in the province. The health center had about 100 people waiting for me, including those affected by leprosy and medical personnel. I encouraged them to join me in solidarity by advocating for their dignity and eliminating discrimination alongside Perhimpunan Mandiri Kusta (PerMaTa, an organization for people affected by leprosy) and Input, while building a nationwide network across Indonesia.

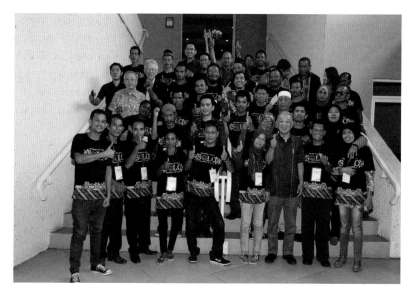

132. With the delegates of PerMaTa, an organization for people affected by leprosy (Indonesia, December 2016)

People affected by leprosy were conducting self-care at the health center that day. I often see such scenes at many of the health centers I visit, but I am aware that it can be performative, put on to impress me, and not something done on a daily basis.

I returned to Jakarta the next day to attend a WHO-sponsored strategy briefing. The objective was to simultaneously eliminate leprosy and yaws in all provinces of Indonesia within five years by 2020. Holding meetings naturally has its role, but unfortunately, the central government's leprosy measures in Indonesia, an archipelagic nation with a population of 300 million, have been communicated to the local governments only in a largely formal way. Understanding the current situation is only possible by actually visiting endemic sites.

Health Minister Nila Moeloek told me: "In the twelve provinces where we have not eliminated leprosy, we are taking a community-engaged, family-targeted approach." I expressed my determination, saying, "I would like you to work with PerMaTa to promote their efforts. I will return to Indonesia as often as possible to help eliminate the disease at the provincial level by 2020."

MAKING THE IMPOSSIBLE POSSIBLE

During my stay in Jakarta, I visited the office of Muhammadiyah, one of Indonesia's most prominent Islamic religious organizations, and met with Dr. Sudibyo Markus, its vice president. Indonesia is the largest Muslim country in the world, where about 88 percent of the population adheres to Islam. Muhammadiyah has the largest network of private schools in Indonesia, with over 10,000 campuses, from kindergartens to universities, and around 30 million members. When I asked Dr. Markus to spread accurate information about leprosy among Muhammadiyah's network, he readily agreed. Bolstering my cooperative relationship with this organization may lead to some positive developments in Indonesia's elimination efforts, which seem so stalled.

The next day, I left Jakarta at 6 a.m. and drove the four hours to Subang Regency in West Java province. Horns blared on the heavily congested highway, and emergency braking was frequent. Some of my companions got carsick, but as far as I was concerned, it was also a perfect time to read. I have become quite accustomed to the traffic jams in Indonesia.

I was deep in a book when we arrived, seemingly in no time, at Subang Regency. The health department director frankly admitted that Subang Regency has the most people affected by leprosy by far in West Java. It does not have sufficient patient detection due to a lack of medical personnel and insufficient funds for preventive measures. By way of encouragement, I said: "Many places in the world have no doctors, no human resources, and no budget, but even some of these places have dramatically decreased their case numbers. Of course, a budget is necessary, but if we work hard and passionately, we can eliminate the disease."

On the final day, I left the hotel again at 6 a.m. and flew from Jakarta to Solo in central Java. My trip happened to coincide with a training session PerMaTa was holding, so I decided to stop by before returning home. Leaders of twenty-seven chapters from three provinces had gathered there to hold discussions and provide reports on their activities, including awareness promotion, economic independence, and education. PerMaTa has many young leaders and 3,000 members nationwide. I encouraged them, saying, "One thread is weak, but ten threads together become strong, demonstrating the enormous power of solidarity."

Countries visited in 2017	
January	United States (President Trump inauguration ceremony)
	● India
February	Thailand (Nationwide ceasefire agreement talks)
	Myanmar (Nationwide ceasefire agreement: talks with government personnel)
March	Iran (International symposium on Japan–Iran relations)
	Myanmar (Nationwide ceasefire agreement: talks with government personnel)
	● India
	● Switzerland
April	● United States
May	● Poland (Jagiellonian University, Krakow; SYLFF program twenty-fifth anniversary ceremony)
	Switzerland (World Health Assembly)
	● Spain
	Myanmar (Nationwide ceasefire agreement: talks with government personnel)
June	Switzerland (UN Human Rights Council)
	United States (New York, World Oceans' Day)
July	India (S-ILF board meeting)
	Vietnam (Conference on Japan–Vietnam relations)
	● Indonesia
	Thailand (Myanmar nationwide ceasefire agreement: negotiations with representatives of armed ethnic organizations)
August	Sweden (Scandinavia–Japan Sasakawa Foundation board meeting)
	United Kingdom (England, Scotland: Signing ceremony relating to maritime development)

	Thailand (Myanmar nationwide ceasefire agreement: negotiations with representatives of armed ethnic organizations)
September	United Kingdom (UK–Japan Global Seminar; Great Britain Sasakawa Foundation board meeting)
	Tunisia (Exchange of views on Tunisian National Dialogue Quartet and the Arab Spring)
	Thailand (Myanmar nationwide ceasefire agreement: negotiations with representatives of armed ethnic organizations)
October	China (100 Books project commemorative ceremony)
	France (Fondation Franco-Japonaise Sasakawa)
	Georgia (Exchange of views on World Maritime University-Sasakawa Global Institute scholars and the environmental problems of the Aral Sea)
	● Azerbaijan
November	● Indonesia
	Myanmar (Nationwide ceasefire agreement: talks with government personnel)
December	India (Government-sponsored leprosy meeting and visit to Disabled Peoples' International)
	Myanmar (Nationwide ceasefire agreement: talks with government personnel)

● Indicates a trip that features in this section.

SYLFF: Sasakawa Young Leaders Fellowship Fund program.

S-ILF: Sasakawa India Leprosy Foundation.

The Global Appeal and the "mitanin" in action—Delhi and Chhattisgarh, Republic of India, January–February 2017

Route: Narita International Airport → Delhi, India (flight time: 10h 20m)—three nights—Delhi → Raipur, Chhattisgarh (flight time: 3h 15m)—three nights—Raipur → Delhi (flight time: 2h; 8h 30m stopover) → Narita (flight time: 7h 20m)

I began 2017 in India. On 30 January, we announced the Global Appeal 2017 in Delhi. This year, the declaration was sent out as a joint declaration with the Inter-Parliamentary Union (IPU), an alliance of 171 (now 179) member-parliaments worldwide. IPU is a venerable, prestigious organization founded in Paris in June 1889, with non-partisan members from various countries. In his address at the ceremony, IPU President Saber Chowdhury (a member of the Bangladesh Parliament), drawing on his experience of working to repeal a 100-year-old discrimination law in his country, said enthusiastically: "Mr. Sasakawa has given us his motorcycle analogy, wherein the front wheel represents efforts to eliminate leprosy and the rear wheel efforts to eliminate discrimination, but that motorcycle needs a very powerful engine. I hope that parliamentarians are going to be that engine. It is legislators who created and repealed the discriminatory laws against leprosy, and it is legislators who allocate funds to fight leprosy. Parliamentarians have the power not only to repeal discriminatory laws but also to legislate, draft policies, obtain budgets, and implement policies. Our role is to create a world without leprosy and without discrimination. That is the spirit of the IPU."

Prime Minister Modi said in his video message: "Gandhi's dream was to eradicate leprosy. We are now within the last mile of achieving this dream, but it will require all our economic and political efforts to achieve it."

I appealed to the audience to join with governments, international organizations, and above all, people affected by leprosy in moving forward through the final mile toward eliminating leprosy. Around 300 people attended the event, including President Narsappa of the Association of People Affected by Leprosy (APAL), others affected by leprosy, members of parliament from India and other Asian countries, support groups, and members of the press.

After the ceremony, I flew to Chhattisgarh. This state had thirty-four colonies, home to 2,500 people affected by leprosy. I immediately sat down with Chhattisgarh's health minister. I introduced him to Mr. Bhoi, the APAL state leader, who was present at the meeting. Mr. Bhoi appealed directly to the minister about the importance of special subsidies for people affected by leprosy. In response to this impassioned plea, the minister promised to create an inter-ministerial coordination committee to address the issue of leprosy from multiple perspectives.

At the Chief Medical and Health Office in Mahasamund, I received a briefing from health officers and medical personnel on the situation in the area and then visited the village of Katti, where two people had recently been diagnosed with leprosy. One diagnosed person was a thirty-year-old woman living along the main road, and the other was a thin, middle-aged man living in a bright emerald-green house. The two had been found by community volunteers called *mitanin*. These volunteers are commonly known as Accredited Social Health Activists (ASHA) throughout India, but in this region, they seem to be called *mitanin*. The government pays them 250 rupees (about US$3) for each person found to have leprosy, with an additional allowance if the patient is completely cured.

In the afternoon, I heard that there were two people affected by leprosy in Memra, Pithora, which had the highest rate of new cases, so I took the two-hour car ride to see them. It was a quiet village with a population of 1,955, mainly making ends meet through rice cultivation. The new cases were both men, one eighty years old and the other fifty. Both men had the patches on their arms that are seen as the sign of leprosy.

The village had two *mitanin*, and one of them found four cases after going to 175 households, around half the total of 370 in the community. I wondered why a village of fewer than 2,000 people would have an eighty-year-old man whose symptoms had only just been discovered. An eighty-year-old would typically have much more advanced symptoms, but this man was in the early stages of the disease. Just one example of a mystery in a disease about which so much remains to be discovered.

In the evening, I visited the Indra Dharam Dham Kusta leprosy colony in Raipur, the state capital. Extremely noisy, due to its proximity to the main road and railroad tracks, the colony was typical of colonies often found in cities, with rows of shanties side-by-side whose brick walls and tiled roofs look as if they might collapse at any moment, plagued with flies and mosquitoes. According to Mr. Bhoi, the APAL state leader who lives in the colony, 170 people from fifty families lived there, and all of the eighty people affected by leprosy made their living by begging. The government had made eviction demands, and Mr. Bhoi and others had repeatedly petitioned the government. Children from the colony were also subjected to bullying and other discrimination at school, but they told me that discrimination has ceased since Mr. Bhoi became the school principal. When I first met Mr. Bhoi, he was quiet and reserved, but at this meeting with the health and social welfare ministers, he spoke clearly and argued the issues in a dignified manner. I imagined as state colony leader he had developed self-confidence and a sense of responsibility. That was encouraging. Mr. Bhoi also made a powerful speech in front of many of his colony's residents.

On the last day of my trip, I held a press conference attended by fifty media outlets. I introduced the achievements of the *mitanin* and spoke about the importance of spreading accurate information about leprosy with the media's help. More than 100 media outlets reported on the press conference.

Marigolds, nerves, and passion—Delhi and Odisha, India, March 2017

> Route: Narita International Airport → Delhi, India (flight time: 10h)—three nights—Delhi → Bhubaneswar, Odisha, India (flight time: 2h 15m)—two nights—Bhubaneswar → Delhi (flight time: 2h)—one night—Delhi → Narita (flight time: 7h 30m)

Following my January and February trips, I again visited India in March, specifically the states of Odisha and Delhi. Odisha state, in eastern India, was once impoverished but had seen rapid industrial development in recent years, as mines extracting iron ore, coal, and other mineral resources, and major companies, moved into the area. However, leprosy remained a problem, with 10,174 new cases in 2016 and a prevalence rate of 1.35 per 10,000 population.

After flying to Odisha's capital, Bhubaneswar, from Delhi, I was greeted in front of the airport by APAL's state leader Umesh Nayak and a group of others, who beat drums and tambourines and placed countless garlands of marigolds around my neck. When I think of how tough their lives are, along with gratitude, such gifts always produce feelings of sorrow and guilt in me. Together with Mr. Nayak, I went directly from the airport to see Justice B. K. Misra, the chair of the Human Rights Commission. Mr. Nayak submitted a request to improve housing conditions for people affected by leprosy, and Justice Misra invited fifteen female students from the Odisha State Open University Law Department to attend the meeting to learn about the current leprosy issues, demonstrating his keen sincerity in addressing the issue. At a meeting with mobile medical personnel, I received a report on their efforts throughout Odisha state. The government-led Leprosy Case Detection Campaign (LCDC) had run for a period of ten months from September to October 2016 and amazingly had discovered 4,498 new patients. All credit should go to the volunteers known as ASHA who went from house to house in endemic areas carrying out their work.

According to the state's Health Secretary Pramod Kumar Meherda, the state was not only discovering new patients but also promoting efforts to reintegrate people with disabilities into society by providing rehabilitation and restorative surgeries. As one would expect from the country of Gandhi, whose wish was to eradicate leprosy, Indian states are more proactive in their efforts than other countries. It makes every one of my trips there exciting.

The next day, I visited the Dhenkanal area, a three-hour drive from Bhubaneswar, the state capital. At the community health center, the ASHA were waiting for my arrival. They had confirmed ten new people affected by leprosy, who had themselves traveled from their villages to the health center. One of them was an eleven-year-old boy, who thanks to early treatment would not develop any disabilities.

At Rama Krishna Pally leprosy colony near Bhubaneswar, ninety of the 300 residents had disability certificates. To my utter surprise, many of these certificates had the word "Beggar" written in the occupation column. There it was, "Beggar," written clearly for all to see where most would typically write "Unemployed." My dream is to completely eliminate begging in all leprosy colonies, but one beggar told me, "Without us, the rich will not be able to give alms and will not be able to go to heaven. There is a need for us." I was at a loss for a response. While I have not been able to confirm how true it is, I was told that there was once a labor union for beggars in New Delhi.

The leader of Rama Krishna Pally colony told me sadly, "The residents have no land ownership rights, and they are on tenterhooks about being evicted. Also, they cannot feed their families due to inadequate support from the government." I tried to encourage him: "I will convey your requests directly to the prime minister and the governor with Mr. Nayak, the state leader. I will also do my utmost to help."

During my stay in Odisha, my schedule was packed with meetings with many key government officials, including the state chief minister, the principal secretary, the minister of health and family welfare, the undersecretary for social security and disability affairs, and the chair of the Committee on Disability Issues. We made clear that private organizations can only do so much, and that is why we were asking the government to help. Later, I urged Mr. Nayak and the members of APAL to convey their requests directly to the government. Mr. Nayak usually speaks loudly, but he spoke quietly with sweat on his brow due to his nervousness as he explained how colony residents needed to acquire land titles and get support through special subsidies, before handing a report summarizing these points to the dignitaries. Most of them responded positively, saying they would consider the proposal. After the meetings, Mr. Nayak told me: "I couldn't sleep last night

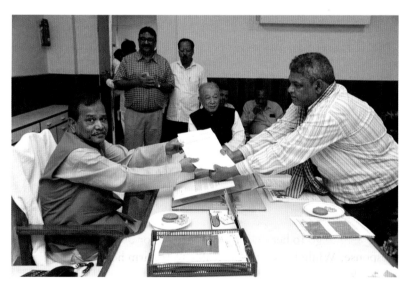

133. APAL state leader Mr. Umesh Nayak submitting the request to Health Secretary Pramod Kumar Meherda (Odisha, India, March 2017)

because I was preparing materials for the meetings. I feel as if I have just completed my exams." He looked relieved, and now he was speaking energetically at his normal volume. We also held a press conference, and the next day, more than twenty articles appeared in various media, as far as I could ascertain.

After my work in Odisha, I went to Delhi, where I informed the WHO India representative, the principal health secretary, and the health minister of state about the situation in Odisha. I said: "There are some vacant leprosy officer posts in rural areas. I would like you to secure the human resources needed to keep grassroots efforts alive." The Union government decided to increase the leprosy elimination budget at the February budget meeting, and the minister of state informed me that the LCDC would continue for three years.

Later, Mr. Nayak e-mailed me to say how pleased he was to have been invited by the state chief minister to have Sunday lunch with him, providing an opportunity to explain in detail the issues facing people affected by leprosy. Amazing: the chief minister and someone affected by leprosy shared a meal together. The chief minister must have understood the quality of person and leadership in Mr. Nayak.

The neglected tropical diseases summit—Swiss Confederation, April 2017

On 19 April, WHO Headquarters hosted a Global Partners Meeting on neglected tropical diseases under the leadership of Director-General Margaret Chan. One billion people worldwide, especially the poor, are severely affected by various diseases collectively known as neglected tropical diseases. I am uncomfortable with this designation, as the word "neglected" has a hurtful ring to it for people who struggle day and night with these diseases.

Nevertheless, measures are being taken. This Global Partners Meeting—based on the slogan "Leave No One Behind" underpinning the 2030 goals—brought together former UN Secretary-General Kofi Annan, Bill Gates, and representatives from the UK, Belgium, and other governments, and from pharmaceutical companies, who all pledged significant sums of money and drugs to fight this category of disease. Bill Gates mentioned the importance of breaking the cycle of poverty, strengthening neglected tropical disease surveillance, and mapping infections, pledging US$335 million over the next four years. A laudable framework for support had been established, but the question was how to put it all into action.

I was given the opportunity to speak at the summit and share my forty years of experience in the fight against leprosy: "As with leprosy, the fight against NTDs [neglected tropical diseases] requires medical solutions and a social approach to ending stigma and discrimination. The road to solving this problem requires three specific milestones: (1) securing the political commitment of leaders; (2) enlisting the cooperation of media to disseminate information about the diseases and encourage people to seek treatment; and (3) forming sustainable initiatives bringing together all stakeholders, including pharmaceutical companies and people affected."

I would also add the necessity to expand the role of people affected as the main actors in awareness-raising, case-finding, and rehabilitation initiatives. They are the people who have actual experience of their diseases. In that sense, it was a shame there were not more

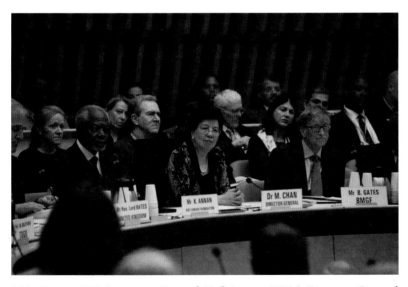

134. Former UN Secretary-General Kofi Annan, WHO Director-General Margaret Chan, and Bill Gates (Geneva, April 2017)

people affected by neglected tropical diseases at the summit of which this meeting was a part. I would like to find some way of enabling the leprosy community to share with those who have suffered from neglected tropical diseases all the experience it has gained in its own struggles and triumphs.

Finally, we must be mindful of what participants at the summit themselves stated—that "we care for people" and that we should "see the faces behind the numbers." It's important that we address not just neglected tropical diseases but engage too with the people who suffer from them. At the conference, I was awarded the WHO Gold Medal for my work on leprosy by WHO Director-General Margaret Chan. It was a great honor, and the standing ovation from the audience encouraged me to continue my efforts.

Touring universities and international organizations—United States of America, Republic of Poland, Swiss Confederation, and Kingdom of Spain, April–May 2017

On 25 April, I attended the Health, Stigma, and Human Rights symposium at the University of Minnesota in Minneapolis, Minnesota, United States. The event was organized by Professor Barbara Frey, director of the university's Human Rights Program. Professor Frey is a vital member of an international working group that researches how to promote the Principles and Guidelines adopted by the United Nations. The symposium featured a wide range of presentations on the relationship between diseases and human rights, including leprosy, tuberculosis, and Ebola. The leprosy panel included me, Professor Yozo Yokota of Chuo University, Executive Director Tatsuya Tanami of the Nippon Foundation, and Mr. José Ramirez Jr., a person who has experienced leprosy himself. During the same event, I also received an honorary doctorate from the University of Minnesota Provost Karen Hanson. The ceremony was attended by former Vice President Walter Mondale, a Minnesota native and UMN alumnus.

In May, I attended the twenty-fifth-anniversary celebration of the Ryoichi Sasakawa Young Leaders Fellowship Fund at Jagiellonian University in Poland. The university was founded in 1364, and it preserves Copernicus's research materials. It also had an impressive globe from before the European discovery of the Americas, which occurred in 1492, 128 years after the university's founding.

I also visited Myanmar to help negotiate a ceasefire and peace, then attended the award ceremony for the Sasakawa Health Prize at the World Health Assembly in Geneva (this year's winner was Dr. Rinchin Arslan for his lifelong contribution to primary health care in Mongolia and in particular his work in combating viral hepatitis). After meeting with health ministers from various countries, I traveled to Barcelona, Spain.

Here I received the Health and Human Rights Award, at the quadrennial general assembly of the International Council of Nurses, representing over 130-member countries. Established in 2000, this award recognizes individuals who have made humanitarian contributions to health and human rights. I was chosen in recognition of over forty years of work with WHO, national governments, international organizations, and NGOs to eliminate leprosy worldwide and end the discrimination and human rights violations faced by people affected by leprosy and their families. In my acceptance speech, I said: "I would like to share this honor with all the nurses working with a sense of mission. I am still only halfway through my work. I accept today's award as encouragement to take on further challenges." I was the fourth award recipient, following three others: Sadako Ogata, former United Nations High Commissioner for Refugees; Stephen Lewis, former United Nations' Special Envoy for HIV/AIDS in Africa; and Mary Robinson, former president of Ireland.

In July, I traveled to Delhi, India, to meet with Javed Abidi, the global chair of Disabled Peoples' International (DPI) and attend a S-ILF board meeting. Afterward, I spoke with Health Minister Jagat Prakash Nadda. Later that month, in Hanoi, Vietnam, I spoke on Japan–Vietnam relations with Japanese Ambassador Kunio Umeda and the director general of the Foreign Affairs Department under Vietnam's Ministry of Defense.

Toumotou, Sorofo, and Nakamura—Republic of Indonesia, July 2017

Route: Haneda International Airport → Jakarta, Indonesia (flight time: 7h 40m; 2h 20m stopover) → Manado, Indonesia (flight time: 3h

25m)—three nights—Manado → Ternate, Indonesia (flight time: 50m)—one night—Ternate → Morotai Island, Indonesia (flight time: 1h)—one night—Morotai Island → Ternate (flight time: 1h)—one night—Ternate → Jakarta (flight time: 3h 30m; 12h stopover) → Haneda (flight time: 7h 25m)

After India and Vietnam, I made my third international trip in July to Indonesia. Here I visited the island of Sulawesi, three hours from Jakarta, in northeastern Indonesia. Manado, the capital of North Sulawesi province, is located on the northern side of the island, about half the size of Japan and just south of Mindanao in the Philippines. The region has many mixed-heritage residents from Dutch colonial rule, and unusually for Muslim-majority Indonesia there are many Christians. Many tourists visit resorts here for diving, and coelacanths have been caught in the nearby waters, so panels of coelacanths were displayed on street corners.

On the morning of my second day, I visited Governor Olly Dondokambey's residence at the foot of Mount Klabat, which looks like a smaller version of Mt. Fuji. The property covers over 10,000 square meters and includes a large pond and fields. According to the governor, a nearby hospital provides treatment for leprosy, and there is little discrimination against patients. However, he said he needed a pamphlet to educate people about leprosy. I promised to send him an Indonesian-language copy of *The New Atlas of Leprosy*, a guide for detecting and treating leprosy produced by the Sasakawa Health Foundation. I had the impression I had already sent it to him before. It may have been left in some warehouse somewhere.

Next, I met with about twenty members of a group of people affected by leprosy called Toumotou (meaning "the most human of human" in the local Minahasa language). According to their leader Fernandez, Toumotou members used their experience to visit patients, give advice, and discuss whether there were any measures the government could take to improve their living conditions. One of my goals in Indonesia was to integrate these groups of people affected by leprosy that have begun working in various regions into a larger organization. Such an entity would greatly influence the central and local governments. Similar attempts in India were already seeing success. I hoped it would not simply be a lobbying group but an organization whose fundamental goal is to help people affected by leprosy become self-reliant.

On the third day, I drove five hours through the forest along the tropical sea coast to visit the Bolaang Mongondow Regency office, where I met with Regent Yasti S. Mokoagow, who had just taken office two months earlier. She then accompanied us to a village where they conducted routine medical checkups to find new cases. About 100 villagers were gathered in a small, tin-roofed hospital in the center of a village of around fifty modest houses. Women wearing hijabs (headcloths used by Muslim women) and children came to receive medical examinations. Fifty-six people were examined that day, with six new cases discovered. That was an extremely high rate, making me doubt whether checkups are conducted regularly. Some people said they were hesitant to go to the hospital because of the severe discrimination they would face if they were diagnosed with leprosy. I reiterated my request to the governor who accompanied me to eliminate this social stigma against the disease. I met a young man here who had been cured of his leprosy, fortunately without any lingering disabilities. When I asked him, with his resilient smile, if I could take his portrait, he replied: "Of course. I am happy to have my picture taken; It feels like it validates my existence." My heart ached as I imagined the harsh experiences the young man with leprosy must have had to endure.

I traveled from Manado Airport to Ternate in North Maluku on the fourth day. After about an hour in the air, a small island appeared. It was the conical island of Ternate, with a steep slope running from the coastline to its peak. Ternate City, the largest town in North Maluku, is located on this island. Female students walking the streets all wore white hijabs, and Islamic mosques were everywhere. From the hotel where I stayed, I had a magnificent view of the steep mountains on the other side of the river. The Tidore Islands are well known for their scenic views, which are depicted on Indonesian banknotes.

The next morning, I visited the Sorofo Self-Care Group in Ternate, where people affected by leprosy live together and care for each other. Sorofo launched in 2010 and had twenty-four members living together when I visited. The members of the group earn money from a farm and a store that they run. I was shown the legs of a man who remains disabled, and they were spotless. The absence of people unable to walk was proof of how well they were maintaining their self-care. One man gave me a bouquet of artificial flowers everyone had made. I said, "This is the first time I've received flowers from a man, but I must say, it feels pretty good," which elicited raucous laughter from the room.

Morotai Island, the last stop on this visit, is located directly south of Okinawa and close to the Palau Islands. Around 50,000 people live on the island, which is 1.5 times the size of the main island of Okinawa. At the regency offices, about 100 people, including village leaders, health authorities, and volunteers, participated in a training program for early leprosy detection. I asked the people affected by leprosy who were scheduled to meet with me separately to attend the training, so that I could demonstrate how I touch the hands and faces of people affected by leprosy to emphasize that leprosy is not a scary disease.

Morotai Island was one of the fiercest battlegrounds between Japan and the United States during the Pacific War, and it has one place I really wanted to visit. I wanted to visit the jungle where Teruo Nakamura, a former Japanese soldier, hid in a cave for more than thirty years after the war ended. I spent more than an hour on a bumpy road in nearly 40-degree temperatures, riding in a car and on a motorcycle to reach my destination, but I gave up as the sun was setting. I visited a nearby village called Nakamura, which was named after Mr. Nakamura. The villagers, who were breaking stones for the road, were surprised at this foreigner's sudden appearance but quickly smiled when I told them I was Japanese. Incidentally, Mr. Nakamura was a Japanese soldier from an ethnic minority in Taiwan during Japanese colonial rule. After he was found, he returned to his home-town in Taiwan, which had since been freed of Japanese control. Mr. Nakamura was still regarded as a hero in the local community. The island had a mural and a splendid bronze statue of him in military uniform, which the local people seem to have erected.

In August, I attended a meeting of the Scandinavia–Japan Sasakawa Foundation Board of Directors in Sweden.

In September, I signed a memorandum of understanding with the Scottish government in the UK for a project to train Japanese marine engineers in cooperation with the Nippon Foundation. After that, I met with Myanmar ethnic minority militia leaders in Mae Sot, Thailand. After briefly returning to Japan from Thailand, I attended a meeting at Chatham House in England and the Great Britain Sasakawa Foundation board meeting. Finally, I went to Tunisia to discuss the Arab Spring with the Tunisian National Dialogue Quartet.

Visiting the Umbaki Leprosarium for the first time in a decade—
Republic of Azerbaijan, October 2017

> Route: Narita International Airport → Paris, France (flight time: 12h 30m)—seven nights (Fondation Franco-Japonaise Sasakawa board meeting)—Paris → Vienna, Austria (flight time: 2h; 2h stopover) → Tbilisi, Georgia (flight time: 3h 25m)—two nights (World Maritime University class reunion and meeting with Prime Minister Giorgi Kvirikashvili)—Tbilisi → Baku, Azerbaijan (flight time: 1h 15m)—two nights—Baku → Dubai, United Arab Emirates (flight time: 2h 50m; 8h stopover) → Narita (flight time: 10h)

In October, I attended the Fondation Franco-Japonaise Sasakawa board meeting in Paris, discussed environmental issues in the Aral Sea with World Maritime University Nippon Foundation scholars in Georgia, and met with the nation's President Giorgi Margvelashvili and Prime Minister Giorgi Kvirikashvili. After that, I traveled to Azerbaijan for the first time in ten years. This country has enjoyed a boom in recent years with the discovery of new oil fields in the Caspian Sea. However, speaking with the local people, I learned that the drop in oil prices had slowed the economic momentum. That said, the skyscrapers lining the main road in the capital city of Baku did not exist a decade ago. The skyscraper-lined Caspian Sea waterfront and the dry, rocky mountains in the background formed a strange contrast. As the country continues to develop, I wondered how the residents at the Umbaki Leprosarium, which I visited ten years prior, were doing. About thirty people were living at the leprosarium, and they treated me to a very large cake in the courtyard. I headed for Umbaki with Japanese Ambassador Teruyuki Katori, carrying photographs from my last trip there.

As we sped along with the car kicking up dust, I looked out at the horizon and recalled how I had felt a decade ago. Many of the world's leprosaria are located in remote areas because they were built to "rid" leprosy from society. Umbaki was no exception. It was built in the capital city of Baku (then in the Soviet Union) in 1926, relocating several times before settling in this desert location in 1957.

After a nearly two-hour drive, the familiar iron gates came into view. They marked the entrance to the leprosarium. On my previous visit, their paint had peeled and there was no sign of its former color, but this time, they had a new coat of blue paint. Inside the gate, I was greeted by the same face as ten years ago. It was Dr. Vidadi Aliyev, the head of the leprosarium. I immediately showed him the photos from my previous visit and asked him about the people depicted in them. He told me that many had died. On my last visit, there were thirty residents, but now there were fifteen, and most were over eighty years old.

I first called on Sayara. The walls of her wooden room were painted blue, with two beds on a soft carpet and warmth emanating from the heater. In the photo of ten years before she was wearing a white coat and I assumed she had been a nurse. But now she told me that she entered the facility in 1969 after a diagnosis of leprosy, and then, once cured, she became a resident caregiver. I asked if we could have another photo taken of us together, but she refused. "Please don't. If my picture appears on the internet, it will only cause trouble to my family." Stigma and discrimination truly are persistent. Nevertheless, Sayara cheered me up when she said: "I heard that a visitor from Japan was coming, and I thought it would be you. It's good to see you again after so many years."

Next, I spoke with Seyidbanu, who was relaxing in the garden. She talked to me while looking nostalgically at the photos I had brought. She was from Lankaran, an area near Iran, and had lived in the facility ever since moving here at fourteen. She said she had kept in touch with her family, but I could not ask why she had not returned to them, as I could only imagine. An elderly man wept at the sight of his late wife when I gave him a photo from ten years ago. A woman told me with a big smile, "My daughter brought my grandchild here to meet me." There used to be residents from Armenia, Georgia, and Tajikistan, but they returned home after 1990.

As we toured the facility, Director Aliyev pointed to the overgrown trees and said: "The immediate surroundings are a desert, but the residents collected soil and planted fruit, making this place a lush oasis." Despite the accomplishment, the leprosarium was a lonely place that could not very well be called an oasis, as its residents endured isolation from their families and wider society.

Answering listeners' questions on a radio program—Republic of Indonesia, November 2017

> Route: Haneda International Airport → Jakarta, Indonesia (flight time: 8h)—one night—Jakarta → Makassar, Indonesia (flight time: 2h 30m; 50m stopover) → Gorontalo, Indonesia (flight time: 1h 30m)—two nights—Gorontalo → Manado, Indonesia (flight time: 50m; 50m stopover) → Jakarta (flight time: 3h 20m)—one night—Jakarta → Haneda (flight time: 7h)

In November, I traveled to Jakarta and the northeastern province of Gorontalo. I had planned to visit Indonesia six times in 2017 and see the many islands of this nation in person. However, due to the circumstances of my hosts, I was ultimately only able to make it there twice: once in July and this trip in November.

I arrived in Gorontalo province on the island of Sulawesi via Jakarta, a journey that took two days from Japan. On my first day there, I appeared on a morning talk show at a local radio station. Joining me in the studio were Dr. Darmiyanty Yahya, head of the provincial health department, and Al Qadri, the vice chairman of PerMaTa, an organization of persons affected by leprosy. The program started with Dr. Yahya explaining the current status of leprosy in Gorontalo province. I showcased the global leprosy situation with the following appeal: "Don't be afraid of leprosy. If you discover a patch on your skin, promptly see a doctor. Treatment is free, and you will be cured. I urge everyone listening to check your family members for patches." Vice Chairman Qadri spoke of his experience of being diagnosed with the disease at age six but not going to the hospital because he was too embarrassed, leaving him with a hand disability. He then stressed the importance of going to the hospital as soon as possible. His story was compelling. A unique feature of this program was that the host took questions directly from listeners, including: Can I catch leprosy by eating a meal with a leprosy patient?

I am affected by leprosy and pregnant, but will my child inherit the disease? And are all white patches leprosy? The panel provided detailed responses to each inquiry. While I had appeared on many foreign TV and radio talk shows, this was the first time I appeared on a program to directly answer questions from local residents. This idea was the brainchild of Sasakawa Health Foundation Executive Director Takahiro Nanri, who decided to focus future educational activities on TV and radio appearances. This was the first of many such appearances, and the program answered many more questions from viewers than I'd ever imagined.

In the afternoon, I visited a hospital that treats leprosy. It was built by the Japanese army in 1942 as an armory and used as a leprosy hospital. However, it now serves as a community general hospital providing medical care to 17,000 patients annually. Behind the hospital was an old yellow-walled building where people affected by leprosy lived. I hugged and greeted each of the residents who welcomed me. I told the local media who accompanied me that I had shaken hands with and hugged thousands of people and never caught leprosy, explaining that leprosy is not a disease to be

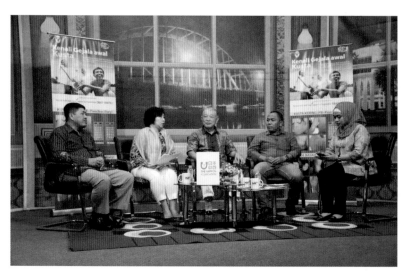

135. The author in a live TV broadcast, taking questions from the audience (Indonesia, November 2017)

feared. Across the road were fields, and beside the grazing cattle were rows of thatch-roofed huts. The huts were used as workshops to make brick braziers, and the residents earned cash income from selling them.

In the evening, a representative from the local health department, Vice Chairman Qadri of PerMaTa, and I appeared on a live TVRI TV program. As with the radio program in the morning, we answered questions from the audience. The health official explained about leprosy, and I told the audience that we must all address problems raised by the disease and discrimination simultaneously. Viewers asked questions such as "What should I do if I get leprosy?" and "If a woman affected by leprosy gets pregnant, will there be any problems with her unborn child?" I emphasized that leprosy is not a genetic disease and is not easily transmitted.

The next day, I observed a trial leprosy awareness program being conducted at Limboto Elementary School. Around 200 children were gathered in the schoolyard of a small campus along the main road. I asked them to tell their parents that leprosy is a curable disease and

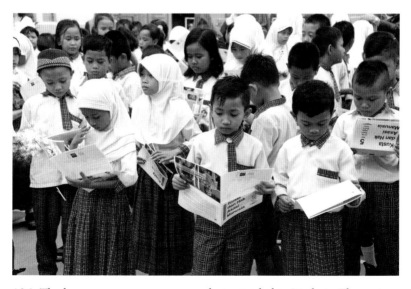

136. The leprosy-awareness program being trialed in Limboto Elementary School (Indonesia, November 2017)

not a punishment from God, despite what they may have heard to the contrary. They replied in a loud voice: "We promise we will." Next, I visited a family of people affected by leprosy living in a fire-ruined mosque about a ten-minute drive from the school. A widowed mother and her three children had just moved there a week earlier from another province. The mother had a disability in her left hand because she had put off going to the hospital. Another elderly woman, who lived deep in a labyrinthine neighborhood, said she took the medication once but stopped halfway through because the side effects were hard to bear, so she relapsed. I asked the woman's grandson, who said he dreamed of becoming a carpenter, to see that his grandmother takes her medicine correctly.

I returned to Jakarta on the third day and met with Governor Anies Rasyid Baswedan. He is an up-and-coming US-educated political scientist turned politician and is thought to be a strong candidate to be the future president. I asked PerMaTa Chairman Paulus Manek and Vice Chairman Qadri to attend the meeting and speak directly with the governor. The meeting was a great success—it was covered by far more television and newspaper outlets than I expected.

This was followed by a meeting with Vice President Jusuf Kalla. It was my first with him since 2005 when I asked him to secure the safety of the Malacca–Singapore Strait and cooperate in measures to combat leprosy. The vice president owns a shipping company and is familiar with the Nippon Foundation's efforts to ensure safe passage in the Malacca–Singapore Strait. He is also from Makassar, a leprosy-endemic area. When I told him that I wanted to visit as many places as possible to help eradicate leprosy in Indonesia, he replied: "My hometown is also affected by leprosy, and there used to be many facilities there. I thank you from the bottom of my heart for your work."

Finally, I visited a prosthetic limb technician training school that the Nippon Foundation had been supporting for ten years. The school is one of the Nippon Foundation's major projects to support people with disabilities. It trains technicians to produce high-quality prosthetic arms and legs, garnering high regard internationally. Around fifteen to twenty prosthetists graduate from the school annually. In the summer of 2018, the Nippon Foundation's support ended, and the Indonesian government took over operations. Graduates are active in many countries, including in Southeast Asia. Some of them were even part of the group that welcomed me on my visit. In addition to this school in Indonesia, the Nippon Foundation has built prosthetist training schools in Cambodia, Thailand, Sri Lanka, the Philippines, and Myanmar.

In December, I visited Delhi, India, to attend the National Leprosy Conference 2017. The following year, I also visited the office of DPI, which jointly issued the Global Appeal calling for the elimination of discrimination against people affected by leprosy and their families, where I spoke with Global Chair Javed Abidi.

Countries visited in 2018	
January	Thailand (Myanmar nationwide ceasefire agreement: negotiations with representatives of armed ethnic organizations)
	Myanmar (Nationwide ceasefire agreement: talks with government personnel)
	● India
February	Myanmar (Nationwide ceasefire agreement: talks with government personnel)
	Thailand (Myanmar nationwide ceasefire agreement: negotiations with representatives of armed ethnic organizations)
March	● Indonesia
	Singapore (Asia Pacific Celebration of Artists with Disabilities)
	Jordan (Prince Hassan, International Conference for Peace)
April	Cambodia (Ceremony to mark textbook delivery for English-language radio program)
	Palau (Palau governing body confers honorary citizenship of Palau)

	• India
	China (Meetings with key persons)
	United States (DeepStar technology development project signing ceremony)
May	Sweden (World Maritime University Sasakawa Global Institute opening ceremony)
	China (Meetings with key persons)
	South Korea (Meetings with key persons)
	Switzerland (Sasakawa Health Prize award ceremony; talks with health ministers)
	Myanmar (Nationwide ceasefire agreement; talks with government personnel)
June	Switzerland (Concert in commemoration of the seventieth anniversary of the UN's Universal Declaration of Human Rights)
	China (Peking University SYLFF twenty-fifth anniversary)
July	China (Lanzhou University, Jilin University, Nanjing University, Fudan University SYLFF twenty-fifth anniversary ceremonies)
	Myanmar (Third Panglong Conference)
	Ethiopia (Sasakawa Africa Foundation)
	• Comoros
	• Mozambique
September	Thailand (Myanmar nationwide ceasefire agreement: negotiations with representatives of armed ethnic organizations)
October	• Indonesia
	Myanmar (Nationwide ceasefire agreement: talks with government personnel)

November	China (Yunnan University SYLFF twenty-fifth anniversary ceremony)
	Thailand (Myanmar nationwide ceasefire agreement: negotiations with representatives of armed ethnic organizations)
	Myanmar (Nationwide ceasefire agreement: talks with government personnel and national conference on combating leprosy)
December	Myanmar (Nationwide ceasefire agreement: talks with government personnel)
	Thailand (Myanmar nationwide ceasefire agreement: negotiations with representatives of armed ethnic organizations)

● Indicates a trip that features in this section.

SYLFF: Sasakawa Young Leaders Fellowship Fund program.

The brave decision to increase case numbers—Delhi and Jharkhand, India, January 2018

> Route: Narita International Airport → Delhi, India (flight time: 10h 20m)—four nights—Delhi → Ranchi, Jharkhand, India (flight time: 1h 40m)—three nights—Ranchi → Delhi (flight time: 1h 50m; 5h stopover) → Shanghai, China (flight time: 5h 30m)—one night (paid my respects to an ill dignitary)—Shanghai → Haneda International Airport (flight time: 4h)

In early 2018, I spent nine days in India. My primary purpose was to present our Global Appeal 2018 in the capital city of Delhi, calling for the elimination of discrimination against people affected by leprosy and their families. I also aimed to lobby the state government in Jharkhand state for an increase in pensions for needy people affected by leprosy while simultaneously conducting an awareness campaign to eliminate discrimination.

That year's Global Appeal was a joint declaration with DPI, an alliance of organizations of people with disabilities from ninety-one countries worldwide. Around 300 people attended the event, including President Narsappa of APAL, others affected by leprosy from colonies near Delhi, organizations of people with disabilities from India and other Asian countries, support groups, and members of the press. In my address, I declared that the Nippon Foundation and DPI were working together toward the goal of realizing an inclusive society where everyone's rights are respected. DPI's Global Chair Javed Abidi expressed his determination: "People affected by leprosy have been the most neglected, marginalized, stigmatized, and discriminated against by society. I would like to uphold and promote this challenge."

At this point, my companion Natsuko Tominaga, who had seen the sign-language interpreter bend five fingers to sign the word leprosy, indicated to Mr. Abidi that she thought it was a little discriminatory. He called the sign-language interpreter and asked them to put what he was about to say into sign language. He then said, "My mother had leprosy," and observing the interpreter confirmed that the finger-bending gesture was being used. Mr. Abidi immediately agreed that we had to do something about it. He was a very friendly person who combined frankness and leadership, and I was extremely sorry that he passed away soon after this event. We lost a valuable comrade.

In the evening, I had an opportunity to explain leprosy issues to President Ram Nath Kovind. Cell phones and other electronic devices were not allowed in the presidential palace, and after a rigorous physical search, I was finally allowed to enter. After passing through a corridor with high stone ceilings, I reached a luxurious room. In a moment, the president appeared. He is a hard worker who has risen from the lowest caste to his current position. In the limited time available, I explained the leprosy issues that pertain in India and our Global Appeal and introduced President Narsappa of APAL.

The next day, I flew to Jharkhand state and set out directly from the Ranchi airport in the state capital for a meeting with state Health Minister Ramchandra Chandravanshi. Accompanying me were APAL Vice President Guntreddy Venugopal and Jharkhand state leader Mr. Jainuddin. Mr. Jainuddin submitted a written request to the minister to improve colony living conditions. He had surveyed all fifty-six colonies in Jharkhand since last November to collect detailed data in time for my visit. The minister, stoutly built with short gray hair and a beard, decided on the spot to form a coordinating committee and include people affected by leprosy on it. He also promised to attend the stakeholders' meeting scheduled for the afternoon.

As promised, the state health minister took time out of his busy schedule to attend the afternoon stakeholders' meeting. Dr. Anil Kumar, deputy director general for leprosy, Ministry of Health and Family Welfare, spoke about eliminating leprosy, saying that even if case numbers temporarily increase, it is vital that we find the hidden patients to prevent disabilities. I told the assembled media and the health minister: "India's work to reduce the number of patients to zero is highly respected globally. Dr. Kumar is the only doctor in the world who has had the courage to say outright that early detection is essential even if it means a temporary increase in the case numbers. Such a temporary increase proves that our work is generating results, and I would like you to feel proud with short-term gains in case numbers." Early leprosy detection is of paramount importance, as delays in detection increase the likelihood of residual disabilities. However, an increase in case numbers is inconsistent with the goal of reducing patient numbers, which lies at the core of elimination. That is why global case numbers have remained flat for nearly ten years. I call this phenomenon "elimination trauma." Dr. Kumar's decision was a direct challenge to this trauma.

Later, I met with the state's Chief Minister Raghubar Das at the state government offices. With his magnificent mustache, the chief minister, having just visited Japan the previous year, was enthusiastic about attracting tourists to Jharkhand. Here again, Mr. Jainuddin made his presence felt. He made a strong appeal: "Let me show you the results of my survey of all colonies in the state. We would like to receive assistance, especially for those with severe disabilities." The chief minister's response: "We intend to create a system in line with the frameworks devised by other states."

On my second day in Jharkhand, I headed for Ramgarh district in the north. About an hour and a half from Ranchi, the provincial capital, I arrived at Ramgarh colony, a noisy place sandwiched between the main road and railroad tracks, with klaxons and whistles blaring in the background. The roofs were made of tin and fabric, and puddles were seething with mosquito larvae. When I visited, a four-year-old boy was performing the dangerous task of sorting electrical items into functional components and scrap metal with a hammer. It was not a child's work, as some of the items were sharp metal and glass. I thought it was not something a little child should be doing, but when I called out to him, he ignored me and continued to work silently. About fifty people, mostly women, had gathered in the common. I told them: "I want to help your children get an education and find proper jobs in the future." I also introduced Rakesh Jha, who handles employment support and scholarships at S-ILF.

On the third day, I visited Nirmal Gram colony in Bokaro District, about a three-hour drive northeast of Ranchi. At the village entrance, I was surrounded by a marching band of uniformed schoolgirls playing drums and flutes and led into the square, marching about 100 meters. There, around 300 people—the entire village—welcomed me with singing and dancing. S-ILF had provided employment support in this colony, which had a cheerful atmosphere. The women had organized

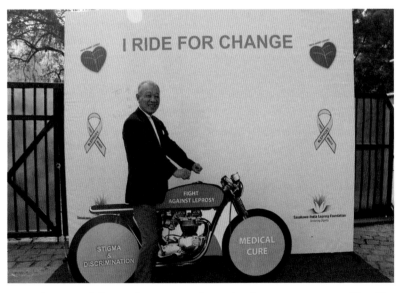

137. The motorbike used to convey the author's message, inspired by Che Guavara's *Motorcycle Diaries*. The front wheel is medical cure, the back wheel stigma and discrimination, symbolizing the author's areas of concern. (India, January 2018)

a self-help group to make ends meet. Their system was to collect members' money and use it for loans and business expenses. On the day of my visit, there were four groups of twenty people. They each planned to set up small-scale businesses selling jewelry, candles, soap, and more.

I encouraged the villagers, saying that the state health minister and chief minister had also promised to improve living conditions in the colonies. S-ILF Chairman Tarun Das and Mr. Jha, my companions, were eager to interview the villagers about their current challenges and desired businesses.

Finding patients in inaccessible places—Republic of Indonesia, March 2018

> Route: Haneda International Airport → Jakarta, Indonesia (flight time: 8h)—one night—Jakarta → Makassar, Indonesia (flight time: 2h 30m)—three nights—Makassar → Palu, Indonesia (flight time: 1h 20m)—three nights—Palu → Jakarta (flight time: 2h 30m; 8h stopover) → Singapore (flight time: 1h 45m)—two nights (Festival of Artists with Disabilities)—Singapore → Dubai, United Arab Emirates (flight time: 7h 40m; 3h 30m stopover) → Amman, Jordan (flight time: 3h 40m)—three nights (attended a summit and met with Prince Hassan)—Amman → Doha, Qatar (flight time: 3h; 2h 30m stopover) → Narita International Airport (flight time: 10h 20m)

During my March visit to Indonesia, I worked in the capital Jakarta and South and Central Sulawesi provinces. On the first day, I spoke with the WHO Indonesia representative and Dr. Anung Sugihantono, the Ministry of Health's director-general of disease control. I explained that I had visited numerous regional leaders to conduct awareness-raising activities and ensure that leprosy does not fall down their policy priority lists. That evening, I flew out of Jakarta, taking three hours to reach Makassar, the capital of South Sulawesi in east central Indonesia. Located on the south side of Sulawesi Island, the city is also the central city of Eastern Indonesia, and as a trading port played a major role in the area's prosperity.

The next day started early. I first arrived at Kanjilo Health Center after an hour-long drive. People gathered in front of the green building and welcomed me with singing and dancing. A female member of

PerMaTa gave an address recounting the stigma she faced due to leprosy. However, with the organization's help, she had been able to reintegrate into society. With complete confidence, she said she longed to show her late mother how she was doing, bringing everyone in the audience to tears. I told them that I wanted them to talk about how *kusta* (Indonesian for "leprosy") can easily be cured in the village by taking medicine so that people affected by the disease would not be ostracized.

A young woman with white patches on her legs, an early sign of leprosy, looked gloomy, so I told her: "It's great you found it quickly. It is easier to cure than the common cold if you take medicine. You won't have any disabilities either." Her expression softened a bit.

The third day began with an appearance on a local radio program. I asked the listeners to look for white patches on each other's bodies once the show ended. Then, Vice President Qadri of PerMaTa talked about his own experience, saying, "My wife is also affected by leprosy, yet our two children are healthy. All that talk about leprosy being hereditary is just superstition."

In the afternoon, I visited the Jongaya neighborhood, where people affected by leprosy and their families live. This is where Vice President Qadri lived. Members of PerMaTa gathered in the pouring rain, and Ms. Yuri, a leader of the organization, introduced their work. She said they take patients who have stopped treatment for financial reasons to clinics and have people affected by leprosy conduct training and awareness-raising efforts. It is a new trend for leprosy-affected organizations to actively work toward eliminating the disease to compensate for the lack of local government initiatives, and I keenly felt my responsibility to provide support.

On the fourth day, I met with the vice-regent and members of the regency parliament at the Gowa Regency government building. One of the parliamentarians explained how the regency parliament and local assemblies worked together to reduce case numbers and end discrimination. Afterward, I flew to Palu, the capital of Central Sulawesi province.

During a meeting on the fifth day at the Sigi Regency government building with Regent Mohamad Irwan and other regency parliamentarians, I told them that we would eliminate the disease if they would join village leaders in discussing leprosy in regular conversations to inform the populace that it is a curable disease and not God's punishment. The regent replied: "I understand the importance of partnering with concerned parties. I will cooperate with the Health Department to convey to each village that there is no shame in being affected by leprosy."

I then accompanied the regent to the Biromaru Health Center. The Health Department director reported, "Case numbers are dwindling, but early detection is crucial. However, five of the nineteen health centers are difficult to access, and child case numbers are on the rise." The villagers had to move about a lot during the busy periods of harvest time and for work in coal mines, which made for difficulties in detection. I offered words of encouragement. Even in an age of smart phones, I said, there was still a lack of knowledge about leprosy. Clearly, my efforts had been insufficient. Join me, I said, in doing all we can. To bring light to just one more person's life is a feat worth achieving.

In the evening, I appeared on a talk show on the state-run TV broadcaster TVRI. The program provided a chance to take questions from the audience. A local man who had experience of leprosy and who appeared with me recounted: "I had white patches on my elbows and legs and could no longer walk. My family accepted me, but the village ostracized me."

In April, I went to Cambodia to attend a ceremony gifting English textbooks before traveling to Palau to visit the Palau National Congress and receive the Palau honorary national award.

Understanding leprosy through photography—Delhi, India, April 2018

In April, I visited Delhi for two days and one night. I arrived on the morning of 19 April and met with Dr. Kumar of India's Ministry of Health and Family Welfare. I expressed my respect for the progress in finding patients through the LCDC, which the Indian government had conducted for two years. In the afternoon, after a meeting with the director of S-ILF, I met with Kailash Satyarthi, who won the Nobel Peace Prize in 2014 for his work as a child rights activist.

In the evening, I attended the opening ceremony of Natsuko Tominaga's photo exhibition, *OUR LIVES*, which was the main purpose of this visit. Ms. Tominaga is a staff photographer for the Nippon Foundation who has traveled the world with me to take photographs of people affected by leprosy and their families. The exhibition was held at the prestigious India International Center in central Delhi from 20 April to 1 May. The opening ceremony was attended by government, WHO, NGOs and other officials, members of the media, and individuals affected by leprosy, as well as many representatives of Japanese companies, thanks to the full cooperation of the Embassy of Japan in India. I hoped the gathering would be an opportunity for Japanese companies to learn about the reality of leprosy, a national issue in India, and the Nippon Foundation's efforts to address it, potentially gaining their cooperation in the future.

During the ceremony, Anita Bhavre from Madhya Pradesh, one of the people who featured in the photos, shared her painful experiences.

The photo exhibition received a great deal of media coverage and brought the issue of leprosy to a broad audience. Ms. Tominaga is the only photographer in the world who has photographed people affected by leprosy for several decades. When leprosy disappears from the face of the earth decades from now, her photographs will remain a valuable asset to global history.

From April to May, I traveled to the United States for the DeepStar (a global offshore technology development consortium) signing ceremony in Houston, Texas, and threw out the first pitch at a Major League Baseball game between the Houston Astros and New York Yankees.

In May, I again visited Malmö, Sweden (for the World Maritime University-Sasakawa Global Ocean Institute opening ceremony at the World Maritime University) and Geneva, Switzerland (for the Sasakawa Health Prize award ceremony and meetings with global health ministers).

In June, I was again in Geneva to address the concert commemorating the Seventieth Anniversary of the Universal Declaration of Human Rights, co-hosted by the Nippon Foundation and the UN Human Rights Council. I also attended the twenty-fifth-anniversary ceremony for SYLFF (for five universities) in China.

HOPE AND COURAGE LEADING THE WAY TO THE FUTURE

Toward reducing case numbers among children—Union of the Comoros, July 2018

> Route: Haneda International Airport → Dubai, United Arab Emirates (flight time: 10h 45m; 5h stopover) → Addis Ababa, Ethiopia (flight time: 4h)—one night—Addis Ababa → Comoros (flight time: 3h 50m)—four nights

In July, I attended the third Twenty-First Century Panglong Conference (a peace conference between the Myanmar government and ethnic minority militia groups) in Myanmar. After a brief return to Japan, I traveled to Comoros in the Indian Ocean off the east coast of Africa. I flew from Haneda via Dubai to Ethiopia for two days before heading to Comoros. The Union of the Comoros is an island nation located north of Madagascar, consisting of three islands: Grande Comore (home to the capital Moroni), Anjouan, and Mohéli. Its primary industries are vanilla and other spice production, agriculture, and fishing. After gaining independence from France in 1975, the country was subject to frequent coups d'état and political instability, resulting in poor economic development and low living standards.

Leprosy case numbers in Comoros exceed the elimination benchmark of less than one case per 10,000 population. The WHO list of countries that have not eliminated leprosy as a public health problem generally includes countries with a population of more than 1 million. However, leprosy is also an issue in countries with small populations, such as the Union of the Comoros, with around 800,000. Furthermore, 40 percent of new cases are children, much higher than the world average. Of the country's three main islands, Anjouan had a remarkably high number of cases. The island is poorer than the others and has a high population density. Malnutrition is thought to be one of the reasons for leprosy's prevalence. According to Dr. Alexander Tiendrebeogo, the WHO focal person for leprosy at the Regional Office for Africa (AFRO), WHO recommended that the Union of the Comoros introduce the leprosy drug MDT in 1981, but it did not do so until 2001. As WHO's Goodwill Ambassador for Leprosy Elimination, I decided to visit the country to assess its current situation and take improvement measures.

MAKING THE IMPOSSIBLE POSSIBLE

From the air, Grande Comore looked like a tranquil paradise surrounded by cobalt blue waters. On the road from the airport to the city, I saw women in hijabs and men with white hats and clothes passing by and realized that this was a Muslim country. I had just met Minister of Health, Solidarity, and Gender Promotion Dr. Rashid Mohamed Mbarak Fatma at the WHO World Health Assembly in Geneva the previous May. I told him I was worried about the many children developing the disease in Comoros, to which he replied that the government was also very concerned. He was formulating a plan to eliminate leprosy as a public health problem by 2030, and he promised he would accompany me on my site visits starting the next day.

The next morning, with Health Minister Fatma and the WHO representative in Comoros, we headed for Anjouan Island, where many cases of children had been detected. We took to the air in a small, thirty-passenger aircraft. After about thirty minutes, we arrived at Anjouan. From the airport, we headed directly to the meeting with the autonomous republic's president. The island has many more tall mountains than I expected, and the houses are densely clustered on their slopes. The seaside market was lined with stores selling freshly caught fish and colorful fabrics. About a twenty-minute drive from the airport, a large white Islamic-style building appeared on top of a hill. The governor's palace is said to be the most magnificent building on the island. It was where our meeting with the president took place. Governor Abdou Salami Abdou was a doctor and had an accurate understanding of the problems associated with leprosy, so I couldn't understand why the situation had got so dire.

At any rate, the next day, we headed for the field. Up a hill toward the center of the island was Hombo Hospital, with its bright yellow and green walls. The hospital was filled with residents who had learned through a radio broadcast that the hospital would be offering free skin disease diagnoses. The broadcast used the phrasing of "skin disease diagnoses" because the residents would not come for fear of discrimination if they heard "leprosy." As I had heard, many young people affected by leprosy were among those who had traveled there, and a high percentage of children. Based on my many years of experience, I could tell that this was not a regular event. It was clearly occurring only to mark my visit.

686

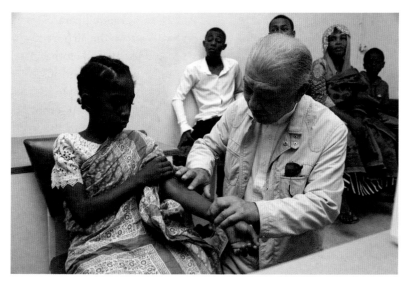

138. Checking a child's skin for the tell-tale patches (Union of Comoros, July 2018)

Leaving the hospital, we crossed the deep green forest to visit the health center in the village of Mahale on the other side of the island. The village had many simple, traditional houses made of leaves and bamboo. The sanitary conditions were deplorable, with garbage strewn in puddles by the side of the road and filled with mosquito larvae. At the small health center, a university student from another village, a boy of about ten years old, and a man with a leprosy-related wound on his sole were among those who had come for a medical exam. I learned firsthand about the harsh situation on Anjouan, where nearly 400 people are found to have leprosy annually, in a population of around 300,000. The leprosy prevalence rate was eleven per 10,000 people. I was at a loss for words about this tragic situation in the face of such widespread leprosy elimination efforts, especially by the WHO. As someone who has traveled around the globe to fight leprosy, it was indeed a shocking reality.

After visiting the site, we held a press conference with the island's media. At the press conference, the Anjouan Island health secretary explained that the high prevalence rate among children is thought to be due to their significant malnutrition and weakened immunity. I

687

noted, "If a child develops the disease, so long as medicine is taken as prescribed at an early stage, leprosy will leave no disabilities: the child will be completely cured. Early detection and treatment are essential. I urge everyone involved in the media to get informed."

After my two-day visit to Anjouan, I returned to Grande Comore and reported to the minister of foreign affairs and international organization representatives on the severity of the leprosy situation. Finally, I told President Azali Assoumani that I was concerned about the high leprosy prevalence among children on Anjouan Island and wanted him to consider what roles WHO and the Nippon Foundation could play. He replied: "The government will do all it can. I would like to accelerate our target date for eliminating the disease to 2025." However, considering the nation's finances and human resource shortages, I could only see his response as lip service. There is no doubt that Comoros needs our support and cooperation. I decided to launch a full-scale effort to eliminate leprosy on this island nation.

Leveraging patient discovery—Republic of Mozambique, July 2018

> Route: Union of the Comoros → Nairobi, Kenya (flight time: 5h 30m; 5h stopover) → Johannesburg, South Africa (flight time: 4h 15m; 3h stopover) → Maputo, Mozambique (flight time: 1h)—four nights— Maputo → Johannesburg (flight time: 1h; 5h stopover) → Dubai, United Arab Emirates (flight time: 8h; 2h 40m stopover) → Narita International Airport (flight time: 10h)

In July, I visited the Republic of Mozambique for the first time in a long time, following a circuitous route from the Comoros via Nairobi, Kenya, and Johannesburg, South Africa. My visit was primarily to see areas where case numbers had been rising since eliminating the disease as a national public health problem and to understand the current situation. I also wanted to ask the government and health institutions to step up measures against leprosy, which tends to receive a lower priority than malaria and tuberculosis. The day after I arrived in the capital Maputo, I met with Health Minister Dr. Nazira Abdula who expressed concern about the increase in case numbers. I encouraged her: "An increase in case numbers is no cause for shame. It is a sign that patient detection efforts are working." I suggested she further bolster these activities.

The next day, I headed to the northeastern province of Nampula, a formerly endemic area where I had experienced the most challenges in my annual visits. It was a two-and-a half-hour flight from the capital city of Maputo. I asked Governor Victor Borges to inform everyone in the province, especially schoolteachers, that leprosy is a curable disease and that disabilities can be avoided through early detection and treatment. I then set out to the village of Namaita, home to many people affected by leprosy and about an hour away by car. At the village entrance, about 200 villagers in colorful ethnic garb gathered to welcome me, playing drums, singing, and dancing, an experience I frequently have in Africa. A stage was set up in the center of the square, creating the atmosphere of a concert hall. A representative of those affected by leprosy in Namaita introduced me, so I took the stage. "I have come from the far-away nation of Japan. I came to eliminate leprosy from this village. Make no mistake: leprosy is not a curse or a punishment from God. You can cure it with medicine." After my address, the villagers, who had been in a festive mood, turned serious and became quiet. I took off my shirt, pointed to my naked chest, and said: "Go home and have your families check your

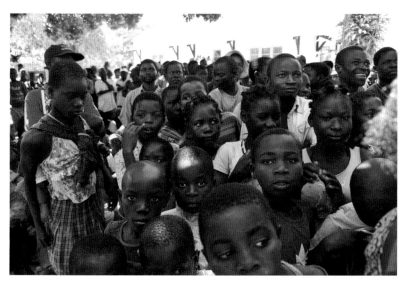

139. Villagers listening carefully (Mozambique, July 2018)

bodies, and if you see white patches, you may have leprosy. I want you to promise that you'll check each other thoroughly." They erupted into loud applause.

I then returned to Nampula and again spoke on a Muslim radio station, telling listeners that there was no need to be afraid of leprosy because it could be cured, and that they should go to the hospital if their families found any spots when examining their skin. The next day, in the capital Maputo, I appeared on Televisão de Moçambique, the national broadcaster, to properly inform the government and the people about leprosy.

From Mozambique, I flew to Tanzania via Johannesburg, but six pieces of luggage (cardboard boxes and suitcases) did not arrive. They arrived the next day, but the suitcases were a mess inside. Incidentally, we carry a large amount of material with us, so we frequently carry lots of cardboard boxes. At customs, they open luggage to inspect it. We naturally have no problem with this, but it is a waste of time and effort, so we use a little trick to get through customs: We place the cardboard boxes in among our suitcases so as not to draw attention.

Transcending ministerial boundaries—Republic of Indonesia, October 2018

> Route: Haneda International Airport → Jakarta, Indonesia (flight time: 7h 40m)—three nights—Jakarta → Ambon, Indonesia (flight time: 3h 40m)—two nights—Ambon → Jakarta (flight time: 3h 25m; 3h 30m stopover) → Haneda (flight time: 7h 25m)

From 1 to 6 October, I was in Indonesia's capital Jakarta and Ambon, Maluku. However, just before my visit, on 28 September, an earthquake and tsunami hit the island of Sulawesi in central Indonesia. I visited Sulawesi in March and was impressed by its beautiful towns surrounded by lush nature, and when I saw the reported devastation, I was left speechless. I would like to thank the Indonesian government for keeping a focus on leprosy elimination and allowing my visit.

Early in the morning of 2 October, Chairman Paulus Manek and Vice Chairman Qadri of PerMaTa came to meet me at my hotel. They had been supportive partners who would once again accompany me on this trip. As of my trip, PerMaTa had four branches in Indonesia, with plans to open a fifth branch in Ambon, Maluku, our scheduled destination. Having celebrated our reunion, we departed from the hotel to attend a leprosy awareness meeting at the Coordinating Ministry for Human Development and Cultural Affairs. It was less than 10 kilometers from the hotel to the ministry, but Jakarta is well known for its traffic jams, so it took over an hour by car to arrive.

The Coordinating Ministry is an administrative structure unique to Indonesia that oversees several ministries, including the Ministry of Religious Affairs; Ministry of Health; Ministry of Social Affairs; Ministry of Education and Culture; Ministry of Research and Technology; and Ministry of Villages, Development of Disadvantaged Regions, and Transmigration. As the name implies, the Coordinating Ministry "coordinates" to ensure smooth cooperation among its ministries and agencies. The Coordinating Ministry for Human Development and Cultural Affairs, in its leading role of the national leprosy program, hosted this first leprosy awareness meeting.

Dr. Sigit Priohutomo, deputy secretary of the Coordinating Ministry, is well versed in leprosy, having worked at a leprosy clinic for five years. He explained, "*Kusta* [leprosy] is not only a medical issue. It is also accompanied by discrimination and stigma. To tackle it, we need the cooperation of not only the health ministry but of other ministries too. That's why I have brought together the relevant people for this meeting." As Goodwill Ambassador, I have traveled to many countries over the years promoting leprosy elimination activities, but very few of my meetings have involved high-level bureaucrats drawn from different ministries and agencies, making this a progressive initiative.

The leprosy awareness meeting was packed with officials from the Coordinating Ministry for Human Development and Cultural Affairs and its ministries of Religious Affairs; Health; Social Affairs; Education and Culture; and Villages, Development of Disadvantaged Regions, and Transmigration, as well as the ministries of Home Affairs, Communication and Information Technology, and Manpower under the jurisdictions of other coordinating ministries. The meeting began with an explanation from the Ministry of Health on the current leprosy situation in Indonesia. The officials shared their concerns that efforts were not progressing as they would have wished. Some officials preferred to avoid doing anything that would increase case numbers, even though they understood the need to find and treat as many patients as possible, out of the fear that it would make them look as if they hadn't been doing their job properly. On the patients' side too, there was a deep-seated fear of receiving a diagnosis of leprosy, they said, based on a misconception that having the disease is shameful. Deputy Secretary Priohutomo commented that discovering new patients is not a shame but an honor, and I made clear my agreement, reiterating the importance of such cross-agency efforts, and promised to attend the next meeting.

In the late afternoon, I was interviewed by the *Jakarta Post*. The English-language newspaper's youthful managing editor was Mr. Ary Hermawan. His mother is affected by leprosy, and he was eager to spread accurate information about leprosy to society at large. I told him about Deputy Secretary Priohutomo's initiative to advance leprosy elimination policies through cross-ministerial efforts and shared our three messages—leprosy is a curable disease, medicine is available free of charge worldwide, and discrimination against leprosy is unacceptable. I also said we could bring case numbers down to zero if everyone affected by leprosy went to the hospital.

The next day, I left the hotel at 5:30 a.m. and traveled by air to Ambon in Maluku province, located about 250 kilometers east of Jakarta. Ambon is the largest city in eastern Indonesia, with a population of 370,000. In 1999, many people died in the Maluku Islands' sectarian conflict between Christians and Muslims. Although the situation had not yet been completely settled, I thought the city was relatively secure on the surface. However, this town's prevalence rate (the number of cases per 10,000 population) was 2.49 in the 2017 statistics, showing a noticeable delay in efforts against leprosy.

In the early morning of 4 October, I entered the governor's office to attend a meeting hosted by the governor of Maluku, but the governor was nowhere to be found. After a while, the local officials became flustered, and Governor Said Assagaff appeared. The officials were more concerned about the governor than the meeting, making me feel a little uneasy about the leprosy elimination efforts in the region. The meeting was attended by about thirty people, including personnel from the health department and other related departments, as well as military and police officials, for some reason. No one had a single document in front of them, and they had no clue about the day's meeting or why they were in attendance. I have experienced such encounters that are nothing more than formalities countless times worldwide. And experience has enabled me to pick up immediately that they are usually a formal demonstration against me. Nevertheless, I intend to visit again and again until I see a serious, full-fledged conference. I visited Africa's Mozambique three years in a row before finally succeeding in making progress in leprosy elimination.

In the afternoon, I appeared on Indonesian state-run television with PerMaTa Chairman Paulus Manek and Dr. Ritha Tahitu, head of disease control at Maluku's provincial health department. While I was speaking, the Islamic prayer time started, and there was a three-minute interruption in the live broadcast, which made me realize Islam's significant influence in this country. The program conveyed that families must check each other's skin for early detection and treatment; that leprosy is not a divine punishment, a curse, a genetic disease, or a highly contagious disease; and that it can be wholly cured with medicine.

The next day began with an appearance on a morning program on Indonesia's public radio station. We took a total of six questions from listeners. One question showed an awareness of international relationships, asking, "How can Japan contribute to eliminating *kusta* in Indonesia?" As part of my elimination efforts, I had recently started to place emphasis on TV and radio appearances.

After that, I planned to attend a leprosy awareness meeting with Ambon's mayor present. However, he did not show up for forty minutes, and without any explanation as to why he was late, those present had no choice but to simply wait. In the end, the meeting began as a mere formality with no outcome, without the mayor's attendance. It made me a little angry, but on the other hand, I felt my passion to do whatever I could to reduce the number of cases in this area grow even stronger.

Countries visited in 2019	
January	Myanmar (Nationwide ceasefire agreement: talks with government personnel)
	Thailand (Myanmar nationwide ceasefire agreement: negotiations with armed ethnic organizations)

	Indonesia (Jakarta School of Prosthetics and Orthotics handover ceremony)
	• India
February	Thailand (Myanmar nationwide ceasefire agreement: negotiations with armed ethnic organizations)
	Bangladesh (Talks with Prime Minister Sheikh Hasina)
	Myanmar (Nationwide ceasefire agreement: talks with government personnel)
	• India
	United States (New York: talks with UN Secretary-General António Guterres)
March	China (Talks with key persons)
	Myanmar (Nationwide ceasefire agreement: talks with government personnel)
April	• Marshall Islands
	• Molokai (Hawaii)
	Thailand (Myanmar nationwide ceasefire agreement: negotiations with armed ethnic organizations)
May	India (Visit to Imphal Peace Museum site)
	United Kingdom (Japan–UK Global Seminar, Chatham House)
June	China (Xinjiang University, Inner Mongolia University SYLFF twenty-fifth anniversary)
	India (Imphal Peace Museum inauguration ceremony)
	Thailand (Myanmar nationwide ceasefire agreement: negotiations with armed ethnic organizations)
	• Brazil
July	Myanmar (Nationwide ceasefire agreement: talks with government personnel)

September	Philippines
	United States (Princeton, New Jersey: Nippon Foundation Nereus Ocean Science Conference)
	China (Chongqing University and Yunnan University SYLFF twenty-fifth anniversary)
	Thailand (Myanmar nationwide ceasefire agreement: negotiations with armed ethnic organizations)
	Myanmar (Nationwide ceasefire agreement: talks with government personnel)
October	United Kingdom (Seabed 2030 Project symposium)
	Norway (Oslo: Our Ocean 2019 Conference)
November	Thailand (First round Myanmar nationwide ceasefire agreement: negotiations with armed ethnic organizations)
	Myanmar (First round nationwide ceasefire agreement: talks with government personnel)
December	● Bangladesh
	Myanmar (Nationwide ceasefire agreement: talks with government personnel)

● Indicates a trip that features in this section.

SYLFF: Sasakawa Young Leaders Fellowship Fund program.

My shared dream with Gandhi—Delhi, Dadra and Nagar Haveli, and Andhra Pradesh, India January 2019

> Route: Narita International Airport → Delhi, India (flight time: 10h 20m)—four nights—Delhi → Mumbai, Maharashtra, India (flight time: 2h)—four nights—Mumbai → Vijayawada, Andhra Pradesh, India (flight time: 2h) → Delhi (flight time: 2h; 9h stopover) → Narita (flight time: 7h 20m)

In early January 2019, we held a ceremony to hand over to the Indonesian government the Jakarta School of Prosthetics and Orthotics, to which the Nippon Foundation had provided US$11,747,000 in support over the previous ten years.

In late January, I traveled to India to visit Delhi, Dadra and Nagar Haveli, and Andhra Pradesh. On 30 January, we launched the Global Appeal 2019 in Delhi. This year, with the endorsement of the International Chamber of Commerce, a global business organization with 45 million corporate members, we appealed to the business community and society at large to eliminate discrimination against people affected by leprosy and their families and promote their employment. The ceremony was lively, with singing and dancing by children of people affected by leprosy. In addition to the endorsing organization International Chamber of Commerce, attendees also included representatives from the Confederation of Indian Industry, who showed their positive attitude toward promoting employment for people affected by leprosy and their families.

The next day, I went to the Union Territory of Dadra and Nagar Haveli. This is a small government-controlled territory located between the states of Maharashtra and Gujarat. A former Portuguese territory, the area is not well known even to Indians. According to the health department, the territory had no people affected by leprosy with visible disabilities the previous year, thanks to an early patient detection campaign and the distribution of preventive medicines to families. According to Dr. Anil Kumar from the Union Ministry of Health and Family Welfare, who accompanied me, the area had no leprosy colonies, which was unusual for India, and no discrimination either. And yet the prevalence rate of 6.7 was six times higher than the national average. I was soon to find out why.

The next day, I attended a meeting with eighty ASHA, female health workers who were working to detect patients in the Union territory. By discovering new patients, they had temporarily increased case numbers. In other words, the high prevalence rate resulted from their work. This higher figure was not a cause for pessimism, as early detection allows treatment before disabilities appear.

Afterward, I flew to Vijayawada in Andhra Pradesh on the east coast. Here, APAL and S-ILF offer support for people affected by leprosy. I met with Chief Minister N. Chandrababu Naidu, but the overriding objective of that meeting was to ask him to raise the special pension for people affected by leprosy. When I made that request, he immediately promised to increase the amount from

1,500 to 4,000 rupees (around US$50) per month. Increasing pensions for people affected by leprosy is one of the main purposes of my work in India. To be honest, leaders among those affected by leprosy are often not taken seriously on their own. As a Japanese national, I can apply gentle pressure to make officials more willing to listen to what these leaders say. Moreover, improving trust by submitting more accurate data than the government on the conditions people affected by leprosy experience has successfully raised pensions in many states. That is an essential step in achieving my dream of eliminating begging in India.

The next day, I visited the Bunni Nagar leprosy colony, where S-ILF provides support. There were forty-two people affected by leprosy among the 140 residents. The state government provided land and housing in 2009, and most of those affected by leprosy were receiving disability pensions, so none worked as beggars. Of the 750 colonies across India we surveyed, this was one of the most fortunate. Rakesh Jha, the head of S-ILF's self-support project, introduced me to the beneficiaries. One man kept buffaloes and sold their milk; another made a living by selling general merchandise. Other beneficiaries were raising goats and selling vegetables.

The year 2019 was the 150th anniversary of Mahatma Gandhi's birth. During my stay in India, I received word from the Indian Ministry of Culture that I had been selected to receive the 2018 Gandhi Peace Prize. They said that the award recognized my efforts to eliminate leprosy. I consider that I received the award not for myself but for my comrades who have worked with me. Gandhi included resolving the leprosy issue in his manifesto for nation-building. Gandhi did not realize his dream of an India free of leprosy and its discrimination during his lifetime. The news of the Gandhi Peace Prize award reinforced my desire to realize his dream.

In February, after holding ceasefire and peace talks with Myanmar's ethnic minority militia groups in Chiang Mai, Thailand, I went to Bangladesh to speak with Prime Minister Sheikh Hasina on leprosy issues and the Rohingya refugee problem. I then visited the Cox's Bazar refugee camp, which is said to have 700,000 refugees, to inspect conditions on the ground, and returned to Myanmar to report the situation to dignitaries. Later, the Nippon Foundation decided to construct fifty schools and vocational training schools in the refugee camps and surrounding areas.

Receiving the Gandhi Peace Prize—Delhi, India, February 2019

On 26 February, at the Gandhi Peace Prize award ceremony hosted by the Indian government and held at the Indian presidential palace in Delhi, I received the Gandhi Peace Prize plaque from President Ram Nath Kovind and a commemorative shawl and a cheque for 10 million Indian rupees (about US$120,000) from Prime Minister Narendra Modi. I received the award in recognition of my global efforts to eliminate leprosy. It was the first time a Japanese national had received the prize, making it a great joy and honor for me. In awarding the prize, President Kovind praised my work, saying: "You have given great strength to our struggle to eliminate leprosy and the discrimination and stigma associated with it." Prime Minister Modi posted on his personal Twitter account: "Individuals like Mr. Yohei Sasakawa motivate millions of people. He is at the forefront of many philanthropic initiatives. His compassionate nature can be seen in the manner in which he has worked to eliminate leprosy." In my acceptance speech, I said: "I receive [this award] together with all who have worked with me over the years. We consider that this award is an encouragement from Mahatma Gandhi." I also declared, "Together, we can realize a world where no one needs to suffer from leprosy or its associated stigma and discrimination. This is not an impossible dream." I conveyed our determination to fulfill the dream that Gandhi could not. I split the prize money into two donations to APAL and S-ILF in the hope that they would use it for their leprosy-related activities.

The Indian government established the Gandhi Peace Prize in 1995 to commemorate the 125th anniversary of Gandhi's birth. The prize jury includes Prime Minister Modi, the chief justice of India, the speaker of the Lok Sabha, and the leader of the opposition in the Lok Sabha. Considered one of the most prestigious peace prizes in the world, the Gandhi Peace Prize has been awarded to foreign nationals and foreign organizations, including former President Nelson Mandela of South Africa, former Archbishop Desmond Tutu of South Africa, former President Václav Havel of the Czech Republic, and the Grameen Bank.

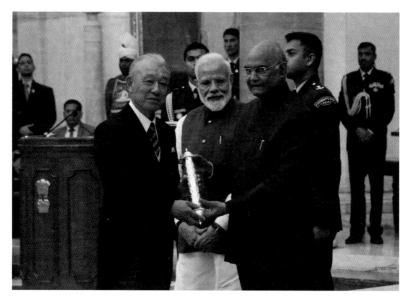

140. The author receiving the 2018 Gandhi Peace Prize from Prime Minister Narendra Modi (left) and President Ram Nath Kovind (right) (India, February 2019)

After attending the Gandhi Peace Prize ceremony, I participated in a meeting to discuss maritime human resource development programs at the Division for Ocean Affairs and the Law of the Sea at UN Headquarters in New York.

Problems and solutions on the ground—Republic of the Marshall Islands, April 2019

> Route: Haneda International Airport → Honolulu, Hawaii (flight time: 7h 20m; overnight stopover) → Majuro, Marshal Islands (flight time: 5h)—one night.

In April, I visited the Marshall Islands and Molokai, Hawaii. The Marshall Islands are a nation of about 50,000 people in the Pacific Ocean, about 4,500 kilometers southeast of Japan. They comprise twenty-nine atolls and five islands and are known collectively as the "Pearl of the Pacific." My first impression was that this was indeed a peaceful tropical country.

MAKING THE IMPOSSIBLE POSSIBLE

After arriving in Majuro, the capital of the Marshall Islands, via Hawaii, there was one place I wanted to go first: the Majuro Peace Park Memorial for those who died in the Pacific War. The Marshall Islands came under Japanese mandate in 1914, and about 19,000 Japanese soldiers died here during the Gilbert and Marshall Islands campaign in the Second World War. In a park along the coast, a cenotaph was erected facing in the direction of Japan. The Japanese and Marshall flags fluttered on either side. I offered my condolences to the spirits of the dead who had fallen in battle for their country.

That evening, I attended a dinner hosted by President Hilda Heine, which was also attended by many cabinet ministers, including the minister of foreign affairs and trade; the minister of health and human services; the minister of finance, banking, and postal services; and the minister of works, infrastructure, and utilities. The dinner was held at a small hotel and was casual, with some ministers wearing sandals. I was grateful that I had the opportunity to meet the various ministers all at once because I believe that leprosy, with its associated discrimination and stigma, must be addressed by health ministries in cooperation with other ministries, including education and welfare. I took this opportunity of an ad hoc cabinet meeting to emphasize that the Marshall Islands could eliminate leprosy if all citizens had correct information on leprosy and checked their skin. Achieving that goal requires the cooperation of all the country's leaders.

The next morning, President Heine told me: "The government will do what's necessary to eliminate leprosy. I ask for your cooperation, Mr. Sasakawa." I naturally agreed to help.

The field holds both problems and their solutions. I am convinced of that. After I met with the president, I received word that a recently discovered person affected by leprosy was living near the hotel where I was staying. I immediately headed to the site. The house was located on the corner of a busy residential area. A woman was sitting on a chair in front of her house. Her name was Monica Thomas. Very early signs of leprosy had appeared on her left leg. I asked Merida, a nurse accompanying me, how she found these early symptoms. In the Marshall Islands, the Ministry of Health and Human Services, WHO, and the US Centers for Disease Control and Prevention had been cooperating to conduct a nationwide screening program for leprosy and tuberculosis, with teams visiting each household to conduct checkups. As a result, they had already covered 80 percent of the population, with new patients being found one after another. When I told Monica that she would be cured without any problems if she took her medicine properly, she nodded her head as though my words had reassured her.

To learn more about the country's efforts, I headed to the Ministry of Health and Human Services, where the leprosy clinic was located. There, I met a young man who had just received medicine from a staff member. He came to the clinic because he suspected he had leprosy. When I asked him what had happened, he told me that his mother had experience of leprosy and recognized the symptoms because they were similar. He had already completed his treatment but was receiving a prescription for a drug called prednisone because he was experiencing mild side effects from the medication. When I asked him if he had any other family members with leprosy besides his mother, he told me that the screening had found two others with leprosy. It seemed that the screening process was finding many new leprosy cases.

Monica had temporarily moved in with her daughter to receive treatment, while the young man at the clinic came to get a leprosy exam without hiding it. According to Health and Human Services Minister Kalani Kaneko, the Marshallese culture had always emphasized family and mutual aid. That may be why there was less prejudice and discrimination in the Marshall Islands compared to other countries. He also gave me a detailed explanation of the status of the nationwide screening program. While it had found many people affected by leprosy, I learned that it faced budget and human resources challenges. I told him that the Nippon Foundation, Sasakawa Health Foundation, and WHO are fully committed to the government's plan to make the Marshall Islands a leprosy-free country.

At a press conference with Health and Human Services Minister Kaneko, I said that no other country had as much potential to become leprosy-free as the Republic of the Marshall Islands, and that with the nationwide screening program, plus skin checks within families on all family members, the dream of zero leprosy cases may soon be a reality. I appealed to the media to join me in raising awareness of our fight.

MAKING THE IMPOSSIBLE POSSIBLE

Father Damien and Japanese-American people affected by leprosy—Hawaii, United States of America, April 2019

Route: Majuro, Marshall Islands → Honolulu, Hawaii, United States (flight time: 4h 45m)—one night—Honolulu → Hoʻolehua, Molokai, Hawaii (flight time: 30m)—day trip—Hoʻolehua → Honolulu (flight time: 30m)—one night—Honolulu → Haneda International Airport (flight time: 8h 30m)

The history of the Kalaupapa Leprosy Settlement on Molokai, Hawaii, dates back to 1866 when twelve people affected by leprosy were isolated there. Over the next 103 years, until the isolation law was repealed in 1969, around 8,000 people were sent to the colony. Initially, while they had practically no support, they took it upon themselves to set up their new lives, organizing a church and securing foodstuffs. Then, in 1873, Father Damien arrived from Belgium. The Catholic priest devoted himself to caring for those affected by leprosy and became known as a saint for helping them. His life has been made into several films.

After completing my work in the Marshall Islands, I visited the Kalaupapa Leprosy Settlement. I'd had several prior opportunities to visit before this but had been unable to do so. That was mainly because I had prioritized my work in countries where leprosy was endemic. Molokai Island, where Kalaupapa is located, is only about a thirty-minute flight from Honolulu, Hawaii's capital, but it isn't easy to get from Molokai Airport to Kalaupapa, my destination. The leprosy settlement is on the Kalaupapa Peninsula, on the north side of Molokai Island. Surrounded by the ocean on three sides, the peninsula is isolated from the rest of the island by 600-meter cliffs. The cliff had a path leading to Kalaupapa Peninsula, but it was unusable due to a landslide. In other words, I could not reach it by land. I urgently arranged a Cessna plane. The flight time was only four minutes.

I was welcomed at Kalaupapa by Ka'ohulani McGuire of the Kalaupapa National Historical Park. The Kalaupapa Peninsula itself was designated as a national historical park in 1980, in accordance with the wish of the residents of the Kalaupapa Leprosy Settlement to keep the history of leprosy from fading away. Surrounded by beautiful forests, the place abounded with silence. According to Ms.

McGuire, the ship that brings supplies still comes once a year, but there are sometimes shortages.

The settlement had ten people affected by leprosy living quiet lives. All of them were elderly; some continued to live in their own homes in the community, while others lived in a care facility. I met one Japanese-American who was living in the care facility. His name was Hashimoto, and he was eighty-eight. His parents, who were born in Toyama prefecture, emigrated to Hawaii, and at the age of eleven he contracted leprosy and was sent to the Kalaupapa Leprosy Settlement. He had since spent seventy-seven years here. Since the mid-1900s, nearly 220,000 Japanese immigrated to Hawaii, and many Japanese-Americans, including Mr. Hashimoto, were forcibly sent to the Kalaupapa Settlement when they developed leprosy.

When I visited a cemetery not far from the care facility, I found many gravestones with Japanese names engraved on them. The site of a Buddhist temple also remains, and paintings and other objects painted by Japanese-Americans were in the archives. The Kalaupapa Leprosy Settlement has a close relationship with Japan, and Valerie

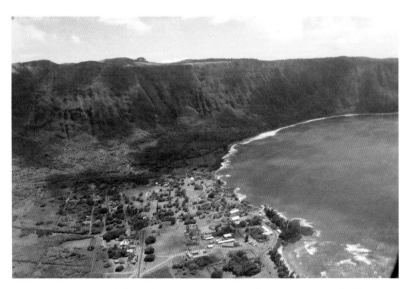

141. An overview of the Kalaupapa Leprosy Settlement surrounded by soaring cliffs (Hawaii, April 2019)

Monson, the executive director of Ka 'Ohana o Kalaupapa, (Association of Family Members of Kalaupapa) and other similar organizations, gave me further details. According to her, a 1996 workshop discussed the future of the Kalaupapa Leprosy Settlement, and people affected by leprosy from Japan were invited to share their opinions. Even now, they conduct exchanges with many Japanese leprosaria, including the National Sanatorium Tama Zenshoen. Ka 'Ohana o Kalaupapa was established through these activities and exchanges in 2003.

Ka 'Ohana o Kalaupapa had pushed through the Kalaupapa Memorial Act and was working to build a monument inscribed with the names of all 8,000 people who were sent to live here. Their project is to realize the wish of their predecessors to leave living proof of the people affected by leprosy sent to the settlement. The monument will be located near St. Philomena Roman Catholic Church. The church was where Father Damien was active from the time of his arrival until his death. A native of Belgium, Father Damien had cared for people affected by leprosy on Molokai since 1873, when he was diagnosed with leprosy, and died in 1889. The Vatican canonized him in 2009.

Built in 1872, St. Philomena Church was later expanded by Father Damien in 1888, becoming the stone structure it remains today. Until the early 1930s, there was a two-story house behind the church where Father Damien lived, but there is no sign of it now. After paying a visit to Father Damien's tomb outside, I entered St. Philomena Church. In the church, I noticed something. There were 2-centimeter square holes in the floor below the pews. I heard Father Damien wanted those affected by leprosy to attend Mass at the church, but many of them had tracheotomies and were hesitant to enter because their phlegm would drip onto the floor. So he made holes in the floor and inserted conical tubes made of long tropical leaves into them so those who needed to could expectorate during Mass. This episode illustrates one aspect of Father Damien's concern for those affected by leprosy.

Finally, when I asked Ms. McGuire about the future plans for the Kalaupapa Leprosy Settlement, she replied: "When no one affected by leprosy lives here anymore, the area will be opened as a park

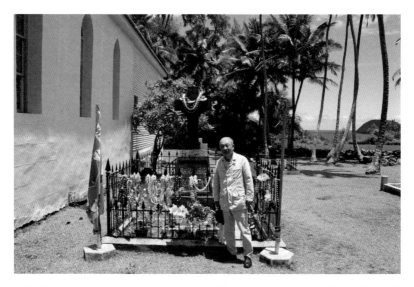

142. Father Damien's tomb, situated right next to the church (Hawaii, April 2019)

where children can learn about the history of leprosy under the management of the National Park Service." Having been isolated from the outside world for so long and remaining quiet in its grief, the settlement will no doubt be filled with the voices of healthy children in due course.

In May, I visited India to observe the construction of the Imphal Peace Museum and London, UK, to attend the UK–Japan Global Seminar at Chatham House. In June, I attended the twenty-fifth-anniversary ceremony of the SYLFF in China and the Imphal Peace Museum opening ceremony in India.

The president's resolve spread through social media—Federative Republic of Brazil, July 2019

Route: Haneda International Airport → Frankfurt, Germany (flight time: 11h 40m; 2h 30m stopover) → São Paulo, Brazil (flight time: 11h 50m; 2h 30m stopover) → Brasília, Brazil (flight time: 1h 45m)—one night—Brasília → Belém, Brazil (flight time: 2h 30m) → Marabá, Brazil (flight time: 1h)—two nights—Marabá → Belém (flight time: 1h; 3h stopover) → São Luís, Brazil (flight time: 1h 10m)—two

nights—São Luís → Brasília (flight time: 2h 30m)—four nights—
Brasília → Rio de Janeiro, Brazil (flight time: 1h 45m; 7h stopover) →
Frankfurt (flight time: 11h 20m; 3h 40m stopover) → Haneda
International Airport (flight time: 11h)

During my visit to Brazil in August 2015, Health Minister Ademar
Arthur Chioro dos Reis publicly declared that Brazil would officially
announce that it had eliminated leprosy as a public health problem by
the end of the fiscal year, which turned out to be a statement made in
error. Since then, Brazil's fight against leprosy had stagnated due to
political instability, among other reasons. I was finally able to visit Brazil
again in June 2019. It was my first visit in four years. The itinerary for
the trip had me fly through Frankfurt on the way there and back.

Brazil remains the only country that has not eliminated leprosy as
a public health problem, and around 25,000 cases are found annually.
People affected by leprosy are mainly in the central west and northeast regions, where the economy is poor and access to medical care
inconsistent. While the government has acknowledged its mistakes in
forcibly isolating people affected by leprosy, discriminatory systems
and ordinances against leprosy still exist at both the state and municipal levels. Healthcare workers and educators also report stigma and
discrimination against people affected by leprosy and their families.

In the capital Brasília, I met with Health Minister Luiz Henrique
Mandetta. The minister is from Mato Grosso state, which has many
people affected by leprosy, and has experience as an orthopedic surgeon treating those affected by the disease. His appointment had
strengthened the leprosy elimination department. I anticipated that
having a minister with enthusiasm at the top would boost the morale
of the entire Ministry of Health and accelerate the efforts to eliminate leprosy.

Pará state in northern Brazil—the second largest in Brazil and
home to the Amazon rainforest—has to close off transportation when
it floods. It is the fifth most endemic state in the country, with 2,678
new cases per year, due no doubt to geographical factors and economic disparities. This trip included my second visit to this state. In
Belém, the state capital, I visited the Marcello Candia Hospital,
guided by Dr. Claudio Salgado, president of the Brazilian Hansen's
Disease Association. Established in the 1930s, it is now the largest

health center in the state, equipped with facilities for rehabilitation and making special footwear for people affected by leprosy. Those with severe disabilities and who cannot be treated at other municipal clinics, as well as those with severe leprosy reactions (a type of allergic reaction in which the immune system reacts to dead leprosy bacteria in the body during or after treatment), come to the hospital.

I then visited Pará Governor Helder Barbalho and urged him to make efforts to eliminate leprosy in the state and make skin checks a habit at home to prevent disabilities in children.

My next stop was in Marabá in Pará, about 500 kilometers south of Belém. Like Belém, Marabá had many leprosy cases, but because of its lack of well-equipped medical facilities, people with severe disabilities have to travel many hours to the health center in Belém. Under the initiative of Mayor Sebastião Miranda Filho, Marabá recently formulated an ordinance to provide food assistance to incoming patients so that they don't interrupt their treatment. I was invited to a ceremony to celebrate the passage of this ordinance. About 100 people attended, including the mayor, city councilors, medical and health professionals, and media representatives. I told them: "Leprosy is difficult to contract, but it is true that it is common among people with poor nutritional status. This ordinance is an act of love," expressing my praise for this step. I joined recordings for TV and radio programs after the ceremony. I then moved on to my next destination, São Luís, in Maranhão state.

This northeastern state had 3,436 new cases per year. It is the third most endemic state in Brazil. The night I arrived in São Luís, I was invited to a dinner party by Governor Flávio Dino. The governor had visited a leprosy community when he was a federal delegate and had interacted with people affected by leprosy and their families. He had vowed to address the problem when he became governor. And indeed, after he took office, leprosy had become an important issue in the state, with active promotion of efforts to detect patients and prevent disability. After hearing the strength of the governor's commitment, I told him: "If Maranhão eliminates leprosy as a public health problem, it will become a beacon for Brazil. With dedicated effort, you and the health department director could reduce nine-tenths of leprosy cases in this state."

The following day, I attended a leprosy conference bringing together 280 medical health workers and social workers in the endemic areas of Maranhão. At the conference, the health director, the public policy director, and the head of the public affairs bureau explained the leprosy situation and their efforts from their respective perspectives. I encouraged the participants, saying, "With your help, we can eliminate leprosy from Maranhão." I then returned to Brasília after observing a clinic and recording TV and radio programs.

In Brasília, I met with President Jair Messias Bolsonaro. He assumed the presidency in January 2019 after being in the military, a councilor of Rio de Janeiro, and a federal deputy. He was joined by his ministers of health, women, family, and human rights, and foreign affairs. When I mentioned Brazil's past efforts against leprosy, especially the previous administration's failures, the president said: "Eliminating leprosy is a significant challenge for Brazil. We should not hide the fact that there are many patients." He then took his smartphone out of his suit pocket and instructed an aide to prepare a

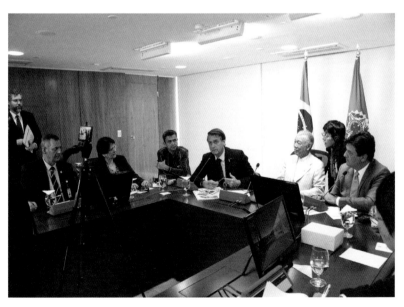

143. Giving a live broadcast on social media with President Jair Messias Bolsonaro (Brazil, July 2019)

live broadcast on social media. I spoke first, and then the president addressed the public directly about eliminating leprosy. The response was swift, with 730,000 views and 19,000 comments.

A national convention was scheduled, to take place in March 2020 under the president's leadership. I was thrilled that a national convention might take place, under direction of the president of the country of Brazil. A great stride would be made toward my life's dream of eliminating leprosy worldwide.

Postscript

I was preparing for the national leprosy convention in Brazil, which the president was scheduled to attend. However, on 10 March 2020, it was discovered that a deputy spokesperson for the Brazilian government was infected with a new type of coronavirus. Just before my departure, the conference was canceled. This was a great disappointment, as I was scheduled to hold individual meetings with the governors of Mato Grosso, Tocantins, Maranhão, Pará, Pernambuco, and Piauí, which are particularly endemic states. With the cooperation of the president's wife, who is very enthusiastic about social work, I had hoped that in a few years, we would be able to declare leprosy eliminated in Brazil and consequently the world. However, the COVID-19 situation continued to deteriorate in Brazil, and my hopes have since come to naught. All plans have been dashed, and there is still no indication as to when we will be able to start over at step one. As long as the COVID-19 pandemic continues, my work is impossible. All I can say is that this outcome was utterly disappointing.

The disease we must not neglect—Republic of the Philippines, September 2019

Route: Haneda International Airport → Manila, Philippines (flight time: 4h 45m)—three nights—Manila → Haneda (flight time: 4h 20m)

In September, I visited Manila, Philippines, to attend the Global Forum of People's Organizations on Hansen's Disease organized by the Nippon Foundation and the Sasakawa Health Foundation. I also joined the Twentieth International Leprosy Congress (ILC), an event that happens every three years, and the conferment ceremony for an honorary doctorate from the prestigious Ateneo de Manila University.

Organizations for people affected by leprosy were springing up worldwide. The Global Forum was held for four days, starting 7 September, and brought together more than eighty attendees, including leaders from organizations of people affected by leprosy from twenty-three countries. Never before had such a conference, on such a grand scale, been held for people with lived experience of leprosy. I made my usual speech, offering my encouragement to all the participants. I told them what a significant thing it was for people affected by leprosy to organize on a national level, but also on an international level too.

A pleasant surprise awaited me at the Global Forum dinner. Alberto Lopez, a man affected by leprosy, had painted my portrait, and he presented it to me. He also performed a song about leprosy that he had written and composed. Like the multitalented Mr. Lopez, people affected by leprosy can change the world. I again encouraged the attendees: "You are the doctors who cure stigma and discrimination. Let us fight them together in solidarity!"

The next day, I was awarded an honorary doctorate from the prestigious Ateneo de Manila University in recognition of my contributions to the fight against leprosy and the elimination of discrimination. Ateneo de Manila University had previously cooperated with the Global Appeal 2007 for the elimination of discrimination against people affected by leprosy and their families. I vividly remember that Global Appeal because an eleven-year-old girl affected by leprosy strongly voiced her belief that discrimination was never justified. In my introductory video produced by the university, I received words of support and appreciation from Dr. Arturo C. Cunanan Jr., a leprosy specialist in the Philippines, and Dr. Takeshi Kasai, regional director of the WHO Western Pacific Regional Office. I hoped that the video would serve as a catalyst for understanding the disease for the many attendees unfamiliar with leprosy.

On the last day of my stay, I attended the twentieth ILC, a gathering of people fighting against leprosy from around the world. I delivered the following keynote address:

HOPE AND COURAGE LEADING THE WAY TO THE FUTURE

Yohei Sasakawa

Chair of the Nippon Foundation and WHO Goodwill Ambassador
for Leprosy Elimination

Keynote Address at Twentieth International Leprosy Congress

Manila, Philippines

This congress is unique because it is open to doctors and health personnel, and many other stakeholders, including NGOs and persons affected by leprosy. This is probably the only academic conference in the world in which persons affected by the disease actively participate. I would like to express my sincere respect to all those involved in the tireless work of the congress.

The first time I met persons affected by leprosy was over forty years ago when I visited a leprosarium with my late father, Ryoichi Sasakawa. I have always been healthy, and it came as a shock to me to learn that there were such people who were struggling against the disease.

They were abandoned by their families.

They were rejected by society.

They were deprived of their freedom.

All that was just because of leprosy.

My father took their hands, spoke with them, held them tight, and cried out loud. That was the first time I ever saw him in tears. I was moved by my father who came face to face with them so seriously. That was when I decided to devote my life to carrying on his work.

Since then, I have been committed to the struggle against leprosy and its associated stigma and discrimination around the world. My only weapons in this struggle have been passion, perseverance, and endurance. My "battlefield" was where the problems lay, as that is where the solutions lie. I have met countless persons affected by leprosy in the jungles of Africa, arid deserts, the Amazon rainforest, and other remote areas. I am eighty years old now, and over a period of forty years, I have visited 120 countries and regions.

MDT must be delivered to the very last patient!

This is what I felt as I continued to visit many places and patients. With this in mind, the Nippon Foundation and WHO co-hosted an international conference in 1994 in Hanoi, Vietnam. There, I made an official announcement that the Nippon Foundation would donate

711

50 million US dollars and distribute MDT for free, for five years, around the world. As a result, in five years, 3.32 million patients were cured. Since 2000, thanks to Novartis, MDT has continued to be supplied for free even now. I would like to take this opportunity to express my gratitude to Novartis for their generous support.

I was confident of a brighter future. However, the situation was completely different from what I had originally imagined. Even though free medication was given, there were some patients who did not come forward to receive the treatment, and also, there were still many undiscovered patients.

I had simply assumed everything would be solved if the disease were cured. But I was wrong. While leprosy became curable, there was no cure for prejudice and discrimination, which I consider a disease that affects society.

Persons affected were abandoned by families.

They could no longer go to school.

And they could no longer work.

They all suffered from discrimination, and all just because of leprosy. Some feared discrimination and avoided getting any treatment, lead-

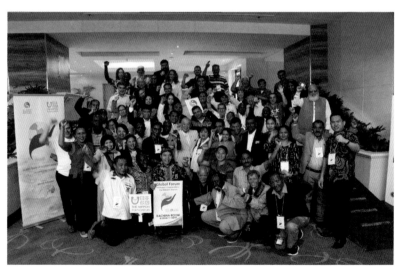

144. Global Forum of People's Organizations on Hansen's Disease confirming the unity of people affected by leprosy worldwide (The Philippines, September 2019)

ing to further disease progress. I realized that leprosy was not a simple medical problem, but that it was clearly a human rights problem.

I decided to take the matter to the United Nations, where global issues are discussed and actions proposed by all the member countries. In 2003, I visited the Office of the United Nations High Commissioner for Human Rights in Geneva for the first time alone to ask for leprosy to be put on the human rights agenda. But to my disappointment and surprise, leprosy had never once been considered a human rights issue. After many visits, I was given an opportunity to speak at a seminar for the officers of the UN Human Rights Council.

However, only five people attended the first seminar. This gave me a clear answer as to how little attention was given to the issue of leprosy. After that, the Nippon Foundation hosted a series of seminars during human rights sessions in Geneva. In order to get the interest of many, we even enticed them with a simple light lunch, hoping they would listen to our presentations. However, they just left as soon as they got hold of the free lunch. Only ten people came to the venue, which had a capacity of fifty.

But I was not a man to give up. We worked hard for seven years with repeated improvements in implementation. Meanwhile, many influential people became our supporters, and finally, in December 2010, the United Nations General Assembly unanimously adopted the resolution on the elimination of discrimination. This was a huge step for us to move forward.

Whenever I go abroad, I always meet with the national leaders of the countries. We cannot solve the issue of leprosy without their understanding and support. Without their cooperation we cannot secure the budget for activities to eliminate leprosy and the associated discrimination.

In July this year, when I visited Brazil, I met President Bolsonaro and received his strong support for my work to eliminate leprosy and its associated stigma. I told him that Brazil has the second-highest number of cases of leprosy in the world, and that it needs to make further efforts against the disease. The president suggested that we reach out to the nation right away. He took his mobile phone and started a live broadcast on Facebook. During the live broadcast, he firmly stated that leprosy is an issue that the government of Brazil needs to be involved in and that he will work with me. I also stressed to the audience the importance of early detection for Brazil to aim for "Zero Leprosy." This thirteen-minute-long video has been viewed more than 700,000 times and attracted countless comments. It is very reassuring to have countries' leaders supporting our activities.

In my opinion, persons affected by leprosy are the most active people of all those who are affected by diseases. In 2006, I supported the establishment of an organization of persons affected by leprosy in India. To date, I continue to fight against the associated issues with the persons affected by leprosy from around the world. There are many organizations around the world in which the persons affected by leprosy play key roles. Thanks to their continuous hard work, I believe that we have opened a new chapter in our history.

There are three important roles the organizations by and for persons affected by leprosy play. First, they remove social constraints, such as abolishing discriminatory laws. Second, they improve the quality of life of those affected by leprosy. And finally, they raise awareness that leprosy is curable, treatment is free, and discrimination has no place. All those here today are focusing on achieving their three important missions.

The Nippon Foundation and the Sasakawa Health Foundation have hosted a series of Regional Assemblies for the organizations of persons affected by leprosy in Asia, Africa, and Latin America, discussing the issues and solutions within each region.

And over the last few days, as a concluding session, we have hosted this Global Forum of People's Organizations on Hansen's Disease. We have had over sixty participants from twenty-three countries worldwide, the biggest forum we have ever organized. We provided practical training, and I am confident that fruitful discussions were had. Later today, I believe Jennifer from CLAP, the Coalition of Leprosy Advocates of the Philippines, will be representing to speak about the forum's achievements. I sincerely hope that you will listen to their collective voice. With us today, there are representatives of organizations of persons affected by leprosy from twenty-three countries. Will all of you please stand? Ladies and gentlemen, please give them a huge round of applause.

To date, many individuals and organizations have worked hard for the elimination of leprosy. I believe the elimination of leprosy has been an important milestone in my life journey. I welcome heartily that a new network of many stakeholders, the "Global Partnership for Zero Leprosy," has now been established. This collaboration will greatly enhance our work toward achieving "Zero Leprosy."

Parenthetically, I would like to make clear that I am one of those opposed to leprosy being considered one of the neglected tropical diseases. Leprosy has never been neglected, even for a moment, either by the persons affected or the people who have worked hard for their betterment. In my opinion, this medical terminology gives the impression that it is looking down on the patients and lacks respect toward those still fighting against leprosy today.

Leprosy is an ongoing issue.

I would like to request all the medical stakeholders here today to continue working on discovering the causes of the transmission of leprosy, developing vaccination, and creating prosthetics and orthotics for those with impairments. With globalization and migration, there are new cases, even in countries that used to see few cases. None of the countries is an exception.

However, the number of leprosy medical specialists is decreasing rapidly worldwide.

In closing, I would like to make a special request to you, leprosy medical doctors, to devote your time to educating the next generation who will have the skills and knowledge to diagnose and treat leprosy.

Now, Ladies and Gentlemen,

Let us unite towards "Zero Leprosy," a historical challenge for all humankind!

Thank you very much.

In September, I visited Princeton, United States (for the Nippon Foundation Nereus Ocean Science Conference) and China (for the SYLFF twenty-fifth anniversary at Chongqing and Yunnan Universities). In October, I visited London, UK (for Seabed 2030, a marine topography mapping symposium) and Norway (for the Our Ocean International Conference), and in November, Myanmar (for Myanmar ceasefire and peace negotiations and a meeting with government officials).

National Leprosy Conference in Bangladesh—People's Republic of Bangladesh, December 2019

Route: Haneda International Airport → Singapore (flight time: 7h 40m; 2h stopover) → Dhaka, Bangladesh (flight time: 4h)—two nights—Dhaka → Bangkok, Thailand (flight time: 2h 30m; 2h 20m stopover) → Narita International Airport (flight time: 5h 50m)

On 12 December, the Bangladesh capital Dhaka hosted the National Leprosy Conference. There was a bit of a story behind this event. As the Japanese government's Special Envoy for National Reconciliation in Myanmar, I had been working behind the scenes as a mediator between ethnic minority militia groups, the Myanmar government, and the national army. However, in Myanmar's Rakhine state, the Rohingya issue had reached a flash point, and more than 700,000 Rohingya refugees flooded across the border into Bangladesh's Cox's Bazar to be housed in refugee camps. During my meeting with Prime Minister Sheikh Hasina on this issue, I explained the need for a national leprosy conference in Bangladesh, which she agreed to immediately. She also readily assented to attend and speak at the conference.

In my keynote presentation to the conference, I described its background and significance as follows:

Yohei Sasakawa

Chair of the Nippon Foundation and WHO Goodwill Ambassador for Leprosy Elimination

Keynote Presentation at National Leprosy Conference

Dhaka, Bangladesh

12 December 2019

This conference came about after I called on Prime Minister Sheikh Hasina in February and received her support. It is very reassuring—and pleasing—to receive such strong commitment from the country's leader.

Over the past forty years, I have traveled the world in my activities to disseminate correct information about leprosy.

Today, leprosy is curable with effective medicine, which is available for free, and early diagnosis and prompt treatment can prevent physical impairment.

It is of utmost importance to detect and treat leprosy early in children to never repeat the tragedy that suffering from leprosy has brought upon the lives of those affected by the disease.

However, even though it is easily curable, many think that leprosy is a disease to be ashamed of. Often, this makes patients reluctant to go to clinics and hospitals for fear of being diagnosed with leprosy.

Furthermore, in the early stage of the disease, there are hardly any noticeable symptoms except for discolored skin patches. This is one of the reasons that delay the diagnosis of patients.

In order that these early symptoms are not overlooked, I use the media worldwide and personally broadcast through radio and television to always check for these skin patches in their homes.

In addition, there are the issues of prejudice and discrimination. These I consider to be diseases of society that we have also to contend with.

Because of leprosy, there are many people who are forced to leave their families and cannot go to school or get a job. Persons affected by leprosy are labeled as "former patients" even after they are cured and continue to suffer from discrimination.

I have met many people suffering from such discrimination around the world. It is very clear that leprosy is not just a medical issue but also an issue of human rights.

So I decided to take this matter to the United Nations. In 2003, I visited the Office of the UN High Commissioner for Human Rights for the first time to have leprosy put on the human rights agenda. But to my disappointment and surprise, leprosy had never once been considered a human rights issue.

On that first visit, we had the opportunity to give a presentation to the High Commissioner's office staff. However, only five people attended. This showed the low level of interest in the issue at the time.

But I was not a man to give up. As a result of a repeated annual appeal for seven years at the general assembly of the UN Human Rights Council in Geneva, finally, the UN General Assembly unanimously adopted a resolution on the elimination of discrimination against persons affected by leprosy and their family members in December 2010.

Over the years of our work against leprosy and its associated stigma and discrimination, persons affected by leprosy around the world have joined us to become our strong partners.

With us today, there are persons affected by leprosy who have traveled long distances to be here. I thank you for coming here from all over Bangladesh. You are motivated by a desire to realize a world without leprosy so that the next generation does not have to experience the hardships you did. I look forward to participating in the national meeting of persons affected by leprosy that will take place for the first time in Bangladesh tomorrow.

Ladies and gentlemen. Due to the government placing high priorities on measures against leprosy, the national prevalence of leprosy has been declining here in Bangladesh in recent years. Yet it is an undeniable reality that many new cases are still discovered nationwide today.

Therefore, I am greatly encouraged by your further activities against leprosy.

Through the active discussions during this conference, I urge everyone to work together to accelerate the actions needed to achieve Zero Leprosy in Bangladesh by 2030. Both the Nippon Foundation and Sasakawa Health Foundation are ready to work with you.

I conclude by wishing you a successful conference, and I hope that the outcome will serve as a model for other countries.

Thank you very much.

Countries visited in 2020	
January	● India
February	Myanmar (First round Myanmar nationwide ceasefire agreement: negotiations with armed ethnic organizations; talks with government personnel)
	Thailand (Myanmar nationwide ceasefire agreement: negotiations with armed ethnic organizations)
March	Taiwan (Talks with President Tsai Ing-wen)
October	Myanmar (First Myanmar general election: head of Japanese election observer team)
November	Myanmar (Myanmar nationwide ceasefire agreement: talks with government personnel)

● Indicates a trip that features in this section.

In Mahatma Gandhi's hometown—Delhi and Gujarat, India, January 2020

Route: Narita International Airport → Delhi, India (flight time: 10h 25m)—three nights—Delhi → Ahmedabad, Gujarat, India (flight time: 1h 35m)—four nights—Ahmedabad → Delhi (flight time: 1h 40m; 8h stopover (meeting with the Japanese ambassador)) → Narita (flight time: 7h 20m)

On 27 January 2020, we presented our Global Appeal 2020 in Tokyo with the International Paralympic Committee in the presence of Prime Minister Shinzo Abe. The next day, I left for India, on my sixtieth visit to that country.

In Delhi, I attended two leprosy awareness events sponsored by S-ILF. The first was an event marking Anti Leprosy Day, held on Leprosy Day (30 January), and the second was an event commemorating the publication of the English edition of my book, *No Matter Where the Journey Takes Me*.

At the Leprosy Day event, the Confederation of Indian Industry (CII) announced that it would work with S-ILF to encourage member companies across India to promote the employment of people affected by leprosy and their families. The CII had proposed this initiative at the Global Appeal 2019 ceremony in Delhi, which it and the International Chamber of Commerce had sponsored. I was delighted to see how they had made concrete progress over the past year. At the event celebrating the publication of my book in English, I was honored to have Foreign Minister Subrahmanyam Jaishankar in attendance. He promised that the Indian government would make serious efforts to realize a society free of leprosy and the discrimination associated with it.

During my stay in Delhi, I called on Dr. Harsh Vardan, minister of health and family welfare, and Thawar Chand Geholot, minister of social justice and empowerment. I asked them for further effort from the Indian government to establish an inter-ministerial coordination committee to eliminate discrimination and stigma alongside leprosy and to enable people affected by the disease to live their lives with dignity. Prime Minister Modi, driving India's development with his strong leadership, had pledged to achieve an Indian society free of leprosy and discrimination by 2030. It was extremely encouraging to learn that the ministries concerned were willing to get to grips with the challenge.

A two-hour flight from Delhi took me to Ahmedabad, the largest city in Gujarat, which faces the Arabian Sea. The birthplace of Mahatma Gandhi and Prime Minister Modi, this state has produced many prominent politicians and businesspeople. The state accounts for almost 40 percent of India's industrial production, and I got the impression that its infrastructure is much better developed than other regional cities.

The number of registered leprosy cases in Gujarat from April to December 2019 was 3,410. Though the state had achieved the WHO benchmark in 2004, leprosy remained endemic in twelve districts. A multifaceted program combining patient detection, awareness-raising, special activities in remote areas and a single dose of the therapeutic drug rifampicin had resulted in eight of the districts reaching the benchmark. The goal was to have all districts do so by 2022.

There were fourteen leprosy colonies in Gujarat state, and at the urging of APAL, whom the Nippon Foundation had supported for more than ten years, they had been collaborating in awareness-raising activities to bring about improvements in their lives. However, the state had no special pension for people affected by leprosy with disabilities, and most of the elderly among them were living in difficult circumstances, with no means of survival other than begging.

I visited a suburban clinic about an hour's drive from Ahmedabad. There, I met with ASHA, female health workers active on the front lines. Dressed in beautiful orange saris, behind their gentle demeanor these women clearly had a fierce determination to help the people in the region. I shared with them words of gratitude and encouragement: "Your efforts are invaluable because both those affected by leprosy and those around them want to hide the disease. I want you to take pride in your work."

The following day, I traveled to the Gandhi Kusta Seva Ashram in Ahmedabad. Formed in the 1960s by people affected by leprosy who had migrated from other areas of the country, the colony was home to sixty-five people affected by leprosy and their families. Since it is located next to an industrial area, many young people work outside the colony. Every Sunday, the young people share news and hold study sessions and are enthusiastic about improving their living conditions as much as possible. On the day I visited, many people from the surrounding colonies gathered to meet me, and the meeting hall was filled with more than 300 people.

The children performed a beautiful welcome dance that alleviated the fatigue from my long trip. I was impressed and moved by the happy expressions on the faces of the parents watching over their children. I encouraged them, saying: "One thread is weak, but ten or 100 threads together become strong. Let's work with APAL and the government and win you the right to live with dignity as Indian citizens."

On my last day in India, I met with state government officials who play an essential role in the fight against leprosy, including B. G. Nainvale, commissioner for persons with disabilities; Dr. Jayanti S. Ravi, principal secretary of health; and Anil Mukim, chief secretary of Gujarat. The government's help was crucial, I told them, in eliminating beggary from the colonies. I then urged APAL Vice President Guntreddy Venugopal and the other representatives who were there with us to state their demands directly to the officials. Since opportunities for people affected by leprosy to speak directly to government officials are limited in India, where caste consciousness is strong, the APAL representatives were tense as they pleaded for special assistance payments, land ownership, and other pressing issues.

In 2019, I had received the 2018 Gandhi Peace Prize from the Indian government in recognition of my efforts to eliminate leprosy.

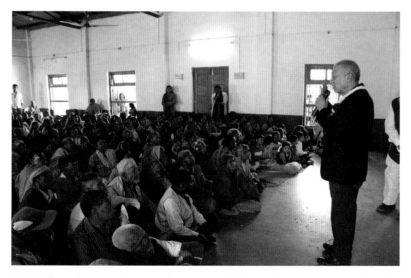

145. "Please live your lives with courage." Words of support to people who have recovered from leprosy, and their family members (Gujarat, India, January 2020)

Unfortunately, Gandhi had not been able to realize his dream of an India free of leprosy and discrimination during his lifetime. My visit to Gandhi's hometown made me even more determined to carry on his dream and make it a reality. Until then, I am determined to visit India as often as possible and fight leprosy with all concerned.

AFTERWORD

THE LAST MILE

The 1980s saw a dramatic decrease in the number of people affected by leprosy, thanks to the development of multidrug therapy (MDT) and to the distribution from 1985 of MDT blister packs free of cost. The countries where leprosy is endemic (that is to say, countries where there are one or more persons affected by leprosy per 10,000 population), which numbered 122 in 1985, are now greatly reduced. Only a single nation remains, Brazil—and even here, in recent years it has seemed that elimination was within reach. Now, however, there is a new reality: the worldwide COVID-19 pandemic. Sadly, the appearance of this new disease has cast a pall on our hopes of seeing the elimination of leprosy throughout the world.

We are now seeing a resurgence of leprosy, both in countries that had met the official World Health Organization (WHO) target and in certain pockets, for example in mountain ranges, or areas that are far off the beaten track, referred to as "hotspots," where despite all best efforts it has remained stubbornly endemic. Despite these tough circumstances, I am determined to continue my efforts, using every means at my disposal, undauntedly and tenaciously, to stick to my original intention of making sure that no country on earth remains where leprosy is endemic, and working toward a world in which not a single person can catch leprosy ever again. What concerns me is the possibility that we might let our efforts lag, in a false sense of security, since the official target has ostensibly been reached in the majority of countries. We have to remember that though we are in a much better position than we were forty years ago—undoubtedly walking the last mile of our 100-mile journey—elimination is but a milestone. Our ultimate target is eradication. Other challenges remain: We have to prevent children catching the disease, and somehow to alleviate the experience of individuals who have recovered from the disease but are left with permanent conditions or disabilities due to delays in treatment. Early diagnosis and treatment are absolutely essential.

And that is only to look at leprosy from a medical point of view. There is also the important issue of the psychosocial aspect to the disease. As I have noted throughout this book, the distinguishing characteristic of leprosy, the thing that marks it off from all other diseases, has to do with the discrimination, based on prejudice, shown by many in society toward people who have been affected by it—even when they have been treated and are completely cured. This discrimination leaves deep emotional scars. For as long as historical records can attest, leprosy has been seen as shameful and impure, and the people affected by it socially shunned and reviled. In many countries, this is a situation that has shown little change. The stigma of ancient times still pertains to the present day.

Sadly, all too often laws and regulations have only worked to deepen discrimination. National and local governments frequently issue regulations that treat people affected by leprosy as a group apart—and the world's religions too have tended to talk of leprosy in terms of innate defilement or impurity, implying that leprosy is a disease visited on people for the sins of their forefathers. Families and partners also come in for discrimination. Sometimes people go so far as to drive their own children, their own siblings, out of the family home for fear that they will be ostracized by their community for having a person with leprosy living with them. In many countries, people diagnosed as having the disease see themselves as having caught it because of some sin they or their ancestors must have committed, and they internalize the blame, in what is known as self-perceived stigma. The psychosocial conditions surrounding leprosy have the same effect whether we are talking about small communities of pygmies deep in the forest, as featured in one episode in this book, or in nations that are generally considered developed. My friend José

Ramirez, who had leprosy in the past and is now a clinical social worker in the United States, told me how when he was diagnosed with leprosy he was taken to the National Leprosarium in Carville, Louisiana not in an ambulance but in a hearse. Fortunately, he managed to get a college education, but at one point he was told by his fellow-students at gunpoint that he should not show up on the campus. This was in the 1960s, during the peak of the American civil rights movement led by the Reverend Martin Luther King Jr., when the issue of human rights was in the air.

It is true that much more knowledge about leprosy is available nowadays than ever before. Many more people now know that leprosy is curable, and that discrimination is unacceptable. Nevertheless, a considerable amount of deep-seated discrimination still exists in modern-day society, and misguided notions about the disease—circulating in society for thousands of years—continue to be deeply entrenched. It isn't unusual to see people who think of themselves as tolerant and enlightened betray a shocking closed-mindedness when they have to deal face-to-face with persons with lived experience of the disease.

The discrimination shown toward people who are affected by leprosy causes those who suspect that they or someone else in their vicinity might have the disease feel fearful about coming forward, so preventing early detection and treatment. This only creates one more impediment to our endeavor to complete this last mile of our 100-mile journey of making sure that leprosy disappears from the face of the earth.

On my travels to countries around the world, I make a point of repeating three key messages. The first is that leprosy is curable. The second is that free treatment is available. And the third is that social discrimination has no place. I do my utmost to make as many people as possible aware of these messages, using whatever methods are available to me, whether it is with government campaigns, mass media, songs, plays, and anything else that is effective and appropriate, so that the messages reach whomever they need to, including those who can't read or write, and those who live far away from the cities and who have no access to telecommunications.

In 2010, on the world stage, my efforts to persuade the human rights organizations of the United Nations, and with the support and collaboration of the government of Japan, the General Assembly at the United Nations, led to a resolution on the elimination of discrimination against persons affected by leprosy and their family members, which included a set of "Principles and Guidelines" explaining how to go about eradicating such discrimination. I am particularly concerned to get the Principles and Guidelines as widely disseminated and implemented as possible, using mass media to persuade national governments as well as frontline workers. In order to publicize the realities that people who have lived experience of the disease have to face in their daily lives, in 2006 I launched my Global Appeal initiative, in which every year I gather together people of influence from various spheres of life and related key players, all of whom sign an announcement, with much fanfare. As a result, in recent years WHO has begun to pay serious attention to the issue of discrimination in its programs to tackle the disease.

Another very important area of concern is getting people who are either currently or previously affected by leprosy, as well as their family members, back into society and employment, able to support themselves. Here too it is prejudice and discrimination that pose the obstacles. In some countries, people with experience of leprosy have taken a stand and formed alliances in the fight against discrimination and in the quest for ways toward social reintegration, and they have been heroic in their efforts. People with lived experience of the disease are by far and away in the best position to grasp and understand the realities people with leprosy have to face, which is why it is right that they lead in the efforts to support those affected by leprosy. Nevertheless, in the grand scheme of things, their power can only go so far. They still need and deserve a good deal of support.

The history of leprosy is a history that involves tragedies and despair, but it is also a history of courage and hope—the courage and hope that people affected by the disease have maintained despite all odds. At this moment, the history of their heroic struggle seems to be slipping away from our attention, and perhaps even slipping away from memory. It is incumbent on us, I firmly believe, to continue to tell the stories of the people involved in this history, and to continue to remember all their achievements.

There is a saying that the last mile of a 100-mile journey is the part that requires the most endurance. We are walking that last mile right now. We cannot afford to relax in the slightest in our efforts to eradicate leprosy completely. We must eradicate it as a medical problem and as a psychosocial problem as well. Our endeavors to solve the biggest problem of leprosy, which is the discrimination associated with it, necessitates that we achieve zero discrimination and zero stigma. And in that endeavor, I would say that the journey has just begun.

As I intimated above, in the spring of 2020 the world was taken over by the COVID-19 pandemic. One consequence of this was that the effort to eliminate leprosy had to be suspended as everyone turned their efforts toward tackling the immediate emergency. All the initiatives we had lined up as we aimed to finally see the whole world rid of leprosy—and specifically in the one country where leprosy still remains an endemic problem, Brazil—had to be shut down. The curtailment of all except the most essential travel in 2020 and 2021 meant that any activities on the front lines directed toward leprosy elimination in countries around the globe were cancelled. Our sixteenth Global Appeal in 2021, scheduled to take place in Tokyo, in the end, sadly, had to take place virtually.

During that Global Appeal, we held a series of online seminars. One of them had the theme of "Zero Leprosy for Whom in the Post-COVID World?" and centered broadly on the importance of people affected by leprosy coming together and forming alliances. I delivered the opening address. Here are just a few passages from my speech:

> Hello, everyone. My warmest greetings to you all. Even though present circumstances mean we are only able to connect online, I am overjoyed that, given these difficult times, I can still connect with everyone in this way, more-or-less directly, and in real time.

> I am well aware of the worry and hardship that persons affected by leprosy and their families will be experiencing at this extraordinary time when the whole world finds itself in the turmoil of a pandemic. I am very grateful to you all, as leaders of organizations of people affected by leprosy, for finding the time to come together and share your concerns.

> In our efforts to work toward zero leprosy, a single statement from leaders of organizations of persons affected by leprosy such as yourselves carries 100 times as much weight as any statement from me.

This is why it is so important that you continue to take a central role in our efforts. I am confident, given how much you have achieved already, that you have the strength to overcome all the difficulties you face, and I hope that you will continue to devote yourselves with undaunted determination to our cause. …

In these difficult times, in many countries around the globe, ongoing efforts at leprosy case detection and treatment have had to be reduced, and in some cases suspended; access to medical care has become difficult; and we continue to see many cases where people continue to experience discrimination and prejudice because of the disease. Nevertheless, we must not allow the issue of leprosy to be pushed aside. I am determined that we will resume our efforts and activities in the struggle against leprosy in all parts of the world at the earliest possible opportunity.

Even amid our concern that the issue of leprosy remains as worthy of concern and vigilance as ever, we at the Nippon Foundation do not see COVID-19 as something we should or indeed can ignore. We have done all we can to support the activities of doctors, nurses, and others engaged in frontline activities, mainly in Japan, to control the spread of infection and to care for those who have become infected, constructing facilities for people who have contracted the disease, supporting testing efforts, providing transport to medical practitioners to enable them to do their work. Sadly, we are seeing some instances of COVID discrimination toward those who have become infected, their family members, and even medical practitioners. As we have always argued, any violation of the dignity and self-respect of a person on account of illness or disability is unacceptable. In the same way that discrimination poses a huge impediment to ridding the world of leprosy, this COVID discrimination is nothing but an obstacle to dealing with coronavirus. The lessons that humankind has learned in the course of the long struggle with leprosy should be put to use at the present time.

This book comprises an edited and enlarged version of articles I contributed to several journals published in leprosy sanatoria in Japan. A certain amount of basic information is repeated in each of the chapters, which some readers might find tedious, but the idea is to have each section stand as an independent record. Regretfully, partly due to my constitutional disinclination to put pen to paper, I wasn't able to take notes on every trip I made to every country, so inevitably there are a few lacunae here and there, and for this I can only offer my sincere apologies.

This book was originally published in July 2021 by the Kosakusha publishing house as *Chikyu wo Kakeru—Sekai no Hansen-byo no Genba kara*. So many people have helped in its writing. My personal assistant, Ms. Taeko Hoshino, has been diligently keeping my records for over forty-five years and pulled together many of the documents on which I have relied for this work. Mr. Tatsuya Tanami accompanied me all over the world as a close confidant and demonstrated superhuman tenacity as we worked with the UN Human Rights Council to get the General Assembly to pass a resolution for the elimination of discrimination against persons affected by leprosy. Ms. Natsuko Tominaga, my photographer, has faithfully recorded the reality of life for people affected by leprosy around the world. Her stark and moving images will continue to amaze people fifty years hence. I am also grateful to her for her powerful support in pulling off our extremely busy travel itineraries. Indeed, without the help of the whole leprosy team at the Nippon Foundation, and everyone at the Sasakawa Health Foundation, none of my achievements would have been possible. I would also be remiss if I did not give thanks to my editor at Kosakusha, Mr. Kei Yonezawa, for his help in publishing the Japanese version of this book. For this English version, I must thank Ms. Lucy North for her faithful translation of this long, detailed work, as well as Mr. Michael Dwyer of Hurst Publishers in the United Kingdom, for his help in getting it published. Ms. Yuko Tani of the Nippon Foundation similarly deserves my thanks for her careful efforts in supervising the whole process of producing the English version of the book. To be honest, there are too many people to whom I owe a debt of gratitude for their help, and so I hope that they will know who they are and that they are deeply appreciated.

Lastly, to my wife Kazuyo, who over the past forty years has sent me off with nary a complaint on more than 550 trips around the globe, and who has been such a wonderful mother to our four sons, I owe you thanks from the very bottom of my heart.

Yohei Sasakawa
May 2023

THE GLOBAL APPEAL INITIATIVE, 2006–21

A TIMELINE

APPENDIX 1

Initiated in 2006 by the author, the annual Global Appeal draws attention to the stigma and discrimination that persons affected by leprosy and their families continue to face all over the world and calls for the

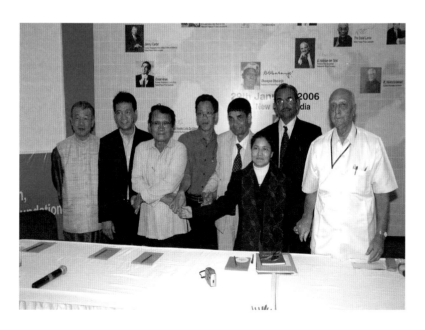

realization of a truly inclusive society in which the fundamental human rights of all people are respected. Held in conjunction with World Leprosy Day in a different city of the world each year, it is endorsed by a different group of individuals and a different organization on each occasion.

First Global Appeal, 2006

New Delhi, India

Endorsed and Co-Signed by:

World Leaders and Nobel Peace Prize Laureates

Óscar Arias
Former President of Costa Rica
Nobel Peace Prize Laureate

Jimmy Carter
Former President of the United States of America
Nobel Peace Prize Laureate

The Dalai Lama
Nobel Peace Prize Laureate

El Hassan bin Talal
Prince of the Jordanian Hashemite Royal Dynasty

Václav Havel
Former President of the Czech Republic

Luiz Inácio Lula da Silva
President of the Federative Republic of Brazil

Olusegun Obasanjo
President of the Federal Republic of Nigeria

Mary Robinson
Former President of Ireland
Former UN High Commissioner for Human Rights

Yohei Sasakawa
Chairman, the Nippon Foundation

APPENDIX 1

Desmond Tutu
Archbishop Emeritus of Cape Town
Nobel Peace Prize Laureate

R. Venkataraman
Former President of India

Elie Wiesel
President, the Elie Wiesel Foundation for Humanity
Nobel Peace Prize Laureate

Second Global Appeal, 2007

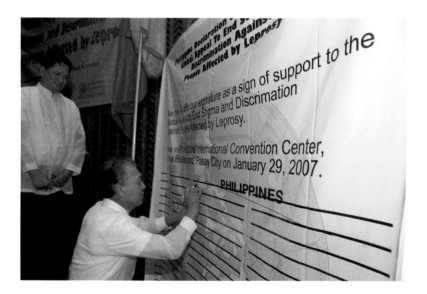

Manila, Philippines
Endorsed and Co-Signed by:
Representatives of People Affected by Leprosy from Eleven
Nations

Third Global Appeal, 2008

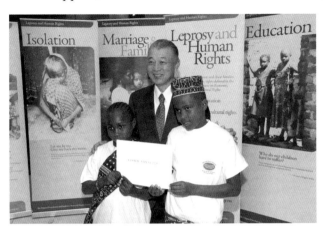

London, United Kingdom

Endorsed and Co-Signed by:

International Human Rights Organizations

Nine NGOs active in human rights around the world, including Amnesty International and International Save the Children Alliance, from six nations

Fourth Global Appeal, 2009

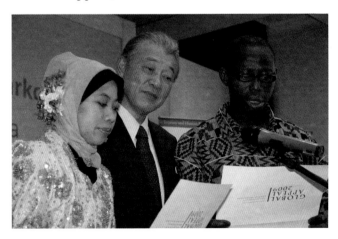

London, United Kingdom

Endorsed and Co-Signed by:

World Religious Leaders

Seventeen religious leaders from sixteen nations around the world, representing Christianity, Islam, Buddhism, Judaism, Hinduism, and other religions

Fifth Global Appeal, 2010

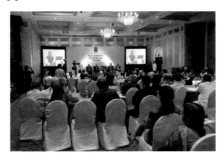

Mumbai, India

Endorsed and Co-Signed by:

World Business Leaders

Fifteen leaders of major corporations from ten nations around the world, including the Tata Group in India, and Japan's Toyota Motor Corporation and Canon Inc.

Sixth Global Appeal, 2011

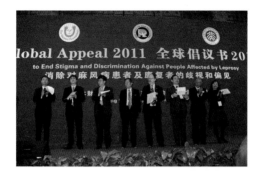

Beijing, China
Endorsed and Co-Signed by:
World-Leading Universities
Presidents, chancellors, and rectors from 110 leading universities
in sixty-four nations around the world

Seventh Global Appeal, 2012

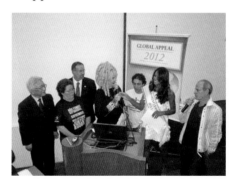

São Paulo, Brazil
Endorsed and Co-Signed by:
World Medical Association
Presidents of fifty member countries of the World Medical
Association

APPENDIX 1

Eighth Global Appeal, 2013

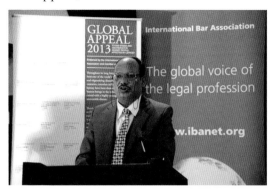

London, United Kingdom
Endorsed and Co-Signed by:
International Bar Association
Forty-six member organizations from forty countries around the world

Ninth Global Appeal, 2014

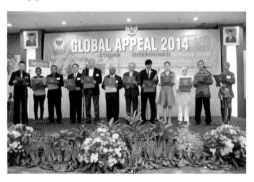

Jakarta, Indonesia
Endorsed and Co-Signed by:
National Human Rights Institutions
Thirty-nine national human rights institutions from thirty-seven nations and two regions

Tenth Global Appeal, 2015

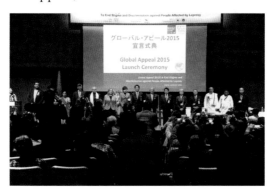

Tokyo, Japan
Endorsed and Co-Signed by:
International Council of Nurses
The International Council of Nurses, and nurse associations and
syndicates from 132 nations

Eleventh Global Appeal, 2016

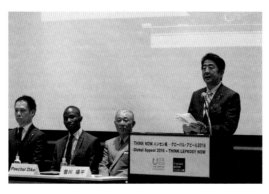

Tokyo, Japan
Endorsed and Co-Signed by:
Junior Chamber International
Junior Chambers from 130 nations

Twelfth Global Appeal, 2017

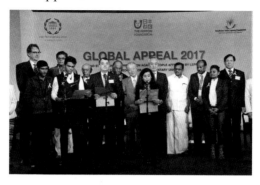

New Delhi, India
Endorsed and Co-Signed by:
The Inter-Parliamentary Union (IPU)
The Executive Committee of IPU and 171 member parliaments of IPU

Thirteenth Global Appeal, 2018

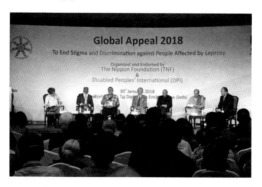

New Delhi, India
Endorsed and Co-Signed by:
Disabled Peoples' International
Member federations of Disabled Peoples' International from around the world

Fourteenth Global Appeal, 2019

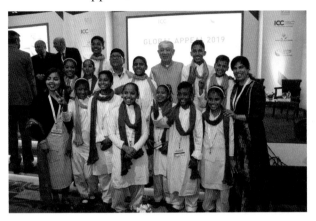

New Delhi, India
Endorsed and Co-Signed by:
International Chamber of Commerce

Fifteenth Global Appeal, 2020

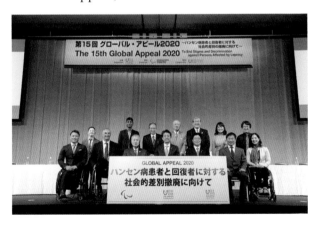

Tokyo, Japan
Endorsed and Co-Signed by:
International Paralympic Committee

APPENDIX 1

Sixteenth Global Appeal, 2021

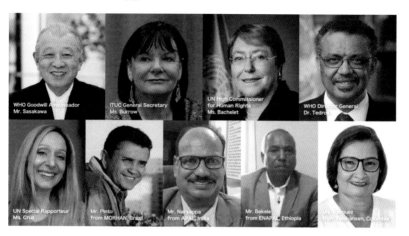

Online

Endorsed and Co-Signed by:

International Trade Union Confederation and its 332 national member organizations representing 200 million workers in 163 countries and territories

Headquarters in Brussels, Belgium

APPENDIX 2

MEETINGS WITH PRINCIPAL LEADERS
OF NATIONS VISITED

1980–2020

* DRC = Democratic Republic of the Congo
* Positions/titles are as of year indicated
* Some meetings with Japanese ministers and prime ministers omitted

Date	Nation/Region	Title/Post	Name
1980			
2 April	Japan	Prime Minister	Tanaka Kakuei
5 August	South Korea	President	Chun Doo-hwan
1981			
June december	United States	Former Secretary of State	Henry Kissinger

	Japan	Prime Minister	Suzuki Zenko
1982			
3 April	UK	Former Prime Minister	Sir Edward Heath
9 May	UK	Former Prime Minister	Sir Edward Heath
2 November	Costa Rica	Former President	Rodrigo Carazo Odio
20 November	United States	Nobel Prize Laureate in Chemistry	Linus Carl Pauling
1983			
22 February	United States	Nobel Prize Laureate in Chemistry	Linus Carl Pauling
9 May	The Vatican	The Pope	John Paul II
18 May	United States	Wife of US General of the Army Douglas MacArthur	Jean Marie MacArthur
24 May	United States	President	Ronald Reagan
3 July	UK	Former Prime Minister	Harold Wilson
22 July	United States	Former President	James "Jimmy" Carter
1984			
17 February	UK	Peer; former leader of SDP	David Owen

20 February	India	Nobel Peace Prize Laureate	Mother Teresa
25 March	United States	Former President	James "Jimmy" Carter
19 June	UK	Prime Minister	Margaret Thatcher
20 June	Sweden	Prime Minster	Olof Palme
3 September	United States	Agronomist; Nobel Prize Laureate	Norman Borlaug
20 December	Peru	UN Secretary-General	Javier Pérez de Cuéllar
20 December	UK	Former Prime Minister	James Wilson
1985			
13 April	Japan	Prime Minister	Nakasone Yasuhiro
13 April	China	Son of Deng Xiaoping	Deng Pufang
30 October	China	Chairman of the Central Military Commission	Deng Xiaoping
1986			
January	United States	Former President	James "Jimmy" Carter
January	Ghana	Head of State	Jerry Rawlings
January	Zambia	President	Kenneth Kaunda

January	Tanzania	President	Ali Hassan Mwinyi
January	Tanzania	Former President	Julius Nyerere
January	Togo	President	(Etienne) Gnassingbé Eyadéma
March	The Philippines	President	Coraz ó n Aquino
March	The Philippines	Former President	Fidel V. Ramos
1987			
24 April	United States	Actor	Dame Elizabeth Taylor
7 August	Sri Lanka	President	Junius Richard ("J. R.") Jayewardene
26 September	China	Vice President	Wang Zhen
26 September	China	Daughter of Deng Xiaoping	Xiao Rong
17 November	France	President	François Mitterrand
1988			
16 March	Kenya	UN Environment Programme Executive Director	Mostafa Tolba
14 April	United States	Actor	Dame Elizabeth Taylor

APPENDIX 2

13 October	United States	President	Ronald Reagan
4 November	Ghana	Head of State	Jerry Rawlings
1989			
3 January	Thailand	Crown Prince	Maha Vajiralongkorn
10 January	Fiji	Former President	Kamisese Mara
22 February	Samoa	Head of State	Malietoa Tanumafili II
22 February	Solomon Islands	Governor General	George Lepping
22 February	Tonga	King	Tāufa'āhau Tupou IV
22 February	Nauru	President	Hammer DeRoburt
22 February	Vanuatu	President	Frederick "Fred" Timakata
22 February	Fiji	President	Penaia Ganilau
30 September	Iceland	President	Vigdis Finnbogadóttir
4 October	Finland	President	Mauno Koivisto
18 November	USSR	Politburo official	Alexander Yakovlev
1990			
13 February	USSR	Politburo official	Alexander Yakovlev

13 February	USSR	Chairman of the Council of the Union of the USSR Supreme Soviet	Yevgeny Primakov
11 June	China	General Secretary of the Communist Party	Jiang Zemin
11 June	China	President	Yang Shangkun
1 July	Japan	Former Prime Minister	Nakasone Yasuhiro
4 July	Ghana	Head of State	Jerry Rawlings
4 July	Japan	Prime Minister	Kaifu Toshiki
11 July	Ghana	First Lady of Ghana	Nana Konadu Agyeman Rawlings
30 July	Japan	Former Prime Minister	Takeshita Noboru
30 July	Japan	Foreign Minister	Abe Shintaro
30 July	Japan	Former Prime Minister	Nakasone Yasuhiro
20 July	Japan	Chief Cabinet Secretary	Obuchi Keizo
6 August	Mongolia	Prime Minister	Dashin Byambasüren
18 September	USSR	President	Mikhail Gorbachev

9 October	USSR	Vice President of the Soviet Union	Gennadii Ivanovich Yanayev
14 November	Togo	President	Etienne Gnassingbé Eyadéma
15 November	Iceland	President	Vigdis Finnbogadóttir
15 November	Bulgaria	President	Zhelyu Zhelev
15 November	Benin	Prime Minister	Nicéphore Soglo
6 December	China	Foreign Minister	Huang Hua
7 December	China	Daughter of Deng Xiaoping	Xiao Rong
7 December	China	Daughter of Yang Shangkun	Li Yang
7 December	Japan	Former Prime Minister	Fukuda Takeo
19 December	USSR	Yakut Autonomous Soviet Socialist Republic President	Mikhail Yefimovich Nikolayev
24 December	USSR	Wife of Soviet President	Raisa Gorbachev
1991			
13 January	Japan	Prime Minister	Kaifu Toshiki
13 February	Nicaragua	President	Violeta Chamorro

28 February	Belarus	Prime Minister	Vyacheslav Kebich
29 August	Israel	Former President	Yitzhak Navon
15 November	Japan	Former Prime Minister	Takeshita Noboru
1992			
27 January	Russia	Former Soviet President	Mikhail Gorbachev
20 March	North Korea	President	Kim Il-sung
April	Russia	Former Soviet President	Mikhail Gorbachev
14 April	United States	Former President	James "Jimmy" Carter
15 October	UK	Prime Minister	Margaret Thatcher
17 November	Japan	Prime Minister	Miyazawa Kiichi
17 November	China	Vice-Chairman of the Central Military Commission	Liu Huaqing
1993			
20 January	United States	President	Bill Clinton
15 April	United States	Former President	James "Jimmy" Carter
1 June	Peru	President	Alberto Fujimori

August	China	Vice-Chairman of the Central Military Commission	Liu Huaqing
25 November	Mongolia	Prime Minister	Puntsagiin Jasrai
1994			
21 February	Benin	Prime Minister	Nicéphore Soglo
15 March	Ecuador	President	Sixto Durán Ballén
21 March	Yakut (Saha)	President	Mikhail Yefimovich Nikolayev
5 June	Peru	President	Alberto Fujimori
4 July	Vietnam	Vice President	Nguyen Minh Triet
4 and 5 July	Vietnam	Prime Minister	Võ Van Kiet
8 July	United States	Former President	James "Jimmy" Carter
11 September	Egypt	UN Secretary-General	Boutros Boutros-Ghali
16 September	Costa Rica	Former President	Óscar Arias Sánchez
20 December	China	Vice-Chairman of the Central Military Commission	Liu Huaqing

21 December	China	General Secretary of the Communist Party	Hu Jintao
1995			
11 April	South Korea	President	Kim Tae-jung
4, 5, 7 September	Djibouti	President	Hassan Gouled Aptidon
14 September	United States	Former President	James "Jimmy" Carter
21 September	Tonga	King	Tāufaʻāhau Tupou IV
25 October	Costa Rica	Former President	Óscar Arias Sánchez
21 December	Bulgaria	President	Zhelyu Zhelev
21 December	Burkina Faso	President	Blaise Compaoré
1996			
8, 9 February	Peru	President	Alberto Fujimori
16 March	Micronesia	President	Bailey Olter
22 April	Iceland	President	Vigdis Finnbogadóttir
26 April	Russia	Former Soviet President	Nursultan Nazarbayev
27 April	Russia	Former Acting President of the Soviet Union	Gennady Yanayev

APPENDIX 2

30 April	Kazakhstan	President	Nursultan Nazarbayev
2 May	Kyrgyzstan	President	Askar Akayev
3 May	Uzbekistan	President	Islam Karimov
23 May	United States	Former President	James "Jimmy" Carter
22 September	United States	Former President	James "Jimmy" Carter
27 September	Haiti	Former First Lady	Mildred Aristide
11 October	India	Prime Minister	H. D. Deve Gowda
18 October	Slovak Republic	President	Michal Kováč
22 October	Belgium	King	Albert II
6 November	Bolivia	President	Gonzalo Sánchez de Lozada Sanchez Bustamante
13 November	Peru	President	Alberto Fujimori
1997			
7 May	Russia	Chairman of Central Committee of Communist Party	Gennady Zyuganov
7 May	Russia	Chairman of Yabloko party	Grigory Yavlinsky

8 May	Russia	Former USSR President	Mikhail Gorbachev
9 May	Russia	Former Soviet Vice President	Gennady Yanayev
30 June	Russia	Head of National Security Council	Aleksandr Lebed
22 July	Russia	Leader of Liberal Democratic Party of Russia	Vladimir Zhirinovsky
3, 4 July	Peru	President	Alberto Fujimori
28 July	Portugal	Former President	Mário Soares
25 August	Ethiopia	Prime Minister	Meles Zenawi Asres
26 August	United States	Agronomist; Nobel Prize Laureate	Norman Borlaug
26 August	United States	Former President	James "Jimmy" Carter
30 August	Ethiopia	Prime Minister	Meles Zenawi Asres
3 September	Czech Republic	President	Václav Havel
12 October	China	Premier	Li Peng
13 October	China	Vice Premier	Zhu Rongji
October	Costa Rica	Former President and Nobel Prize Laureate	Óscar Arias Sánchez

APPENDIX 2

October	Jordan	Prince; Chairman of West Asia–North Africa Institute	Hassan bin Talal
October		Nobel Peace Prize Laureate	Fourteenth Dalai Lama
October	South Africa	Former President and Nobel Peace Prize Laureate	F. W. de Klerk
October	Australia	Foreign Minister	Gareth Evans
14 November	China	Premier	Li Peng
7 December	Sweden	Prime Minister	Göran Persson
1, 2 December	Ghana	President	Jerry Rawlings
1998			
10 February	Slovakia	President	Michal Kovac
13 March	United States	Former President	James "Jimmy" Carter
16 April	China	Premier	Zhu Rongji
20 April	South Korea	Prime Minister	Kim Chung-pil
22, 23 April	China (PRC)	Vice President of PRC	Hu Jintao
14 May	United Staates	First Lady	Hillary Rodham Clinton
14 May	Cuba	President of the Council of Ministers	Fidel Castro

14 May	Cote d'Ivoire	President	Henri Konan Bédié
2 June	Jordan	Prince	Hassan bin Talal
29 June	Peru	President	Alberto Fujimori
3 September	Palau	President	Kuniwo Nakamura
22 September	China	Minister of National Defense	Chi Haotian
10 October	Slovakia	President	Michal Kováč
13 October	Czech Republic	President	Václav Havel
13 October	United States	First Lady	Hillary Rodham Clinton
18 October	Burkina Faso	President	Blaise Compaoré
19 October	Ethiopia	Prime Minister	Meles Zenawi Asres
23 October	Tanzania	Prime Minister	Frederick Sumaye
11 November	Peru	President	Alberto Fujimori
1999			
31 January– 2 February	South Korea	Former President	Chun Doo-hwan
26 February	Cambodia	Prime Minister	Hun Sen
23 March	Malaysia	Prime Minister	Mahathir Mohamad

30 April	United States	President	William "Bill" Clinton
30 April	United States	First Lady	Hillary Rodham Clinton
4 May	Taiwan	President	Lee Teng-hui
5 May	Taiwan	Former Mayor of Taipei	Chen Shui-bian
18–20 May	Peru	President	Alberto Fujimori
10 October	Czech Republic	President	Václav Havel
10 October	United States	Author and Nobel Peace Prize Laureate	Elie Wiesel
10 October	South Africa	Former President, and Nobel Peace Prize Laureate	F. W. de Klerk
10 October	United States	Founder and Chair of Open Society Foundations	George Soros
12 October	South Africa	Former President	F. W. de Klerk
17 October	United States	Former President	James "Jimmy" Carter
15 October	Mali	President	Alpha Oumar Konaré
5 November	South Korea	Former President	Chun Doo-hwan
5 November	South Korea	President	Kim Tae-jung

1 December	Myanmar	Head of State	Than Shwe
2000			
25 March	Nigeria	President	Olusegun Obasanjo
20 May	Taiwan	President	Chen Shui-bian
7 June	Uganda	President	Yoweri Museveni
9 June	Laos	Prime Minister	Sisavath Keobounphanh
12 June	Ghana	President	Jerry Rawlings
10 July	Indonesia	President	Abdurrahman Wahid
1 September	Ghana	President	Jerry Rawlings
11 September	Romania	President	Emil Constantinescu
25 September	China	Vice President	Hu Jintao
15–18 October	Czech Republic	President	Václav Havel
15–18 October		Nobel Peace Prize Laureate	Fourteenth Dalai Lama
16 October	Israel	Foreign Minister	Shimon Peres
27 October	China	President	Jiang Zemin
21 November	Laos	Prime Minister	Sisavath Keobounphanh
2001			
January	India	Health Secretary	Prasada Rao

APPENDIX 2

January	India	West Bengal Minister of Health	Prof. Partha De
January	Indonesia	WHO Regional Director for Southeast Asia	Uton Muchtar Rafei
January	Ghana	Former President	Jerry Rawlings
8 February	Papua New Guinea	Former Prime Minister	Michael Somare
10 February	Palau	Former President	Kuniwo Nakamura
10 February	Fiji	Former President	Kamisese Mara
16 February	Mongolia	Prime Minister	Nambaryn Enkhbayar
17 February	Peru	Former President	Alberto Fujimori
16 May	Madagascar	Minister of Health	Henriette atsimbazafima-hefa (Rahantalalao)
21, 22 May	FR Yugoslavia	President	Vojislav Koštunica
May	India	Former President	Ramaswamy Venkataraman
May	India	Minister of Health	C. P. Thakur
May	Ghana	President	John Agyekum Kufuor

May	Ghana	Minister of Health	Kwaku Afriyie
May	Norway	WHO Director-General	Gro Harlem Brundtland
May	Brazil	Minister of Health	José Serra
May	Myanmar	Minister for Health	Kat Sein
May	Mozambique	Minister of Health	Francisco Songane
3 June	Ghana	President	John Agyekum Kufuor
4 June	Ghana	Former President	Jerry Rawlings
6, 7 June	United States	Former President	James "Jimmy" Carter
June	United States	Agronomist; Nobel Prize Laureate	Norman Borlaug
7 June	Uganda	President	Yoweri Kaguta Museveni
6 August	Malaysia	Prime Minister	Mahathir Bin Mohamad
31 August	Palau	Former Prime Minister	Kuniwo Nakamura
14 September	India	Former President	Ramaswamy Venkataraman
September	India	WHO Regional Director for Southeast Asia	Uton Muchtar Rafei

September	India	Minister of Health	C. P. Thakur
September	India	Maharashtra Minister of Health	Digvijay Khanvilkar
5 October	Czech Republic	President	Václav Havel
15 October	United States	President	William "Bill" Clinton
October	Iraq	Islamic scholar	Sheikh Mohammed Mohammed Ali
October	East Timor	Foreign Minister	José Ramos-Horta
October	Somalia	Supermodel	Waris Dirié
2002			
30 January	Brazil	President	Fernando Henrique Cardoso
13 February	Romania	President	Ion Iliescu
13 May	Latvia	President	Vaira Vike-Freiberga
13 May	Latvia	Prime Minister	Andris Bērziņš
16 May	Norway	WHO Director-General	Gro Harlem Brundtland
May	Myanmar	Minister for Health	Kat Sein
May	India	Minister of Health	C. P. Thakur

May	Mozambique	Minister of Health	Francisco Songane
May	Ghana	Minister of Health	Kwaku Afriyie
4 June	South Korea	Former President	Chun Doo-hwan
3 June	India	Minister of Health	C. P. Thakur
3 June	India	Director General of Health Services, Ministry of Health and Family Welfare	S. P. Agarwal
3 June	India	Bihar Minister of Health	Shakuni Choudhary
3 June	India	Chhattisgarh State Health Secretary	Alok Shukla
3 June	India	Jharkhand State Health Secretary	B. K. Chauhan
3 June	India	Madhya Pradesh Health Secretary	Alka Sirohi
3 June	India	West Bengal Principal Secretary	Ashim Kumar Barman
3 June	India	WHO Regional Director for Southeast Asia	Uton Muchtar Rafei
16 September	Mozambique	Prime Minister	Pascoal Mocumbi

APPENDIX 2

September	Mozambique	Minister of Health	Francisco Songane
16 October	The Vatican	Pope	John Paul II
18 October	Czech Republic	President	Václav Havel
19 October	Hong Kong	Former Governor	Christopher Patten
19 October	United States	Columbia University Professor, Economist	Jeffrey Sachs
19 October	South Africa	Former President	F. W. de Klerk
10 November	Papua New Guinea	Prime Minister	Michael Somore
12 November	Papua New Guinea	Governor General	Sir Silas Atopare
19 November	Philippines	Former President	Corazon Aquino
December	Bangladesh	Foreign Minister	Zillur Rahman
December	Bangladesh	Minister of Health	Khandaker Mosharraf Hossain
2003			
14 February	United States	Former President	James "Jimmy" Carter
17 February	Nicaragua	President	Enrique José Bolaños Geyer
February	Myanmar	Minister of Health	Kyaw Myint

February	Myanmar	First Secretary of State Peace and Development Council	Khin Nyunt
February	Myanmar	Executive Director of WHO Communicable Diseases Cluster	David Heymann
February	Indonesia	WHO Regional Director for Southeast Asia	Uton Muchtar Rafei
February	Nepal	Minister for Health, Science and Technology	Upendra Devkota
17 March	Palau	President	Thomas "Tommy" Remengesau Jr.
1 May	Myanmar	Chair of the State Peace and Development Council	Than Shwe
15 May	Papua New Guinea	Prime Minister	Michael Somare
3 June	Sweden	Prime Minister	Hans Göran Persson
2 July	Guyana	UN Deputy High Commissioner for Human Rights	Bertrand Ramcharan
July	India	Odisha Governor	M. M. Rajendran

July	South Korea	WHO Director-General	Lee Jong-wook
4, 5 September	United States	Former President	James "Jimmy" Carter
15 September	Madagascar	President	Marc Ravalomanana
15 September	Madagascar	Prime Minister	Jacques Sylla
28 September	Guinea	Prime Minister	Lamine Sidimé
28 September	Nigeria	President	Olusegun Obasanjo
28 September	Burkina Faso	President	Blaise Compaoré
28 September	Madagascar	President	Marc Ravalomanana
28 September	Mali	President	Amadou Toumani Touré
28 September	Mozambique	President	Joaquim Alberto Chissano
30 September	Ethiopia	Prime Minister	Meles Zenawi Asres
30 September	Senegal	President	Abdoulaye Wade
September	Angola	WHO Regional Director for Africa	Luis Gomes Sambo
2 October	Mongolia	President	Nambaryn Enkhbayar

6 October	Malawi	President	Bakili Muluzi
18 October	Czech Republic	Former President	Václav Havel
18 October	Jordan	Prince	Hassan bin Talal
18 October	South Africa	Former President	F. W. de Klerk
13 November	India	Minister for Health and Family Welfare	Sushma Swaraj
November	India	Chief Minister of Maharashtra	Sushilkumar Shinde
November	India	Governor of Maharashtra	Mohammed Fazal
November	India	Minister of Health of Maharashtra	Digvijay Khanvilkar
4 December	Cambodia	Prime Minister	Samdech Hun Sen
5 December	Cambodia	King	Norodom Sihanouk
December	Cambodia	Secretary of State for Health	Mam Bunheng
December	Cambodia	Minister of Health	Mam Bunheng
2004			
28 January	India	President	Abdul Kalam
29 January	India	Chief Minister of Chhattisgarh	Raman Singh

29 January	India	State Minister of Health of Chhattisgarh	Krishnamurti Bandhi
February 26	Nepal	Minister of Health	Bhekh Bahadur Thapa
8 March	China	Minister of National Defense	Cao Gang-chuan
26 March	Malta	President	Guido de Marco
23 April	South Korea	WHO Director-General	Lee Jong-wook
15 April	Nepal	Prime Minister	Surya Bahadur Thapa
15 April	Nepal	Minister of Health	Bhekh Bahadur Thapa
18 May	Jordan	Prime Minister	Faisal al Fayez
7 June	Bhutan	King	Jigme Singye Wangchuck
June	Bhutan	Prime Minister	Jigmi Y. Thinley
June	Thailand	WHO Regional Director for Southeast Asia	Samlee Plianbangchang
5 July	Brazil	President	Luiz Inácio "Lula" da Silva
29 July	Guyana	UN Acting High Commissioner for Human Rights	Bertrand Ramcharan

29 July	India	Chairman of UN Sub-Commission on the Promotion and Protection of Human Rights	Soli Sorabjee
26 August	India	Chief Minister of Bihar	Rabri Devi
26 August	India	Minister of Railways	Laloo Prasad Yadav
6 September	Russia	Primate of Russian Orthodox Church	Patriarch Alexy II of Moscow
September	India	Health Secretary	J. V. R. Prasada Rao
10 November	Canada	UN High Commissioner for Human Rights	Louise Arbour
December	India	Governor of Andhra Pradesh	Sushil Kumar Shinde
December	India	Chief Minister of Madhya Pradesh	Babulal Gaur
December	India	Governor of Madhya Pradesh	Balram Jakhar
December	India	Minister for Health	Gauri Shankar Shejwar
13 December	East Timor	President	Kay Rala Xanana Gusmão

2005			
27 January	India	Former President	Ramaswamy Venkataraman
27 January	India	Health Secretary for Delhi National Capital Territory	S. P. Aggarwal
31 January	South Africa	Minister of Health	Manto Tshabalala-Msimang
6 February	Madagascar	Prime Minister	Jacques Hugues Sylla
15 February	Papua New Guinea	Prime Minister	Michael Somare
February	Madagascar	Minister of Health	Jean-Louis Robinson
21 March	India	Prime Minister	Manmohan Singh
21 March	India	Minister of Health and Family Welfare	Anbumani Ramadoss
24 March	Cambodia	Prime Minister	Samdech Hun Sen
21 April	Mozambique	Minister of Health	Ivo Garrido
24 April	Tanzania	Minister of Health	Anna Abdallah
26 April	Tanzania	President	Benjamin Mkapa

April	Angola	WHO Regional Director for Africa	Luis Gomes Sambo
13 May	India	West Bengal Chief Minister	Buddhadeb Bhattacharjee
13 May	India	West Bengal Minister of Health	Surjya Kanta Mishra
15 May	India	Tamil Nadu Minister for Health and Family Welfare	Thiru N Thalavai Sundaram
May	Madagascar	President	Marc Ravalomanana
May	Madagascar	Prime Minister	Jacques Hugues Sylla
6 August	DRC	Minister of Health	Emile Bongeli Yeikelo Ya Ato
8 August	DRC	Vice President	Z'ahidi Ngoma
6 September	East Timor	President	Kay Rala Xanana Gusmão
20 September	East Timor	Minister of Health	Rui Maria de Araújo
20 September	India	Governor of West Bengal	Gopalkrishna Gandhi
20 September	India	West Bengal Minister of Health	Surjya Kanta Mishra
22 September	India	Governor of Bihar	Sardar Buta Singh

5 October	Peru	Former President	Alberto Fujimori
9, 10 October	Czech Republic	Former President	Václav Havel
10 October	Canada	Former Prime Minister	Kim Campbell
28 October	Benin	Former President	Nicéphore Soglo
October	Czech Republic	Former Deputy Prime Minister	Karel Schwarzenberg
1 December	Indonesia	Vice President	Jusuf Kalla
1 December	Indonesia	Minister of Health	Siti Fadilah Supari
December	India	Minister of Justice and Social Empowerment	Meira Kumar
December	India	AICC General Secretary	Oscar Fernandes
[Date unclear]	Malaysia	Former Deputy Prime Minister	Anwar Ibrahim
2006			
29 January	India	Former President	Ramaswamy Venkataraman
January	India	Former Chief Justice	Y. V. Chandrachud
27 February	Ethiopia	Prime Minister	Meles Zenawi Asres
8 March	Palau	Former President	Kuniwo Nakamura

26 April	India	Minister of Health	Anbumani Ramadoss
5 May	Philippines	Former President	Corazon Aquino
22 May	Papua New Guinea	Prime Minister	Michael Somare
25 May	Madagascar	Minister of Health	Jean-Louis Robinson
25 May	Tanzania	Minister of Health	Anna Abdallah
26 May	Nepal	Minister of Health and Population	Giriraj Pokharel
26 May	Myanmar	Minister for Health	Kyaw Myint
26 May	Thailand	WHO Regional Director for Southeast Asia	Samlee Plianbangchang
26 May	Argentina	WHO Regional Director for the Americas	Mirta Roses
26 May	Angola	WHO Regional Director for Africa	Luis Gomes Sambo
May	Jordan	Prince, Chairman of West Asia–North Africa (WANA) Institute	Hassan bin Talal
12 June	Brazil	Minister of Health	José Agenor Álvares da Silva

12 June	Brazil	Head of the Special Secretariat for Human Rights	Rogerio Sotille
June	Brazil	Vice President	Tião Viana
17 July	India	Delhi Chief Minister	Sheila Dikshit
1 August	Lesotho	Minister of Health and Social Welfare	Motloheloa Phooko
3 August	Angola	Minister of Health	Sebastião Veloso
3 August	Angola	WHO Regional Director for Africa	Luis Gomes Sambo
8 August	Mozambique	President	Armando Emílio Guebuza
8 August	Mozambique	Minister of Health	Ivo Garrido
14 September	India	Chhattisgarh Minister of Health	Krishnamurti Bandhi
14 September	India	Chhattisgarh Chief Minister	Raman Singh
15 September	India	President	Abdul Kalam
September	India	Odisha Minister of Health	Duryodhan Majhi
September	India	Odisha Minister for Woman and Child Development	Pramila Mallik

4 October	India	Vice President	Bhairon Singh Shekhawat
4 October	India	Delhi Chief Minister	Sheila Dikshit
9 October	Ireland	Former President	Mary Robinson
9 October	Czech Republic	Former President	Václav Havel
9 October	Republic of Latvia	President	Vaira Vike-Freiberga
9, 10 October		Nobel Peace Prize Laureate	Fourteenth Dalai Lama
31 October	Mali	President	Amadou Toumani Touré
8 October	United States	Author and Nobel Peace Prize Laureate	Elie Wiesel
8 October	Czech Republic	Mayor of Prague	Pavel Bém
8 October	Canada	Former Prime Minister	Kim Campbell
8 October		Nobel Peace Prize Laureate	Fourteenth Dalai Lama
8 October	United States	President of Carnegie Corporation	Vartan Gregorian
8 October	Ireland	Former President	Mary Robinson
8 October	Egypt	Former UN Secretary-General	Boutrus Boutrus-Ghali

8 October	Georgia	Speaker of Georgian Parliament	Nino Burjanadze
23 November	Laos	Prime Minister	Bouasone Bouphavanh
27 November	Nepal	King	Gyanendra Shah
29 November	Nepal	Prime Minister	Girija Prasad Koirala
29 November	Nepal	Former Prime Minister	Sher Bahadur Deuba
November	Nepal	Health and Population Minister	Amik Sherchan
2007			
23 January	Mozambique	President	Armando Emílio Guebuza
31 January	Sri Lanka	President	Mahinda Rajapaksa
January	Zanzibar	President	Amani Abeid Karume
January	Tanzania	Former Minister of Health	Anna Margareth Abdallah
January	DRC	Minister of Health	Victor Makwenge Kaput
12 January	East Timor	Minister of Health/Deputy Prime Minister of Social Affairs	Rui Maria de Araújo
13 February	Indonesia	Minister of Health	Siti Fadilah Supari

13 February	Indonesia	Chair of National Human Rights Commission	Abdul Hakim Garuda Nusantara
13 February	Indonesia	Coordinating Minister for People's Welfare	Aburizal Bakrie
28 February	Mongolia	President	Nambaryn Enkhbayar
7, 13, 14 March	Malaysia	Deputy Prime Minister	Najib Razak
12 April	India	Vice President	Bhairon Singh Shekhawat
3 May	Madagascar	President	Marc Ravalomanana
4 May	Madagascar	Minister of Health	Jean-Louis Robinson
7 May	Mozambique	Former President	Joaquim Chissano
7 May	Mozambique	Prime Minister	Luísa Dias Diogo
7 May	Mozambique	Minister of Health	Ivo Garrido
17 May	Brazil	Minister of Health	José Gomes Temporão
17 May	Nepal	Minister of Health	Govinda Raj Pokharel
17 May	Tanzania	Minister of Health	David Mwakyusa

APPENDIX 2

18 May	Angola	Minister of Health	Anastácio Artur Ruben Sicato
21, 23 August	Mongolia	President	Nambaryn Enkhbayar
19 September	Vietnam	President	Nguyen Minh Triet
September	Canada	UN High Commissioner for Human Rights	Louise Arbour
September	Denmark	Former WHO Director-General	Halfdan Mahler
10 October	India	President	A. P. J. Abdul Kalam
14 October	Nepal	Minister of Health	Govinda Raj Pokharel
19 October	Georgia	Prime Minister	Zurab Nogaideli
7 November	DRC	Minister of Health	Victor Makwenge Kaput
8 November	DRC	Prime Minister	Antoine Gizenga
8 November	DRC	Speaker of the National Assembly	Vital Kamerhe
13 November	Zanzibar	President	Abeid Karume
10 November		Nobel Peace Prize Laureate	Fourteenth Dalai Llama

2008			
4 February	Nepal	King	Gyanendra Shah
4 February	Nepal	Minister of Health and Population	Govinda Raj Pokharel
26 February	Israel	Prime Minister	Ehud Olmert
9 April	Marshall Islands	President	Litokwa Tomeing
21 May	Madagascar	Minister of Health	Jean-Louis Robinson
21 May	Mozambique	Minister of Health	Ivo Garrido
21 May	Brazil	Minister of Health	José Gomes Temporão
21 May	Nepal	Minister of Health	Govinda Raj Pokharel
21 May	DRC	Minister of Health	Victor Makwenge Kaput
21 May	Indonesia	Minister of Health	Siti Fadilah Supari
22 May	Philippines	Secretary of Health	Francisco Tiongson Duque
22 May	Romania	UN Human Rights Council President	Doru Costea
22 May	China	WHO Director-General	Margaret Chan

27 May	Ethiopia	Prime Minister	Meles Zenawi Asres
28 May	Mozambique	Former President	Joaquim Alberto Chissano
29 May	Niger	Prime Minister	Seyni Oumarou
30 May	Madagascar	President	Marc Ravalomanana
30 May	Mali	President	Amadou Toumani Touré
30 May	Mozambique	President	Armando Emílio Guebuza
3 June	Sweden	King	Carl XVI Gustaf
7 June	Switzerland	Former President	Ruth Dreifuss
19 June	Guinea	Minister of Health	Sangare Hadja Maimouna Bah
19 June	Guinea	Vice Foreign Minister	Mohamed II Cisse
20 June	Guinea	Prime Minister	Ahmed Tidiane Souaré
20 June	Guinea	President of the National Assembly	Aboubacar Somparé
8 August	Niger	Minister of Public Health	Issa Lamine
8 August	Niger	Minister of Population and Social Reforms	Zila Manane

9 August	Niger	Prime Minister	Seini Oumarou
13 August	DRC	Minister of Health	Victor Makwenge Kaput
13 August	DRC	Minister of State for Agriculture	Nzanga Mobutu
12 October	Czech Republic	Former President	Václav Havel
13 October	Iraq	Leader of the Islamic Supreme Council Iraq	Ammar Al-Hakim
13 October	UK	President, British Academy	Adam Roberts
15 October	Finland	Former President	Martti Ahtisaari
17 October	Mozambique	Former President	Joaquim Alberto Chissano
13 November	Costa Rica	President	Óscar Arias Sánchez
16 November	Peru	Former President	Alberto Fujimori
18 November	Brazil	President	Luiz Inácio "Lula" da Silva
18 November	Brazil	Minister of Health	José Gomes Temporão
2 December	Nepal	Prime Minister	Pushpa Kamal Dahal
2 December	Nepal	Minister of Health	Govinda Raj Pokharel

2009			
20 April	Finland	Former President	Martti Ahtisaari
21 April	Israel	President	Shimon Peres
24 April	Nepal	Minister of Health	Govinda Raj Pokharel
26 April	Nepal	Former King	Gyanendra Shah
21 May	Philippines	Secretary of Health	Francisco T. Duque III
21 May	Zambia	Minister of Health	Kapembwa Simbao
21 May	China	WHO Director-General	Margaret Chan
21 May	Thailand	WHO Regional Director for Southeast Asia	Samlee Plianbangchang
21 May	Argentina	WHO Regional Director for the Americas	Mirta Roses
21 May	Myanmar	Minister for Health	Dr. Kyaw Myint
21 May	Mozambique	Minister of Health	Ivo Garrido
22 May	South Africa	UN Commissioner for Human Rights	Navanethem Pillay
8 June	China	Minister for National Defense	Liang Guanglie

15 June	Thailand	Former Minister of Foreign Affairs, ASEAN Secretary-General	Surin Pitsuwan
1 July	Zambia	President	Rupiah Bwezani Banda
1 July	Zambia	Minister of Health	Kapembwa Simbao
2 July	Zambia	Former President	Kenneth Kaunda
6 July	Malaysia	Prime Minister	Najib Razak
17 July	Mongolia	Prime Minister	Sanjaagiin Bayar
2 September	Cambodia	Prime Minister	Samdech Hun Sen
21 September	Taiwan	Chairperson of the Democratic Progressive Party	Tsai Ing-wen
22 September	Taiwan	President	Ma Ying-jeou
30 September	United States	Former President	James "Jimmy" Carter
11 October	Czech Republic	Former President	Václav Havel
12 October	Czech Republic	Prime Minister	Jan Fischer
29 October	Philippines	Former President	Fidel Valdez Ramos
7 November	Myanmar	Prime Minister	Thein Sein

APPENDIX 2

2010			
19 January	Nepal	Prime Minister	Madhav Kumar
19 January	Nepal	President	Ram Baran Yadav
19 January	Nepal	Minister of Health	Uma Kanta Chaudhary
20 January	Nepal	Former King	Gyanendra
9 March	Ghana	Former President	Jerry Rawlings
11 March	Mozambique	Former President	Joaquim Alberto Chissano
11 March	Mozambique	Prime Minister	Aires Bonifácio Ali
11 March	Mozambique	Minister of Health	Ivo Garrido
16 March	East Timor	President	José Ramos-Horta
19 April	Papua New Guinea	Prime Minister	Michael Somare
19 April	Malaysia	Prime Minister	Najib Razak
3 May	Sri Lanka	Minister of Health	Maithripala Sirisena
7 May	Sri Lanka	President	Mahinda Rajapaksa
11 May	India	Bihar	Nand Kishore Yadav
19 May	Poland	Former President	Lech Wałęsa

19 May	East Timor	President	José Ramos-Horta
13 July	United States	Former President	James "Jimmy" Carter
13 July	Ethiopia	President	Girma Wolde-Giorgis
14 July	Ethiopia	Minister of Health	Tewodros Adhanom
19 July	Chad	Prime Minister	Emmanuel Nadingar
19 July	Chad	Minister of Health	Toupta Boguena
27 August	Japan	Former Prime Minister	Mori Yoshiro
30 August	Indonesia	Minister of Health	Endang Rahayu Sedyaningsih
31 August	Indonesia	Governor of South Sumatra	Alex Noerdin
10 October	Czech Republic	Former President	Václav Havel
October	Philippines	President	Benigno Aquino III
11 November	Palau	Former President	Kuniwo Nakamura
11 November	Palau	President	Johnson Toribiong
11 November	Micronesia	President	Emanuel "Manny" Mori
16 November	Mongolia	President	Tsakhiagiin Elbegdorj

23 November	Malaysia	Sultan	Mizan Zainal Abidin
16 December	Egypt	WHO Regional Director for Eastern Mediterranean	Dr. Hussein Gezairy
2011			
7 March	Serbia	President	Boris Tadić
26 April	Philippines	President	Benigno Aquino III
9 May	Jordan	Prince, Chairman of WANA Forum	Hassan bin Talal
9 May	Thailand	ASEAN Secretary-General	Surin Pitsuwan
13 May	Malawi	Minister of Health and Population	David Mphande
18 May	Myanmar	Minister for Health	Pe Thet Khin
18 May	Philippines	Secretary of the Department of Health	Enrique Tangonan Ona Jr.
18 May	Nepal	Minister of Health and Population	Shakti Bahadur Basnet
19 May	Malawi	Minister of Health and Population	David Mphande

19 May	Thailand	WHO Regional Director for Southeast Asia	Samlee Plianbangchang
20 May	Angola	WHO Regional Director for Africa	Luis Gomes Sambo
17 July	Central African Republic	Minister of Public Health, Population, and HIV/AIDS Prevention and Control	Jean Michel Mandaba
17 July	Central African Republic	Minister of Social Affairs	Marguerite Petro Koni Zeze
17 July	Central African Republic	Minister for Primary and Secondary Education	Gisèle Annie Nam
19 July	Central African Republic	President	Faustin-Archange Touadéra
19 July	Central African Republic	President of the National Assembly	Célestin Gaombalet
19, 20 July	Central African Republic	Prime Minister	Faustin Archange Touadéra
20 July	Central African Republic	Minister for Higher Education and Scientific Research	Jean Willybiro-Sako

20 July	Central African Republic	Minister for Primary, Secondary Education, and Literacy	Gisèle Annie Nam
20 July	Central Africa Republic	Minister for Technical, Vocational, and Skills Training	Djimrine Sall
22 September	India	Chhattisgarh Minister of Health	Amar Agrawal
23 September	India	Chhattisgarh Human Rights Commissioner	Y. K. S. Thakur
26 September	India	Governor of Andhra Pradesh	Ekkadu Srinivasan Laskshmi Narashimhan
27 September	India	Andhra Pradesh Minister of Social Welfare	Pithani Satyanarayana
27 September	India	Chair of Andhra Pradesh State Human Rights Commission	Kakumanu Peda Peri Reddy
29 September	India	Minister of Law and Justice	Salman Khurshid
September	India	Minister for Minor Irrigation	Sunitha Laxma Reddy
9 October	United States	Nobel Prize Laureate in Economic Sciences	Joseph Stiglitz

9 October	France	Philosopher	André Glucksmann
9 October	Russia	Economist and Politician	Grigory Yavlinsky
9 October	Ghana	Former President	John Agyekum Kufuor
9, 10 October	Czech Republic	Former President	Václav Havel
2 November	Nigeria	Former President	Olusegun Obasanjo
2 November	Mali	President	Amadou Toumani Touré
3 November	Benin	Former President	Nicéphore Soglo
5 November	Mali	Former Prime Minister	Modibo Sidibé
25 November	Burkina Faso	Minister of Health	Adama Traore
28 November	Brazil	Minister of Health	Alexandre Padilha
14 December	Myanmar	President	Thein Sein
13 December	Myanmar	Minister for Border Affairs	Thein Htay
13 December	Myanmar	Minister of Social Welfare, Relief, and Resettlement	Aung Kyi
13 December	Myanmar	General Secretary of the Union Solidarity and Development Party	Htay Oo

15 December	Myanmar	Minister of Foreign Affairs	Wunna Maung Lwin
19 December	Myanmar	Former Minister of Health	Kyaw Myint
19 December	Myanmar	General Secretary of the National League for Democracy; Nobel Peace Prize Laureate	Aung San Suu Kyi
December	Myanmar	Minister for Education	Mya Aye
2012			
19 January	East Timor	President	José Ramos-Horta
27 January	Peru	Former President	Alberto Fujimori
22 February	Mozambique	Prime Minister	Aires Bonifácio Ali
12 April	Bangladesh	Minister of Health and Family Welfare	A. F. M. Ruhal Haque
23 April	Myanmar	President	Thein Sein
22 May	Brazil	Vice Minister for Health Surveillance	Jarbas Barbosa
22 May	Philippines	Minister of Health	Enrique Tangonan Ona Jr.
22 May	South Korea	WHO Regional Director for the Western Pacific	Shin Young-soo

22 May	Myanmar	Minister for Health	Pe Thet Khin
22 May	China	WHO Director-General	Margaret Chan
24 May	Thailand	WHO Regional Director for Southeast Asia	Samlee Plianbangchang
14 June	Benin	Former President	Nicéphore Soglo
21 June	Antigua	Prime Minister	Winston Baldwin Spencer
21 June	Indonesia	President	Susilo Bambang Yudhoyono
21 June	Australia	Prime Minister	Julia Gillard
21 June	Granada	Prime Minister	Tillman Joseph Thomas
26 July	Myanmar	President	Thein Sein
28 July	Myanmar	General Secretary of the National League for Democracy; Nobel Peace Prize Laureate	Aung San Suu Kyi
27 August		Nobel Peace Prize Laureate	Fourteenth Dalai Llama
30 August	India	Chair of National Human Rights Commission of India	K. G. Balakrishnan

30 August	India	Chief Minister of Madhya Pradesh	Shivraj Singh Chouhan
August	India	Minister for Social Justice and Empowerment	Mukul Wasnik
August	India	Chief Minister of Delhi	Sheila Dikshit
August	Thailand	WHO Regional Director for Southeast Asia	Samlee Plianbangchang
August	India	Chairman of the Parliamentary Petition Committee on Integration and Empowerment of Persons Affected by Leprosy	Bhagat Singh Koshiyari
August	Hungary	WHO Regional Director for Europe	Zsuzsanna Jakab
17 September	Myanmar	General Secretary of the National League for Democracy; Nobel Peace Prize Laureate	Aung San Suu Kyi
September	Thailand	WHO Regional Director for Southeast Asia	Samlee Plianbangchang
September	India	Minister of Justice	Salman Khurshid

4 October	India	Minister for Justice and Social Empowerment	Mukul Wasnik
21 October	Nigeria	Former President	Olusegun Obasanjo
21 October	Benin	Former President	Nicéphore Soglo
21 October	Mauritius	Former President	Karl Offmann
28 November	East Timor	Former President	José Ramos-Horta
2013			
3 January	Myanmar	President	Thein Sein
1 March	Benin	President	Thomas Yayi Boni
21 May	Philippines	Minister of Health	Enrique Tangonan Ona Jr.
21 May	Sri Lanka	Minister of Health	Maithripala Sirisena
21 May	Angola	WHO Regional Director for Africa	Luis Gomes Sambo
22 May	Myanmar	Minister of Health	Pe Thet Khin
23 May	Indonesia	Minister of Health	Nafsiah Mboi
23 May	South Africa	UN High Commissioner for Human Rights	Navanethem Pillay

23 May	Ethiopia	Minister of Health	Kesetebirhan Admasu Birhane
23 May	Tanzania	Minister of Health	Hussein Ali Hassan Mwinyi
23 May	China	WHO Director-General	Margaret Chan
23 May	South Korea	WHO Regional Director for the Western Pacific	Shin Young-soo
23 May	Dominica	WHO Regional Director for the Americas	Carissa F. Etienne
26 May	Myanmar	President	Thein Sein
May	Japan	Prime Minister	Abe Shinzo
2 June	Thailand	WHO Regional Director for South-East Asia	Samlee Plianbangchang
2 June	Uganda	President	Yoweri Kaguta Museveni
2 June	Ethiopia	Prime Minister	Hailemariam Desalegn Boshe
2 June	Ghana	President	John Dramani Mahama
2 June	Benin	President	Thomas Yayi Boni
2 June	Mozambique	President	Armando Emilio Guebuza
2 June	Nigeria	Vice President	Namadi Sambo

11 June	Palestinian National Authority	Prime Minister	Rami Hamdallah
4 July	Uzbekistan	Deputy Minister of Health	Alimov Anvar
24 July	Thailand	WHO Regional Director for Southeast Asia	Samlee Plianbangchang
26 July	DRC	Minister of Health	Shodu Lomami Kalema
26 July	Madagascar	Minister of Health	Johanita Ndahimanajara
26 July	Mozambique	Minister of Health	Alexandre Manguele
26 July	Tanzania	Minister of Health	Hussein Ali Hassan Mwinyi
26 July	Bangladesh	Minister of Health and Welfare	A. F. M. Ruhal Haque
26 July	Myanmar	Minister of Health	Pe Thet Kin
26 July	Nepal	Minister of Health	Vidyadhar Malik
26 July	Sri Lanka	Minister of Health	Maithripala Sirisena
August	India	Principal Secretary of Health	Keshav Desiraju
August	India	Union Minister of State, Social Justice, and Empowerment	Balram Naik

August	India	Minister of Petroleum and Natural Gas	Ram Naik
August	India	Former Minister of Railways	Dinesh Trivedi
August	India	Chair Human Rights Commission of India	K. G. Balakrishnan
16 September	Belgium	Princess	Princess Astrid of Belgium
18 September	Ethiopia	Prime Minister	Hailemariam Desalegn Boshe
18 September	Ethiopia	Minister of Health	Kesetebirhan Admasu Birhane
23 September	India	Former Minister of Railways	Dinesh Trivedi
23 September	India	West Bengal Minister for Agriculture	Moloy Ghatak
24 September	India	West Bengal Minister for Health and Family Welfare	Chandrima Bhattacharya
24 September	India	West Bengal Human Rights Commission Chair	Justice Asok Kumar Ganguly
8 October	Serbia	President	Tomislav Nikolić

23 October	India	Uttar Pradesh Governor	Banwari Lal Joshi
23 October	India	Uttar Pradesh Minister for Health and Welfare	Ahmad Hassan
25 November	Myanmar	General Secretary of the National League for Democracy; Nobel Peace Prize Laureate	Aung San Suu Kyi
2, 3 December	Palau	President	Thomas Esang Remengesau Jr.
15, 16 December	Myanmar	President	Thein Sein
18 December	Brazil	Minister of Health	Alexandre Padilha
18 December	Brazil	Minister of Human Rights	Maria do Rosário Nunes
20 December	Brazil	Governor of the Brazilian State of Pará	Simão Robson Oliveira Jatene
20 December	Brazil	Pará State Minister of Health	Helio Franco
2014			
27 January	Indonesia	Minister of Health	Nafsiah Mboi
27 January	Indonesia	Minister for People's Welfare	Agung Laksono

27 January	Jordan	Commissioner-General for the National Centre for Human Rights	Mousa Burayzat
27 January	India	Chair of National Human Rights Commission of India	K. G. Balakrishnan
13 February	Marshall Islands	President	Christopher Jorebon Loeak
12 March	Somalia	President	Xasan Sheekh Maxamuud
20 March		Nobel Peace Prize Laureate	Fourteenth Dalai Lama
23 March	Nepal	Minister of Health and Population	Khagaraj Adhikari
23 March	Nepal	Former Prime Minister	Pushpa Kamal Dahal
25 March	Nepal	Prime Minister	Sushil Prasad Koirala
25 March	Nepal	President	Ram Baran Yadav
16 April	Mongolia	President	Tsakhiagiin Elbegdorj
3 May	Sri Lanka	President	Mahinda Rajapaksa
13 May	Israel	Prime Minister	Benjamin Netanyahu

20 May	Myanmar	Minister for Health	Pe Thet Khin
20 May	DRC	Minister of Health	Felix Kabange Numbi
20 May	Mozambique	Minister of Health	Alexandre Manguele
20 May	Angola	WHO Regional Director for Africa	Luis Gomes Sambo
20 May	India	WHO Regional Director for Southeast Asia	Poonam Khetrapal Singh
20 May	Angola	Minister of Health	Jose Van-Dúnem
20 May	Philippines	Minister of Health	Enrique Tangonan Ona Jr.
21 May	South Korea	WHO Regional Director for the Western Pacific	Shin Young-soo
21 May	Tanzania	Minister of Health and Social Welfare	Seif Seleman Rashidi
22 May	Sri Lanka	Minister of Health	Maijhareepala Sirisena
22 May	China	WHO Director-General	Margaret Chan
22 May	Dominica	WHO Regional Director for the Americas	Carissa F. Etienne

22 May	Iraq	WHO Regional Director for Eastern Mediterranean Region	Ala Alwan
11 June	Israel	President	Shimon Peres
12 June	Palestinian National Authority	President	Mahmoud Abbas
10 July	Uganda	Vice President	Edward Ssekandi
2 September	India	Prime Minister	Narendra Modi
2, 3 October	UK	Former Prime Minister	Sir John Major
7 October	Myanmar	President	Thein Sein
24 October	Georgia	President	Giorgi Margvelashvili
12 November	Myanmar	President	Thein Sein
12 November		Nobel Peace Prize Laureate	Fourteenth Dalai Lama
24 November	India	Prime Minister	Narendra Modi
16, 17 December	Palau	President	Thomas Esang Remengesau Jr.
2015			
28 January	Japan	Emperor	Akihito
28 January	Japan	Empress	Michiko
29 January	East Timor	Former President	José Ramos-Horta

3 February	Myanmar	President	Thein Sein
17 March	Micronesia	President	Emmanuel "Manny" Mori
18 March	Kiribati	President	Anote Tong
3 April	Ethiopia	Minister of Health	Kesetebirhan Admasu
8 April	DRC	Vice President	Victor Makwenge Kaput
7 May	Papua New Guinea	Former Prime Minister	Michael Somare
20 May	Madagascar	Minister of Health	Mamy Lalatiana Andriamanarivo
20 May	South Korea	WHO Regional Director for the Western Pacific	Shin Young-soo
20 May	Indonesia	Minister of Health	Nila F. Moeloek
20 May	DRC	Minister of Health	Felix Kabange Numbi
21 May	Myanmar	Minister for Health	Than Aung
21 May	Mozambique	Minister of Health	Nazira Abdula
21 May	India	Minister of Health	J. P. Nadda
21 May	Botswana	WHO Regional Director for Africa	Matshidio Moeti

APPENDIX 2

21 May	Kiribati	President	Anote Tong
25 May	Malaysia	Prime Minister	Najib Razak
25 May	Mongolia	President	Tsakhiagiin Elbegdorj
May	Mozambique	Vice President	Mouzinho Saide
May	India	WHO Regional Director of Southeast Asia	Poonam Khetrapal Singh
May	Indonesia	Minister of Health	Rasuna Said
4 June	Philippines	President	Benigno Simeon Cojuangco Aquino III
20 June	East Timor	Former President	José Ramos-Horta
3 July	Cambodia	Prime Minister	Samdech Hun Sen
3 July	Thailand	Prime Minister	Prayuth Chan-ocha
3 July	Vietnam	Prime Minister	Nguyen Tan Dung
3 July	Laos	Prime Minister	Thongsing Thammavong
3, 4 July	Myanmar	President	Thein Sein
7 July	Myanmar	President	Thein Sein
9 July	Sri Lanka	President	Maithripala Yapa Sirisena

6 August	Brazil	Minister of Health	Arthur Chioro
21 September	Myanmar	President	Thein Sein
23 September	Myanmar	State Counsellor; Nobel Peace Prize Laureate	Aung San Suu Kyi
21 October	Kiribati	President	Anote Tong
23 October	Fiji	Chief Justice	Anthony Gates
23 October	Fiji	Minister of Health	Jone Usamate
23 October	Fiji	First Lady	Adi Koila Mara Nailatikau
7 November	Ireland	Former President	Mary Robinson
19 November	Nepal	President	Thein Sein
2016			
2 January	Myanmar	President	Thein Sein
17 January	Taiwan	President	Ma Ying-jeou
17 January	Taiwan	Chairperson of the Democratic Progressive Party	Cai Ying-win
3 February	United States	Former President	James "Jimmy" Carter
26 February	Palau	President	Thomas Esang Remengesau Jr.
26 February	Marshall Islands	President	Hilda Heine

26 February	Micronesia	President	Peter Martin Christian
29 March	Slovenia	Former President	Danilo Türk
12 May	India	WHO Regional Director for Southeast Asia	Poonam Khetrapal Singh
12 May	India	WHO Representative to India	Henk Bekedam
19 May	Taiwan	Former President	Lee Teng-hui
20 May	Taiwan	President	Tsai Ing-wen
25 May	DRC	Minister of Health	Felix Kabange Numbi
25 May	Ethiopia	Minister of Health	Kesetebirhan Admasu
26 May	Mozambique	Minister of Health	Nazira Karimo Vali Abdula
26 May	Myanmar	Minister of Health	Myint Htwe
6 June	Bulgaria	Rector of Sofia University	Anastas Gerdjikov
8 June	The Vatican	Head of the Catholic Church	Pope Francis [John Paul II]
11 June	Nigeria	Former Chairperson of the UN Human Rights Council Advisory Committee	Obiora Chinedu Okafor

11 June	Brazil	President of the International Leprosy Association	Marcos Virmond
15 June	Monaco	Prince	Albert II
5 July	Cameroon	Minister of Health	André Mama Omgba Fouda
5 July	Botswana	WHO Regional Director for Africa	Matshidiso Rebecca Moeti
5 July	Cameroon	WHO Representative to Cameroon	Jean-Baptiste Roungou
6 July	Cameroon	Governor of the East Region	Gregoire Mvongo
19 July	Kiribati	President	Anote Tong
19 July	Palau	President	Thomas Esang Remengesau Jr.
26, 27 August	Benin	Former President	Nicéphore Soglo
27 August	Mali	President	Ibrahim Boubacar Keita
31 August	Myanmar	State Counsellor; Nobel Peace Prize Laureate	Aung San Suu Kyi
18 October	Peru	Former President	Alberto Fujimori
26 October	India	Speaker of the Lower House	Sumitra Mahajan

26 October	Bangladesh	President of Inter-Parliamentary Union	Saber Hossain Chowdhury
2 November	Myanmar	State Counsellor; Nobel Peace Prize Laureate	Aung San Suu Kyi
7 November	Kazakhstan	President	Nursultan Nazarbayev
11 November	India	Prime Minister	Narendra Modi
20 November	India	Former Minister of Railways	Dinesh Trivedi
20 November	India	Chair of Disabled Peoples' International (DPI)	Javed Abidi
21 November	India	Speaker of the Lower House	Sumitra Mahajan
21 November	India	WHO Representative to India	Henk Bekedam
15 December	India	Minister of Health	Nila Farid Moeloek
15 December	Indonesia	WHO Representative to Indonesia	Jihane Tawilah
2017			
29 January	India	Minister of Social Justice and Empowerment	Thawar Chand Gehlot

30 January	Bangladesh	President of Inter-Parliamentary Union	Saber Hossain Chowdhury
1 February	India	Chhattisgarh Minister Secretary of Sports and Social Welfare Department, Chhattisgarh	Sonmoni Borah
1 February	India	Chhattisgarh State Minister of Health	Ajay Chandrakar
3 February	India	Chhattisgarh State Minister for Women and Child Development	Ramshila Sahu
17 February	Myanmar	President	Thein Sein
February	India	Minister of Social Justice and Empowerment	Thawar Chand Gehlot
February	India	Deputy Director General (Leprosy) at the Minister of Health and Family Welfare	Anil Kumar
18 March	India	Odisha State Minister of Health and Welfare	Pramod Kumar Meherda

18 March	India	Odisha State Human Rights Commission Chair	B. K. Mishra
20 March	India	Odisha State Commissioner for Persons with Disabilities	Minati Behera
20 March	India	Odisha State Chief Minister	Naveen Patnaik
21 March	India	Odisha State Governor	S. C. Jamir
21 March	India	Deputy Director General (Leprosy) at the Minister of Health and Family Welfare	Anil Kumar
March	India	WHO Representative to India	Henk Bekedam
March	India	WHO Representative to India	Saurabh Jain
19 April	China	WHO Director-General	Margaret Chan
20 April	Ghana	Former UN Secretary-General	Kofi Annan
20 April	United States	Former Vice President; Ambassador to Japan	Walter Mondale

25 April	United States	University of Minnesota Provost	Karen Hanson
25 May	Myanmar	Minister of Health	Myint Htwe
25 May	India	WHO Regional Director for Southeast Asia	Poonam Khetrapal Singh
25 May	South Korea	WHO Regional Director for the Western Pacific	Shin Young-soo
25 May	Mexico	Assistant Director of the Pan American Health Organization and WHO Regional Office for the Americas	Francisco Becerra
26 May	Nepal	WHO Representative to Nepal	Jos Vandelaer
26 May	Ethiopia	WHO Incumbent Director-General	Tedros Adhanom Ghebreyesus
26 May	China	WHO Director-General	Margaret Chan
26 May	Mongolia	Minister of Health	A. Tsogtsetseg
7 June	Kiribati	President	Anote Tong

7 June	Palau	President	Thomas Esang Remengesau Jr.
7 June	Fiji	Prime Minister	Josaie Voreqe Bainimarama
8 June	Fiji	President	Jioji Konrote
3 July	India	DPI Representative	Javed Abidi
4 July	India	Minister of Health and Family Welfare	Jagat Prakash Nadda
24 July	Indonesia	North Sulawesi Governor	Olly Dondokambey
15 September	Palau	President	Thomas Esang Remengesau Jr.
21 September	Tunisia	President of the National Order of Lawyers; Nobel Peace Prize Laureate	Mohamed Fadhel Mahfoudh
21 September	Tunisia	President of the Tunisian League of Human Rights; Nobel Peace Prize Laureate	Abdessattar Ben Moussa
21, 25 September	Tunisia	Secretary General, General Union of Tunisian Workers; Nobel Peace Prize Laureate	Hassine Abassi

22 September	Tunisia	WHO Representative to Tunisia	Yves Souteyrand
24 September	Tunisia	Minister of Culture	Mohamed Zine Elabidine
25 September	Tunisia	President	Beji Caid Essebsi
25 September	Tunisia	Minister of Social Affairs	Mohamed Trabelsi
September	Tunisia	Former Foreign Minister	Habib Beh Yahia
23 October	Georgia	President	Giorgi Margvelashvili
23 October	Georgia	Prime Minister	Giorgi Kvirikashvili
15 November	Indonesia	Governor of Jakarta	Anies Baswedan
15 November	Indonesia	Vice President	Jusuf Kalla
6 December	India	International Chamber of Commerce Chair	Sunil Bharti Mittal
7 December	India	Minister of Health and Welfare	Jagat Prakash Nadda
14–16 December	Myanmar	President	Htin Kyaw
2018			
29 January	India	Minister of Culture	Mahesh Sharma

30 January	India	President	Ram Nath Kovind
1 February	India	Jharkhand State Minister of Health	Ramchandra Chandravanshi
1 February	India	Jharkhand State Minister for Minority Welfare, Social Welfare, and Women and Child Development	Louis Marandi
1 February	India	Jharkhand Prime Minister	Raghubar Das
8, 9 February	Iceland	Former President	Ólafur Ragnar Grimsson
14 March	Sri Lanka	President	Maithripala Yapa Sirisena
21 March	Indonesia	Governor of Central Sulawesi	Longki Djanggola
23 March	Singapore	President	Halimah Yacob
25 March	Ireland	Former President	Mary Robinson
13 April	Palau	President	Thomas Esang Remengesau
25 April	Sweden	King	Carl XVI Gustaf
April	India	Nobel Peace Prize Laureate	Kailash Satyarthi

15 May	South Korea	Former Prime Minister	Kim Chong-pil
16 May	Fiji	Prime Minister	Josaia Vorque Bainimarama
18 May	Kiribati	President	Taneti Mamau
18 May	Solomon Islands	Prime Minister	Rick Houenipwela
18 May	Tuvalu	Prime Minister	Enele Sosene Sopoaga
18 May	Nauru	President	Baron Waqa
18 May	Palau	President	Thomas Esang Remengesau Jr.
18 May	Marshall Islands	President	Hilda Heine
22 May	Kiribati	Minister of Health	Tauanei Marea
22 May	Palau	Minister of Health	Emais Roberts
12 May	Myanmar	Minister of Health	Myint Htwe
22 May	Mongolia	Minister of Health	Tsogtsetseg Ayush
22 May	India	Minister of Health and Family Welfare	Jagat Prakash Nadda
22 May	Marshall Islands	Minister of Health	Kalami Kaneko
22 May	Nepal	Minister of State for Health and Population	Padma Kumari Aryal

22 May	Comoros	Minister of Health	Rashid Mohamed Mbarak Fatma
23 May	Vanuatu	Minister of Health	Norris Jack Kalmet
23 May	Tonga	Minister of Health	Saia Ma'u Piukala
23 May	Ethiopia	Minister of Health	Tedros Adhanom
24 May	Nigeria	Minister of Health	Osagie Ehanire
24 May	India	WHO Regional Director for Southeast Asia	Poonam Khetrapal Singh
7 June	Taiwan	President	Tsai Ing-wen
16 June	Jordan	UN High Commissioner for Human Rights	Zeid Ra'ad Al Hussein
16 June	Portugal	UN Special Rapporteur on the Elimination of Discrimination against Persons Affected by Leprosy and Their Family Members	Alice Cruz
June	Myanmar	Minister for the Office of State Counsellor of Myanmar	Kyaw Ting Swe

11 July	Myanmar	State Counsellor; Nobel Peace Prize Laureate	Aung San Suu Kyi
22 July	Comoros	Minister of Health	Rashid Mohamed Mbarak Fatma
22, 23 July	Comoros	President	Azali Assoumani
27 July	Mozambique	Former President	Joaquim Alberto Chissano
30 July	Malta	Prime Minister	Joseph Muscat
July	Comoros	Foreign Minister	Mohamed El-Alime Souef
July	Mozambique	WHO Representative to Mozambique	Khady Cabral
July	Mozambique	Minister of Health	Nazila Vali Abdula
July	Mozambique	Governor of Nampula Province	Victor Borges
29 August	Comoros	President	Azali Assoumani
30 August– 1 September	Tanzania	Former President	Benjamin Mkapa
30 August– 1 September	Nigeria	Former President	Olusegun Obasanjo
30 August– 1 September	Benin	Former President	Nicéphore Soglo

30 August, 1 September	South Africa	Former President	Thabo Mvuyelwa Mbeki
30 August, 1 September	Mozambique	Former President	Joaquim Alberto Chissano
31 August	Burkina Faso	President	Roch Marc Christian Kaboré
2 October	Indonesia	Deputy Minister for Health Improvement	Sigit Priohutomo
4 October	Indonesia	Governor of Maluku	Said Assagaff
8, 9 October	Myanmar	State Counsellor of Myanmar; Nobel Peace Prize Laureate	Aung San Suu Kyi
19 November	Burkina Faso	President	Roch Marc Christian Kaboré
26 November	East Timor	Former President	José Ramos-Horta
3 December	Jordan	Prince	Ali bin al-Hussein
12 December	Myanmar	Former President	Thein Sein
12 December	Myanmar	State Counsellor; Nobel Peace Prize Laureate	Aung San Suu Kyi

December	Myanmar	Minister of Health	Myint Htwe
December	Myanmar	State Counsellor of Myanmar	Kyaw Tint Swe
December	Myanmar	Minister for Welfare	Win Myat Age
2019			
18 January	Palau	President	Thomas Esang Remengesau Jr.
29 January	India	Director General of the Indian Coast Guard	Rajendra Singh
30 January	India	Minister of Law and Justice	Ravi Shankar Prasad
January	India	Minister of Health and Family Welfare	Jagat Prakash Nadda
January	India	Minister of Social Justice and Empowerment	Thawar Chand Gehlot
2 February	India	Andhra Pradesh State Chief Minister	Nara Chandrababu Naidu
10 February	Bangladesh	WHO Representative to Bangladesh	Bardan Jung Rana
10 February	Bangladesh	Prime Minister	Sheik Hasina Wazed
10 February	Bangladesh	Minister of Health	Zahid Maleque

11 February	Bangladesh	Speaker of the National Parliament	Shirin Sharmin Chaudhury
26 February	India	Prime Minister	Narendra Modi
26 February	India	President	Ram Nath Kovind
28 February	Portugal	UN Secretary-General	Antonio Manuel De Oliveira Guterres
25 March	Myanmar	State Counsellor; Nobel Peace Prize Laureate	Aung San Suu Kyi
26 March	Switzerland	UN Special Envoy on Myanmar	Christine Schreiner Bergner
23 April	Marshall Islands	President	Hilda Heine
23, 24 April	Marshall Islands	Minister of Health and Human Services	Kalani Kaneko
24 April	Marshall Islands	Minister of Foreign Affairs and Trade	John Silk
April	Marshall Islands	Minister of Finance	Brenson Wase
April	Marshall Islands	Minister of Transportation, Communication, and Information of Technology	Jack Ading

April	Marshall Islands	Minister for Works, Utilities, and Infrastructure	Tony Muller
April	Marshall Islands	Minister of Education	Wilbur Heine
18 June	Finland	Former President	Tarja Kaarina Halonen
1 July	Brazil	Minister of Health	Luiz Henrique Mandetta
1 July	Brazil	Minister of Citizenship	Osmar Terra
1 July	Brazil	General Secretary of the National Conference of Bishop of Brazil; Assistant Bishop of Rio de Janeiro	Dom Joel Portela Amado
2, 3 July	Brazil	Pará State Governor	Helder Barbalho
4, 5 July	Brazil	Maranhão State Governor	Flavio Dino
8 July	Brazil	Minister of Family, Women and Human Rights	Damares Alves
8 July	Brazil	President	Jair Messias Bolsonaro
8 July	Brazil	President of the Human Rights and Minorities Committee	Helder Salomão

9 July	Brazil	Chairman of Social Affairs and Family Committee	Antonio Brito
10 July	Colombia	WHO Representative to Brazil	Socorro Gross Galiano
29 July	Palau	President	Thomas Esang Remengesau Jr.
29 August	Ghana	President	Nana Addo Kankwa Akufo-Addo
29 August	Comoros	President	Azali Assoumani
29 August	Sierra Leone	President	Julius Maada Bio
29 August	Burkina Faso	President	Roch Marc Christian Kaboré
29 August	Mali	President	Ibrahim Boubacar Keita
29 August	Mozambique	Former President	Joaquim Alberto Chissano
30 August	Uganda	President	Yoweri Kaguta Museveni
30 August	Ethiopia	Prime Minister	Abiy Ahmed
9 September	Philippines	Minister of Health	Francisco T. Duque
11 September	The Netherlands	International Federation for the Liberation of Anti-Leprosy Associations (ILEP) President	Jan van Berkel

24 October	Norway	Prime Minister	Erna Solberg
24 October	Norway	Crown Prince	Haakon Magnus
24 October	Palau	President	Thomas Esang Remengesau Jr.
29 October	Ireland	Former President	Enda Kennedy
5 November	Japan	Emperor	Naruhito
5 November	Japan	Empress	Masako
12 November	Palau	President	Thomas Esang Remengesau Jr.
14 November	Micronesia	President	David W. Panuelo
11 December	Bangladesh	Prime Minister	Sheik Hasina Wazed
2020			
12 March	Taiwan	President	Tsai Ing-wen
10 November	Myanmar	Commander-in-Chief of the Armed Forces	Min Aung Hlaing
10 November	Myanmar	State Counsellor; Nobel Peace Prize Laureate	Aung San Suu Kyi
10 November	Myanmar	Union Minister for the Office of the State Counsellor	Kyaw Tint Swe
3 December	Myanmar	State Counsellor; Nobel Peace Prize Laureate	Aung San Suu Kyi

3 December	Myanmar	Union Minister of Union Government	Min Thu

INDEX OF COUNTRIES VISITED

Chile [The Republic of Chile]

China [The People's Republic of China]

Colombia [The Republic of Colombia]

Comoros, The [The Union of the Comoros]

Costa Rica [The Republic of Costa Rica]

Côte d'Ivoire [The Republic of Côte d'Ivoire]

Cuba [The Republic of Cuba]

Czech Republic

Denmark

DRC [The Democratic Republic of the Congo]

East Timor [The Democratic Republic of Timor-Leste]

Ecuador [The Republic of Ecuador]

El Salvador [The Republic of El Salvador]

Equatorial Guinea [The Republic of Equatorial Guinea]

Ethiopia [The Federal Democratic Republic of Ethiopia]

Fiji [The Republic of Fiji]

Finland [The Republic of Finland]

France [The French Republic]

Georgia

Germany [The Federal Republic of Germany]

Ghana [The Republic of Ghana]

Greece [The Hellenic Republic]

Guinea [The Republic of Guinea]

Honduras [The Republic of Honduras]

Hong Kong Special Administrative Region of the People's Republic of China

Hungary

Iceland

India [The Republic of India]

Indonesia [The Republic of Indonesia]

Iran [The Islamic Republic of Iran]

Norway [The Kingdom of Norway]

Palau [The Republic of Palau]

Palestine

Papua New Guinea [The Independent State of Papua New Guinea]

Peru [The Republic of Peru]

Philippines [The Republic of the Philippines]

Poland [The Republic of Poland]

Portugal [The Portuguese Republic]

Republic of the Congo

Romania

Russia [The Russian Federation]

Serbia [The Republic of Serbia]

Singapore [The Republic of Singapore]

Slovakia [The Slovak Republic]

South Africa [The Republic of South Africa]

South Korea [Republic of Korea]

Spain [The Kingdom of Spain]

Sri Lanka [The Democratic Socialist Republic of Sri Lanka]

Sudan [The Republic of the Sudan]

Sweden [The Kingdom of Sweden]

Switzerland [The Swiss Confederation]

Taiwan [The Republic of China]

Tajikistan [The Republic of Tajikistan]

Tanzania [The United Republic of Tanzania]

Thailand [The Kingdom of Thailand]

Togo [The Togolese Republic]

Tunisia [The Republic of Tunisia]

Turkey [The Republic of Turkey]

Uganda [The Republic of Uganda]

UK [The United Kingdom of Great Britain and Northern Ireland]

INDEX OF COUNTRIES VISITED

AWARDS AND HONORS

December 2019: Fuji Sankei Communications Group Seiron Taisho Award

November 2019: Jürgen Palm Prize (TAFISA, Association for International Sports for All)

November 2019: Person of Cultural Merit

May 2019: Grand Cordon of the Order of the Rising Sun, Japan

January 2019: Gandhi Peace Prize (awarded in 2018)

April 2018: Honorary Citizenship of the Republic of Palau

April 2018: The Royal Order of Monisaraphon Knight Grand Cross, Cambodia

June 2017: Ocean's 8 Award, the Intergovernmental Oceanographic Commission of UNESCO

May 2017: Health and Human Rights Award (International Council of Nurses)

May 2017: Plus Ratio Quam Vis Medal (Jagiellonian University, Poland)

April 2017: Health for All Gold Medal (WHO)

June 2016: The Award of Distinction of the President of Bulgarian Academy of Sciences

July 2015: International Maritime Prize (IMO) (awarded in 2014)

October 2014: The Rule of Law Award (International Bar Association)

February 2013: Gold Medal for Merits (Republic of Serbia)

January 2013: Friendship Medal (Socialist Republic of Vietnam)

November 2011: Grand Cross of the Royal Order of Sahametrei (Cambodia)

July 2011: Commander of the Order of Recognition (Central African Republic)

November 2010: Commander of the Order of the Defender of the Realm (Paglima Mangku Negara) Tan Sri (Malaysia)

September 2010: Commander of the Royal Norwegian Order of Merit (Norway)

July 2010: Ethiopian Millennium Gold Medal (Ethiopia)

July 2010: Commander First Class of the Royal Order of the Polar Star (Sweden)

May 2010: Order of Timor-Leste (East Timor)

April 2010: The Grand Cross of the Order of the Falcon with Star (Iceland)

April 2010: Knight of the Order of the Dannebrog (Denmark)

April 2010: Dr. Norman E. Borlaug Medallion

February 2010: Commander of the Order of the White Rose of Finland (Finland)

January 2010: The Patriarch's Chart of the Patriarch of Moscow and All Russia Kirill

January 2010: The Diploma of an Academician of the Russian Academy of Natural Sciences

May 2009: Science for Society Award (Hungary Academy of Sciences)

April 2007: International Gandhi Award (awarded in 2006)

February 2007: Order of the Pole Star (Mongolia)

January 2007: Coast Guard Legion of Honor (Philippines)

October 2006: Commander of the National Order of Mali

October 2004: Yomiuri International Cooperation Prize (Japan)

December 2003: Commandeur de l'Ordre Royal du Muniseraphon (Cambodia)

November 2003: National Construction Medal (Cambodia)

September 2003: Officer of the National Order of Madagascar (Republic of Madagascar)

June 2003: The Special Award (Word Maritime University, Sweden)

October 2001: Václav Havel Memorial Medal (Czech Republic)

September 2001: Millennium Gandhi Award (International Leprosy Union)

September 2001: Grand Officer of the Order for Merit (Romania)

September 2000: International Green Pen Award for Pacific Environmental Journalism (Fiji)

May 2000: Decerne la Medaille d'Honneur de Menerbes (France)

June 1998: Al Hussein Bin Ali Decoration for Accomplishment, First Degree (Jordan)

May 1998: WHO Health for All Gold Medal (World Health Organization)

December 1997: China Health Medal (Republic of China)

October 1996: Francysk Skaryna Medal (Belarus)

October 1996: Order of Merit Third Class (Ukraine)

June 1996: Order of Friendship (Russian Federation)

February 1996 Inca Golds Award (Peru)

February 1996: Commander of the Order of Merit for Distinguished Service (Peru)

August 1995: Order of the Grand Star of Djibouti (Republic of Djibouti)

January 1989: Grand Officer of the Order of Mono (Togo)

HONORARY DEGREES

2019   Doctor of Humanities, Ateneo de Manila University, Philippines

2018   Honorary Doctor, Institute of Engineering and Technology, Mongolia

2018   Advisory Professor, Jilin University, China

2017   Doctor of Law, University of Minnesota, United States

2016   Doctor Honoris Causa, Sofia University, Bulgaria

2013   Honorary Degree of the Doctor of the University, University of York, United Kingdom

2012   Honorary Degree of Doctor of Humanities, University of Malaya, Malaysia

2012   Honorary Degree of Doctor of Agricultural Development Honoris Causa, Hawassa University, Ethiopia

2010   Honorary Academician, Russian Academy of Natural Sciences, Russia

2009   Honorary Professorship, Yunnan University, China

2008   Honorary Degree of Doctor in Humane Letters, University for Peace, Costa Rica

2008   Honorary Professorship, Dalian University of Foreign Language, China

2007   Honorary Doctor of Humanity, University of Cambodia, Cambodia

2007   Honorary Professorship, Guizhou University, China

2007   Honorary Doctorate of Humane Letters, Rochester Institute of Technology, United States

2006	Honorary Professorship, Dalian Maritime University, China
2005	Doctor Honoris Causa, Jadavpur University, India
2004	Honorary Professorship, Shanghai Maritime University, China
2004	Doctor Honoris Causa, World Maritime University, Sweden
2004	Honorary Professorship, Heilongjiang University, China
2004	Honorary Professorship, Harbin Medical University, China
2003	Honorary Professorship, China Medical University, China
2000	Doctor Honoris Causa, University of Bucharest, Romania
2000	Doctor Honoris Causa, University of Cape Coast, Ghana
2000	Honorary Professorship, Yanbian University, China

PUBLICATIONS

No Matter Where the Journey Takes Me: One Man's Quest for a Leprosy-Free World, London: C. Hurst & Co., 2019.

My Struggle against Leprosy. Tokyo: Festina Lente, 2019.

Ai suru sokoku e [To my beloved country]. Sankei Shimbun Shuppan. March 2016.

Shinshi no hinkaku 2 Zatsugaku no susume [The mark of a gentleman 2: An encouragement of miscellaneous knowledge]. PHP Kenkyūsho. August 2015.

Zanshin: Sekai no Hansen-byō wo seiatsu suru [Following through: The world-wide elimination of leprosy]. Gentōsha. May 2014.

Shinshi no hinkaku Waga zange-roku [The mark of a gentleman: Some personal jottings]. PHP Kenkyūsho. March 2012.

Rinjin: Chūkokujin ni itte okitai koto [A message for my neighbors in China]. PHP Kenkyūsho. December 2010.

Sore demo tabako wo suimasu ka? [Why you may not want to light up that cigarette]. Co-authored with Kanagawa Prefecture Governor Matsuzawa Shigefumi. Gentōsha. May 2010.

Fukanō wo kanō ni: Sekai no Hansen-byō to no tatakai [Making the impossible possible: The global struggle against leprosy]. Akashi Shoten. January 2010.

Wakamono yo: Sekai ni kake! [Youth of Japan: Go and explore the world!]. PHP Kenkyūsho. August 2009.

Ningen to shite ikite hoshii kara Watakushi ga mita sekai no genba [Because everyone deserves a life. My visits to the frontlines in the fight against leprosy]. Kairyūsha. November 2008.

Sekai no Hansen-byō ga naku naru hi [The day when the world is finally free of leprosy]. Akashi Shoten. November 2004.

Kono kuni, ano kuni Kangaete hoshii Nippon no katachi [A country among many.

Thoughts on the role Japan might play in the world]. Sankei Shimbunsha. July 2004.

Nisennen no rekishi wo kagami to shite [What to learn from 2000 years of history]. Nippon Kyōhōsha. August 2003.

Gaimushō no shiranai sekai no sugao [The world unmasked: Secrets that the foreign office still doesn't know]. Sankei Shimbunsha, April 1998.

Chie aru mono wa chie de tsumazuku [When knowledge can only take you so far]. Kuresto-sha, September 1996.

WORKS CONSULTED

Hansen-byō Forum, ed., *Hansen-byō: Nippon to sekai* [Leprosy: Japan and the World]. Kosakusha, 2016.

Sasakawa Yohei, *Sekai no Hansen-byō ga naku naru hi* [The day when the world is finally free of leprosy]. Akashi Shoten. November 2004.

——— *Ningen to shite ikite hoshii kara Watakushi ga mita sekai no genba* [Because everyone deserves to have the basics of an ordinary human life. My visits to the front lines of the fight against leprosy]. Kairyūsha. November 2008.

——— *Fukanō wo kanō ni: Sekai no Hansen-byō to no tatakai* [Making the impossible possible: The global struggle against leprosy]. Akashi Shoten. January 2010.

——— *Zanshin: Sekai no Hansen-byō wo seiatsu suru* [Following through: The worldwide elimination of leprosy]. Gentosha. May 2014.

——— *Ai suru sokoku e* [To my country, the land of my forebears, the land that I love]. Sankei Shimbun Shuppan. March 2016.

Takayama Fumihiko, *Shukumei no Senki*. Shogakkan, 2017.

AUTHOR PROFILE

Yohei Sasakawa is the chairman of the Nippon Foundation, Japan's largest charitable and grant-making organization. He is also the World Health Organization (WHO) Goodwill Ambassador for Leprosy Elimination, Japan's Goodwill Ambassador for the Human Rights of People Affected by Leprosy, and Special Envoy of the Government of Japan for Peace and Reconciliation in Myanmar. For more than four decades, Sasakawa has spearheaded the global struggle to eliminate leprosy. More recently, he has devoted his energies to tackling the various forms of discrimination associated with the disease. He holds numerous awards from many countries, including the Yomiuri International Cooperation Prize from Japan (2004), the International Gandhi Award (2007), the Rule of Law Award from the International Bar Association (2014), the Health-For-All Award from WHO (2017), the Health and Human Rights Award from the International Council of Nurses (2017), and the Gandhi Peace Prize from the government of India (2019). In 2019, the Japanese government bestowed on him the Grand Cordon of the Rising Sun and designated him a Person of Cultural Merit. His numerous publications include *My Struggle against Leprosy* (Festina Lente, 2019) and *No Matter Where the Journey Takes Me: One Man's Quest for a Leprosy-Free World* (Hurst, 2019). Ambassador Sasakawa has a blog, where he frequently posts information about his activities.

The Nippon Foundation website: https://www.nippon-foundation.or.jp/en/
Leprosy Today website: https://leprosytoday.org
Yohei Sasakawa's Official Blog: https://blog.canpan.info/yoheisasakawa/